AN ATLAS OF

# CLINICAL NUCLEAR MEDICINE

SECOND EDITION

# AN ATLAS OF
# CLINICAL NUCLEAR MEDICINE

## SECOND EDITION

### IGNAC FOGELMAN
BSc, MD, FRCP

**Consultant Physician and
Director of the Department of Nuclear Medicine
Guy's Hospital, London**

### MICHAEL N MAISEY
BSc, MD, FRCP, FRCR

**Professor of Radiological Sciences
United Medical and Dental Schools of
Guy's and St Thomas's Hospitals, London**

### SUSAN E M CLARKE
MSc, FRCP

**Consultant Physician in Nuclear Medicine
Guy's Hospital and
Senior Lecturer in Radiological Sciences
United Medical and Dental Schools of
Guy's and St Thomas's Hospitals, London**

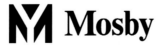 Mosby

St. Louis Baltimore Boston Chicago London Madrid Philadelphia Sydney Toronto

# MARTIN DUNITZ

First published in the United Kingdom in 1994
by Martin Dunitz Ltd, 7–9 Pratt Street, London NW1 0AE

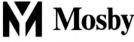

**Mosby**

Dedicated to Publishing Excellence

Distributed in the U.S.A. and Canada by
Mosby–Year Book
11830 Westline Industrial Drive
St. Louis, Missouri 63146

**Library of Congress Cataloging-in-Publication Data**
Fogelman, Ignac, 1948–
    An atlas of clinical nuclear medicine/Ignac Fogelman, Michael N.
  Maisey, Susan E.M. Clarke. -- 2nd ed.
      p.   cm.
    Includes index.
    ISBN 0-8151-3341-3
    1. Radioisotope scanning--Atlases.   2. Nuclear medicine--Atlases.
  I. Maisey, Michael.   II. Clarke, Susan E. M.   III. Title.
    [DNLM: 1. Nuclear Medicine--atlases.   WN 17 F6555a 1993]
  RC78.7.R4F64   1993
  616.07'575--dc20
  DNLM/DLC                     93-23372
  for Library of Congress                     CIP

Composition by Scribe Design, Gillingham, Kent, UK
Origination by Imago Publishing Ltd
Manufacture by Imago Publishing Ltd
Printed and bound in Singapore

# CONTENTS

# ACKNOWLEDGEMENTS

We would like to thank all the contributors of material to the *Atlas*, who are identified by their contributions. We would also like to thank the staff of the Department of Nuclear Medicine at Guy's Hospital who have assisted in obtaining the new material for this second edition. In particular, we acknowledge the valuable contribution made by Dr Petra Lewis to the Brain chapter. She has collated all the new material and assisted in the reconstruction of this chapter. Finally, our thanks again to the staff of Martin Dunitz for their constructive help throughout the preparation of this new edition.

IF
MNM
SEMC

# PREFACE

Although only five years have passed since the first edition of *An Atlas of Clinical Nuclear Medicine* was published, a number of new radiopharmaceuticals have been accepted into routine clinical practice and single photon emission computed tomographic imaging (SPECT) has now become widely available. This edition of the *Atlas* has been fully revised to cover these recent advances, while retaining the best of the material from the previous edition. In addition, there are new chapters on tumour imaging and gastrointestinal studies. Without detracting from the comprehensiveness of the first edition, the book has been completely restructured to enhance its use as a teaching aid. Each chapter is divided into four sections: anatomy and physiology; radiopharmaceuticals; normal scans with variants and artefacts; and clinical applications.

This second edition of *An Atlas of Clinical Nuclear Medicine* retains the emphasis on obtaining functional information and its relationship to solving clinical problems that was so central to the first edition, and it is hoped that it will continue to be a valuable source of information to all those involved in the field of nuclear medicine.

# NOTE ON SINGLE PHOTON EMISSION COMPUTED TOMOGRAPHY (SPECT)

SPECT imaging is used to permit 3D reconstruction of data, increasing the sensitivity and anatomical localization of lesions in the skeleton, brain and heart. The sensitivity of localization of tumours is also increased with the use of SPECT acquisition reconstruction. The use of SPECT is becoming much more widely used and this second edition of *An Atlas of Clinical Nuclear Medicine* includes SPECT images in the Bone chapter for the spine, hips and knees, the Brain chapter, Heart chapter and Tumour chapter.

The standard planes of reconstruction are shown diagrammatically below for use with these SPECT images.

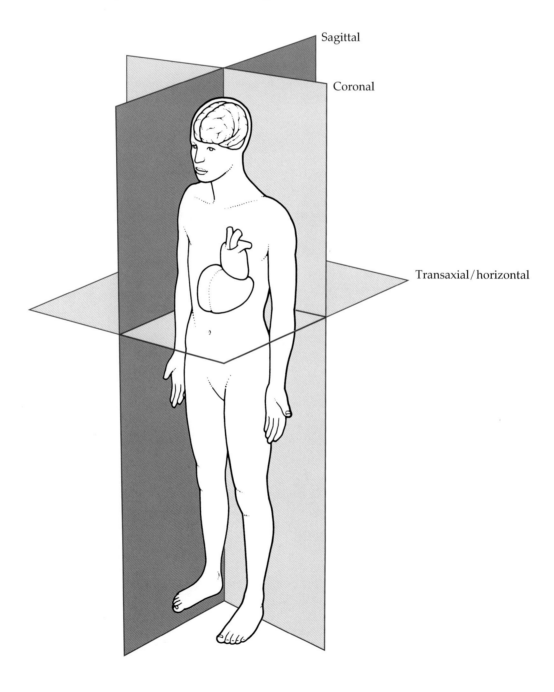

# CHAPTER 1

# BONE

Bone scanning is usually exclusively performed using technetium-99m ($^{99m}$Tc) labelled diphosphonate (Fig. 1.3), which shows exquisite sensitivity for skeletal abnormality. The technique has the limitation that scan appearances may be non-specific; however, in many clinical situations recognizable patterns of scan abnormality are seen, which often suggest a specific diagnosis.

The mechanism of tracer uptake on bone is not fully understood, but it is believed that diphosphonate is adsorbed onto the surface of bone, with particular affinity for sites of new bone formation (Figs 1.1, 1.2). It is thought that diphosphonate uptake on bone primarily reflects osteoblastic activity but is also dependent on skeletal vascularity. Thus bone scan images provide a functional display of skeletal activity. As functional change in bone occurs earlier than structural change, the bone scan will often detect abnormalities before they are seen on an x-ray. Any diphosphonate which is not taken up by bone is excreted via the urinary tract, and in a normal study the kidneys are clearly visualized on the bone scan; indeed there are many examples of renal pathology which have been detected for the first time on the bone scan.

It is also recognized that, on occasion, there may be uptake of $^{99m}$Tc diphosphonate at non-skeletal sites. There have been many situations reported where this can occur, but it is believed that in all cases the common factor is the presence of local microcalcification.

## CHAPTER CONTENTS

# 1.1  ANATOMY/PHYSIOLOGY

## Mechanism of diphosphonate uptake on bone

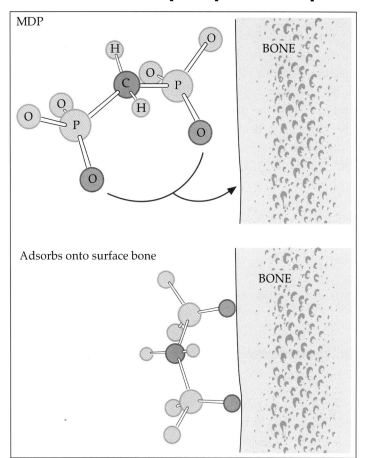

**Fig. 1.1**

*Mechanism of diphosphonate uptake on bone.*

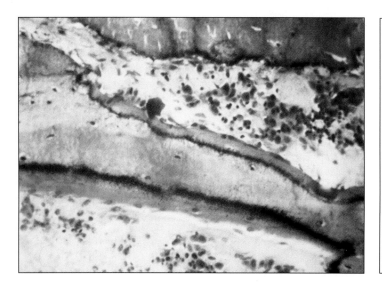

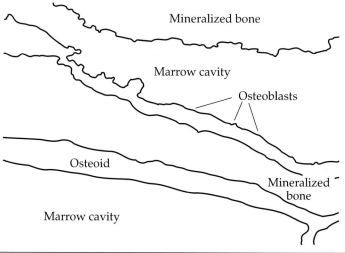

**Fig. 1.2**

*Microautoradiograph of rabbit bone, showing adsorption of [3]H-hydroxyethylidene diphosphonate (hedp) on bone surfaces. The heavy concentration of silver grains is at the interface between osteoid and bone, ie at the site where mineralization occurs. (Courtesy of Dr M.D. Francis, Cincinnati, USA.)*

# 1.2   RADIOPHARMACEUTICALS

## Chemical structures of diphosphonates

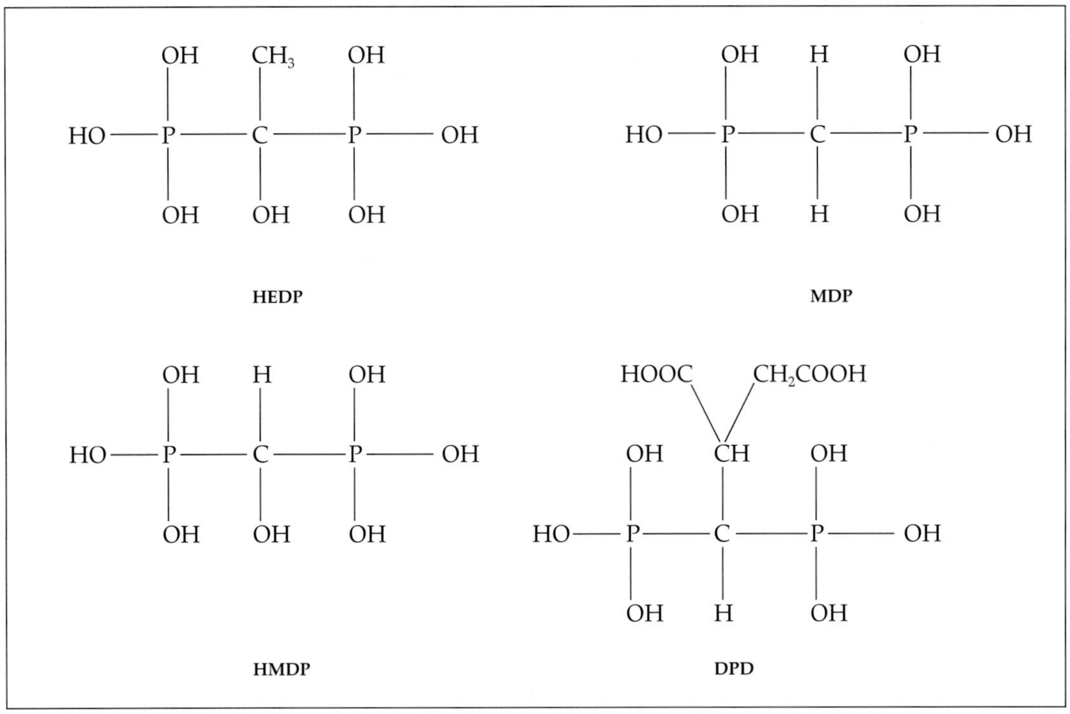

*Fig. 1.3*

*Chemical structures of diphosphonate compounds used for bone scanning.*

*At the present time MDP is the most widely used agent; HEDP, hydroxyethylidene diphosphonate; MDP, methylene diphosphonate; HMDP, hydroxymethylene diphosphonate; DPD, dicarboxypropane diphosphonate.*

# 1.3 NORMAL SCANS WITH VARIANTS AND ARTEFACTS

## 1.3.1 Normal bone scan

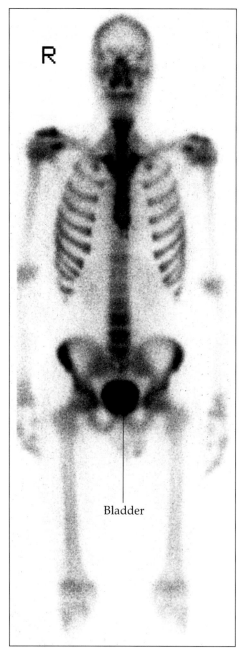

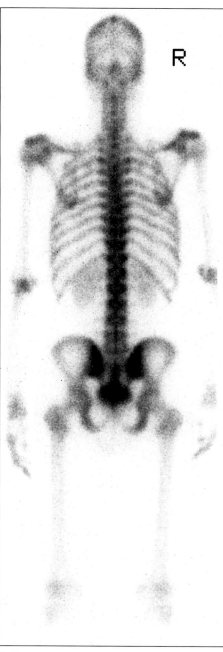

*a Anterior*

*b Posterior*

### Fig. 1.4

*(a, b) An example of a normal bone scan.
Note that there is clear visualization of the whole skeleton. The count rate is highest in those parts of the skeleton which are metabolically most active. These areas generally contain a high percentage of trabecular bone and are subject to considerable stress, eg the axial skeleton. The most important feature in a normal bone scan is symmetry about the midline in the sagittal plane. The left and right halves of the body should be virtually mirror images of each other. There should be uniform uptake of tracer throughout most of the skeleton, but some exceptions do arise, as will be discussed in Section 1.3.8. Note that the kidneys are clearly visualized on a normal bone scan because the diphosphonate which is not taken up by the skeleton is excreted via the urinary tract.*

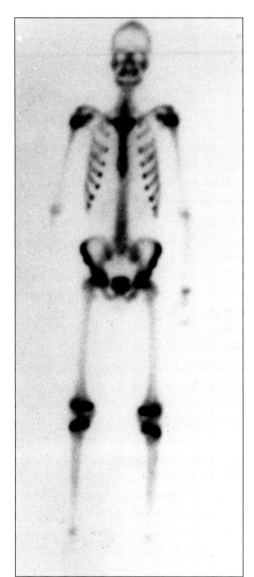

*a Anterior*

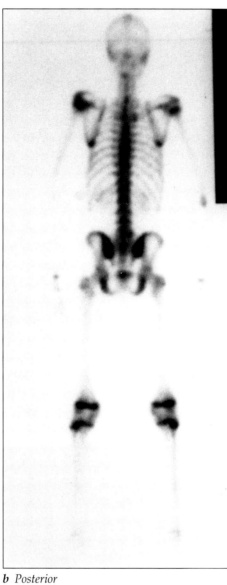

*b Posterior*

### Fig. 1.5

*(a, b) Normal bone scan of a growing 16-year-old boy.*

*Note that there is high uptake of tracer throughout the skeleton, with prominent uptake at the epiphyses. (Courtesy of Drs P Wraight and L Smith, Cambridge, UK.)*

# NORMAL SCANS WITH VARIANTS AND ARTEFACTS

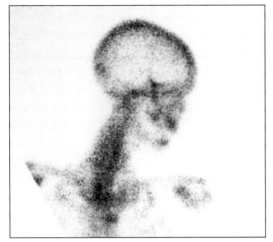

*a* Right lateral

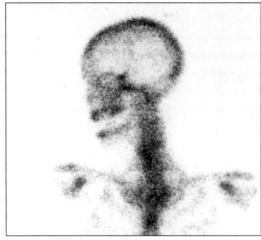

*b* Left lateral

### Fig. 1.6

*Normal spot bone scan views:*
*(a, b) skull; (c, d) thorax;*
*(e) pelvis; (f) thoracic spine;*
*(g) lumbar spine/pelvis;*
*(h) femora; (i) tibiae; (j) feet;*
*(k) lower forearms and hands.*

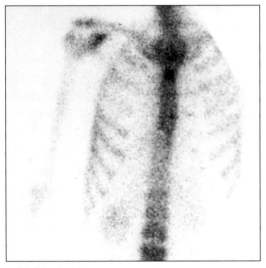

c Right anterior

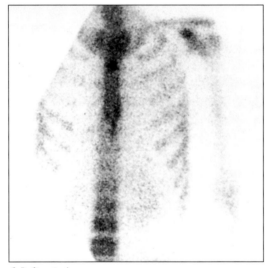

d Left anterior

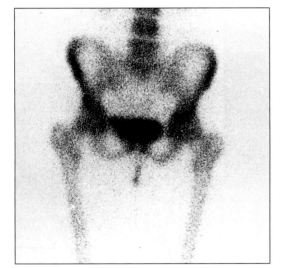

e Anterior

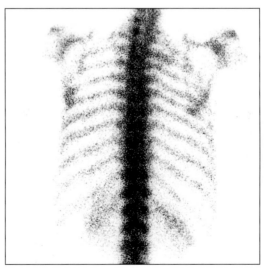

f Posterior

## NORMAL SCANS WITH VARIANTS AND ARTEFACTS

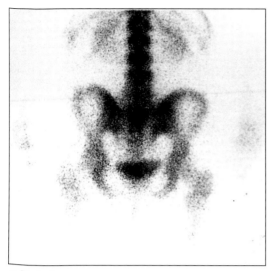

*g* Posterior

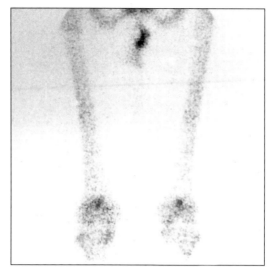

*h* Anterior

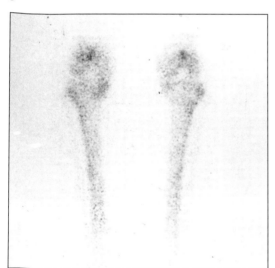

*i* Anterior

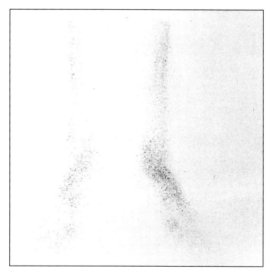

*j* Anterior

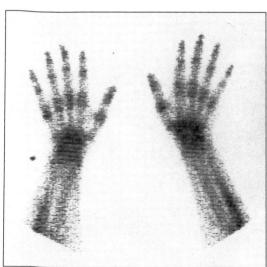

*k*

## 1.3.2   Three-phase bone scan

The timing of bone scan images may depend upon the clinical problem under investigation. There is, at present, no complete agreement as to the optimum time interval between injection and static imaging, but it is customary to obtain images at between 2 and 4 hours. In certain circumstances a three-phase bone scan will provide valuable additional information with regard to the vascularity of a lesion. This involves a dynamic flow study of the area of interest, with rapid sequential images taken every 2–3 seconds for 30 seconds. This is followed by a blood pool image at 5 minutes, when the radiopharmaceutical is still predominantly within the vascular compartment. Delayed static images are then obtained between 2 and 4 hours.

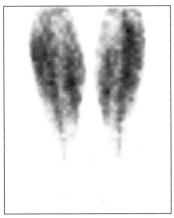 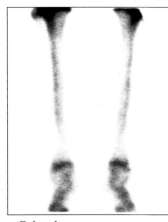 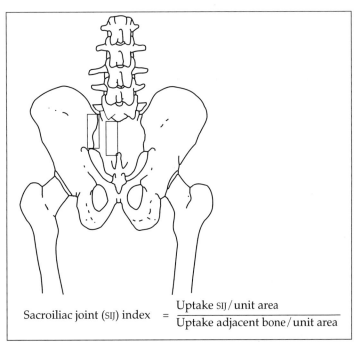

*a  Dynamic*      *b  Equilibrium*      *c  Delayed*

**Fig. 1.7**

*(a–c) Normal three-phase bone scan of the lower limbs. Bone scan views*

## 1.3.3   Bone scan quantitation

Visual assessment of tracer uptake in the sacroiliac joints is difficult, and quantitation is recommended. Several different methods have been proposed, one of which is shown in Fig. 1.8.

**Fig. 1.8**

*Sacroiliac joint quantitation.*

$$\text{Sacroiliac joint (SIJ) index} = \frac{\text{Uptake SIJ/unit area}}{\text{Uptake adjacent bone/unit area}}$$

## 1.3.4    Normal SPECT of the lumbar spine

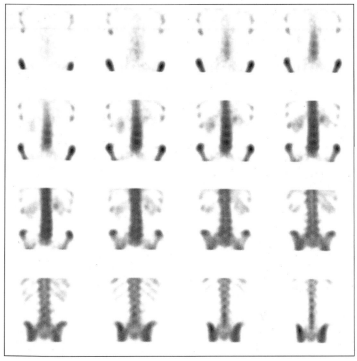

*a  Coronal*

*b  Sagittal*

### Fig. 1.9

*Normal SPECT scans of the lumbar spine: **(a)** coronal sections; **(b)** sagittal sections; **(c)** transaxial sections.*

*The anatomy of the vertebra is best seen on the transaxial view, with the body lying anteriorly, pedicles and facet joints lying laterally and the spinous process lying posteriorly.*

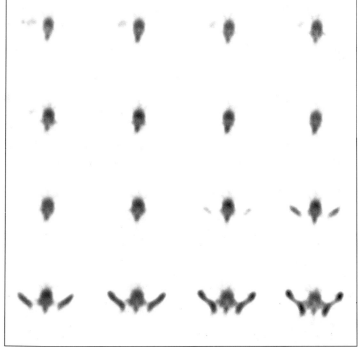

*c  Transaxial*

## 1.3.5 Normal SPECT of the hips and pelvis

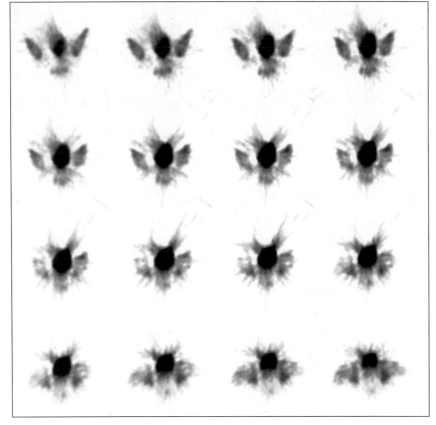

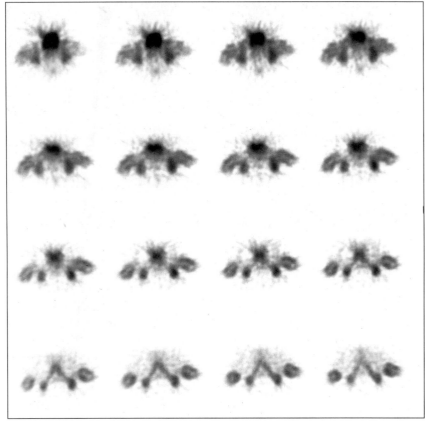

*a Transaxial*

**Fig. 1.10**

*Normal SPECT scans of the hip and pelvis: (a) transaxial sections from the bladder level through to the femoral heads; (b) coronal sections; (c) sagittal sections of the left hip; (d) sagittal sections of the right hip.*

## NORMAL SCANS WITH VARIANTS AND ARTEFACTS

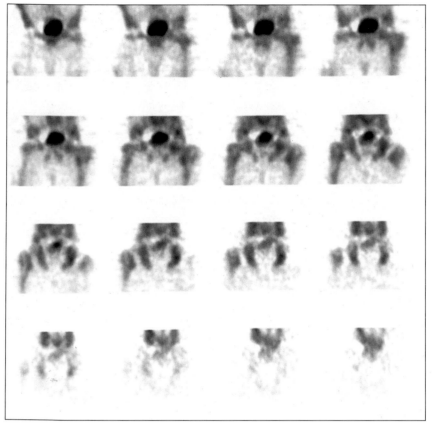

**b** Coronal

A full bladder may produce artefacts on SPECT reconstruction due to high activity levels.

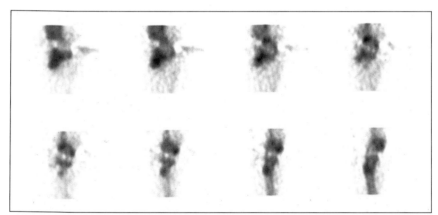

**c** Sagittal, left hip

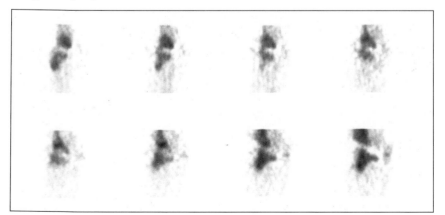

**d** Sagittal, right hip

## 1.3.6    Normal SPECT of the knees

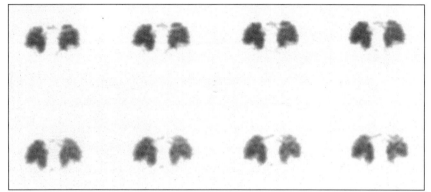

*Femoral level*

### Fig. 1.11

*Normal SPECT scans of the knees: (a) transaxial sections cutting from the lower femoral shaft to the upper tibial and fibula shafts; (b) coronal sections cutting anterior to posterior; (c) sagittal sections of the left knee; (d) sagittal sections of the right knee.*

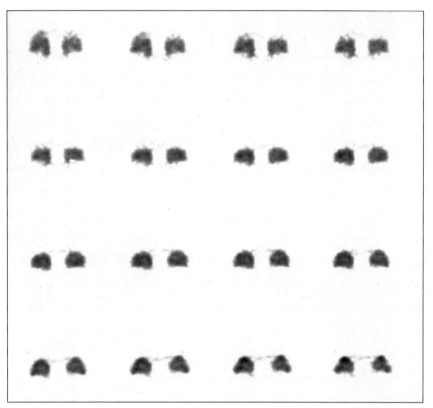

*Tibial plateaux*

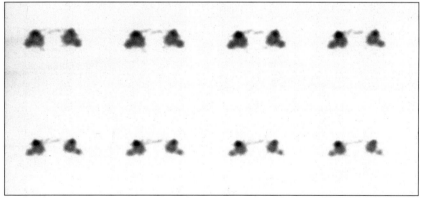

*a  Transaxial*                                    *Tibial and fibular level*

# NORMAL SCANS WITH VARIANTS AND ARTEFACTS

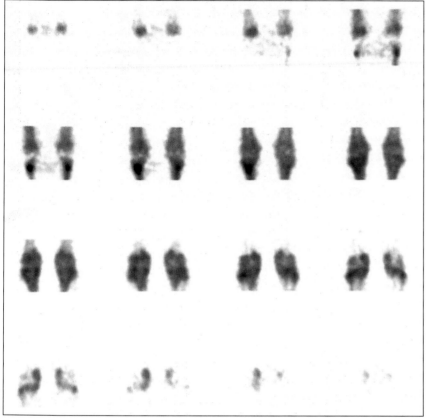

*b* Coronal

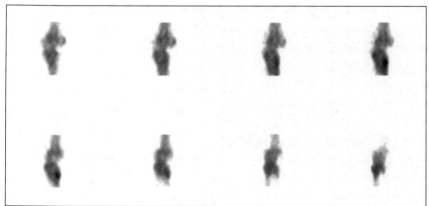

*c* Sagittal, left knee

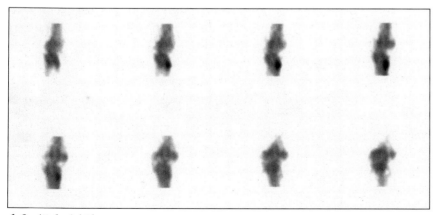

*d* Sagittal, right knee

## *Normal SPECT of the knees in adolescence*

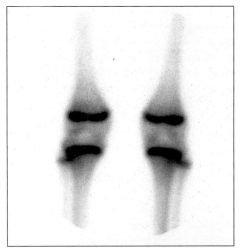

*a  Anterior*

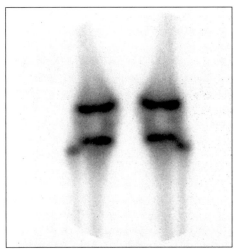

*b  Posterior*

### Fig. 1.12

*Normal SPECT scans of the knees in adolescence: (a) anterior planar view; (b) posterior planar view; (c) transaxial sections; (d) coronal sections; (e) sagittal sections of the left knee; (f) sagittal sections of the right knee.*

*Note the intense uptake in the epiphyses.*

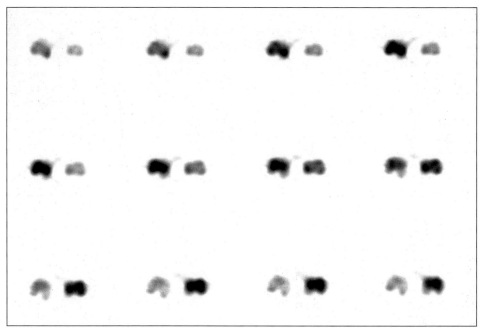

*Femoral level*

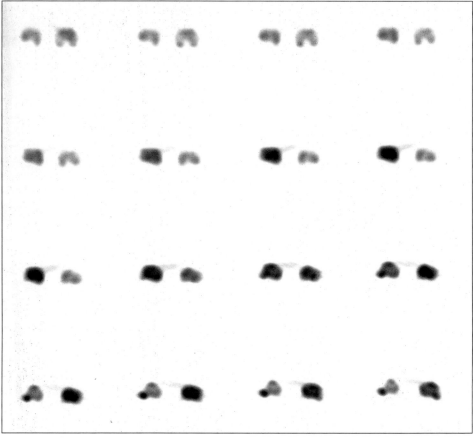

*c  Transaxial*                    *Tibial and fibular level*

## NORMAL SCANS WITH VARIANTS AND ARTEFACTS

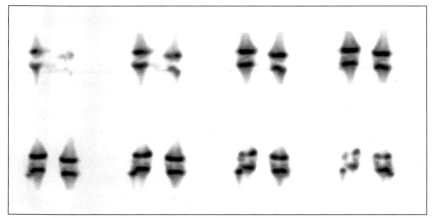

SPECT images must be interpreted with caution in adolescents and young adults as the epiphyses may appear asymmetrical.

**d** *Coronal*

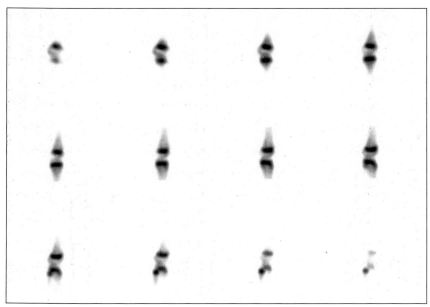

**e** *Sagittal, left knee*

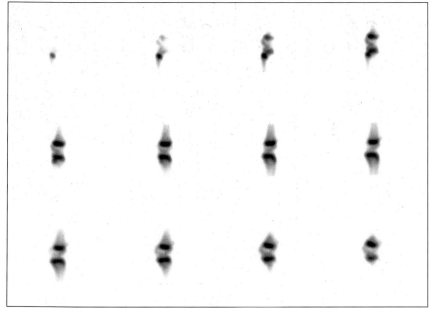

**f** *Sagittal, right knee*

## 1.3.7 Technical points

### *Localization of lesion*

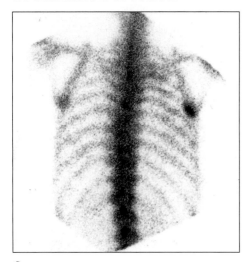 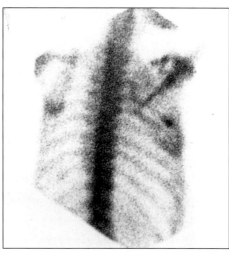

*a* *b*

**Fig. 1.13**

*Lesion of scapula or rib? Bone scan views:*
*(a) thoracic spine; (b) with arm elevated.*
*    On the original study the lesion appears*
*to lie at the tip of the scapula. However,*
*with the arm elevated, it is apparent that*
*the lesion is in a rib.*

### *Bladder*

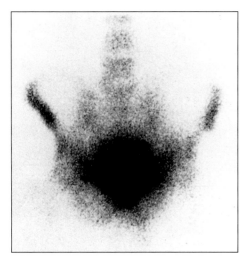

**Fig. 1.14**

*Full bladder partially obscuring pelvis.*

• Prior to skeletal imaging, a patient should empty the bladder, since retained activity may lead to difficulties in scan interpretation.
• It is not possible to exclude abnormalities in the pelvis unless the bladder is empty. If the bladder obscures the pelvic bones, the patient may be catheterized or a pelvic x-ray should be performed.
• A squat view may be useful when bladder activity obscures the pelvis.

# NORMAL SCANS WITH VARIANTS AND ARTEFACTS

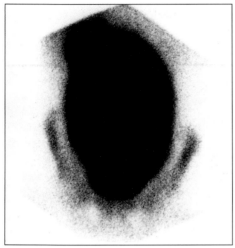 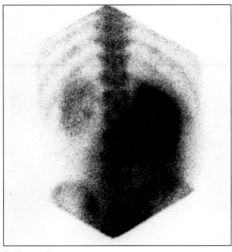 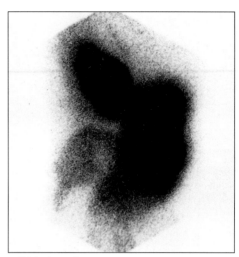

*a* Anterior    *b* Posterior    *c* Right lateral

**Fig. 1.15**

*Massive urinary retention. Bone scan views: **(a)** pelvis; **(b)** lumbar spine; **(c)** abdomen.*
   *The bladder is massively dilated, extending to well above the umbilicus. In addition, there is markedly increased tracer uptake seen in association with the right kidney. The scan findings represent massive urinary retention, with some obstruction of the right kidney.*

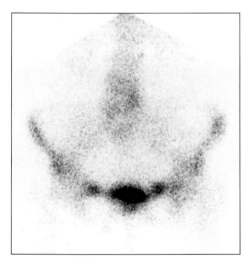 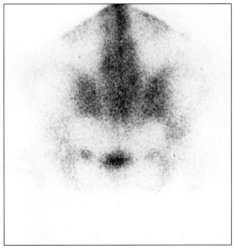 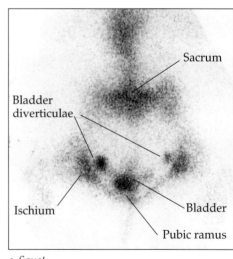

*a* Anterior    *b* Posterior    *c* Squat

**Fig. 1.16**

*Bladder diverticulae. Bone scan views: **(a, b)** pelvis; **(c)** squat view.*
   *On the anterior and posterior views of the pelvis, focal areas of increased tracer uptake are seen on each side of the bladder, overlying the superior pubic rami. The squat view clearly separates these areas from bone and confirms that these represent bladder diverticulae.*

NORMAL SCANS WITH VARIANTS AND ARTEFACTS

## NORMAL SCANS WITH VARIANTS AND ARTEFACTS

## *Skull views*

### Skull sutures

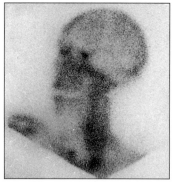

*a Left lateral*

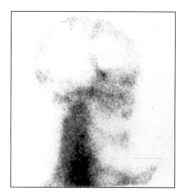

*b Right lateral*

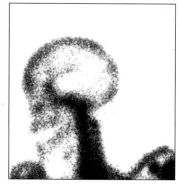

*c Left lateral*

**Fig. 1.17**

*(a–c)* Three examples of tracer uptake in skull sutures.

It is common to see a focal area of increased tracer uptake which corresponds to the pterion, the site of confluence of the frontal, parietal, temporal and sphenoid bones. However, tracer uptake may be seen extending along individual sutures.

### Occipital protuberance

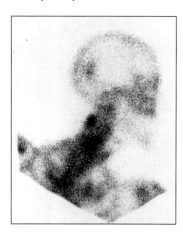

**Fig. 1.18**

The skull is slightly rotated, and a focal area of increased uptake is seen in the occipital region. This is a normal variant and corresponds to tracer uptake at the site of the occipital protuberance. Of course, coexistent pathology at this site cannot be absolutely excluded and, if clinically relevant, an x-ray may be required for further evaluation. Note that in this case there is a focus of increased uptake in the mid-cervical spine. This is a common finding and is most often due to degenerative change.

### Dental disease

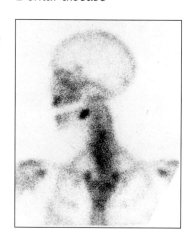

**Fig. 1.19**

A focus of increased tracer uptake is seen at the angle of the left mandible. Focal abnormalities in the mandible and maxilla are common and most often reflect dental disease. In this case the patient had an apical abscess. If clinically relevant, however, an x-ray may be required for further evaluation because, although it is an extremely rare occurrence, patients can present with a solitary metastasis at this site (see Fig. 1.71, page 40).

### Hyperostosis frontalis

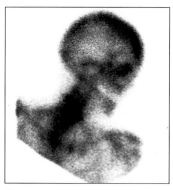

*a*

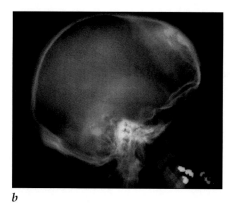

*b*

**Fig. 1.20**

In elderly subjects increased tracer uptake may be seen in the frontal region of the skull *(a)*, and these appearances are typical of hyperostosis frontalis. If clinically relevant, the diagnosis will be confirmed on a skull x-ray *(b)*.

## *The importance of correct contrast*

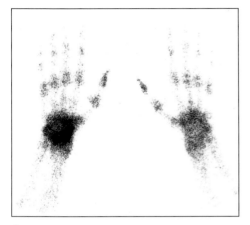 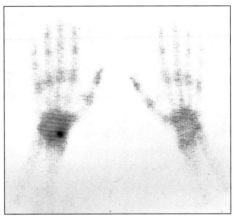

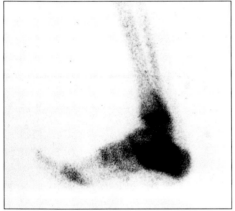 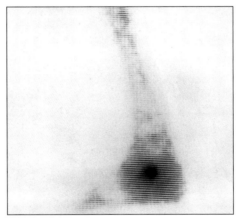

*a*   *b*   *c*   *d*

**Fig. 1.21**

*Two cases where the focal nature of a lesion was not apparent from analogue images: (a,c) analogue; (b,d) digital.*

*In both cases, at higher contrast, generally increased tracer uptake is visualized at the site of abnormality. However, at lower intensity, the discrete nature of the lesions is apparent.*

**If digital images are obtained, the data can be reviewed and the contrast altered if necessary. With analogue images, the correct contrast has to be obtained at the outset; and if the quality of images is inadequate, the study has to be repeated.**

## *Renal*

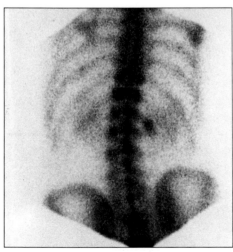 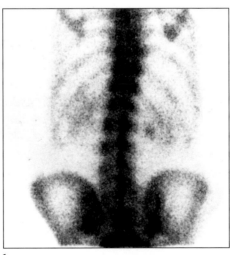

*a*   *b*

**Fig. 1.22**

*Apparent bone lesion accounted for by renal uptake of tracer. Bone scan views: (a) supine; (b) erect.*

*There is a focal area of increased tracer uptake which appears to overlie the right 12th rib posteriorly. However, this moves with position, and it is clear that the lesion was due to pooling of the tracer in the renal pelvis.*

# 1.3.8    Variants

## *Calcification*

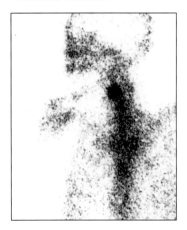

**Fig. 1.23**

*An example of diphosphonate uptake in the thyroid cartilage. The uptake is thought to be due to microcalcification in the cartilage, and this finding is of no clinical relevance.*

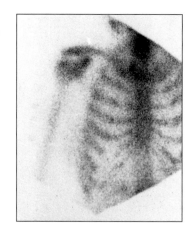

**Fig. 1.24**

*Tracer uptake is seen in the region of the costal cartilages. This is an extreme example, but may be seen in elderly subjects and is thought to be due to calcification of the cartilages.*

## *Hot patella sign*

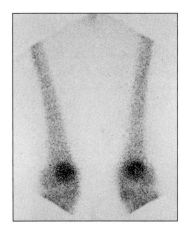

**Fig. 1.25**

*There is increased tracer uptake in both patellae, the so-called hot patella sign. This finding should be considered a normal variant and is of no pathological significance in the absence of symptoms.*

## *Deltoid sign*

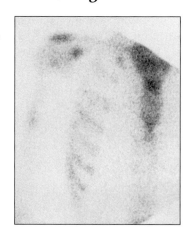

**Fig. 1.26**

*A focal area of increased tracer uptake is seen at the upper third of the right humerus. This corresponds to the deltoid tuberosity and the site of insertion of the deltoid muscle. It should be considered a normal variant; however, when it is pronounced, the physician should be alert to the possibility of coexistent disease, particularly if the patient is known to have a primary malignancy.*

## *Spina bifida*

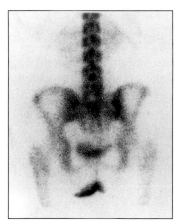

*a*
*b*

**Fig. 1.27**

*Bone scan views: (a) lumbar spine; (b) pelvis.*
*There is a small photon-deficient area associated with the L5/S1 region which, on the x-ray, was attributable to incomplete partial fusion of the spinous processes.*

## 1.3.9    Artefacts

### *Free pertechnetate*

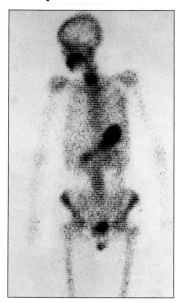

*Fig. 1.28*

*Tracer uptake is seen in the mouth, salivary glands, thyroid and stomach. These are the typical appearances found in the presence of free pertechnetate.*

### *Activity at site of injection*

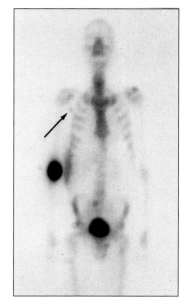

*Fig. 1.29*

*A right-sided injection has been tissued. Note that an axillary lymph node is visualized on that side (arrow). There is no clinical significance associated with this finding.*

### *Urine contamination*

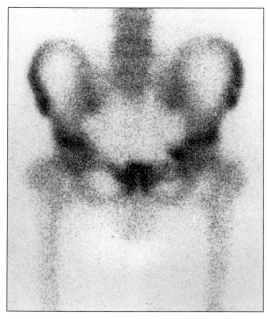

*a*

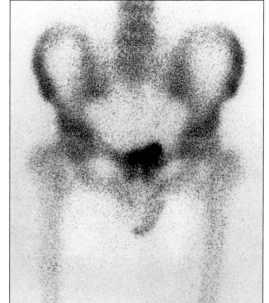

*b*

*Fig. 1.30*

*Bone scan view of anterior pelvis.*

*A focal area of increased tracer uptake is seen medial to the left acetabulum (**a**). This does not appear to be in bone, and is caused by urine contamination. The repeat study (**b**) was normal.*

## *Other artefacts*

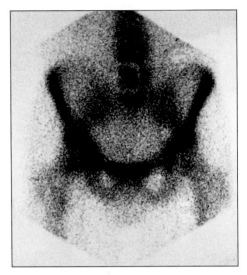

**Fig. 1.31**

*Artefact caused by a belt buckle.*

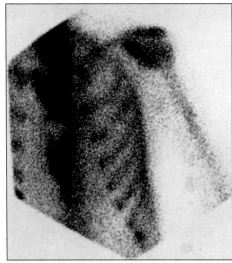

**Fig. 1.32**

*Artefact caused by a medallion.*

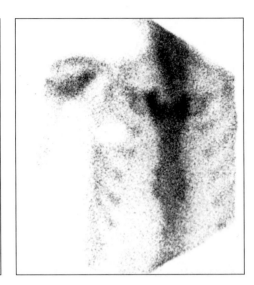

**Fig. 1.33**

*Artefact caused by a pacemaker.*

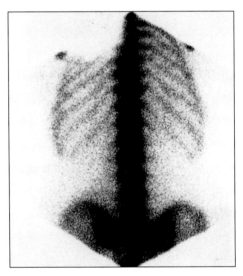

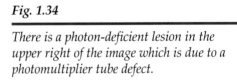

**Fig. 1.34**

*There is a photon-deficient lesion in the upper right of the image which is due to a photomultiplier tube defect.*

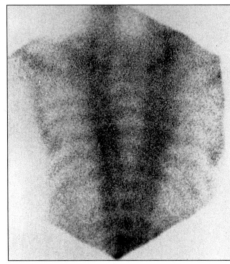

**Fig. 1.35**

*Motion artefact.*

# 1.4 CLINICAL APPLICATIONS

The bone scan is widely used in clinical practice, and is the most commonly requested investigation in any nuclear medicine department because of its sensitivity for lesion detection. The indications for a bone scan are continually being extended, but fall into four main categories:

- Investigation of bone pain
- Investigation of malignancy
- Investigation of benign bone disease
- Miscellaneous

The clinical applications of bone scanning are listed below, and examples of the various clinical problems are given on subsequent pages.

**1.4.1 Investigation of bone pain**
Metastatic tumour
Benign bone tumour
Trauma
Avascular necrosis
Infection
Osteomalacia
Paget's disease
Unexpected findings

**1.4.2 Investigation of malignancy**
Initial staging
Discordant scan/x-ray findings
Assessment of extent of disease
Monitoring progress of disease and response to therapy
Hypertrophic pulmonary osteoarthropathy
Primary bone tumours

**1.4.3 Investigation of benign bone disease**
Orthopaedic disorders
Benign bone tumours
Infection
Fracture
Exercise-related trauma
Surgical trauma
Degenerative disease
Metabolic bone disease
Paget's disease
Assessment of significance of x-ray lesions

**1.4.4 Miscellaneous**
Soft tissue accumulation of diphosphonate
Vascular abnormalities
Abnormalities of the renal tract
Abnormalities of the urinary tract

# 1.4.1 Investigation of bone pain

## *Metastatic tumour*

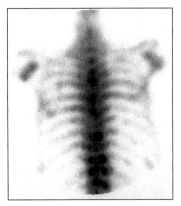 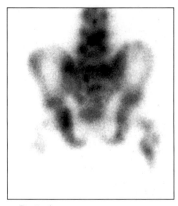 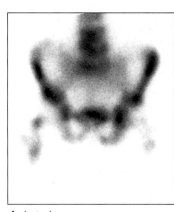

*a Posterior*          *b Posterior*          *c Posterior*          *d Anterior*

**Fig. 1.36**

*A 79-year-old man who complained of low back-ache.*

*The bone scan of (a) the posterior thoracic spine, (b) the posterior lumbar spine, (c) the posterior pelvis and (d) the anterior pelvis shows multiple areas of increased uptake throughout the ribs, vertebrae, pelvis and femora. There is poor visualization of the kidneys consistent with a developing superscan of malignancy. The scan findings are those of multiple metastases. The patient was later diagnosed as having cancer of the prostate.*

## *Benign bone tumour*
### Osteoid osteoma

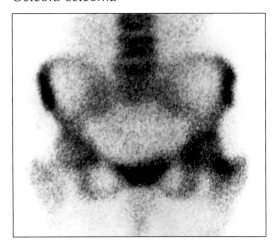 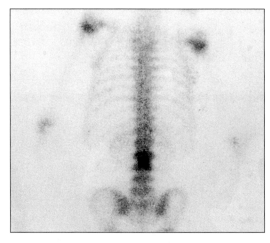

**Fig. 1.37**

**Fig. 1.38**

*A 14-year-old boy who complained of pain in the left hip.*

*The bone scan view of the anterior pelvis shows a discrete focus of strikingly increased tracer uptake in the left femoral neck. The scan appearances are strongly suggestive of osteoid osteoma: this was confirmed at surgery. The x-rays were normal.*

*A 6-year-old boy who complained of back pain.*

*X-rays identified a lesion at L2, the nature of which was uncertain. The bone scan shows an intense discrete focus of increased tracer uptake at that site, an appearance which is strongly suggestive of osteoid osteoma. This was confirmed at surgery.*

## CLINICAL APPLICATIONS

# Trauma

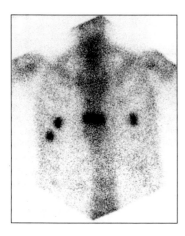

### Fig. 1.39

*A 66-year-old woman who complained of pain in her anterior chest, caused by a fall while getting out of the bath.*

*The bone scan view of the anterior chest shows marked linearly increased tracer uptake in the mid-sternum with further focal abnormalities present in the right 3rd and 4th, and left 3rd ribs anteriorly, close to the costochondral junctions. The scan findings are typical of fracture at the above sites.*

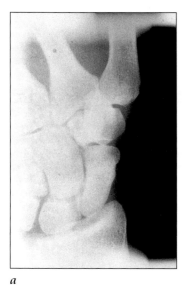

*a*

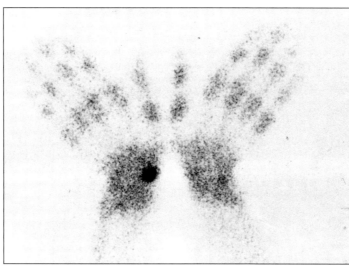

*b*

### Fig. 1.40

*A 50-year-old man who had fallen on to his outstretched hand and was experiencing tenderness over the anatomical snuff-box area.*

*Although a scaphoid fracture was clinically suspected, the x-ray (a) was thought to be normal. The bone scan (b) clearly shows a focal bone lesion, typical of a scaphoid fracture.*

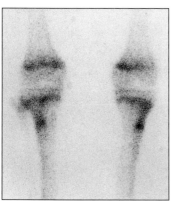

*a  Anterior*

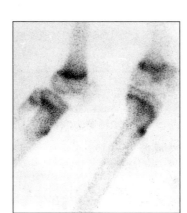

*b  Lateral*

### Fig. 1.41

*(a, b) Bone scan views of knees in an 18-year-old male who complained of pain in his knees.*

*There are symmetrical focal lesions just below, and lateral to, the tibial tuberosity. The scan findings are likely to represent small stress lesions, which are metabolically active and relate to the site of muscle insertion. The area of abnormality on the scan corresponded with the site of the patient's symptoms.*

## Stress fracture

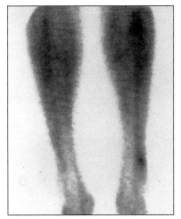
*a  Equilibrium*

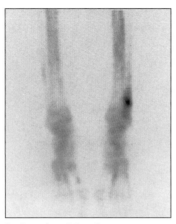
*b  Anterior, delayed*

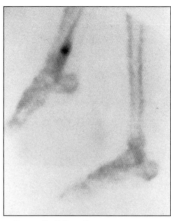
*c  Lateral, delayed*

*Fig. 1.42*

*(a–c) Bone scan view of lower limbs in a 17-year-old dancer who complained of pain in her left lower leg.*

*There is a focus of intensely increased tracer uptake present at the lower end of the left fibula. This is vascular. Although the initial x-rays were normal, this area corresponded to a stress fracture seen on subsequent x-rays.*

## Non-accidental injury

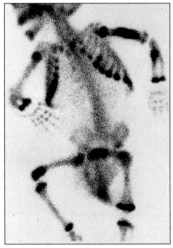
*a  Anterior*

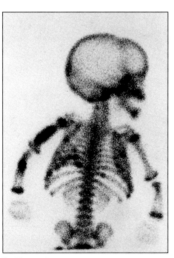
*b  Posterior*

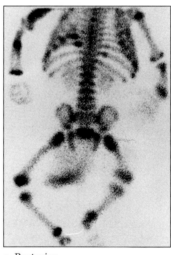
*c  Posterior*

*Fig. 1.43*

*(a–c) Bone scan views of the skeleton in a 9-month-old male infant with bony tenderness.*

*Focal abnormalities are present in the right 11th and left 9th and 10th ribs posteriorly, left 5th rib anteriorly, left humerus, left radius, left mid-femur and right knee. Thus there are multiple lesions throughout the skeleton, and the scan appearances are strongly suggestive of non-accidental injury.*

- In non-accidental injury the bone scan may occasionally miss skull fractures, so a skull x-ray should be obtained routinely.
- Sometimes, pinhole views of the epiphyses may be of value, since this is a common site of fracture; a lesion may not be apparent on the initial study.
- Rib fractures at different stages of healing may be visualized, confirming repeated injury.

## CLINICAL APPLICATIONS

### *Reflex sympathetic dystrophy syndrome*

The reflex sympathetic dystrophy syndrome is poorly understood, and is often forgotten in clinical practice. It is seen most commonly following trauma, and symptoms include pain and tenderness, swelling and dystrophic skin changes. Other terms applied to this syndrome include:

- Causalgia
- Sudeck's atrophy
- Acute atrophy of bone
- Post-traumatic osteoporosis
- Shoulder–hand syndrome

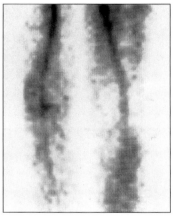 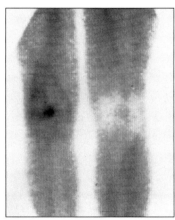 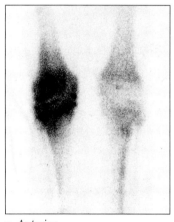

*a Dynamic*  *b Equilibrium*  *c Anterior*

**Fig. 1.44**

*(a–c)* Bone scan views of knees in a 20-year-old man who continued to complain of pain in the right knee following an injury to that site.

*The bone scan study shows diffusely increased tracer uptake associated with all three bones involving the knee joint. There is increased vascularity to the area. These findings are typical of reflex sympathetic dystrophy syndrome. Two arthroscopies were performed, which both gave negative results. The clinical diagnosis was one of reflex sympathetic dystrophy syndrome following trauma.*

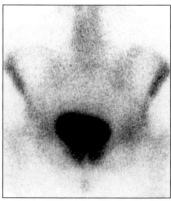 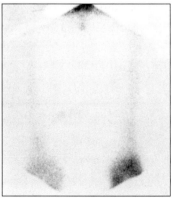 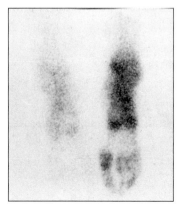

*a Anterior*  *b*  *c*

**Fig. 1.45**

*Bone scan views: (a) pelvis; (b) femora; (c) feet.*

*There is increased tracer uptake present in all the bones of the left leg, but it is most marked at the femoral neck, knee, ankle and forefoot. The scan findings are typical of reflex sympathetic dystrophy syndrome and are commonly seen in patients who have been immobilized, eg following a stroke.*

## CLINICAL APPLICATIONS

### *Avascular necrosis*

Causes of avascular necrosis

- Sickle cell disease
- Osteochondritis dissecans
- Trauma
- Steroid therapy

- Vascular injury
- Caisson disease
- Radiation
- Gaucher's disease

### Sickle cell disease

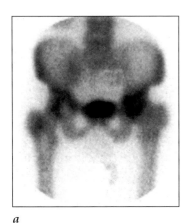
*a*

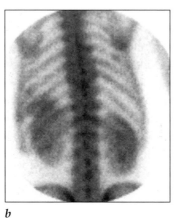
*b*

**Fig. 1.46**

A 22-year-old man with sickle cell disease and pain in the hips.

    The bone scan **(a)** shows increased uptake in both hips and the right femoral greater trochanter due to avascular necrosis of the femoral heads and a femoral trochanteric infarct. Diphosphonate accumulation is noted in the region of the spleen in a splenic infarct **(b)**.

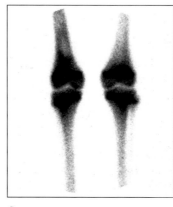
*a*

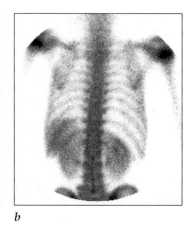
*b*

**Fig. 1.47**

A 12-year-old boy with sickle cell disease and pain in the right knee.

    The bone scan **(a)** shows uptake in the lower shaft of the right femur consistent with a sickle cell bone infarct. There is diphosphonate uptake in a splenic infarct **(b)**.

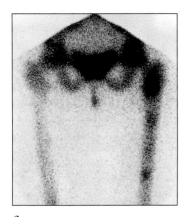
*a*

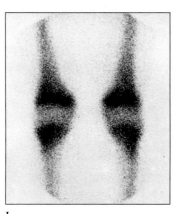
*b*

**Fig. 1.48**

A 71-year-old woman with sickle cell disease who complained of pain in her left thigh. Bone scan views: **(a)** upper femora; **(b)** lower femora/upper tibiae.

    Several focal areas of increased tracer uptake are seen in the left upper and mid-femur. In addition, there is increased tracer uptake at the ends of the long bones. The scan appearances are those of multiple bone infarcts involving the left femur, together with marrow hyperplasia.

 **While avascular bone is represented by a photon-deficient area on a bone scan, in practice this is seldom seen unless images are performed early in the disease process. The most frequent finding is increased tracer uptake; this reflects the healing response by surrounding bone.**

## CLINICAL APPLICATIONS

## *Osteochondritis dissecans*

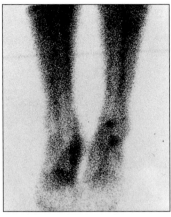

*a Anterior*

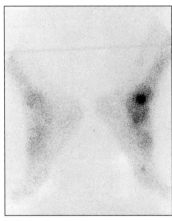

*b Lateral*

### Fig. 1.49

***(a, b)*** *Bone scan views of feet in a 22-year-old man who complained of pain in his left ankle.*

*Static images show a small intense focus of increased tracer uptake in the region of the left lower tibia. This is vascular. The initial x-rays were normal. It was felt that the bone scan appearances were likely to be due to an osteoid osteoma, but at surgery a small defect in the posterior surface of the articular cartilage covering the talus was seen. The diagnosis was osteochondritis dissecans.*

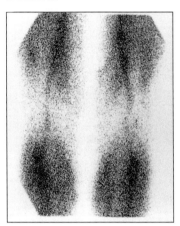

*a Equilibrium*

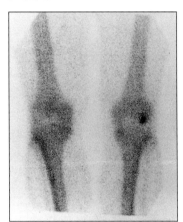

*b Delayed*

### Fig. 1.50

*A 20-year-old man with pain in the left knee.*

*The equilibrium image **(a)** shows a small area of increased blood pool. The delayed image **(b)** shows metabolic activity in the lateral femoral condyle. This was subsequently demonstrated to be due to osteochondritis dissecans of the left femur.*

## *Trauma*

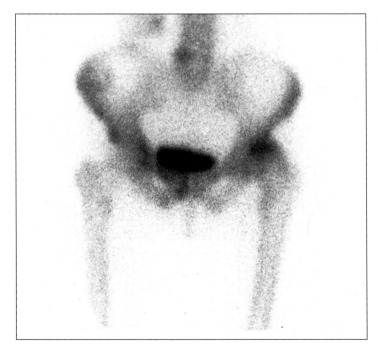

### Fig. 1.51

*An 82-year-old woman with known breast cancer and pain in the left hip. The patient was also known to have fractured the hip 10 years previously.*

*The bone scan shows focal uptake in the lower lumbar spine, right ilium and right pubic ramus due to metastases. The appearances in the left hip, however, are those of avascular necrosis secondary to femoral neck fracture.*

## CLINICAL APPLICATIONS

*Steroid therapy*

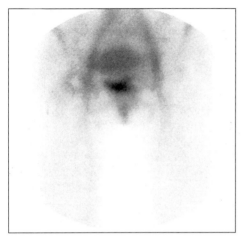

*a  Equilibrium*

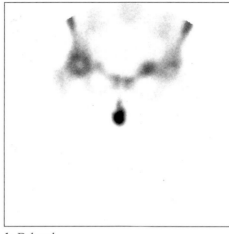

*b  Delayed*

*Fig. 1.52*

*A 42-year-old woman with a history of systemic lupus erythematosus treated with steroids presented with pain in the right hip.*

*The equilibrium image (a) shows a ring of increased blood pool surrounding an area of reduced blood pool in the region of the right femoral head. The delayed image (b) shows a ring of metabolic activity surrounding an area of reduced metabolic activity in the region of the right femoral head, diagnostic of avascular necrosis.*

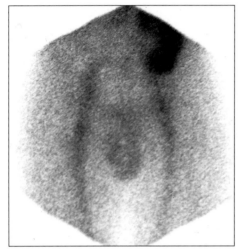

*a  Equilibrium*

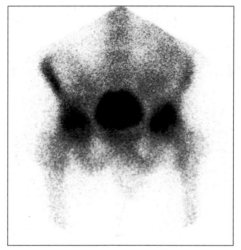

*b  Anterior, delayed*

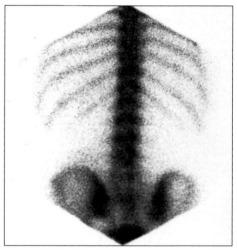

*c  Posterior, delayed*

*Fig. 1.53*

*A 40-year-old man with a renal transplant taking steroids for immunosuppression. The equilibrium image (a) shows a perfused transplant in the left pelvis. The delayed image (b) shows bilateral increased uptake in the femoral heads and the delayed image (c) confirms absent renal images. The features of these scans are those of bilateral femoral head avascular necrosis in a patient with a renal transplant on steroids.*

## CLINICAL APPLICATIONS

## *Infection*

*Fig. 1.54*

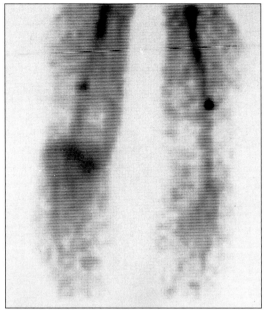

*a Dynamic*

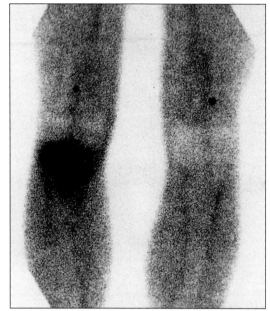

*b Equilibrium*

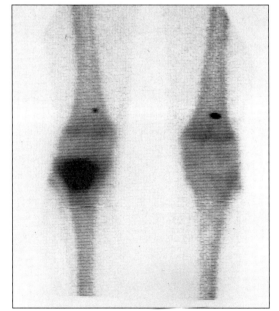

*c Anterior*

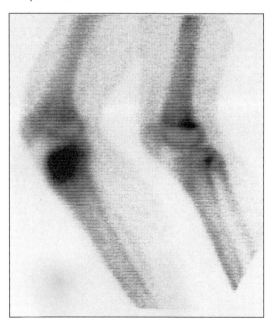

*d Right lateral*

**(a–d)** *Bone scan views of lower limbs in an 19-year-old boy who presented with pain in the right tibia.*

*There is a large vascular, metabolically active lesion present in the right upper tibia. At operation a Brodie's abscess (chronic, low-grade osteomyelitis) was found at that site.*

**Markers may help in the evaluation of a dynamic study, since it is frequently difficult to know if a vascular blush corresponds exactly to a metabolically active lesion.**

## Osteomalacia

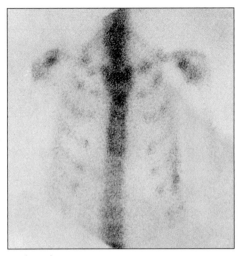

*a Anterior*

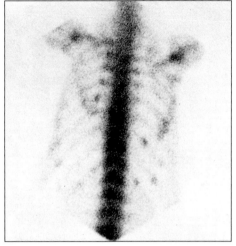

*b Posterior*

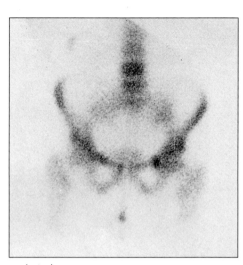

*c Anterior*

**Fig. 1.55**

*A 71-year-old woman who complained of generalized musculo-skeletal pain. Bone scan views: (a) chest; (b) thoracic spine; (c) pelvis.*

*The bone scan study shows generally good uptake of tracer throughout the skeleton, with high contrast between bone and soft tissue. There are multiple focal abnormalities in the ribs and left superior pubic ramus near to the acetabulum. This patient was shown to have osteomalacia with multiple pseudofractures.*

## Paget's disease

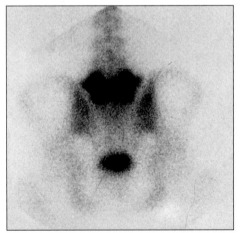

*Posterior*

**Fig. 1.56**

*A 61-year-old man who complained of low back pain.*

*The bone scan shows strikingly increased tracer uptake throughout the whole of L5, and the bone appears expanded. No other abnormality was present throughout the skeleton. This patient had monostotic Paget's disease involving L5.*

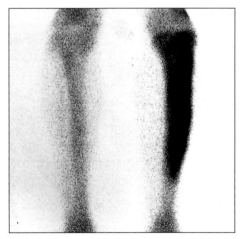

*a Anterior*

**Fig. 1.57**

*A further example of Paget's disease.*

*There is strikingly increased tracer uptake involving most of the left tibia. The scan appearances (a) are typical of Paget's disease, which is confirmed on the x-ray (b).*

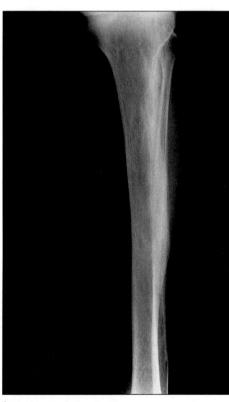

*b*

## Unexpected findings

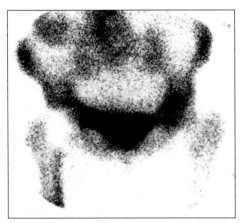

*a* Anterior

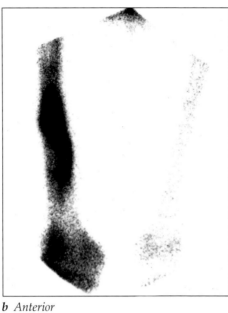

*b* Anterior

### Fig. 1.58

*A 78-year-old woman who complained of pain in her right hip. Bone scan views: (a) pelvis; (b) femora.*

*The woman had had a total right hip replacement performed several years previously. The prosthesis is clearly identified on the bone scan, with no associated abnormality. However, there is strikingly increased tracer uptake in mid-shaft below the prosthesis, with the appearances suggestive of fracture. An x-ray confirmed spiral fracture at that site.*

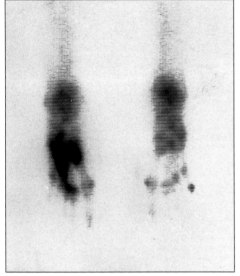

*a* Anterior

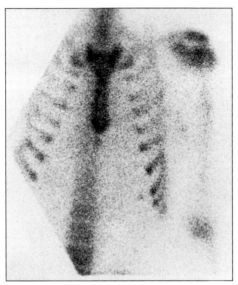

*b* Anterior

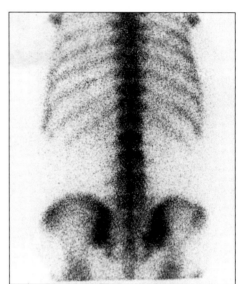

*c* Posterior

### Fig. 1.59

*A 42-year-old woman who sustained trauma to her left forefoot. Bone scan views: (a) feet; (b) thorax; (c) lumbar spine.*

*The x-rays were not thought to be typical of fracture, and the possibility of primary bone tumour or infection was suggested. In addition to abnormality in the left forefoot, the scan appearances were thought to be strongly suggestive of metabolic bone disease. Although the patient felt well, with no other bone-related symptoms, biochemistry revealed chronic renal failure and significant renal osteodystrophy.*

## 1.4.2 Investigation of malignancy

Although a bone scan lesion is a non-specific finding, characteristic scan appearances of multiple asymmetrical 'hot spots' throughout the skeleton are virtually diagnostic of metastases.

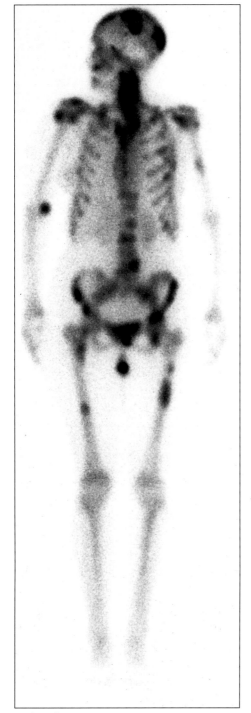 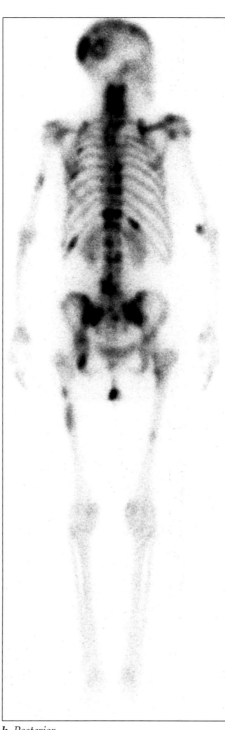

*a Anterior*  *b Posterior*

**Fig. 1.60**

*(a, b) Whole-body scan in a patient with bone metastases, confirming multiple focal areas of increased uptake at metastatic sites.*

## Initial staging

The bone scan is important in the initial evaluation of patients with malignancy, since the knowledge that metastases are or are not present may alter subsequent management. The bone scan is extremely sensitive for lesion detection, and, in the case of carcinoma of the breast, when compared with routine radiography, has a lead time of up to eighteen months (on average four months) for identification of metastases.

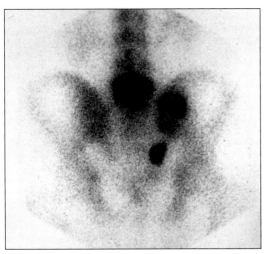

*a Posterior*

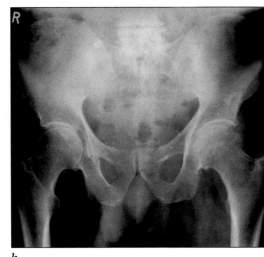

*b*

**Fig. 1.61**

*A 66-year-old man with carcinoma of the prostate: (a) bone scan view of pelvis; (b) x-ray of pelvis.*

*On the bone scan there is markedly increased tracer uptake involving L5, with further focal abnormalities in the right ilium and right border of the sacrum. The scan appearances are those of metastatic disease, and this is confirmed on the x-ray.*

## Recommended protocol for investigation of malignancy

(1) Bone scan
(2) Obtain x-rays of abnormal sites to exclude benign cause
(3) If x-rays are normal, malignancy is likely
(4) Depending on clinical relevance, further investigation such as CT, MRI or occasionally biopsy may be indicated
(5) Proceed to further imaging investigations if clinically indicated.

## CLINICAL APPLICATIONS

### Multiple myeloma

Multiple myeloma is the classic situation in which a false negative bone scan may be obtained. This occurs when the lesions are purely lytic, with no osteoblastic response. An example of this is shown in Fig. 1.62 where the bone scan views appear essentially normal, but the x-rays show multiple lytic lesions throughout the skeleton. In practice, however, it is rare to see a completely normal bone scan in multiple myeloma when skeletal involvement is present.

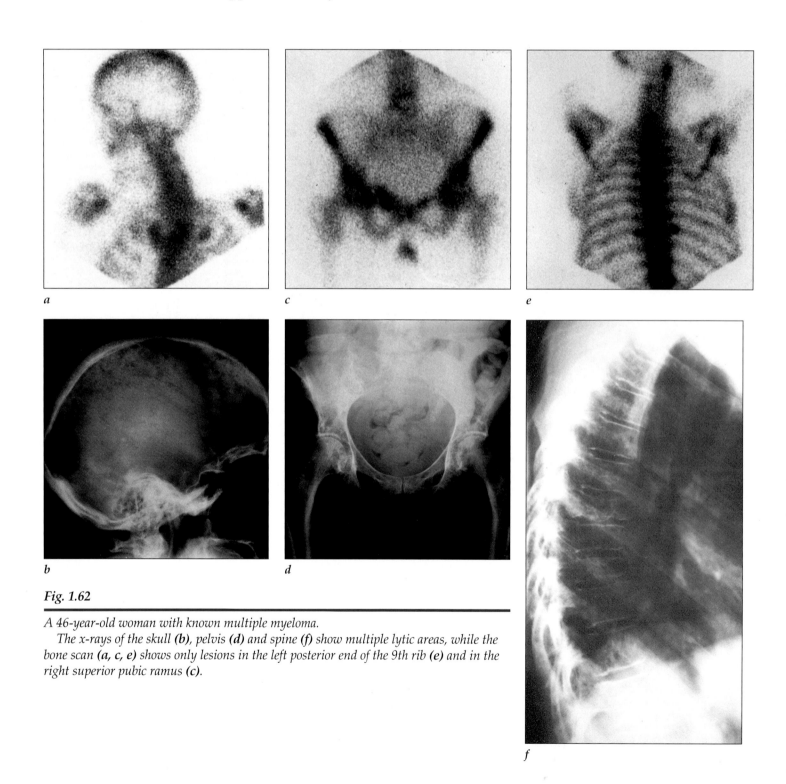

*a*

*c*

*e*

*b*

*d*

**Fig. 1.62**

*A 46-year-old woman with known multiple myeloma.*
  *The x-rays of the skull (b), pelvis (d) and spine (f) show multiple lytic areas, while the bone scan (a, c, e) shows only lesions in the left posterior end of the 9th rib (e) and in the right superior pubic ramus (c).*

*f*

## CLINICAL APPLICATIONS

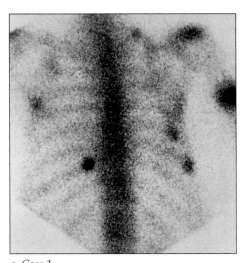
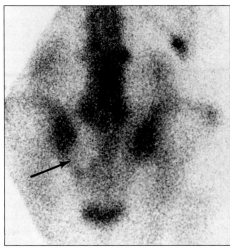
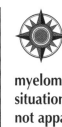

*a  Case 1*          *b  Case 2*

*Fig. 1.63*

*Two further cases of multiple myeloma.*

*(a) In this first case several focal abnormalities are present throughout the ribs, with a large intense area of increased uptake in the mid-shaft of the right humerus. The scan findings represent bony involvement secondary to myeloma and pathological fracture of the right humerus.*

*(b) In this second case a large photon-deficient area is seen in the left border of the sacrum (arrow). In addition, focal areas of increased tracer uptake are present in the right 12th rib and L3.*

While the bone scan may underestimate the extent of disease in multiple myeloma, it may, as in other situations, identify disease which is not apparent on x-rays. Radiography and bone scanning can be considered as complementary investigations, when accurate documentation of all skeletal disease is required.

## Photopaenic lesion

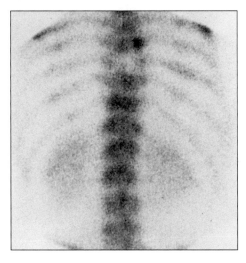
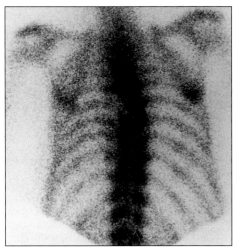
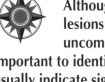

Although photopaenic lesions are relatively uncommon, it is important to identify them since they usually indicate significant bony destruction. Photopaenic areas are seen in association with aggressive lytic disease, which does not induce an osteoblastic response.

*Fig. 1.64*

*In this case of carcinoma of the lung the bone scan shows a photon-deficient area at T9. In addition, there is a focal area of increased tracer uptake at the right border of T8 and there is generally patchy tracer uptake throughout the ribs. The scan appearances are those of metastatic disease.*

*Fig. 1.65*

*A case of carcinoma of the breast with a lytic area seen in the mid-thoracic spine to the left of the midline.*

## CLINICAL APPLICATIONS

## Discordant scan/x-ray findings

### Solitary metastasis

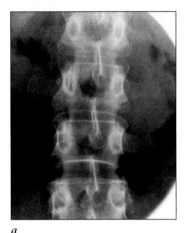

*a*

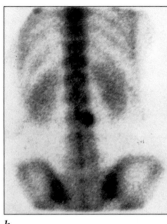

*b*

**Fig. 1.66**

*A patient with carcinoma of the breast who complained of severe low back pain.*

*An x-ray (**a**) of the lumbar spine was normal. However, the bone scan (**b**) showed a discrete focal area of increased tracer uptake at the right border of L3. This was caused by a metastasis.*

### Extensive metastases on scan with normal x-rays

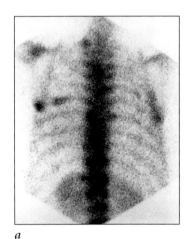

*a*

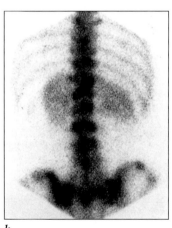

*b*

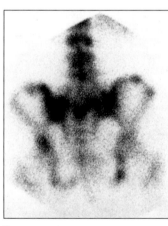

*c*

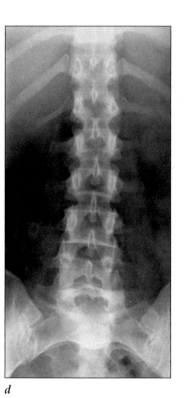

*d*

**Fig. 1.67**

*A patient with carcinoma of the breast who had a bone scan for staging purposes.*

*Multiple focal abnormalities representing metastases were seen throughout the skeleton (**a–c**). The radiographic skeletal survey (**d**) was normal at that time.*

**The bone scan may detect metastatic disease before any abnormality is seen on x-rays. The knowledge that skeletal metastases are present may significantly alter patient management.**

## *Assessment of extent of disease*

*Significance of solitary lesions*

*Table 1.1   Incidence of solitary metastases by site in order of frequency*

Spine
Pelvis
Sternum (in breast cancer)
Ribs
Long bones
Skull

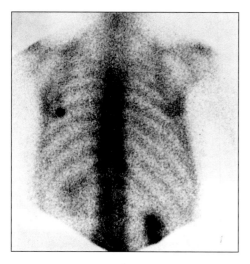

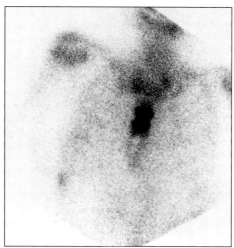

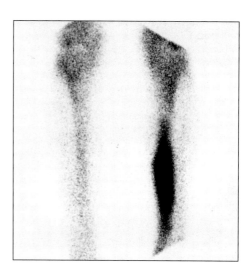

**Fig. 1.68**

*A patient with carcinoma of the breast who complained of pain in her back.*

*The bone scan showed a focal area of increased tracer uptake in the right 7th rib posteriorly. No other abnormality was present. While a single, metabolically active lesion in a rib has only a 10% probability of representing malignancy, in this case an x-ray of the area revealed a destructive lesion in the rib caused by a metastasis.*

**Fig. 1.69**

*A patient with carcinoma of the breast who had intensely abnormal radionuclide accumulation throughout the upper half of the sternum.*

*No other abnormality was present in the skeleton. The findings indicated a solitary metastasis involving the sternum, and this was confirmed by radiography.*

**Fig. 1.70**

*Solitary metastasis in tibia.*

## CLINICAL APPLICATIONS

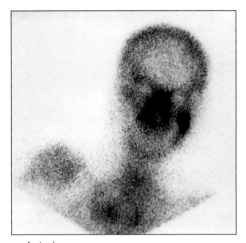

*a Anterior*

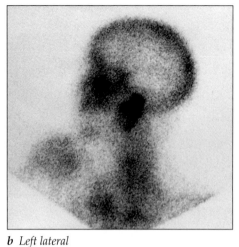

*b Left lateral*

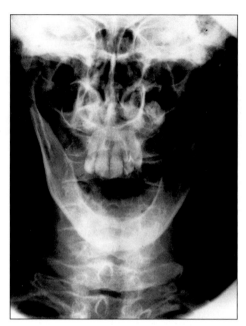

*c*

### Fig. 1.71

*(a, b) Bone scan views of the skull in a patient with carcinoma of the breast. (c) X-ray of mandible.*

*There is an intense focus of increased tracer uptake in the left mandible (a, b). No other lesion was present elsewhere in the skeleton. The x-ray of the mandible (c) revealed a lytic lesion, which corresponded to the abnormality on the bone scan. Biopsy revealed a metastasis from carcinoma of the breast.*

- While solitary peripheral metastases are relatively uncommon, they do occur. There has been some controversy as to whether routine views of the skull and lower limbs are necessary; however, if they are not obtained, some lesions will be missed.
- Sites such as the sternum, ribs and scapula can be difficult to evaluate on routine radiography, whereas a bone scan will provide clear visualization of these areas.

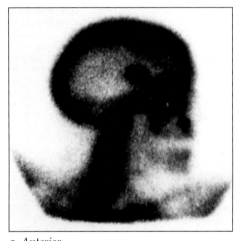

*a Anterior*

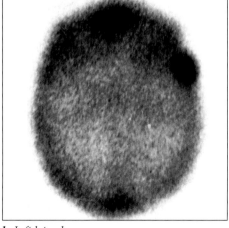

*b Left lateral*

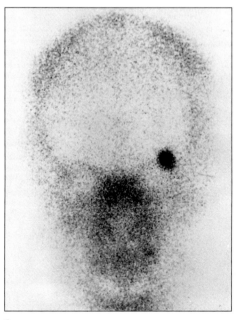

*c*

### Fig. 1.72

*Further examples of patients with carcinoma of the breast who each presented with a single peripheral metastasis.*

*(a, b) Solitary skull metastasis. (c) Solitary metastatic deposit in supraorbital ridge bone.*

## Localization problems
### Shine through

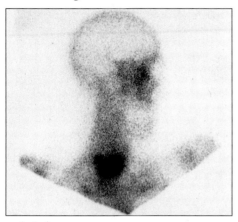

*a* Anterior

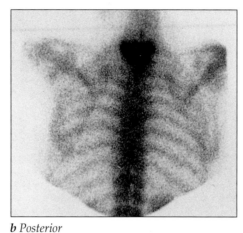

*b* Posterior

• Lesions should be visualized in two views whenever possible
• On occasion, the precise localization of an abnormality may not be apparent, but will often be clarified if additional views are obtained.

**Fig. 1.73**

*An elderly man with known carcinoma of the prostate. Bone scan views: (a) skull and anterior cervical spine; (b) posterior cervical and thoracic spine.*

*On the anterior view the appearance might suggest avid tracer accumulation in the thyroid. However, on the posterior view it is apparent that the lesion lies posteriorly and represents a metastasis in the thoracic spine.*

### Pelvic lesion

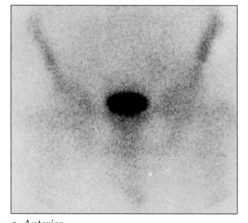

*a* Anterior

*b* Posterior

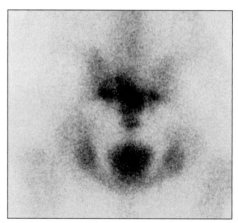

*c* Squat

**Fig. 1.74**

*(a–c) Bone scan views in a 66-year-old man with sacral metastasis.*

*There is intensely increased tracer accumulation in the lower sacrum extending throughout the coccyx and the lower portions of both sacro-iliac joints. An x-ray confirmed a metastatic deposit at that site. No other lesion was seen throughout the skeleton.*

Although the scans in Fig. 1.74 are obviously abnormal, the study emphasizes the potential importance of obtaining a 'squat' view to separate the bladder from bone. It is possible to imagine a situation where an abnormality is attributed to 'shine through' from the bladder.

# CLINICAL APPLICATIONS

## Localization

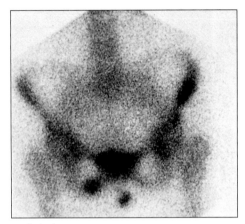

*a* Anterior

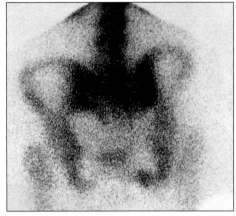

*b* Posterior

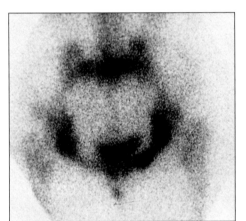

*c* Squat

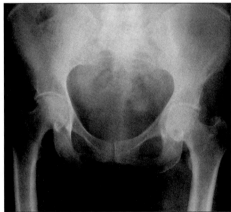

*d*

### Fig. 1.75

*(a–c) Bone scan views of pelvis in a patient with known carcinoma of the breast.(d) X-ray of pelvis.*

*The bone scan shows a focal area of increased tracer uptake in the right inferior pubic ramus. In addition, there is increased tracer uptake in the region of the left anterior superior iliac spine. The squat view shows that the lesion overlying the pubic ramus is indeed in bone (it is common to see urine contamination). The scan appearances reflect metastatic disease involving the pelvis. The lesion in the right inferior pubic ramus is confirmed on the x-ray.*

## Overlying scapula and rib

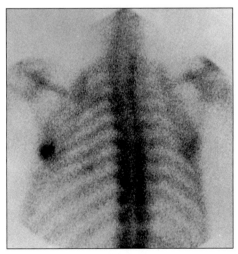

*a*

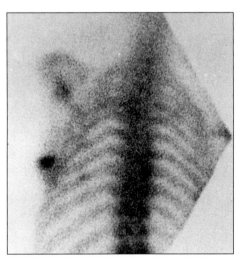

*b*

### Fig. 1.76

*Lesion of scapula or rib? Bone scan views: (a) posterior thorax; (b) with arm elevated.*

*A lesion is seen in the left chest on (a), but it is not clear whether it is associated with a rib or the scapula. With the arm elevated, it is apparent that the lesion is in the scapula.*

## CLINICAL APPLICATIONS

*Superscan*

**Table 1.2   The 'superscan'**

| Causes | Helpful features |
| --- | --- |
| Malignancy | Irregularity of tracer uptake<br>Focal lesions<br>Often skull and long bones poorly visualized |
| Hyperparathyroidism | Metabolic features<br>Hypercalcaemia |
| Osteomalacia | Metabolic features<br>Pseudofractures |
| Delayed imaging in normal subject | |

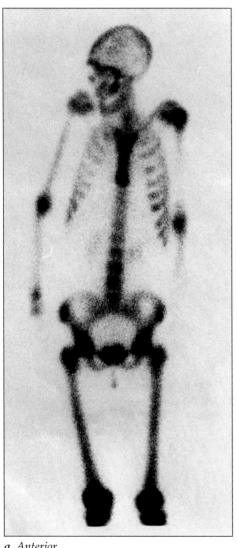

*a Anterior*

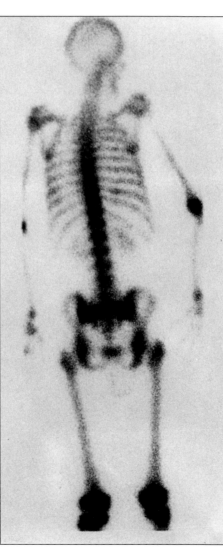

*b Posterior*

**Fig. 1.77**

*(a, b) Bone scan.*

*An example of the 'super scan' of malignancy, where scan appearances are much more difficult to evaluate. There is high uptake of tracer throughout the axial skeleton, with the kidneys only faintly visualized, but there is also increased tracer uptake in the skull and long bones — features shared with metabolic bone disease. However, there is also more focally increased tracer uptake in the left shoulder, and uptake in the region of the left anterior superior iliac spine is slightly irregular.*

## Monitoring progress of disease and response to therapy

The bone scan may be used to monitor progression of disease and response to therapy, since reliance on symptoms alone can be misleading. Furthermore, radiographic evidence of healing is slow to manifest, and not possible in the presence of sclerotic metastases.

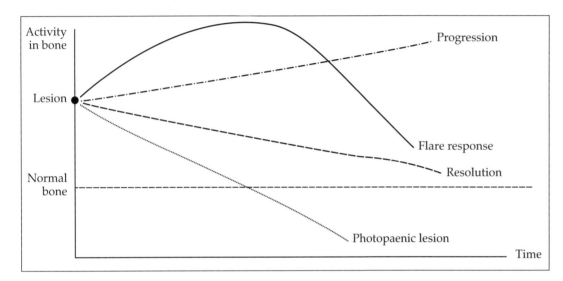

**Fig. 1.78**

*Bone scan patterns seen on serial studies*

## Progression of disease

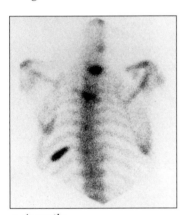

*a 4 months*

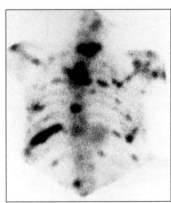

*b 8 months*

**Fig. 1.79**

*Carcinoma of the prostate.*
   *The original bone scan showed evidence of metastatic disease in the upper thoracic spine and left 8th rib posteriorly. On subsequent studies obtained 4 months later (a) and 8 months later (b) there is clear progression of disease.*

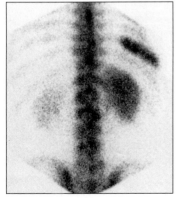

*a 0 months*

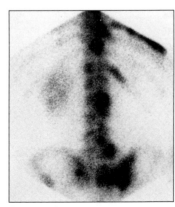

*b 3 months*

**Fig. 1.80**

*Progression of metastases with loss of function in the kidney.*
   *On the original study (a) of the posterior lumbar spine there is evidence of metastatic involvement of the skeleton, with some increased uptake of tracer seen in association with the right kidney. On the repeat study (b) obtained 3 months later there has been a dramatic progression of disease and the right kidney is no longer visualized. This patient had carcinoma of the prostate, with skeletal metastases. On the original study the right kidney was probably obstructed, with subsequent loss of function.*

# CLINICAL APPLICATIONS

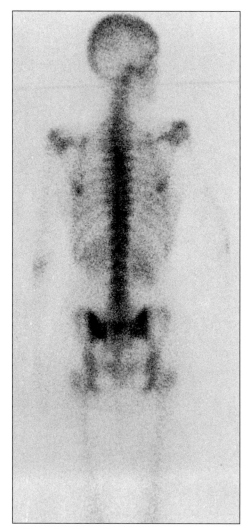

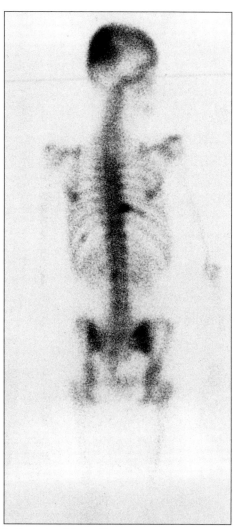

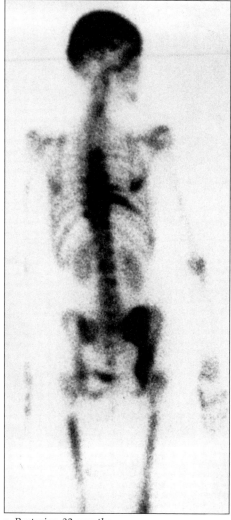

*a  Posterior, 0 months*      *b  Posterior, 24 months*      *c  Posterior, 32 months*

*Fig. 1.81*

A 37-year-old woman with carcinoma of the breast.

  The initial bone scan *(a)* is normal.  However, the repeat bone scan *(b)* obtained 2 years later shows evidence of metastatic disease, and there is dramatic progression of disease shown in the subsequent study *(c)* obtained after a further 8 months.

## *Resolution of disease*

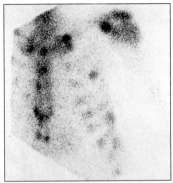

*a Before treatment*

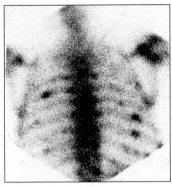

*b Before treatment*

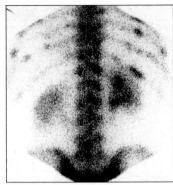

*c Before treatment*

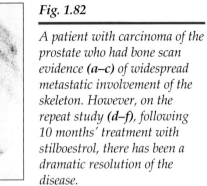

### *Fig. 1.82*

*A patient with carcinoma of the prostate who had bone scan evidence **(a–c)** of widespread metastatic involvement of the skeleton. However, on the repeat study **(d–f)**, following 10 months' treatment with stilboestrol, there has been a dramatic resolution of the disease.*

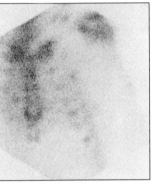

*d After treatment*

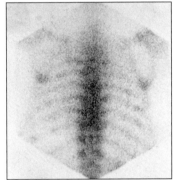

*e After treatment*

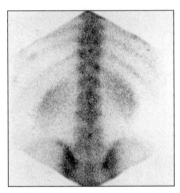

*f After treatment*

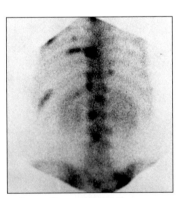

*a 0 months, pre-chemotherapy*

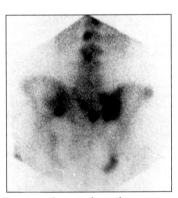

*b 0 months, pre-chemotherapy*

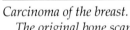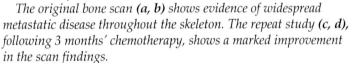

### *Fig. 1.83*

*Carcinoma of the breast.*
   *The original bone scan **(a, b)** shows evidence of widespread metastatic disease throughout the skeleton. The repeat study **(c, d)**, following 3 months' chemotherapy, shows a marked improvement in the scan findings.*

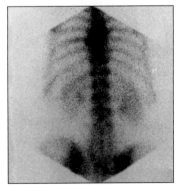

*c 3 months, post-chemotherapy*

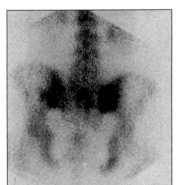

*d 3 months, post-chemotherapy*

## Flare response to therapy

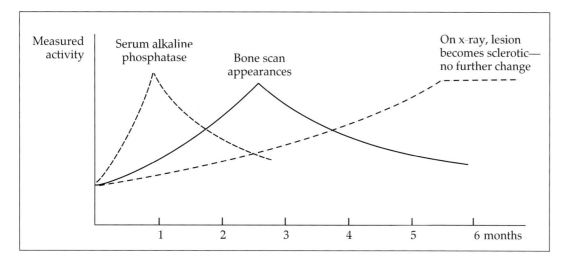

Measured activity

Serum alkaline phosphatase

Bone scan appearances

On x-ray, lesion becomes sclerotic— no further change

1   2   3   4   5   6 months

**Fig. 1.84**

*Flare response with successful therapy.*

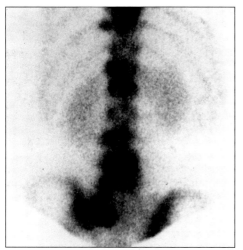

*a  0 months*

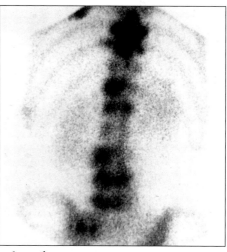

*b  3 months*

*c  6 months*

**Fig. 1.85**

 A further case of carcinoma of the breast, in which there was a good response to chemotherapy.

The initial scan (a) shows widespread metastatic involvement, but the repeat scan (b) obtained 3 months later was thought to show progression of disease, since individual lesions appeared more intense and a new focal abnormality was present in the left 10th rib. However, a subsequent scan (c) obtained after a further 3 months showed some evidence of improvement. This is an example of the 'flare' response to therapy, where a scan obtained shortly after instigation of treatment may show an apparent deterioration caused by an intense osteoblastic response reflecting healing. In order to evaluate therapy adequately, there should be a delay of at least 6 months, and perhaps a little longer, between scans.

**In a patient with metastatic disease it may not be possible to evaluate response to therapy in the initial months, since apparent deterioration in scan findings may reflect bone healing.**

## Bone scan response to radiotherapy

Bone scan appearances in patients who have received radiotherapy are often characteristic.

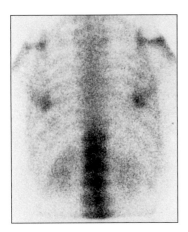

### Fig. 1.86

*An example of the characteristic bone scan appearance after radiotherapy.*

*There is generally reduced tracer uptake throughout the thoracic spine, with a sharp cut-off between abnormal and normal bone.*

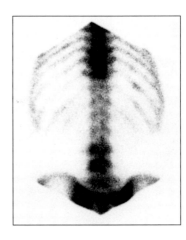

### Fig. 1.87

*A patient who received radiotherapy because of severe pain in the lumbar spine.*

*However, there is widespread metastatic disease involving the whole skeleton, and the scan appearances dramatically show the effect of radiotherapy in a patient with a 'superscan' of malignancy.*

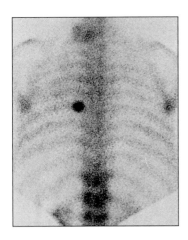

### Fig. 1.88

*A patient with carcinoma of the lung who received radiotherapy for a metastasis in the thoracic spine.*

*A bone scan was requested for reassessment of the disease. Marked differential uptake of tracer between the thoracic and lumbar spine is seen, characteristic of previous radiotherapy. However, there is a discrete focus of increased tracer uptake in the left 7th rib posteriorly, which was due to fracture. Appearances are, however, non-specific and x-ray confirmation is necessary.*

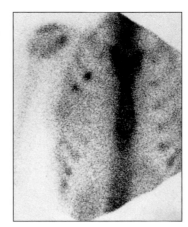

### Fig. 1.89

*Fractured ribs following radiotherapy in a patient with carcinoma of the breast. Bone scan view: right anterior chest.*

*There are focal areas of increased tracer uptake in the right 2nd and 3rd ribs anteriorly. X-ray confirmed fractures at these sites. These are pathological fractures secondary to radiation necrosis.*

**Following radiotherapy, fracture of the ribs may occur spontaneously. This is seen most often in carcinoma of the breast.**

## Increased renal uptake of diphosphonate

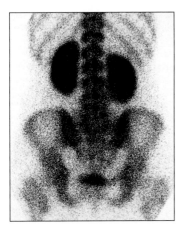

### Fig. 1.90

*A patient with carcinoma of the lung being treated with chemotherapy.*

*On the bone scan image high uptake of tracer is seen in both kidneys. This reflects the renal cytotoxic effect of chemotherapy. However, similar appearances may be seen, on occasion, in patients who are significantly hypercalcaemic.*

**CLINICAL APPLICATIONS**

## Hypertrophic pulmonary osteoarthropathy

*Four cases of hypertrophic pulmonary osteoarthropathy associated with carcinoma of the lung*

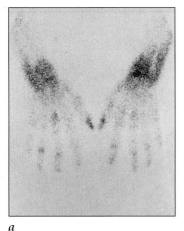
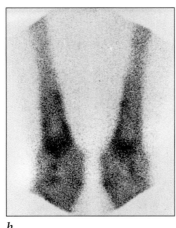
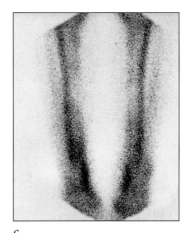

*a*　　　　*b*　　　　*c*

**Fig. 1.91**

*(a–c) On the bone scan images there is diffusely increased tracer uptake, with more focal areas also present, in the cortical aspects of the lower ends of the radius and ulna, the tibiae and lower femora. The scan findings are typical of hypertrophic pulmonary osteoarthropathy.*

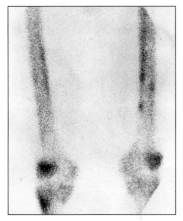
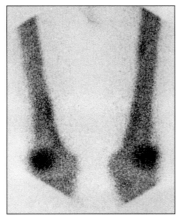
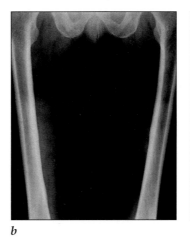
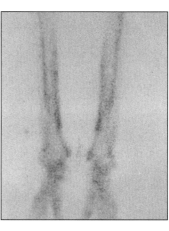

*a*　　　　*b*

**Fig. 1.92**

*There is increased tracer uptake peripherally in both femoral shafts and the right upper tibia. The scan appearances are typical of a periosteal reaction, and in this case were due to hypertrophic pulmonary osteoarthropathy. Note also that there is increased patellar uptake. This is of no real significance, but has been observed in approximately 50% of cases of hypertrophic pulmonary osteoarthropathy.*

**Fig. 1.93**

*The bone scan (a) shows slight, diffusely increased tracer uptake in the medial aspect of both lower femora, with more focal areas of increased tracer uptake in the left upper femur and lower right femur. The x-ray (b) confirms periosteal reaction at these sites.*

**Fig. 1.94**

*Bone scan view of tibiae, showing increased tracer uptake, particularly associated with the cortical margins. The scan findings are typical of hypertrophic pulmonary osteoarthropathy in association with carcinoma of the lungs. This is a good example of the so-called tramline or parallel stripe sign.*

## Primary bone tumours

*Table 1.3   Classification of malignant primary bone tumours*

| Site of origin | Tumour |
|---|---|
| Skeletal connective tissues | Osteogenic sarcoma |
| | Chondrosarcoma |
| | Fibrosarcoma |
| | Giant-cell tumour |
| | |
| Other skeletal components | Sarcoma |
| | Liposarcoma |
| | |
| Unknown | Ewing's tumour |

### Ewing's tumour

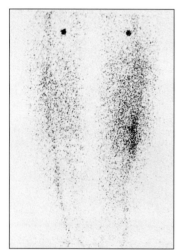

*a  Dynamic*

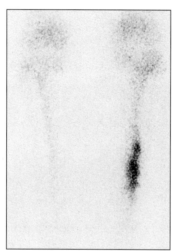

*b  Delayed*

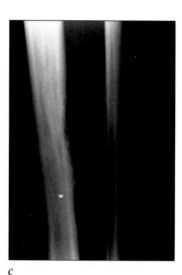

*c*

**Fig. 1.95**

*A 20-year-old woman with Ewing's tumour. (a,b) Bone scan views of anterior tibiae.*
*There is increased vascularity and increased tracer uptake at the left mid-tibia. The tumour is shown on the x-ray.*

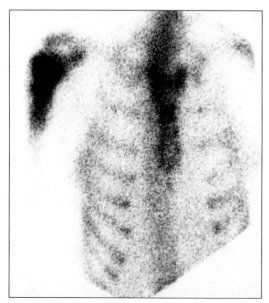

*a  Anterior*

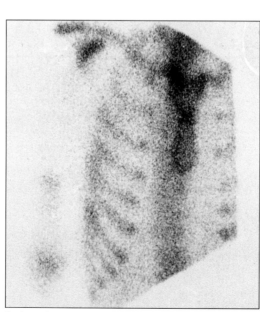

*b  Anterior*

**Fig. 1.96**

*A 29-year-old man with Ewing's tumour involving the right upper humerus. Bone scan views of chest: (a) pre- and (b) post-surgery.*
*On the original study there is markedly increased tracer uptake involving the right upper humerus at the site of a known Ewing's tumour. On the repeat study following surgery, a right humeral prosthesis can be seen. In addition, there is some increased tracer uptake associated with the right coracoid, which was presumably related to surgical intervention.*

## CLINICAL APPLICATIONS

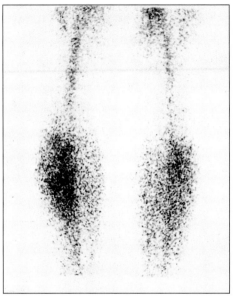 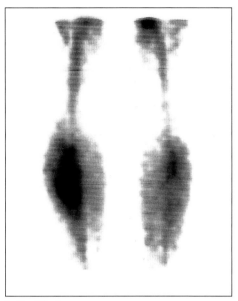 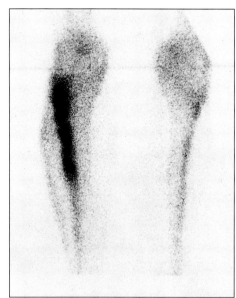

*a Dynamic*  *b Equilibrium*  *c Delayed*

**Fig. 1.97**

*(a–c) Three-phase bone scan in a 17-year-old male with Ewing's tumour.*
*There is a massively increased blood flow to the right fibula and associated soft tissue.*
*Delayed images show intense metabolic activity at the upper two-thirds of the right fibula.*

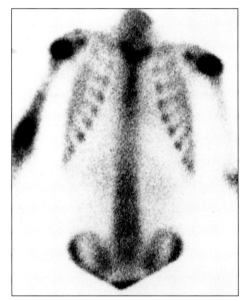

**Fig. 1.98**

*Bone scan showing massively increased tracer uptake in the right lower humerus caused by a Ewing's tumour.*

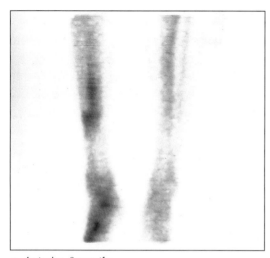

*a Anterior, 0 months*

### Fig. 1.99

*A 30-year-old man with a history of swelling in the right lower leg.*

*The bone scan (a) shows increased uptake in the region of the right tibia. An x-ray confirmed a Ewing's sarcoma. Three years later the patient developed severe pains in the back. The bone scan (b–e) shows metastatic spread of Ewing's sarcoma to the left scapula (b), spine (c) and pelvis (d,e).*

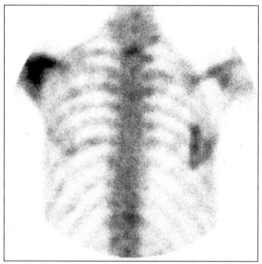

*b Posterior, 36 months*

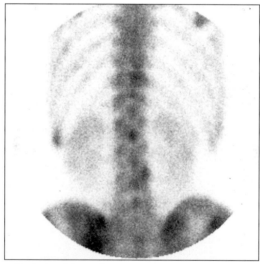

*c Posterior, 36 months*

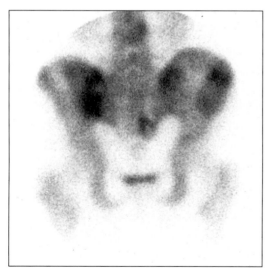

*d Posterior, 36 months*

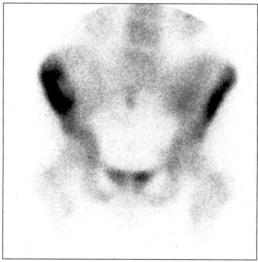

*e Anterior, 36 months*

## CLINICAL APPLICATIONS

## Osteogenic sarcoma

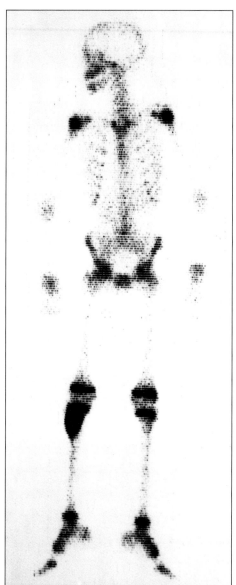

*a  Anterior*

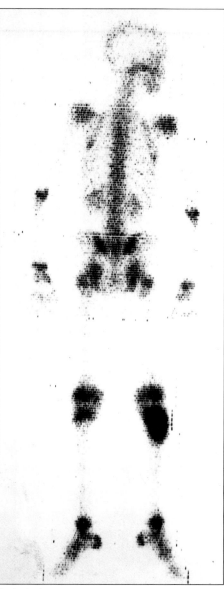
*b  Anterior*

### Fig. 1.100

*(a, b) Bone scan views of osteogenic sarcoma of the right upper tibia.*

*There is no evidence of metastatic disease elsewhere in the skeleton. Skeletal metastases are relatively uncommon at the time of presentation with osteogenic sarcoma, and occur more frequently with Ewing's tumour.*

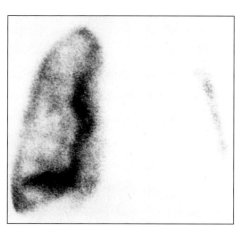

### Fig. 1.101

*Osteogenic sarcoma with lung metastases.*

*In this case there is massive uptake of MDP throughout the right lung caused by pulmonary and pleural deposits.*

 **It is well recognized that pulmonary deposits of osteogenic sarcoma may take up diphosphonate.**

# CLINICAL APPLICATIONS

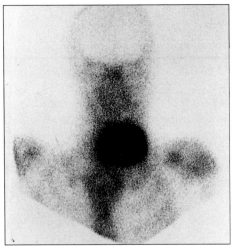
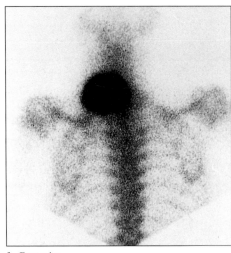
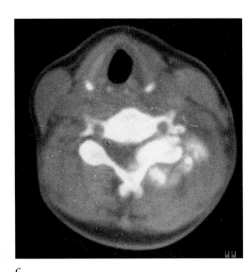

*a Anterior*　　　　　*b Posterior*　　　　　*c*

**Fig. 1.102**

*(a, b) Bone scan views of the upper thorax representing an unusual case of osteogenic sarcoma in a 28-year-old woman. (c) CT scan.*

　*The bone scan images show massive focal tracer accumulation in the region of the cervical spine, extending out to the left. The CT scan confirms a destructive lesion involving the cervical spine and extending into soft tissue. This was subsequently shown to be an osteogenic sarcoma.*

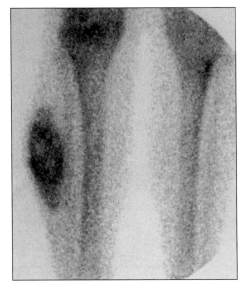
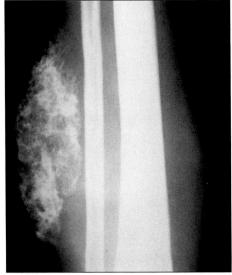
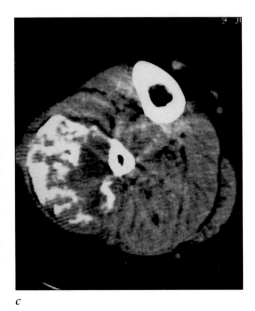

*a*　　　　　*b*　　　　　*c*

**Fig. 1.103**

*A 52-year-old woman with a hard swelling of the right calf.*

　*The bone scan (a) shows diphosphonate accumulation lateral to the right fibula. The x-ray (b) demonstrates calcification within the mass, and the CT scan (c) confirms that this osteogenic sarcoma arises from the fibula.*

## Chondrosarcoma

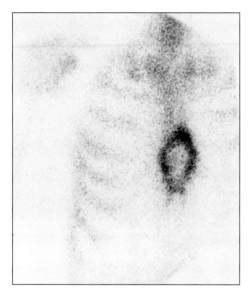

**Fig. 1.104**

*An elderly man who presented with a sternal mass.*

*The bone scan image of the anterior chest shows increased tracer uptake in the sternum, particularly at the peripheral borders, with a relative photon-deficient area at its centre. Biopsy of the sternal mass revealed chondrosarcoma.*

## Giant cell tumours

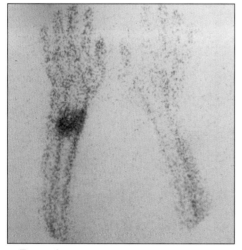 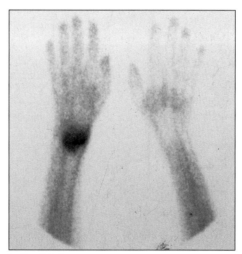 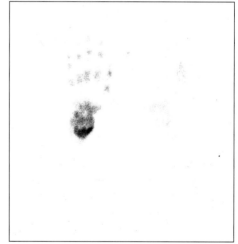

*a Dynamic*  *b Equilibrium*  *c Delayed*

**Fig. 1.105**

*A 32-year-old woman with a rapidly growing swelling of the right wrist and a large lytic lesion seen in the distal radius on x-ray.*

*The bone scan shows a vascular lesion (a,b) which accumulates diphosphonate (c) on delayed imaging. A giant cell tumour was identified at biopsy.*

## CLINICAL APPLICATIONS

### Histiocytosis x

Histiocytosis x describes a triad of diseases in which there are focal accumulations of macrophages in various organs, including bone. The triad is:

- Letterer–Siwe disease
- Hand–Schüller–Christian disease
- Eosinophilic granuloma of bone

### Hand–Schüller–Christian disease

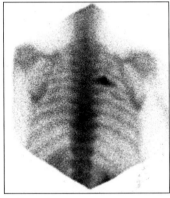

*a Posterior*

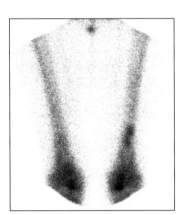

*b Anterior*

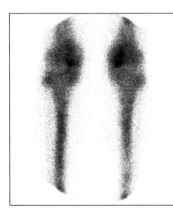

*c Anterior*

***Fig. 1.106***

*A 45-year-old woman with known Hand–Schüller–Christian disease and diabetes insipidus.*

*The bone scan shows abnormal tracer uptake in the right posterior 5th and 6th ribs (a), left lower femur (b) and both tibiae (c), confirming histiocytic lesions in the bone marrow at those sites.*

### Eosinophilic granuloma

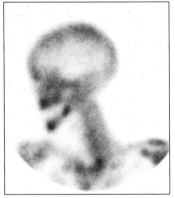

*a Anterior*

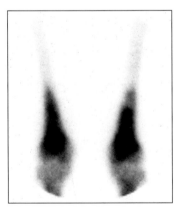

*b Anterior*

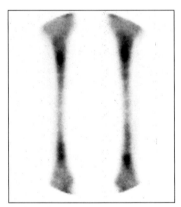

*c Anterior*

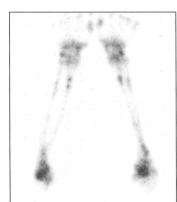

*d Anterior*

***Fig. 1.107***

*A young female with known eosinophilic granuloma.*
*The bone scan shows sites of disease in the mandible (a), lower femora (b), tibiae (c), and radii and ulnae (d).*

# 1.4.3 Investigation of benign bone disease

## *Orthopaedic disorders*

### *Causes of a painful prosthesis*

- Loosening
- Infection
- Fracture
- Heterotopic ossification
- Development of metastases

### *Hip prostheses*

### *Loosening*

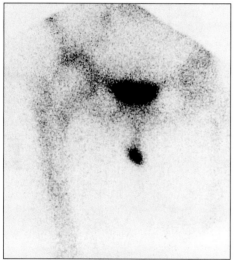

*a  1 year post-operation*

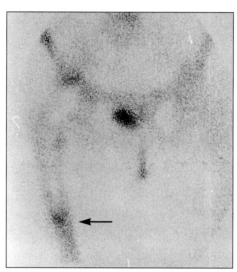

*b  2 years post-operation*

**Fig. 1.108**

*(a, b) Bone scan views of anterior right hip and upper femur.*

*On the original study, the scan appearances 1 year after insertion of a right hip prosthesis are normal. However, 1 year later the patient complained of recurrence of pain in the right hip, and the repeat scan shows a focus of increased activity at the tip of the prosthesis. The scan findings are typical of loosening of a prosthesis.*

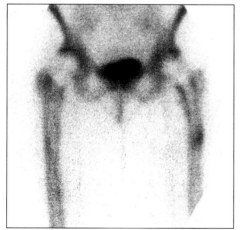

*a  Anterior*

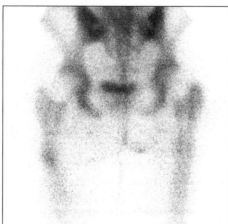

*b  Posterior*

**Fig. 1.109**

*A 63-year-old woman with bilateral hip prostheses and pain in the left hip.*

*The bone scan (a, b) indicates uptake around the right prosthesis, which is within normal limits. There is increased uptake at the top of the left femoral component consistent with loosening.*

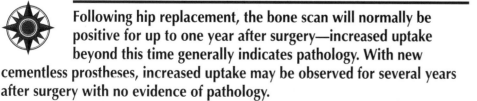

**Following hip replacement, the bone scan will normally be positive for up to one year after surgery—increased uptake beyond this time generally indicates pathology. With new cementless prostheses, increased uptake may be observed for several years after surgery with no evidence of pathology.**

## CLINICAL APPLICATIONS

*Differentiation between loosening of a prosthesis and infection*

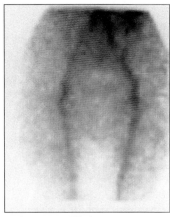

*a  Case 1, equilibrium*

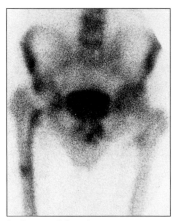

*b  Case 1, delayed*

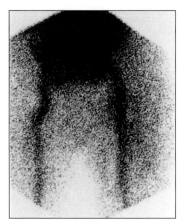

*c  Case 2, equilibrium*

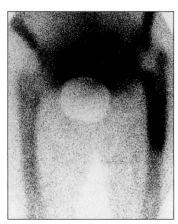

*d  Case 2, delayed*

**Fig. 1.110**

**Case 1** *Loosening.*
  *There is a discrete focus of increased tracer uptake at the tip of the femoral prosthesis **(b)**. The blood pool image **(a)** is normal.*

**Case 2** *Infected prosthesis.*
  *There is markedly increased tracer uptake associated with the femoral component of the prosthesis **(d)**. The blood pool image **(c)** indicates increased vascularity at that site.*

**In some cases it will not be possible to differentiate between infection and loosening on the basis of the bone scan alone, and a repeat study with either gallium- or indium-labelled white cells should provide additional information.**

*Metastatic involvement around a prosthesis*

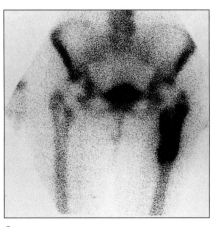

*a*

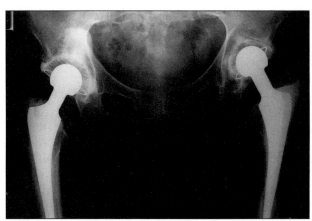

*b*

**Fig. 1.111**

*A 68-year-old woman with bilateral hip prostheses and cancer of the breast.*

  *The bone scan **(a)**, which was performed as the patient developed pain in the left hip, shows the bilateral hip prostheses, with intense uptake surrounding the shaft of the left femoral prosthesis. The x-ray **(b)** demonstrates bone destruction consistent with metastatic involvement of the left femur.*

*Heterotopic ossification*

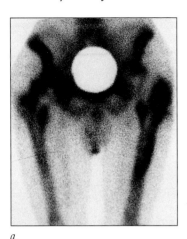

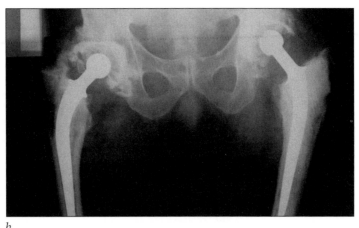

*a*                    *b*

**Fig. 1.112**

*Heterotopic ossification. Bilateral hip prostheses are present.*

*The bone scan **(a)** shows increased uptake of tracer on the right, in the region of the femoral neck, bridging the acetabulum and greater trochanter. These appearances are typical of heterotopic ossification, which is confirmed on the x-ray **(b)**. The scan findings on the left are quite abnormal, with markedly increased tracer uptake in the region of the left greater trochanter and along the lateral border of the femoral component of the prosthesis. Infection cannot be excluded.*

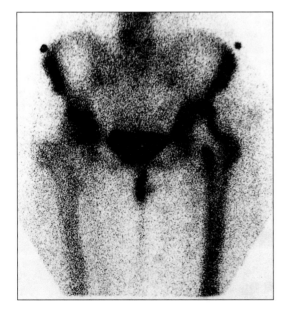

**Fig. 1.113**

*A further case of heterotopic ossification associated with a left femoral prosthesis.*

### Knee prostheses

Increased diphosphonate uptake is normally seen for a varible time interval following knee replacement surgery and does not necessarily indicate pathology. A $^{67}$Ga scan or white cell scan will be helpful in diagnosing infection in these cases.

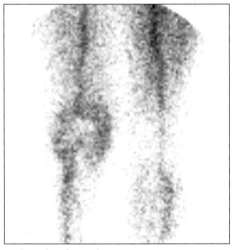

*a  Anterior, dynamic*

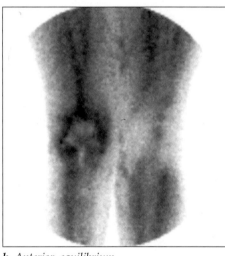

*b  Anterior, equilibrium*

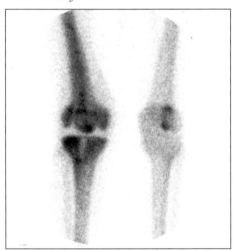

*c  Anterior, delayed*

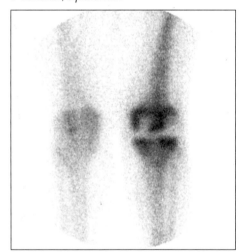

*d  Posterior, delayed*

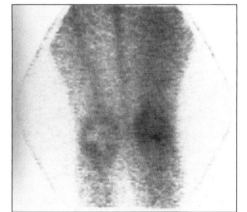

*e  Anterior, $^{67}$Ga*

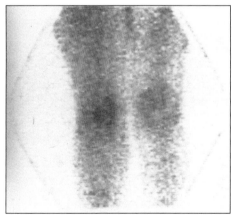

*f  Posterior, $^{67}$Ga*

**Fig. 1.114**

*A 78-year man with severe osteoarthritis and a one-year history of right-sided knee replacement. The patient presented with continuing pain and swelling of the right knee.*

*The bone scan shows increased blood flow and blood pool activity (a,b) around the prosthesis, and some uptake is seen in bone adjacent to the prosthesis, particularly in the region of the lateral tibial plateau (c,d).*

*A $^{67}$Ga scan performed in this patient showed increased $^{67}$Ga accumulation in the right knee (e,f), corresponding to the abnormal blood pool activity. Uptake in the tibial plateau was not significantly increased. Uptake was also noted in the left knee.*

*The scan findings were those of septic arthritis with no evidence of an osteomyelitis. Uptake in the left knee identified an inflammatory component of this patient's osteoarthritis.*

## Avascular necrosis
### Steroid-induced

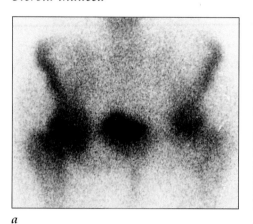

a

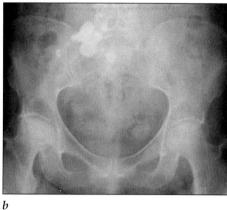

b

**Fig. 1.115**

*(a) Bone scan view of anterior pelvis and hips. (b) X-ray of pelvis.*

*This patient was taking steroid therapy for nephrotic syndrome. The bone scan shows intensely increased tracer uptake in the region of both hips. The scan findings are compatible with avascular necrosis, which is confirmed on the x-ray.*

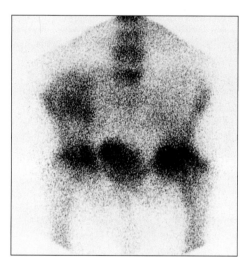

**Fig. 1.116**

*A further case of avascular necrosis of the hips caused by steroid therapy.*

*The bone scan shows increased tracer uptake in both hips, which is more pronounced on the left. This patient has a renal transplant, which is seen on the scan in the right iliac fossa.*

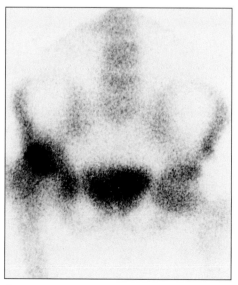

a

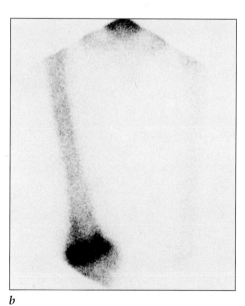

b

**Fig. 1.117**

*A 30-year-old man who was receiving steroids for hepatitis. Bone scan views: (a) pelvis; (b) femur.*

*It is apparent that there is strikingly increased tracer uptake in the region of the right femoral head (a), which corresponds with avascular necrosis and dislocation seen on x-ray. There is also diffusely increased tracer uptake throughout the shaft of the right femur, with focal increased uptake at the lower femur (b).*

*Avascular necrosis of lunate*

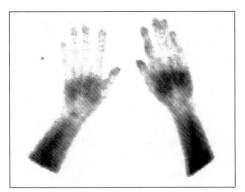 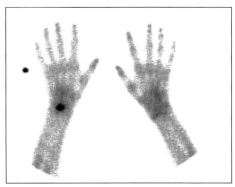

*a* Equilibrium  *b* Delayed

*Avascular necrosis following fracture*

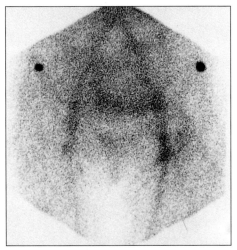 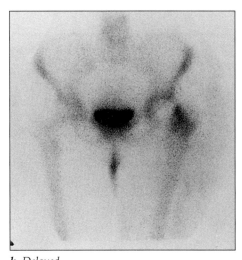

*a* Equilibrium  *b* Delayed

**Fig. 1.118**

*(a, b) Bone scan views of hands in a patient who complained of pain in the right hand.*

X-rays suggested avascular necrosis of the lunate bone. The bone scan confirms a discrete focus of increased tracer uptake associated with the lunate. There is also increased blood flow to that site.

**Fig. 1.119**

Bone scan views of anterior pelvis and femora.

This patient sustained a subcapital fracture of the left femur, which was fixed with compression screws. The blood pool image (a) shows reduced vascularity to the left femoral head. On the delayed image (b) there is an obvious photon-deficient area in the region of the left femoral head, together with some increased tracer uptake at the greater trochanter, which presumably reflects surgical intervention. The scan appearances indicate that the left femoral head is no longer viable.

## CLINICAL APPLICATIONS

*Perthes disease*

Perthes disease is a form of osteochondritis dissecans caused by an infarct in the capital femoral epiphysis. This results in abnormal growth and reduced mobility in the affected hip.

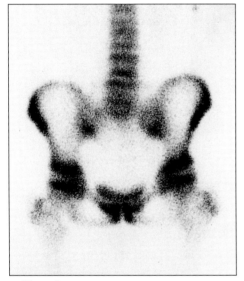

*a Normal*

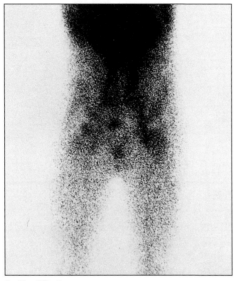

*b Equilibrium*

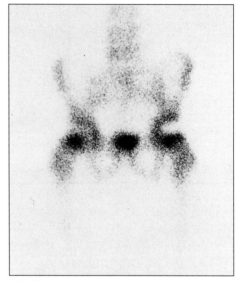

*c Delayed*

**Fig. 1.120**

**(a)** *Normal comparative bone scan.* **(b, c)** *Bone scan views of anterior pelvis and femora in a 14-year-old boy with Perthes disease.*

*Although the resolution is poor on the blood pool study, there is probably reduced blood flow in the region of the left femoral head. On the delayed images there is a clear photon-deficient area in the femoral epiphysis on the left.*

## CLINICAL APPLICATIONS

## *Benign bone tumours*

*Osteoid osteoma*

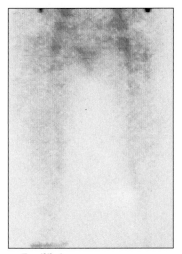 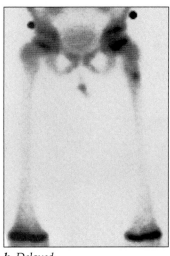 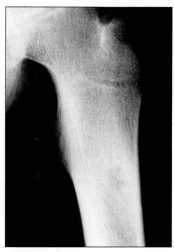

*a  Equilibrium*          *b  Delayed*          *c*

**Fig. 1.121**

*(a, b) Bone scan views of femora. (c) X-ray of upper left femur.*

    There is a discrete focus of increased tracer uptake seen in the upper third of the left femur. The lesion is vascular. This corresponds with lucency seen on the x-ray, representing a central nidus. The overall appearances are typical of osteoid osteoma.

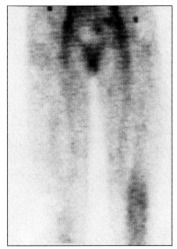 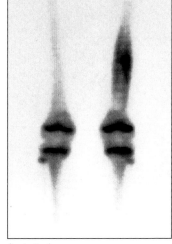 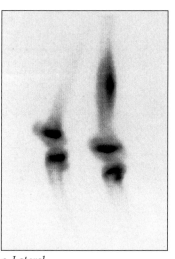

*a  Equilibrium*          *b  Anterior*          *c  Lateral*

**Fig. 1.122**

*(a–c) Bone scan views of lower femora and knees in a further case of osteoid osteoma involving a femur.*

    There is increased blood flow and increased tracer uptake in the left lower femur, which corresponded to an area of intense periosteal reaction seen on an x-ray. On the bone scan it is apparent that a more focal area of increased tracer uptake is seen within the generalized lesion. When an osteoid osteoma arises in the mid-shaft of a long bone, there may be an intense cortical reaction which can occasionally be confused with a malignant bone tumour.

# CLINICAL APPLICATIONS

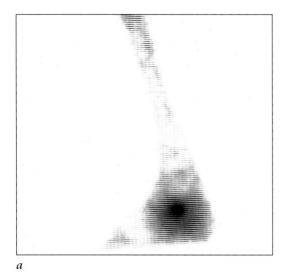

*a*

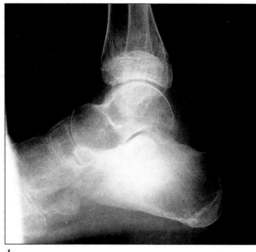

*b*

### Fig. 1.123

**(a, b)** *A further case of osteoid osteoma: osteoid osteoma of the left calcaneus.*

## Osteoid osteoma of the spine

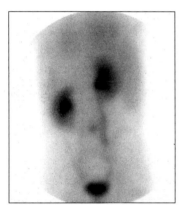

**a** *Posterior, equilibrium*

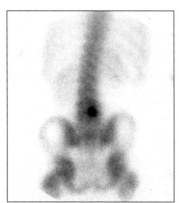

**b** *Posterior, delayed*

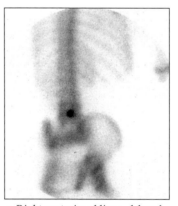

**c** *Right posterior oblique, delayed*

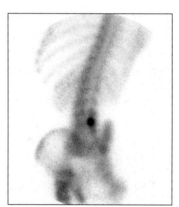

**d** *Left posterior oblique, delayed*

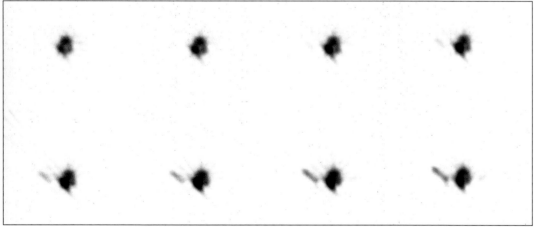

**e** *Transaxial,* SPECT

### Fig. 1.124

*A 12-year-old boy with a two-year history of back pain and normal x-rays.*

*The equilibrium view of the bone scan **(a)** shows a vascular lesion in the region of the lower lumbar spine. The delayed bone images **(b–d)** show an intense uptake of tracer in the right side of L4.*

*The transaxial* SPECT *scan **(e)** localizes the lesion to the right posterolateral elements of L4.*

*The findings were typical for an osteoid osteoma.*

## *Ivory osteoma*

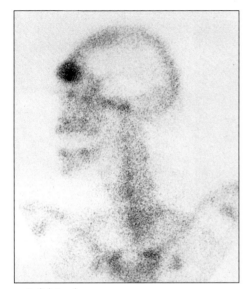

*a  Left lateral*

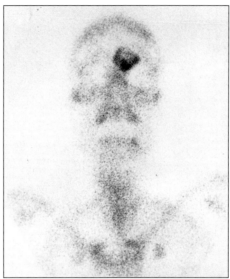

*b  Anterior*

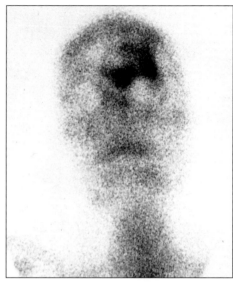

*c  Anterior*

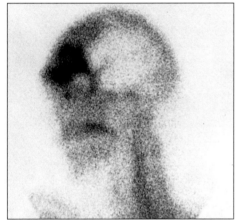

*d  Left lateral*

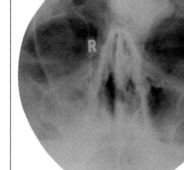

*e  Anterior*

### *Fig. 1.125*

*(a–d) Bone scan views of skull in a 32-year-old male acromegalic with an ivory osteoma.*
*(e) X-ray of anterior skull.*

   *An intense focus of increased tracer uptake is seen in the left supraorbital area (a, b)*
*This appearance is typical of an ivory osteoma, which was confirmed on x-ray (e). This*
*patient subsequently complained of severe pain in the left frontal region of the skull. The*
*repeat bone scan (c, d) showed, in addition to the above, increased tracer uptake extending*
*upwards and laterally, involving the frontal sinus. The scan findings were due to*
*sinusitis.*

## CLINICAL APPLICATIONS

### Haemangioma of spine

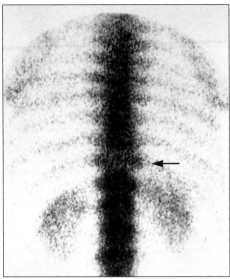

a  Posterior

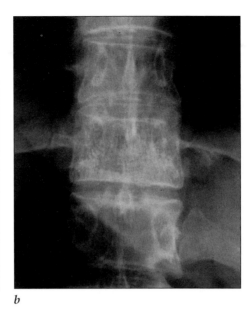
b

**Fig. 1.126**

*A 34-year-old man with haemangioma of the spine: (a) bone scan view of posterior thoracic spine; (b) corresponding x-ray.*

*There is a slight reduction of tracer uptake diffusely throughout the body of D11. This corresponds to the changes seen on the x-ray, which are those of haemangioma.*

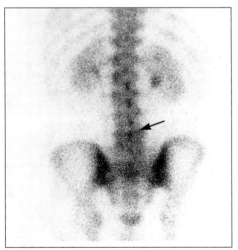

a  Posterior

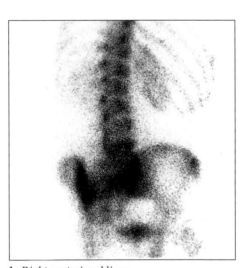

b  Right posterior oblique

**Fig. 1.127**

*(a, b) Bone scan views of lumbar spine in a 37-year-old man with haemangioma. (c) X-ray.*

*There is slightly increased tracer uptake throughout L4 corresponding to the changes of haemangioma seen on the x-ray.*

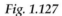

**Haemangioma of the spine may appear either photon-deficient or show slightly increased tracer uptake on the bone scan study.**

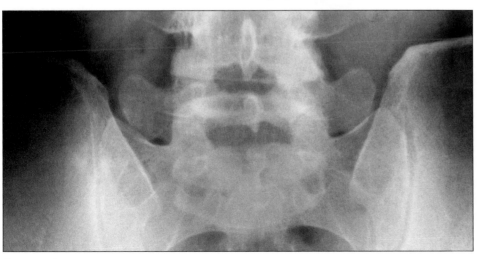

c

## Infection

The standard diphosphonate bone scan and imaging with gallium-67 ($^{67}$Ga) or labelled white cells have been used to identify osteomyelitis and to differentiate it from septic arthritis and cellulitis. A triple-phase bone scan should always be obtained in cases of suspected infection. Acute osteomyelitis is characterized by increased vascularity and enhanced activity in the delayed skeletal images, whereas septic arthritis and cellulitis show increased vascularity but normal or low-grade bone uptake on delayed images.

In some cases the diagnosis may still be in doubt, and a $^{67}$Ga or labelled white cell scan will provide additional information. Opinions vary as to which is the most sensitive. A white cell study will identify the sites of active white cell migration and, while more specific for infection, has a higher false negative rate, particularly in patients being treated with antibiotics or with chronic disease. $^{67}$Ga has bone-seeking properties in its own right and will show uptake at any areas of increased metabolic activity. This study should be read in conjunction with the bone scan image; the following features strongly favour infection:

• focally increased uptake greater than that seen on the corresponding bone scan image

• focally increased uptake which does not correspond precisely to a discrete lesion on the bone scan.

Although indium-111 ($^{111}$In) labelled white cells have been widely used to investigate the presence of bone sepsis, technetium-99m ($^{99}$Tc) labelled white cells are now being evaluated. These yield higher-resolution images, but poorer 24-hour data in view of the 6.4-hour half-life.

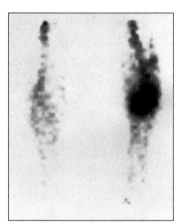

*a Dynamic*

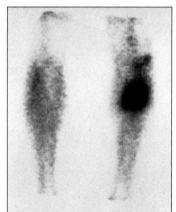

*b Equilibrium*

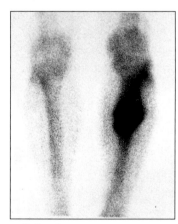

*c Delayed*

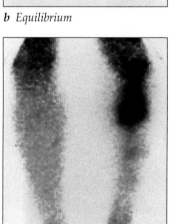

*d $^{67}$Ga*

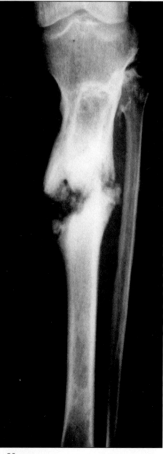

*e X-ray*

### Fig. 1.128

*(a–d) Bone scan views of tibiae in a 44-year-old man with fractured tibia, non-union and infection. (e) X-ray.*

*On the bone scan views there is marked vascularity to the upper third of the left tibia, and on the delayed image there is strikingly increased tracer uptake at that site corresponding to both ends of the fracture. On the $^{67}$Ga scan there is strikingly increased tracer uptake in the region of the non-united fracture.*

## CLINICAL APPLICATIONS

## *Osteomyelitis involving the foot*

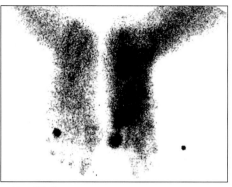

*a Equilibrium*

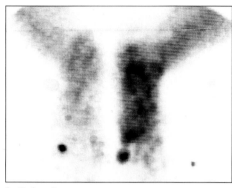

*b Delayed*

**Fig. 1.129**

*(a, b) Bone scan views of both feet in an elderly diabetic patient who had previous amputation of the right great toe. The right foot was painful and swollen.*

*The bone scan shows intense metabolic activity with increased vascularity at the site of amputation. Subsequent investigations confirmed osteomyelitis.*

## *Osteomyelitis involving the second metacarpal*

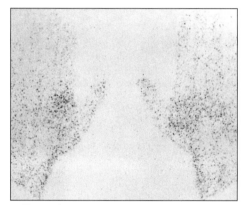

*a Dynamic*

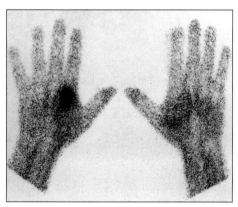

*b Equilibrium*

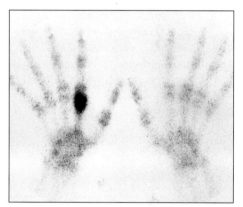

*c Delayed*

**Fig. 1.130**

*(a–c) Bone scan views of hands.*

*There is an intense focus of increased tracer uptake seen in the proximal second metacarpal. There is increased vascularity at this site, and an x-ray showed a periosteal reaction. The scan findings were due to osteomyelitis.*

## *Osteomyelitis of the right femur*

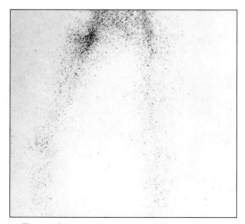

*a Dynamic*

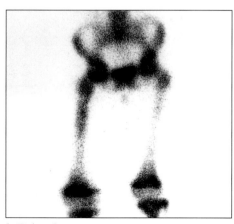

*b Delayed*

**Fig. 1.131**

*(a, b) Bone scan views of femora in a 6-year-old girl who complained of pain in her right thigh.*

*There is increased tracer uptake in the right upper femur. This area is vascular. The child had confirmed osteomyelitis of the right femur.*

*Acute exacerbation of chronic osteomyelitis*

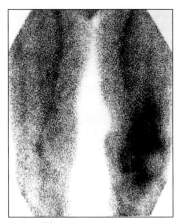

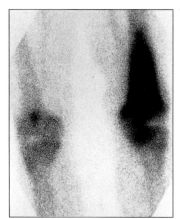

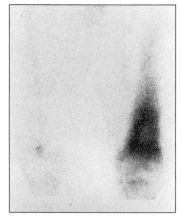

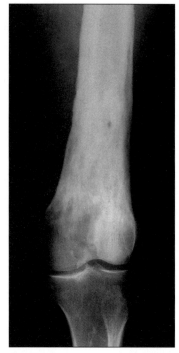

*a Equilibrium*    *b Delayed*    *c Following antibiotic therapy*

**Fig. 1.132**

*d*

*(a–c) Bone scan views of femora. (d) X-ray of left femur.*

    *There is strikingly increased tracer uptake to the lower third of the left femur, and also in the medial aspect of the left tibial plateau. These areas are highly vascular. Following antibiotic therapy, the scan appearances show marked improvement, with resolution of the tibial abnormality. The initial bone scan appearances in isolation are suggestive of Paget's disease, but are in fact due to an acute exacerbation of chronic osteomyelitis. Once again, this case illustrates that the bone scan is sensitive but the appearances are non-specific.*

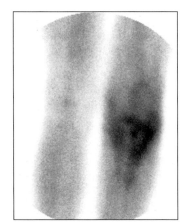

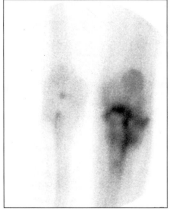

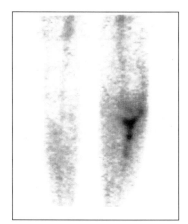

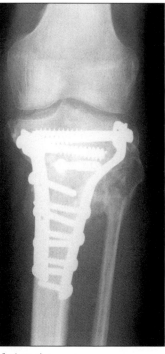

*a Anterior, equilibrium*    *b Anterior, delayed*    *c Anterior, $^{99m}$Tc WBC*

**Fig. 1.133**

*A 68-year-old man who had undergone internal fixation (d) for a fractured left tibia following a road accident. Six months later the patient complained of increasingly severe pain in left leg.*

    *A bone scan showed increased blood pool (a) and metabolic activity (b) in the region of the left upper tibia, raising the possibility of osteomyelitis. A $^{99m}$Tc white cell scan (c) at 3 hours showed intense white cell accumulation at fixation sites, confirming infection.*

*d Anterior, x-ray*

**CLINICAL APPLICATIONS**

# *Fracture*

## Fractured ribs

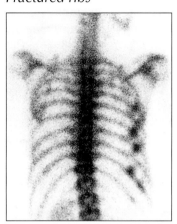
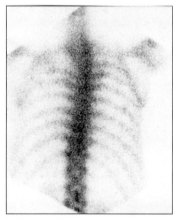

*a* 0 months

*b* 11 months

### Fig. 1.134

**(a, b)** *Bone scan views of posterior thoracic spine in an elderly woman who had suffered a fall.*

*On the original bone scan multiple focal abnormalities are present in a linear pattern in the right posterior ribs. The scan appearances are diagnostic of fracture. On the repeat study there is almost complete resolution, indicating healing of the fractures.*

## Fractured neck of the femur

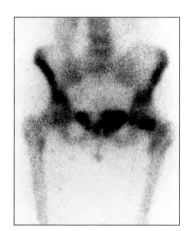

### Fig. 1.135

*A 65-year-old woman who complained of pain in her left hip following a fall. The x-rays were normal, but the bone scan showed increased tracer uptake in the left femoral neck, with appearances suggestive of fracture. Subsequent x-rays confirmed an impacted fracture of the left femoral neck.*

## Fractures from non-accidental injury

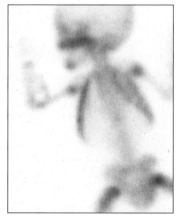
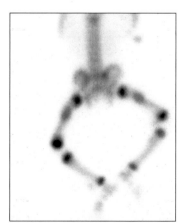
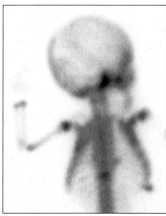

*a* Anterior

*b* Anterior

*c* Anterior

### Fig. 1.136

**(a–c)** *Bone scan in a 2-month old girl with a history given by the mother of cracking sounds in legs during bathing.*

*The scan identifies uptake in both femora, anterior ribs and the lower thoracic spine. The features are typical of fractures from non-accidental injury.*

## Scaphoid fracture

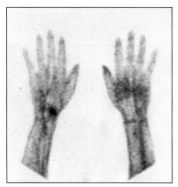 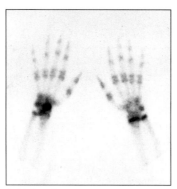 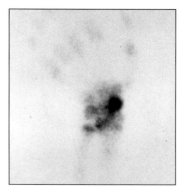

*a Dynamic*       *b Delayed*       *c*

**Scaphoid fracture may be missed on early x-rays. A bone scan with dynamic views is a sensitive method of diagnosing scaphoid fracture.**

**Fig. 1.137**

*(a, b) Bone scan views of hands in a 16-year-old boy who sustained a right-sided scaphoid fracture while boxing. (c) Magnified image of right wrist and hand.*

*There is a clear focus of increased tracer uptake in the region of the right scaphoid. This area is highly vascular.*

## Non-union of fracture

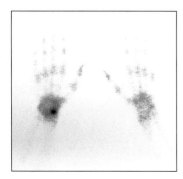

**Fig. 1.138**

*A patient who sustained a fracture of the scaphoid and was still experiencing persistent pain 4 months later.*

*The bone scan shows an intense focus of increased uptake in the region of the scaphoid, attributable to failed union of the fracture.*

## Registration of bone scan and x-ray

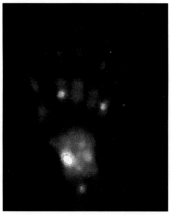 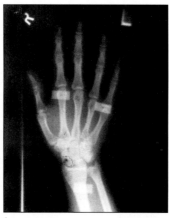

*a*       *b*

**Fig. 1.139**

*(a) Registered bone scan. (b) X-ray of the hand.*

*The region of interest (black lines) is drawn around the intense bone scan lesion and displayed on the digitized x-ray, confirming that the tracer uptake is located in the region of the scaphoid. The markers used to register the study are visualized on the bone scan and x-ray.*

**• The accurate, anatomical localization of bone scan lesions may not be possible.**

**• By incorporating the bone scan and the x-ray image, accurate anatomical localization of the lesion identified on the bone scan can be obtained.**

## Exercise-related trauma

With the increasing popularity of jogging and other forms of exercise, it is common for patients to complain of pain in a lower limb. While radiography remains the primary diagnostic procedure for identification of skeletal trauma, often the initial x-rays may fail to diagnose an injury. The bone scan may provide valuable information in such cases. Pain in a lower limb may be caused by any of the following:

- Fracture
- Stress fracture
- Shin splints
- Periosteal reaction
- Knee trauma
- Joint abnormalities
- Skeletal muscle injuries

### Stress fracture

*Table 1.4   Response of bone to increasing stress*

| | Normal | Bone | Bone scan/x-ray | Symptoms | Remodelling |
|---|---|---|---|---|---|
| S | + | | Normal/Normal | — | Normal: Resorption = Formation |
| T | | | | | (R)      (F) |
| R | ++ | | ?+ve/Normal | Pain | Accelerated R > F |
| E | +++ | | +ve/Normal | Pain | Fatigue R ≫ F |
| S | | | | | Cortex weakened |
| S | ++++ | | +ve/+ve | Pain | Exhaustion R ⋙ F |
| | FRACTURE | | | | |

(Adapted with permission from Roub LW, Gumerman LW, Hanley EN et al, Bone stress: a radionuclide imaging prospective I, *Radiology* **132**: 431–8, 1979.)

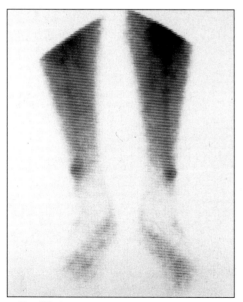

*a Equilibrium*

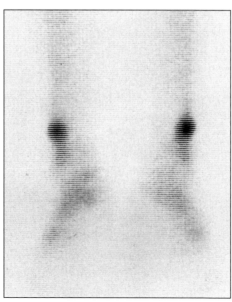

*b Delayed*

**Fig. 1.140**

*(a, b) Bone scan views in a 20-year-old female ballet dancer with bilateral stress fractures of the fibulae.*

*There are focal areas of increased tracer uptake in both lower fibulae just above the ankle. The lesions are highly vascular.*

## CLINICAL APPLICATIONS

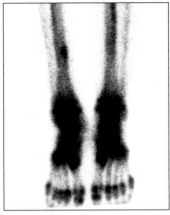 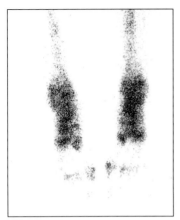 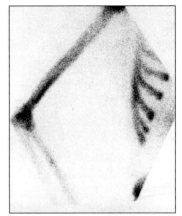 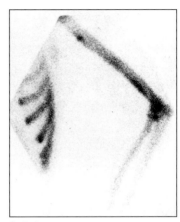

*a  0 months*          *b  10 months*          *a  Right*          *b  Left*

**Fig. 1.141**          **Fig. 1.142**

*(a, b) Bone scan views of lower legs in a 16-year-old ballet dancer with stress fracture.*

*There is a focal lesion present at the medial aspect of the right lower tibia, caused by a stress fracture. On the repeat study the lesion has resolved.*

*(a, b) Bone scan views of the arms in a 24-year-old male weight-lifter with a stress fracture of the humerus.*

*There is increased tracer uptake throughout both humeri, particularly at the medial aspect of the lower third. The linear changes at this site are typical of periosteal reaction, and the scan appearances in the humeri presumably reflect cortical hypertrophy. In addition, there is a focus of more intense increased tracer uptake at the medial aspect of the upper third of the left humerus, indicating a stress fracture.*

## Shin splints

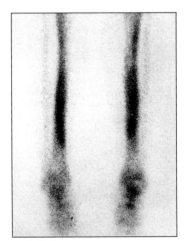 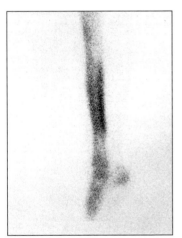 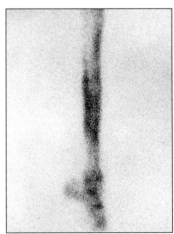

*a  Anterior*          *b  Right lateral*          *c  Left lateral*

**Fig. 1.143**

*(a–c) Bone scan views of tibiae in a 26-year-old aerobics teacher with shin splints.*

*There is strikingly increased tracer uptake diffusely along the posterior third of both tibiae, and in addition there is some increased tracer uptake throughout the rest of the tibiae. Note also slightly increased tracer uptake in the left forefoot. The scan appearances of the posterior tibiae are typical of shin splints. The more generalized increased tracer uptake in the tibiae presumably reflects cortical hypertrophy. The scan appearances in the left forefoot are non-specific, but are likely to represent minor degenerative change.*

• **Differentiation between shin splints and stress fracture is important. Shin splints is a syndrome due to a periosteal reaction at the site of muscle insertion at the lower third of the posterior tibia. Patients can continue with exercise as long as they feel comfortable. However, patients with stress fracture must avoid exercise for at least six weeks, since they are at risk of sustaining complete fracture.**
• **It is important to obtain lateral views in patients who are complaining of pain in a lower limb, since otherwise the diagnosis of shin splints will be missed.**

**CLINICAL APPLICATIONS**

## Knee trauma: meniscal tears

A common sequel of trauma to the knees is a torn meniscus. The bone scan using tomography and dynamic imaging will assist in the diagnosis of the meniscal tear. Meniscal tears appear as a crescentic area of increased uptake at the site of the tear. This uptake is presumed to reflect on osteoblastic response following trauma to the meniscal attachment to the bone.

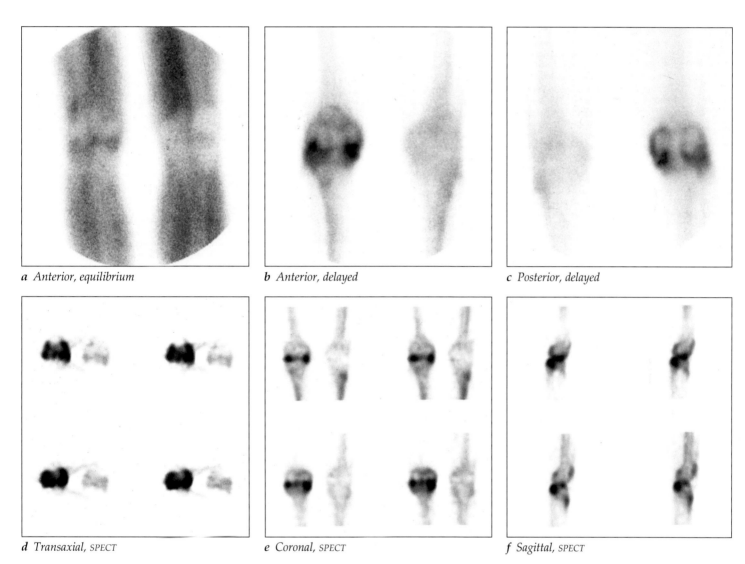

*a Anterior, equilibrium*

*b Anterior, delayed*

*c Posterior, delayed*

*d Transaxial, SPECT*

*e Coronal, SPECT*

*f Sagittal, SPECT*

**Fig. 1.144**

*(a–c) Bone scan in a 32-year-old man following a football injury. There is increased blood pool activity in the right knee (a) with intense uptake in the medial and lateral compartments of the right knee seen on delayed imaging (b, c). Uptake appears to involve both the femur and tibia.*

*This finding is confirmed on SPECT imaging (d–f), which shows crescentic uptake patterns in the medial and lateral right tibial plateau on the transaxial slices (d) and uptake also in the lower femur on the coronal and sagittal slices (e, f).*

*These findings are typical of medial and lateral meniscal tears.*

## CLINICAL APPLICATIONS

# Surgical trauma

## Thoracoplasty

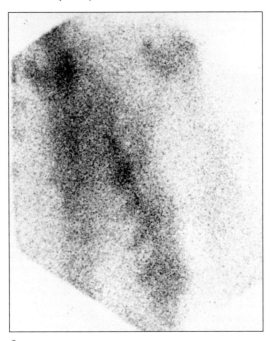

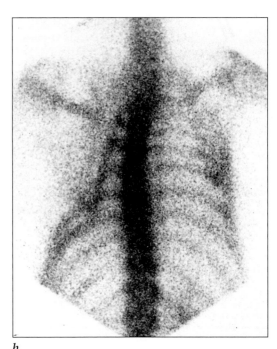

*a*                                    *b*

### Fig. 1.145

*Bone scan views: **(a)** left anterior chest; **(b)** anterior thoracic spine.*

   *Typical scan appearances of previous thoracoplasty are seen in the left upper ribs.*

## Rib resection

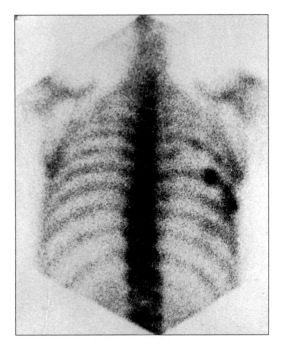

### Fig. 1.146

*Bone scan of a patient who had rib resection for plasmacytoma.*

   *Note the absence of the right 6th rib posteriorly. Focal abnormalities are seen in the right 5th and 7th ribs posteriorly. There are metabolically active lesions of ribs, which most probably represent fractures following surgery.*

**CLINICAL APPLICATIONS**

## Degenerative disease

Degenerative disease is a feature in the elderly. The differentiation between degenerative disease and metastatic disease in elderly patients with known malignancy may be impossible from a single bone scan, but serial imaging will frequently identify progression if metastatic disease is present. Comparison with a current x-ray may also aid differentiation

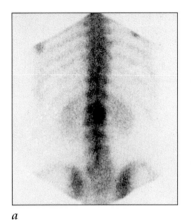

*a*

### Fig. 1.147

*(a)* Bone scan view of lumbar spine in a 70-year-old woman who complained of pain in her back. *(b)* Corresponding x-ray.

There is a focal area of increased tracer uptake at the right border of L1/2. The scan appearances are non-specific, but represent degenerative change, which is confirmed on the x-ray.

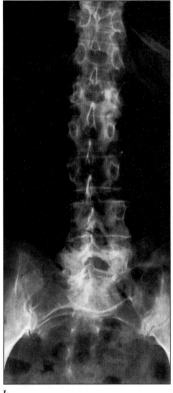

*b*

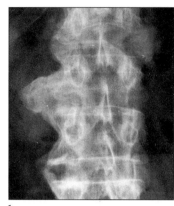

*a Posterior*   *b*

### Fig. 1.148

*(a)* Bone scan of lumbar spine. *(b)* Corresponding x-ray.

There is a focus of increased tracer uptake seen at the left aspect of L2/3, which extends beyond the normal anatomical border. The x-ray reveals a large osteophyte at that site.

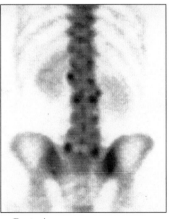

*a Posterior*

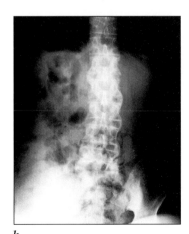

*b*

### Fig. 1.149

*(a)* Bone scan of lower thoracic and lumbar spine. *(b)* Corresponding x-ray.

In this case multiple focal areas of increased tracer uptake are present in the lumbar spine at the following sites: left border of L1/2, corresponding to a large osteophyte seen on the x-ray; right L2/3 junction, again corresponding to an osteophyte; L3 pedicles; L5/S1 articulations bilaterally and symmetrically. This patient had carcinoma of the breast, and had a bone scan as part of routine evaluation. Although focal abnormalities are present in the spine, they are all attributable to degenerative change, with no evidence of metastatic disease.

Note that not all sites of degenerative change are seen on the bone scan. A positive scan result depends on metabolic activity, and inactive lesions, ie 'burnt-out' disease, will not be visualized.

## Degenerative disease of the spine: SPECT imaging

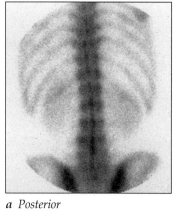
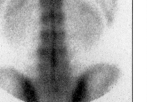

*a Posterior*

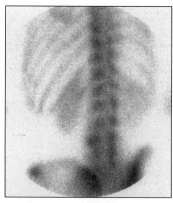

*b Right posterior oblique*

*c Left posterior oblique*

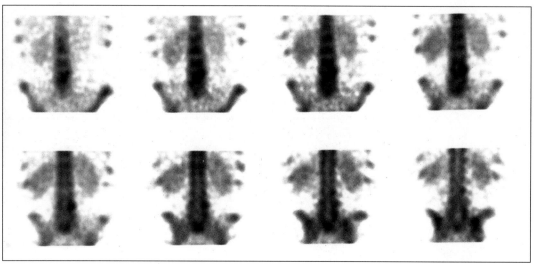

*d Coronal*

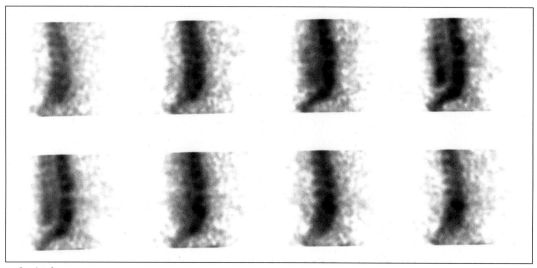

*e Sagittal*

### Fig. 1.50

*A 54-year-old man with a history of chronic back pain.*

*The planar bone scan (**a–c**) is within normal limits. The SPECT bone scan (**d–g**) identifies several foci of abnormal uptake in the body and lateral elements of L3 and L4. The findings are typical of degenerative disease.*

## CLINICAL APPLICATIONS

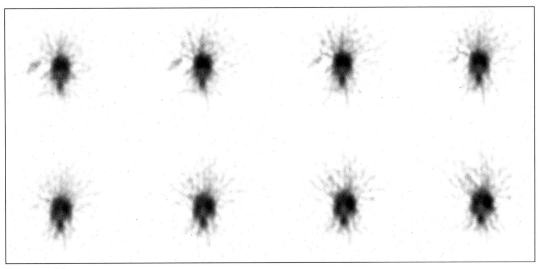

*f Transaxial*

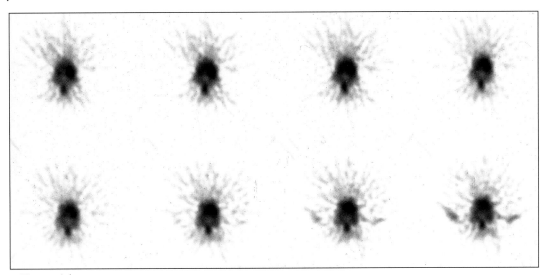

*g Transaxial*

*Degenerative disease of the hips: SPECT imaging*

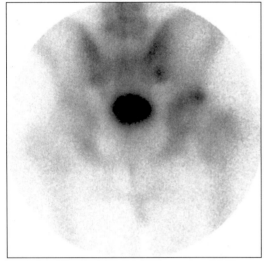

*a Posterior*

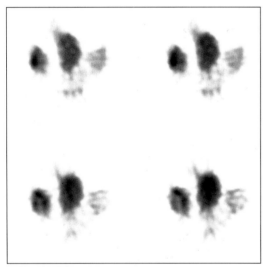

*c Transaxial*

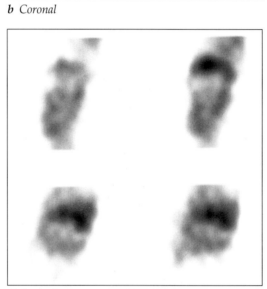

**Fig. 1.151**

**(a)** *Posterior planar view of pelvis in a 72-year-old male with pain in the right hip. The planar imaging identifies uptake in the acetabular region of the left hip, and this is confirmed on SPECT imaging* **(b–d)**. *The findings are those of degenerative disease.*

*b Coronal*

*d Sagittal*

## Degenerative disease of the knees: SPECT imaging

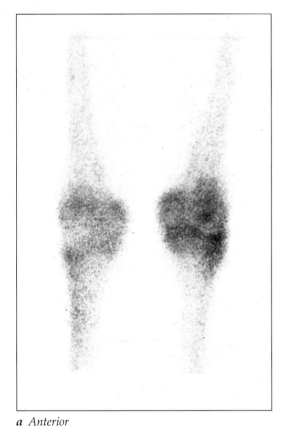

*a Anterior*

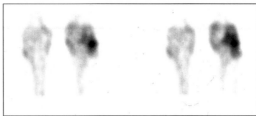

*b Coronal*

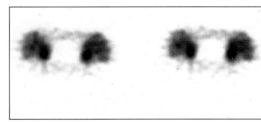

*c Transaxial, femora*

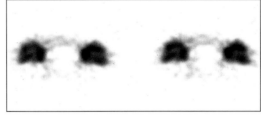

*d Transaxial, tibiae*

**Fig. 1.152**

*(a) Anterior planar view of the knees in a 57-year-old woman with bilateral knee pain. The planar imaging shows patchy uptake in both knees. The SPECT imaging (b–d) confirms the patchy nature of the abnormality involving the femora and tibiae consistent with degenerative disease only.*

## Degenerative disease and poliomyelitis

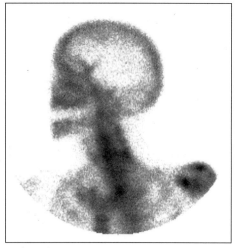

*a Anterior*

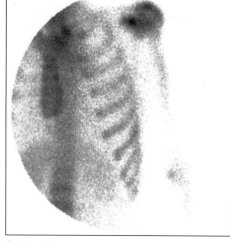

*b Anterior*

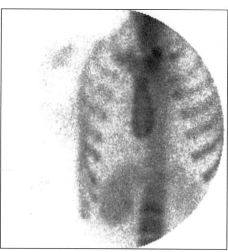

*c Anterior*

**Fig. 1.153**

*A 62-year-old woman with degenerative disease of the cervical spine (a) and left shoulder (b).*
*Low uptake in the region of the right humerus (c) is due to past poliomyelitis, resulting in a profoundly wasted right arm.*

## 'Hot' patella sign

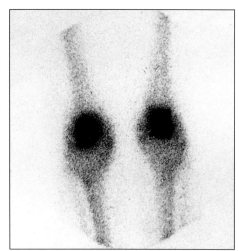

*a Anterior*

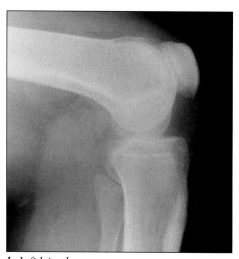

*b Left lateral*

**Fig. 1.154**

*(a) Bone scan of knees. (b) X-ray of left lateral knee.*

*Both patellae show marked uptake of tracer on the bone scan images. The x-ray reveals that increased uptake is due to degenerative change.*

## Arthritis
### Osteoarthritis

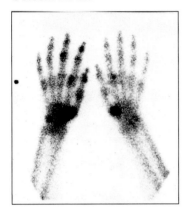

**Fig. 1.155**

*Multiple focal areas of increased tracer uptake are present in the interphalangeal joints, particularly involving the distal joints. There is bilaterally increased tracer uptake at the first carpometacarpal joint. The scan appearances are typically those of osteoarthritis.*

### Pseudogout

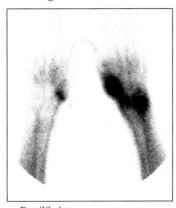 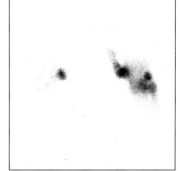

*a Equilibrium*  *b Delayed*

**Fig. 1.156**

*Marked increase in blood pool (a) and metabolic activity (b) at the base of the left thumb, medial carpus and distal ulnar in a patient with pseudogout.*

### Rheumatoid arthritis

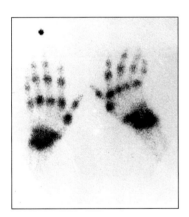 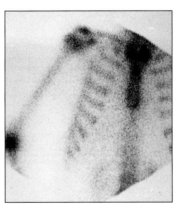 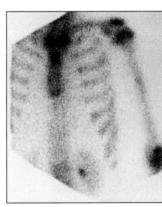 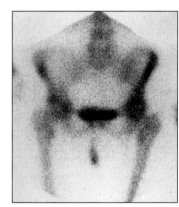

*a Right anterior*  *b Left anterior*  *c Anterior*

**Fig. 1.157**

*There is increased uptake of tracer in both wrists, with more focally increased uptake in many small joints of the hands. Ulnar deviation is apparent. The scan appearances are typical of rheumatoid arthritis.*

**Fig. 1.158**

*Bone scan views: (a, b) chest; (c) pelvis; (d) knees.*

*There is increased tracer uptake in association with both shoulders, elbows and knees (more marked on the left), and the left hip. Scan findings were attributable to rheumatoid joint disease.*

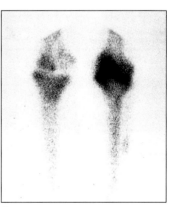

*d*

## Sacroiliitis

The bone scan is more sensitive than routine radiography for the detection of early sacroiliitis, as illustrated in Fig. 1.159.

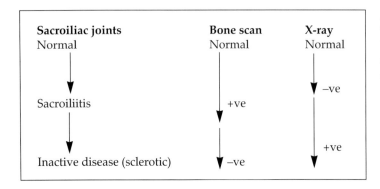

| Sacroiliac joints | Bone scan | X-ray |
|---|---|---|
| Normal | Normal | Normal |
| ↓ | | ↓ −ve |
| Sacroiliitis | ↓ +ve | |
| ↓ | | ↓ +ve |
| Inactive disease (sclerotic) | ↓ −ve | ↓ |

**Fig. 1.159**

*Comparison of the use of bone scanning and x-rays in the detection of early sacroiliitis.*

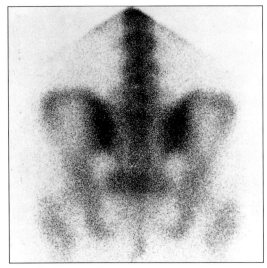

*a* Posterior

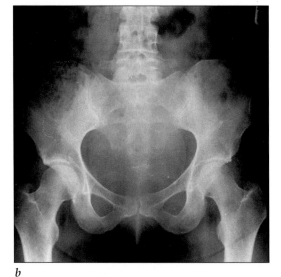

*b*

**Fig. 1.160**

**(a)** *Bone scan view of pelvis in a 37-year-old woman with sacroiliitis.* **(b)** *X-ray of pelvis.*
*Sacroiliac quantitation: left SIJ index 142, right SIJ index 148 (normal range 105–136). Both of these results are elevated, and support the diagnosis of active sacroiliitis, which is confirmed on the x-ray.*

## CLINICAL APPLICATIONS

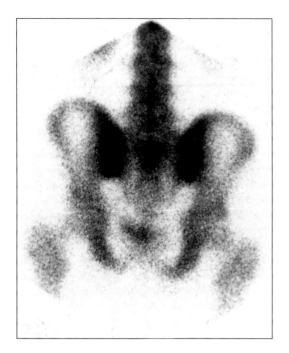

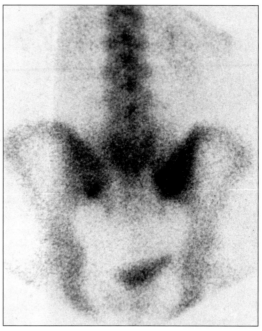

**Fig. 1.161**

*A 27-year-old man with sacroiliitis.*
*Sacroiliac quantitation: left SIJ index 149, right SIJ index 144 (normal range 105–136).*

**Fig. 1.162**

*A 41-year-old woman with Crohn's disease and unilateral sacroiliitis.*
*The right sacroiliac joint shows increased tracer uptake relative to the left. Sacroiliac quantitation: right SIJ index 144, left SIJ index 110 (normal range 105–136).*

## Psoriatic arthropathy

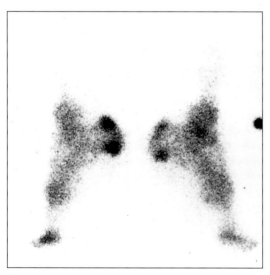

a

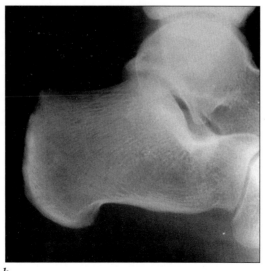

b

**Fig. 1.163**

*(a) Bone scan of feet. (b) X-ray of left heel.*
*The bone scan shows increased tracer uptake at the sites of insertion of the Achilles tendon and plantar fascia. The calcaneal changes are more marked on the left than on the right. The x-ray shows an erosion on the posterior aspect of the left calcaneus, with some overlying soft tissue thickening. This patient has psoriatic arthropathy with left-sided sacroiliitis, in addition to the calcaneal changes.*

## Metabolic bone disease

*Table 1.5   Bone scan in metabolic bone disease (MBD)*

| Disease | Cause +ve bone scan | Differentiating features | Comment |
|---|---|---|---|
| Renal osteodystrophy | Hyperparathyroidism | Metabolic features<br>Absence of tracer in bladder | May find the most dramatic images seen in MBD |
| Primary hyperparathyroidism | Hyperparathyroidism | Metabolic features<br>Uncommon:<br>  brown tumours<br>  ectopic calcification | Bone scan usually normal |
| Osteomalacia | Hyperparathyroidism<br>Uptake in osteoid | Metabolic features<br>Pseudofractures (PF) | May not be possible to differentiate PF and metastases |
| Aluminium (Al)-induced osteomalacia | — | Low bone uptake<br>High background activity | Al is a bone poison which blocks mineralization |
| Osteoporosis | Fracture | Intense linear uptake at site of vertebral fracture<br>May be low/patchy uptake in axial skeleton | Bone scan usually normal<br>When there is fracture the bone scan cannot differentiate other causes, eg tumour, on basis of scan alone<br>Activity at site of fracture fades over subsequent 1–2 years |

## Individual metabolic features

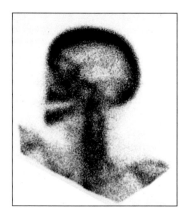 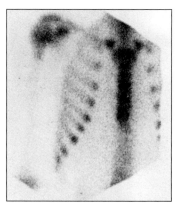 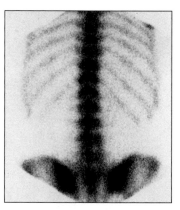 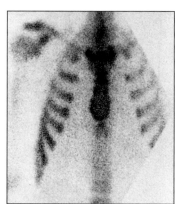

*Fig. 1.164*

*Increased tracer uptake throughout the calvaria and mandible.*

*Fig. 1.165*

*Increased tracer uptake at costochondral junctions (beading).*

*Fig. 1.166*

*Increased uptake of tracer in the axial skeleton, with high contrast between bone and soft tissue. The kidneys are not visualized.*

*Fig. 1.167*

*Increased tracer uptake throughout the sternum, the so-called tie sign.*

## Renal osteodystrophy

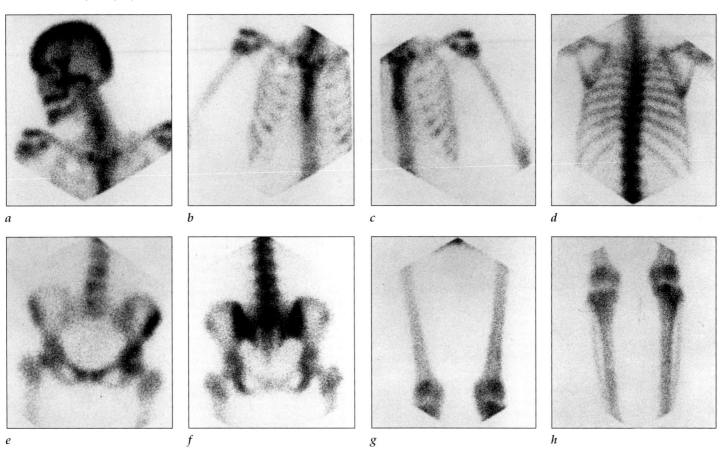

*Fig. 1.168*

*(a–h) A 45-year-old woman with chronic renal failure.*

*There is markedly increased tracer uptake throughout the whole skeleton and strikingly increased uptake in the calvaria and mandible; these appearances are typical of hyperparathyroidism. In addition, the kidneys are not visualized. The scan findings are typical of metabolic bone disease and, in this case, represent severe renal osteodystrophy. Note that there is no activity present in the bladder.*

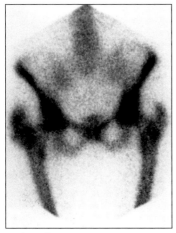

*a Anterior*

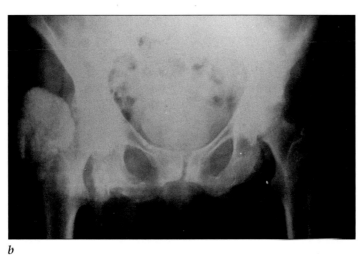

*b*

*Fig. 1.169*

*(a) Bone scan view of a 71-year-old woman with ectopic calcification. (b) X-ray of pelvis.*

*There is markedly increased tracer accumulation in the region of the greater trochanter and extending upwards, which is more pronounced on the right. This patient had severe renal bone disease with ectopic calcification, which is obvious on the x-ray. The patient also had avascular necrosis in both hips.*

## Osteomalacia

### Causes of osteomalacia

- Poor exposure to ultraviolet light and low intake of dietary vitamin D
- Vitamin D malabsorption, eg coeliac disease
- Abnormal vitamin D metabolism, eg chronic renal failure
- Peripheral resistance to vitamin D, eg vitamin D dependent rickets
- Hypophosphataemia, eg X-linked hypophosphataemic (or vitamin D resistant) rickets
- Hypophosphatasia
- Inhibition of mineralization, eg by sodium fluoride.

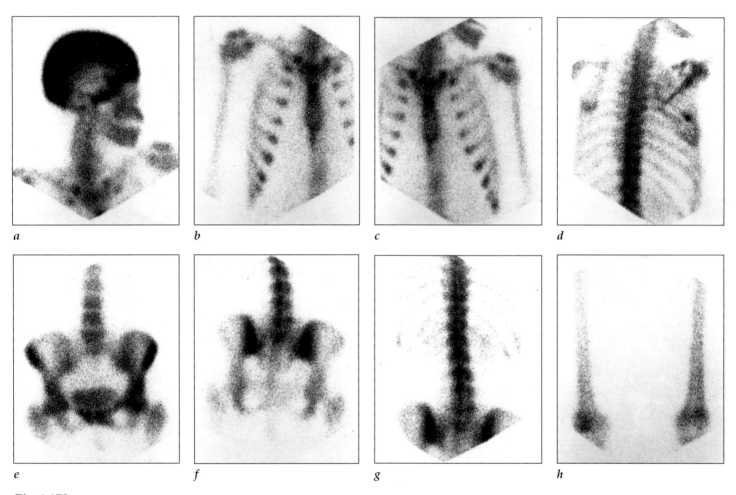

*a*  *b*  *c*  *d*

*e*  *f*  *g*  *h*

**Fig. 1.170**

*(a–h) An Asian woman with osteomalacia.*
*There is high uptake of tracer throughout the skeleton, with several metabolic features present. In addition, there is a focal lesion in the right 4th rib posteriorly caused by a pseudofracture.*

## CLINICAL APPLICATIONS

### Pseudofractures

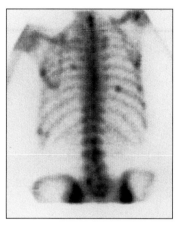
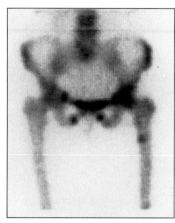

a                                    b

*Fig. 1.171*

*Bone scan views of (a) posterior spine and thoracic cage and (b) pelvis and femora in a 50-year-old Asian woman with osteomalacia who complained of pain in her ribs and difficulty in walking.*

*The bone scans show multiple focal lesions in the ribs, pubic rami, left upper femur and neck of the right femur. There is generally high uptake of tracer throughout the skeleton, and the renal images are not visualized, in keeping with metabolic bone disease. Focal lesions in this case represent pseudofractures.*

*Table 1.6    Most common sites at which pseudofractures are seen on bone scan*

| Ribs | 90% | Scapula | 20% |
|------|-----|---------|-----|
| Femur | 70% | Forearm | 10% |
| Pelvis | 40% | Fibula | 10% |

### Resolution of metabolic features

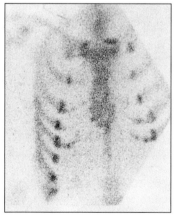
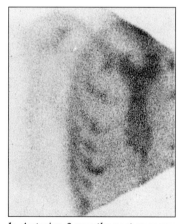

*a  Anterior, 0 months*         *b  Anterior, 2 months post-surgery*

*Fig. 1.172*

*(a, b) Bone scan views of chest. At the time of the original study the patient had active acromegaly, and increased tracer uptake is seen at the costochondral junctions. Following the transphenoidal removal of a pituitary tumour, the scan appearances are essentially normal, with a clear reduction in the avidity of the tracer uptake at the costochondral junctions.*

**Metabolic features are non-specific and may be seen where there is increased skeletal metabolism, from whatever cause.**

## Brown tumour in primary hyperparathyroidism

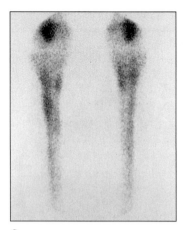

*a*

**Fig. 1.173**

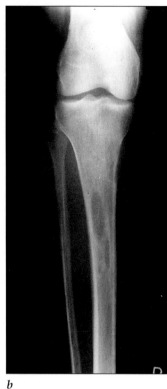

*b*

**(a)** *Bone scan view of tibiae.*
**(b)** *X-ray of right tibia.*
   *Focal areas of increased tracer uptake are present in both upper tibiae caused by brown tumours, which are shown on the x-ray.*

## Aluminium-induced bone disease

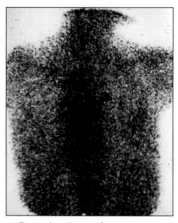

*a  Posterior, 0 months*

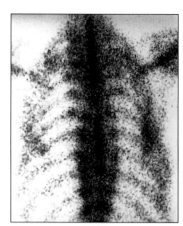

*b  Posterior, post-therapy*

**Fig. 1.174**

*Bone scan views of thoracic spine:* **(a)** *original study;* **(b)** *following desferrioxamine therapy.*
   *On the original study there is very high background activity with poor delineation of bone. These findings are accounted for in this patient with chronic renal failure by aluminium-induced osteomalacia, where aluminium acts as a bone poison, blocking mineralization. There is a dramatic improvement in the quality of the bone scan image following therapy. (Courtesy of Dr A. Schoutens.)*

## Vertebral collapse associated with osteoporosis

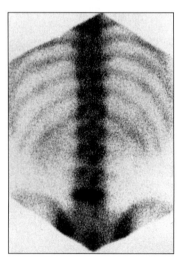

**Fig. 1.175**

*There is intense linearly increased tracer uptake in the region of L4. The scan appearances are typical of benign vertebral collapse, but the presence of coexistent pathology cannot be excluded.*

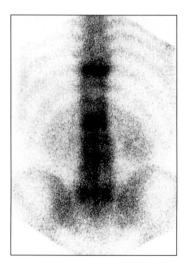

**Fig. 1.176**

*There are several areas of increased tracer uptake present at T10, L1 and L5, with non-homogeneity of tracer uptake throughout the remainder of the spine. Such scan appearances are often seen in patients with severe osteoporosis with multiple collapsed vertebrae.*

## CLINICAL APPLICATIONS

### Resolution of osteoporotic collapse

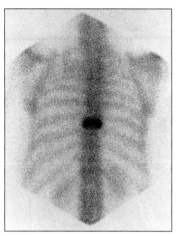

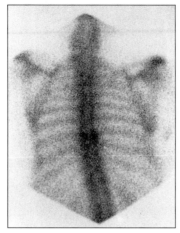

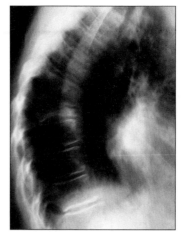

*a  Posterior, 0 months*

*b  Posterior, 8 months*

*c  Lateral*

**The bone scan may be of value in patients with** known osteoporotic collapse in assessing the time interval since collapse occurred.

**Fig. 1.177**

*(a, b) Bone scan views of thoracic spine in an 82-year-old woman who experienced a sudden onset of severe back pain. (c) X-ray of spine.*

*On the original study there is markedly increased tracer uptake in a linear pattern associated with the collapsed vertebra seen on the x-ray at T8. On the repeat study the abnormality is largely resolved. More often, a longer interval of 1–2 years is required before there is scan resolution in this situation.*

### Thyroid acropachy

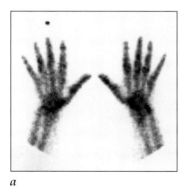

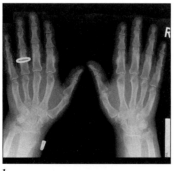

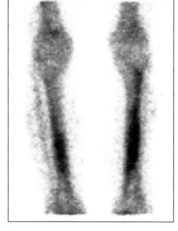

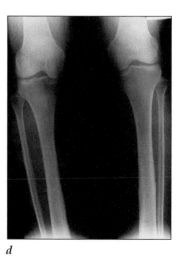

*a*

*b*

*c*

*d*

**Fig. 1.178**

*(a) Bone scan view of hands. (b) X-ray of hands. (c) Bone scan view of tibiae. (d) X-ray of tibiae.*

*The bone scan in thyrotoxicosis is most often normal but, depending on the severity of disease, may show metabolic features. In this patient with severe Graves' disease increased patchy tracer accumulation is present in both hands, with more markedly increased uptake seen in the mid-tibiae. The scan findings are in keeping with the x-ray changes of thyroid acropachy, an uncommon complication of this disease. The patient also had severe eye disease and pretibial myxoedema.*

## CLINICAL APPLICATIONS

## Paget's disease

*Bone scan features of Paget's disease*

- Intense uptake of tracer
- Diffuse involvement of bone
- Emphasis of anatomical features, eg transverse processes in spine
- Ends of long bones affected, rather than diaphyseal disease

- Bone expansion
- Deformity, eg bowing of a long bone
- Gradual change only over years
- Polyostotic disease usually present
- Spine and pelvis are the most commonly involved sites.

**Table 1.7  Incidence of Paget's disease on bone scans**

| Spine | 78% | Clavicle | 9% |
|---|---|---|---|
| Pelvis | 70% | Ribs | 9% |
| Femur | 65% | Metacarpal | 9% |
| Tibia | 44% | Patella | 4% |
| Skull | 39% | Mandible | 4% |
| Scapula | 26% | Forearm | 4% |
| Humerus | 17% | | |

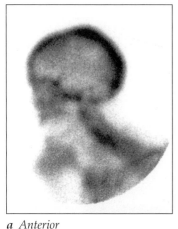

*a  Anterior*          *b  Anterior*

**Fig. 1.179**

*(a, b) Bone scan views in a 65-year-old woman with Paget's disease.*
*There is increased tracer uptake seen throughout the skull and left humerus. The scan findings are typical of Paget's disease.*

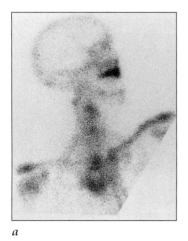 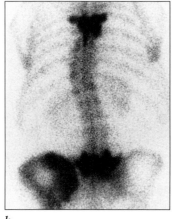 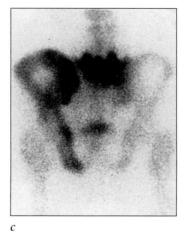 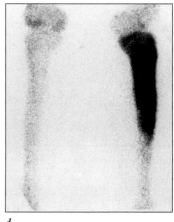

*a*          *b*          *c*          *d*

**Fig. 1.180**

*(a–d) A further case of polyostotic Paget's disease.*
*There is increased tracer uptake in the left tibia, left hemipelvis, L5, T7, maxilla and left clavicle.*
*The scan findings are typical of Paget's disease involving the above sites.*

## CLINICAL APPLICATIONS

*Further examples of Paget's disease*

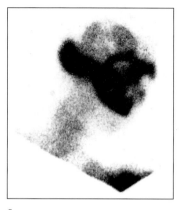

*a*

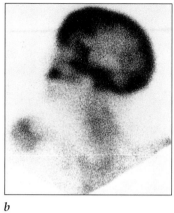

*b*

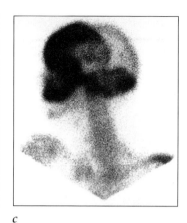

*c*

### Fig. 1.181

*(a–c) Three cases of Paget's disease involving the skull.*

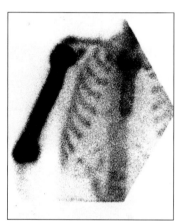

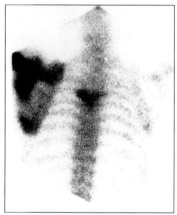

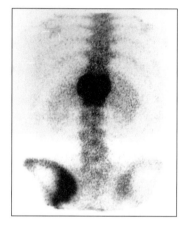

### Fig. 1.182

*Paget's disease involving the right humerus.*

### Fig. 1.183

*Paget's disease involving the left scapula and T5.*

### Fig. 1.184

*Paget's disease involving L1 and the left hemipelvis.*

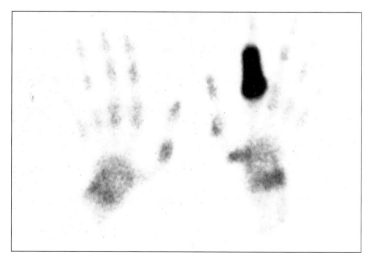

### Fig. 1.185

*Paget's disease involving the left first proximal phalynx.*

## Vascularity of pagetic bone

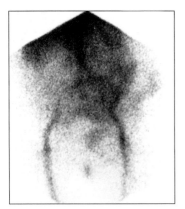

*a* *Anterior, dynamic*

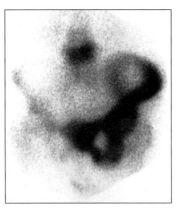

*b* *Anterior, delayed*

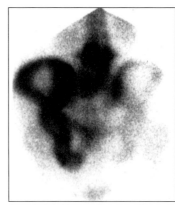

*c* *Posterior*

### Fig. 1.186

***(a–c)*** *Bone scan views.*
*There is strikingly increased tracer uptake throughout the whole of the left hemipelvis and throughout the body of L5. The left hemipelvis is intensely vascular on the dynamic study. The scan appearances are typical of Paget's disease.*

## Monostotic Paget's disease

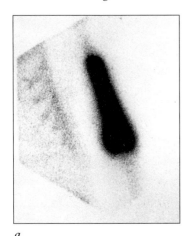

*a*

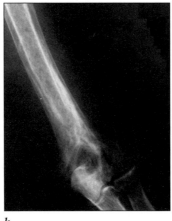

*b*

### Fig. 1.187

***(a)*** *Bone scan view of left chest and humerus in an 84-year-old man with monostotic Paget's disease involving the left humerus.* ***(b)*** *X-ray of left humerus.*
*On the bone scan image there is strikingly increased tracer uptake throughout the left lower humerus. The scan appearances are typical of Paget's disease; this is confirmed on the x-ray.*

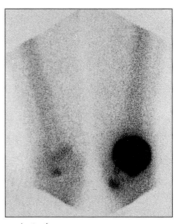

*a* *Anterior*

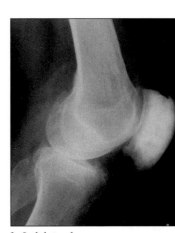

*b* *Left lateral*

### Fig. 1.188

***(a)*** *Bone scan view of lower femora and knees in a 75-year-old man with monostotic Paget's disease involving the patella.* ***(b)*** *X-ray of lateral left knee.*
*The bone scan image shows strikingly increased tracer uptake throughout the left patella. The x-ray confirms Paget's disease at this site. The bone scan is otherwise normal; thus this is a most unusual case of monostotic Paget's disease involving the left patella.*

 **Monostotic Paget's disease is not uncommon, and accounts for approximately 20% of cases.**

## Progression of Paget's disease

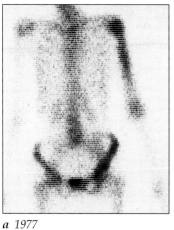

*a* 1977

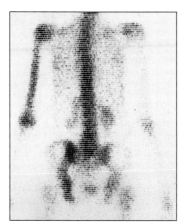

*b* 1977

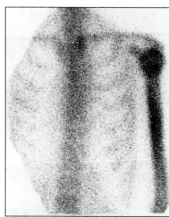

*c* 1979

### Fig. 1.189

*On the original study **(a, b)** in 1977 the typical scan appearances of Paget's disease involving the left humerus and left hemipelvis are seen. Further scans in 1979 **(c, d)** and 1985 **(e, f)** showed little change in these findings. However, the latter show involvement of the sacrum, which was not apparent in 1977. It is most unusual to be able to document the development and progression of Paget's disease.*

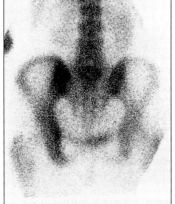

*d* 1979

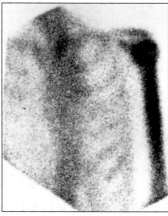

*e* 1985

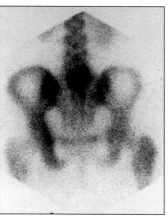

*f* 1985

**If changes occur in a bone scan over a relatively short period of time, they should not be attributed to Paget's disease, and other pathology should be considered.**

## Response to therapy

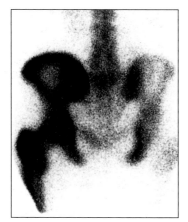

*a* Pre-therapy

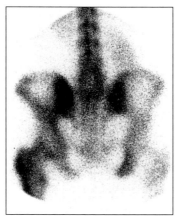

*b* Post-therapy

### Fig. 1.190

***(a, b)** Bone scan views of posterior pelvis and upper femora in a 63-year-old woman with Paget's disease.*

*There is markedly increased tracer uptake throughout the left hemipelvis and upper femur. These scan appearances are typical of Paget's disease. Following 9 months' treatment with oral diphosphonate, there has been a striking resolution of disease.*

## Complications of Paget's disease

### Fracture

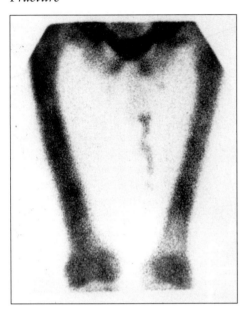

**Fig. 1.191**

*Bone scan view of femora in an elderly man with known extensive Paget's disease who complained of pain in his right leg.*

*There is increased but patchy tracer uptake in both femora, which is most pronounced on the right due to multiple stress fractures.*

**The bone scan is not adequate to exclude fracture in patients with Paget's disease. This is because increased tracer uptake associated with fracture may not be recognized against high background activity.**

### Osteogenic sarcoma

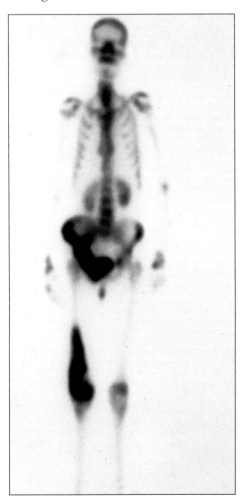

**Fig. 1.192**

*A patient with known Paget's disease of the pelvis and right femur who presented with pain in his right leg.*

*The bone scan shows a focal defect at the medial aspect of the right lower tibia, and destructive changes were identified at this site by radiography. This patient had an osteogenic sarcoma associated with Paget's disease. (Courtesy of Drs P Wraight and L Smith, Cambridge, UK.)*

## CLINICAL APPLICATIONS

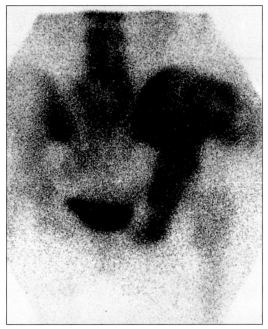

*a Posterior*

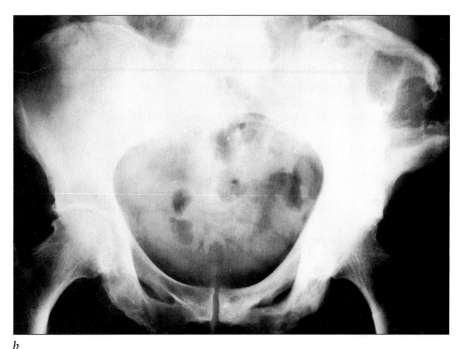

*b*

### Fig. 1.193

*(a) Bone scan view of pelvis. (b)X-ray of pelvis.*
*The bone scan shows extensive abnormal tracer accumulation throughout the right hemipelvis, with gross disruption of the anatomical borders in the lateral portion of the iliac wing. Note also that there is tracer uptake in associated soft tissue. The x-ray shows evidence of gross destruction at the corresponding site, together with the changes of Paget's disease. The scan appearance and x-ray findings are attributable to known Paget's disease, with the expanded destructive appearance caused by sarcomatous change.*

• **If sarcomatous change is suspected in a patient with known Paget's disease, radiographic investigation is required for evaluation, because, as with fracture, increased uptake may not always be apparent.**

• **While sarcomatous change normally appears 'hot' on the bone scan, this is not always the case.**

## CLINICAL APPLICATIONS

*Coexistent Paget's disease and metastatic disease*

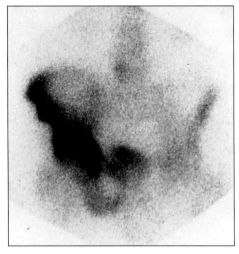

*a*

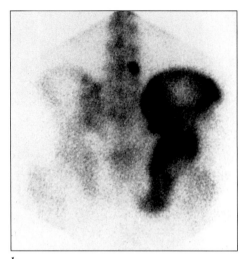

*b*

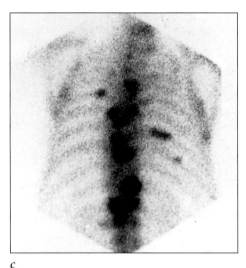

*c*

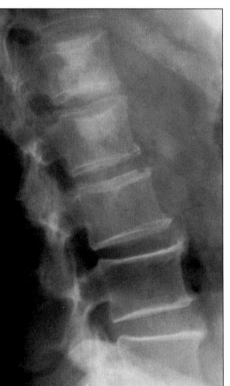

*d*

*e*

**Fig. 1.194**

*The bone scans (a, b) show the typical features of Paget's disease involving the right hemipelvis. In addition, however, multiple focal abnormalities are present in the spine and ribs which are typical of metastases (c). The x-ray of the pelvis (d) confirms Paget's disease, while the x-ray of the spine (e) confirms the presence of metastases.*

**Although Paget's disease and metastases usually show characteristic scan patterns of abnormality and can be easily differentiated, radiographic examination is still required for confirmation, because on occasion each of these conditions can mimic the other.**

# CLINICAL APPLICATIONS

## *Assessment of significance of x-ray lesions*

*Metabolic activity of a lesion*

*Bone island*

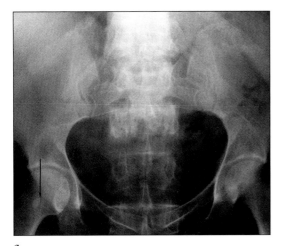

*a*

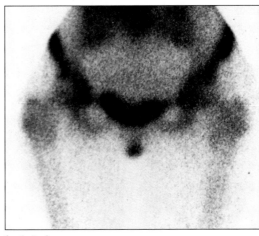

*b  Anterior*

**Fig. 1.195**

*(a)* X-ray of pelvis. *(b)* Bone scan image of pelvis and upper femora.

On the x-ray a sclerotic lesion (arrow) was noted in the right femoral neck. It was thought that this was probably a bone island and of no clinical significance. The bone scan image is normal, and, in particular, there is no increased activity in the right femoral neck.

**While a bone island usually appears normal on a bone scan, this is not always the case.**

*Bone infarct*

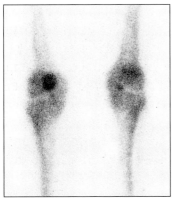

*a  Anterior*

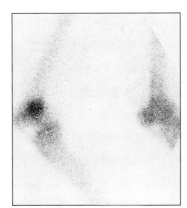

*b  Right medial*

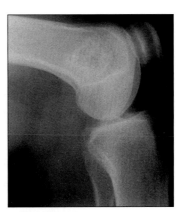

*c  Right lateral*

**Fig. 1.196**

*(a, b)* Bone scan views of knees. *(c)* X-ray of right lateral knee.

There is a single area of increased radionuclide accumulation between the condyles of the right femur which corresponds to the sclerotic lesion seen on the x-ray. It was felt that the lesion represented a bone infarct. Note that on the anterior view alone the scan appearances could be mistaken for the 'hot' patella sign.

## 1.4.4  Miscellaneous

### *Soft tissue accumulation of diphosphonate*

There are many situations in which diphosphonate may localize in soft tissues, and the common factor for these appears to be the presence of microcalcification.

Soft tissue accumulation may occur in the following sites:

- Infarcts
- Muscle
- Tumour
- Amyloid
- Fibroids
- Systemic sclerosis

### *Infarct accumulation*

*Diphosphonate uptake in cerebrovascular accident*

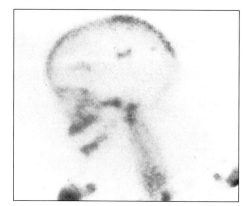

**Fig. 1.197**

*Bone scan view of lateral skull, showing three foci of diphosphonate accumulation in the left hemisphere, corresponding to a known cerebral infarct.*

### *Splenic infarct*

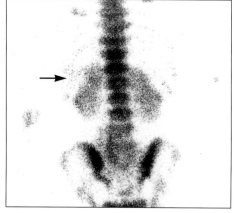

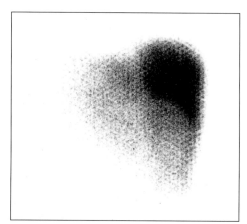

a *Posterior*          b *Anterior*          c *Posterior*

**Fig. 1.198**

*(a) Bone scan view of lumbar spine in a case of sickle cell disease. (b, c) Liver scan.*
   *On the bone scan there is faint tracer uptake by the spleen (arrow). On the liver scan the spleen is not visualized. This patient therefore has functional asplenia caused by previous splenic infarction.*

## CLINICAL APPLICATIONS

### *Ectopic calcification related to hypercalcaemia*

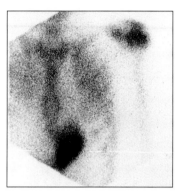 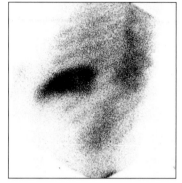 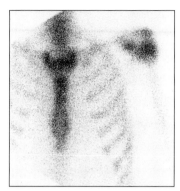

*a Anterior, 0 months*    *b Left lateral, 0 months*    *c Anterior, 1 month*

**Fig. 1.199**

*(a–c) Bone scan views of chest in a 57-year-old man with severe hypercalcaemia caused by milk–alkali syndrome.*

*This patient presented in acute renal failure, and serum calcium was found to be significantly elevated at 4 mmol/litre. The initial bone scan study shows strikingly increased tracer uptake in the stomach and lungs which is presumably related to microcalcification in these organs. Following rehydration and dialysis, this patient made a good recovery. The subsequent bone scan (c) is normal.*

> **Scan features of ectopic calcification may be reversible in the short term.**

### *Muscle accumulation*
#### *Repeated intramuscular injections*

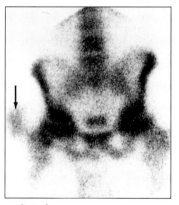 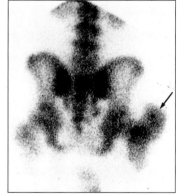

*a Anterior*    *b Posterior*

**Fig. 1.200**

*(a, b) Bone scan views of pelvis.*

*There is a large area of abnormal tracer uptake lateral to the right hip (arrows) which is caused by repeated intramuscular injections.*

#### *Myositis ossificans*

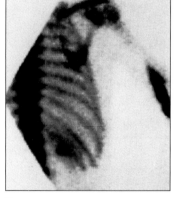

*a*

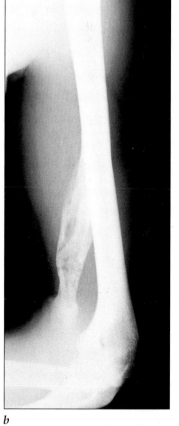

*b*

**Fig. 1.201**

*(a) Bone scan of thorax and arm in a 22-year-old man with myositis ossificans.*
*(b) Corresponding x-ray.*

*There is increased tracer accumulation lying within the brachialis muscle, corresponding to the soft tissue calcification seen on the x-ray. The scan appearances represent continuing active bone turnover associated with myositis ossificans.*

## Muscle necrosis

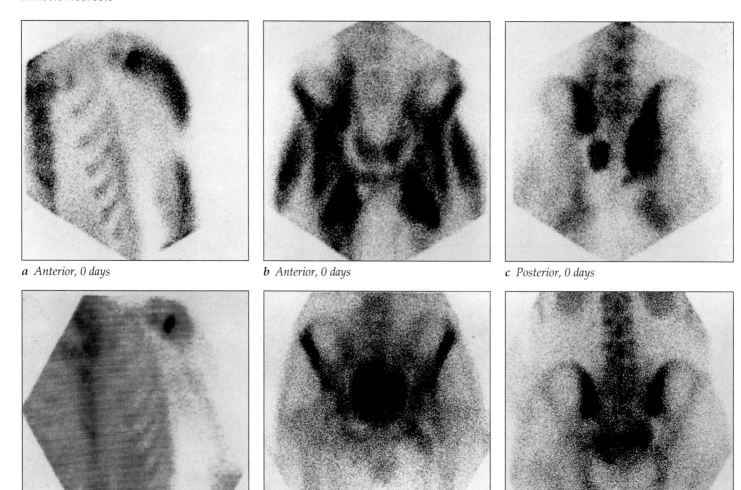

*a  Anterior, 0 days*    *b  Anterior, 0 days*    *c  Posterior, 0 days*

*d  Anterior, 11 days*    *e  Anterior, 11 days*    *f  Posterior, 11 days*

**Fig. 1.202**

*A 34-year-old man who presented with acute renal failure secondary to rhabdomyolysis.
Bone scan view: (a) chest; (b, c) pelvis; (d–f) corresponding views on repeat study 11 days
later.*

*On the original study there is massive accumulation of tracer in muscle, particularly in
the hip girdle muscle. On the repeat study there is dramatic resolution of the scan
appearances, although the background tracer activity is slightly increased.*

## Tumour accumulation
### Neuroblastoma

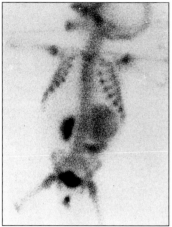
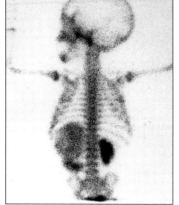

*a* Anterior          *b* Posterior

**Fig. 1.203**

*(a, b) Bone scan views.*

There is massive abnormal tracer accumulation associated with a left-sided adrenal tumour (neuroblastoma). Note that the left kidney is markedly rotated by the adrenal mass. No abnormality was present in the skeleton.

### Oesophagus

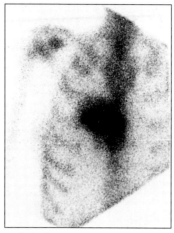
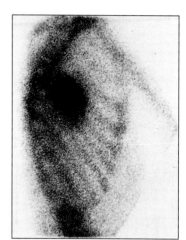

*a* Anterior          *b* Right lateral

**Fig. 1.204**

*(a, b) Bone scan views of chest in a 61-year-old woman with carcinoma of the oesophagus.*

There is massive abnormal accumulation of tracer in the right posterior mediastinum. No focal abnormalities were seen in the skeleton. The tracer uptake in this case is associated with primary oesophageal malignancy.

### Meningioma

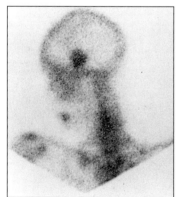
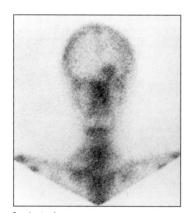

*a* Left lateral          *b* Anterior

**Fig. 1.205**

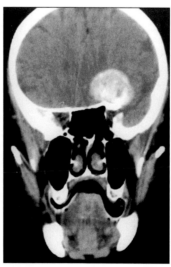

*c*

*(a, b) Bone scan views of the skull. (c) CT brain scan.*

On *(a)* an intense focus of increased tracer uptake is seen. This patient was known to have carcinoma of the breast and, based on a lateral view alone, the physician would be justified to conclude that a skull lesion was present, most probably a metastasis. But *(b)* clearly shows that the lesion is intracerebral. A skull x-ray was not considered to be helpful, but the CT scan confirmed the presence of a meningioma. There were no lesions anywhere else on the skeleton on bone scan.

'Peau d'orange'

Ascites

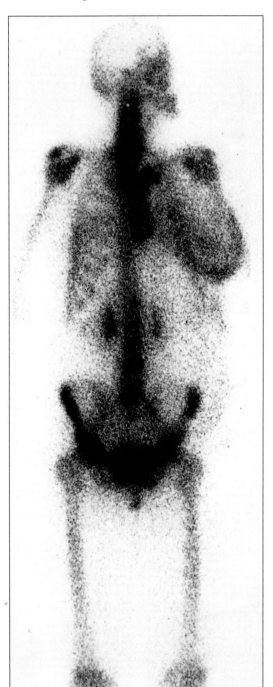

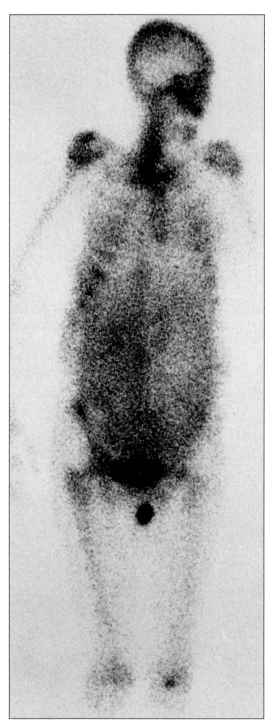

**Fig. 1.206**

Lymphoedema in the breast. A patient with carcinoma of the left breast and associated 'peau-d'orange' changes.

**Fig. 1.207**

Ascites in the abdomen.

Increased tracer uptake is seen diffusely throughout the abdomen, related to known malignant ascites. No discrete focus is seen throughout the skeleton.

*Metastases*

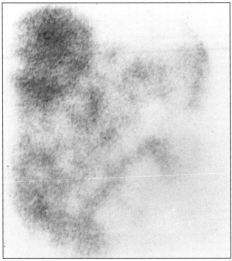

*a  Anterior*

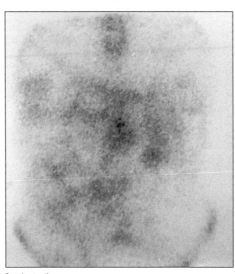

*b  Anterior*

**Fig. 1.208**

*(a) Liver scan. (b) Bone scan view of abdomen.*

This patient with medullary carcinoma of the thyroid had known hepatic metastases. The liver scan shows the liver to be markedly enlarged, with multiple focal defects throughout. On the bone scan image there is tracer uptake in the liver, corresponding to the tumour.

*Pleural effusion*

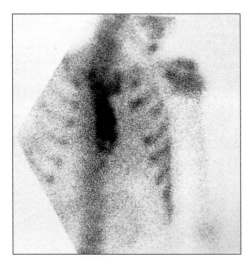

*a  Anterior*

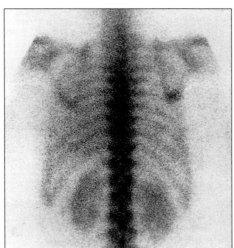

*b  Posterior*

**Fig. 1.209**

*Bone scan views: (a) chest; (b) thorax. (c) X-ray of chest.*

The tracer uptake in the left hemithorax is related to a malignant pleural effusion, as seen on the x-ray. Also note focal abnormalities due to metastases in the sternum, the tip of the right scapula, and the left ribs anteriorly.

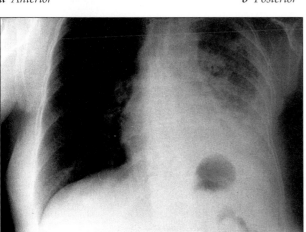

*c*

## CLINICAL APPLICATIONS

### Amyloid

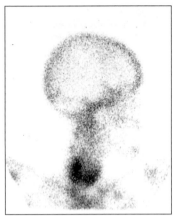
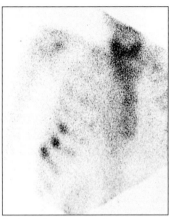
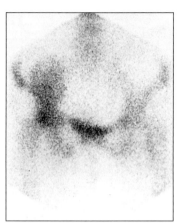
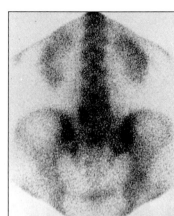

*a Right*  *b Anterior*  *c Anterior*  *d Posterior*

**Fig. 1.210**

*A 63-year-old woman with a renal transplant for amyloid kidney. Bone scan views: (a) skull; (b) chest; (c) pelvis; (d) lumbar spine and pelvis.*

*Although this patient had a functioning renal transplant, which is seen in the right iliac fossa, tracer uptake is visualized in the host kidneys and there is also increased uptake present in the thyroid. There was no radiopharmaceutical problem, and the stomach was not visualized. These findings are due to uptake in the amyloid tissue. In addition, focal abnormalities are noted in the right anterior ribs caused by fracture following trauma. The uptake in the right femoral neck is accounted for by avascular necrosis.*

### Fibroid

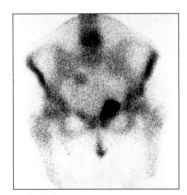

*a Anterior*  *b*

**Fig. 1.211**

*(a) Bone scan view of pelvis. (b) Corresponding x-ray.*

*On the bone scan image a focal area of increased tracer uptake is seen in the right pelvis which is not related to bone. Note also that the bladder is displaced to the left. The x-ray confirms calcification within the right pelvis. The scan and radiographic findings are due to a calcified fibroid. The bladder was being displaced by a large, bulky uterus.*

### Systemic sclerosis

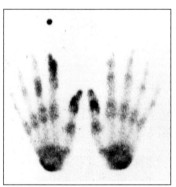
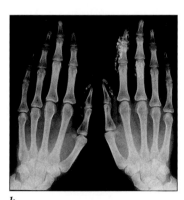

*a*  *b*

**Fig. 1.212**

*(a) Bone scan and (b) x-ray of hands in a patient with systemic sclerosis and calcinosis.*

## Vascular abnormalities

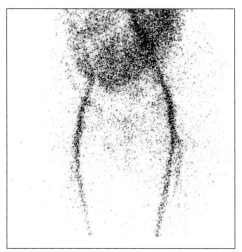

*a* Dynamic

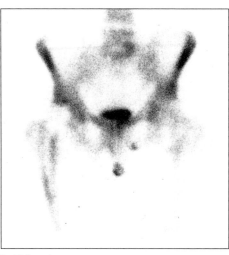

*b* Delayed

### Fig. 1.213

*(a, b) Bone scan views of anterior pelvis and upper femora in a 54-year-old man who presented 2 years after right total hip replacement complaining of pain in the region of the right groin and greater trochanter.*

*On the dynamic study the right common iliac artery is not visualized, but there appears to be symmetrical perfusion in the femoral arteries. On static imaging the appearance of the right prosthesis are unremarkable, with no evidence of infection or loosening. An arterial block was subsequently confirmed, and the patient's symptoms were attributed to claudication.*

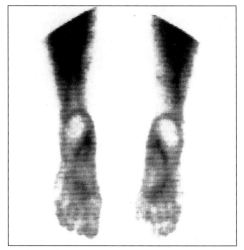

*a* Dynamic

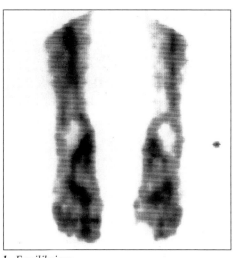

*b* Equilibrium

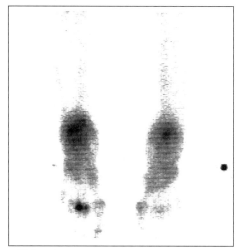

*c* Delayed

### Fig. 1.214

*(a–c) Bone scan views of feet in a 22-year-old woman with systemic lupus erythematosus and vasculitis.*

*On the dynamic and blood pool images there is reduced flow to the right 1st and 2nd toes, but on the delayed image tracer uptake is seen at these sites. However, there are two focal areas of increased uptake seen on the delayed views in the left 2nd and 3rd metatarsophalangeal joints. In the light of the clinical history, the reduced blood flow almost certainly reflects vasculitis. The significance of more focal areas of increased uptake is uncertain, but is likely to represent arthritis/degenerative change in the absence of trauma.*

## CLINICAL APPLICATIONS

## *Abnormalities of the renal tract*

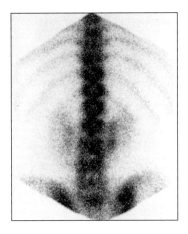

**Fig. 1.215**

*Horseshoe kidney.*

**Fig. 1.216**

*Cyst in right kidney.*

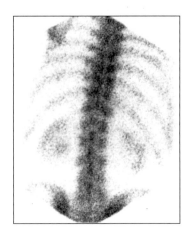

**Fig. 1.217**

*Renal defect (right kidney) caused by stag-horn calculus.*

> ✦ It is important to remember that abnormalities of the kidney may be diagnosed on a bone scan.

### *Pelvic kidney*

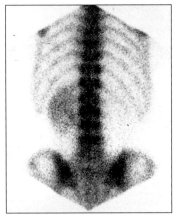

*a Posterior*

*b Anterior*

**Fig. 1.218**

*Bone scan views: (a) lumbar spine; (b) pelvis.*

*On the posterior view the right kidney is not visualized, and increased tracer uptake is seen in the region of the right sacroiliac joint. The anterior view, however, clarifies these findings, and there is a right-sided pelvic kidney which is contributing to the 'shine-through' seen on the posterior view. In this case there is also increased tracer uptake in the left hip, which is due to degenerative disease.*

### *Increased renal uptake of diphosphonate caused by hypercalcaemia*

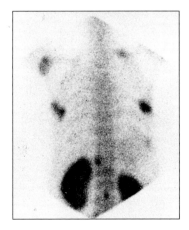

**Fig. 1.219**

*A 67-year-old woman with carcinoma of the breast and hypercalcaemia.*

*There are multiple focal abnormalities seen throughout the skeleton, attributable to metastases. In addition, there is high uptake of tracer in the kidneys, which in this case reflects nephrocalcinosis but may also be found in patients receiving chemotherapy.*

## CLINICAL APPLICATIONS

## Abnormalities of the urinary tract
### Obstructed urinary tract

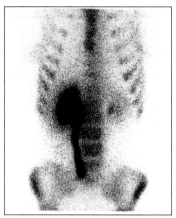

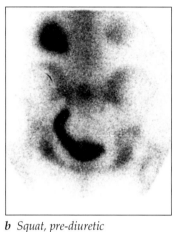

*a Posterior, pre-diuretic*

*b Squat, pre-diuretic*

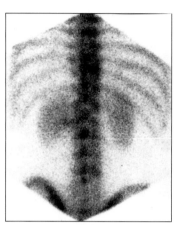

*c Posterior, post-diuretic*

**Fig. 1.220**

*Anterior bone scan view of lower thorax and abdomen.*

*There is markedly increased tracer uptake in the right kidney and ureter, indicating obstruction in the right ureter. This was an incidental finding on an otherwise normal bone scan.*

**Fig. 1.221**

*Bone scan views of thoracic spine: (a, b) before; (c) after diuretic.*

*Tracer accumulation is seen in the left renal pelvis, and the lower ureter is prominent. These appearances would be consistent with obstruction at the level of the vesicoureteric junction. However, following diuretic, the tracer is seen to clear. Therefore, there is a dilated pelvi-ureteric system which is not obstructed.*

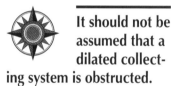
**It should not be assumed that a dilated collecting system is obstructed.**

### Urinary diversion

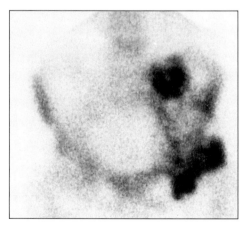

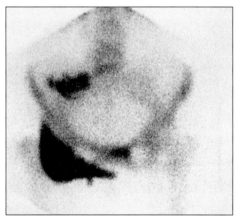

*a Anterior*

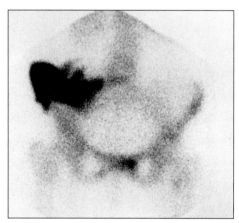

*b Anterior*

**Fig. 1.222**

*Anterior bone scan view of pelvis.*

*Tracer uptake is noted in the region of the ileostomy, relating to urinary diversion. Tracer is also seen in the urine bag.*

**Fig. 1.223**

*(a) Bone scan view of pelvis in a patient who had urinary diversion carried out for carcinoma of the bladder. (b) Same view with urinary collecting bag elevated.*

*In this case, there is a focal lesion in the left pubic ramus caused by a metastasis, and the scan appearances in the left anterior superior iliac spine are also suspicious.*

## Acute renal failure

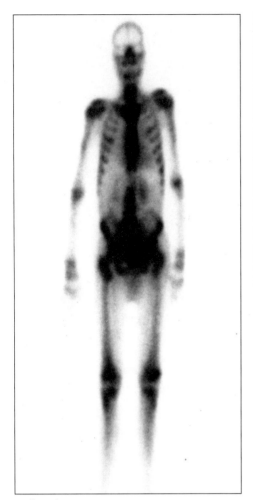

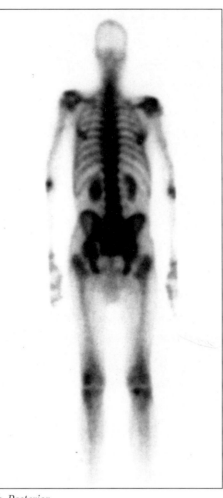

**Fig. 1.224**

Bone scan views: **(a)** anterior; **(b)** posterior.

There is high background tracer activity and the scan appears to be of poor quality. This patient was in acute renal failure at the time of the study. (Courtesy of Drs P Wraight and L Smith. Cambridge, UK.)

*a* Anterior

*b* Posterior

# CHAPTER 2
# ENDOCRINE

## Thyroid

The thyroid gland's main function is to concentrate and organify inorganic iodine, to store the iodinated compounds and then release them as active hormones into the circulation. As a result of this, radioactive iodine compounds, in particular $^{131}$I, have been used for many years to investigate thyroid function. More recently, technetium-99m pertechnetate ($^{99m}TcO_4$) has been shown to be concentrated by the thyroid but is not organified into the thyroid hormones. When thyroid imaging is performed with $^{99m}TcO_4$, the scan appearances essentially provide a display of tracer uptake which is dependent on the trapping mechanism of the thyroid gland, but in practice it is possible to obtain the same information as with radioiodine, with a few rare exceptions. As $^{99m}Tc$ has near ideal physical properties, it is the agent used most often for thyroid scanning. However, as cyclotron-produced isotopes are becoming more available, $^{123}$I, which has considerable advantages over $^{131}$I for routine imaging, may also be used for thyroid scanning although it is significantly more expensive.

## Adrenal

Imaging the adrenal glands with radionuclides is dependent on the metabolic activity of the adrenal cortex or the adrenal medulla. Such tests are only undertaken when biochemical investigations have confirmed the diagnosis, and are performed in conjunction with an anatomical imaging technique, which is usually the CT scan. Positive imaging with the compound $^{131}$I/$^{123}$I *meta*-iodobenzylguanidine (MIBG) is a prerequisite before this agent can be used for therapy.

## Parathyroid

A parathyroid adenoma may be imaged using combined thallium-201 ($^{201}$Tl) and $^{99m}TcO_4$ subtraction scanning. $^{201}$Tl localizes in glandular tissue according to regional blood flow and ATPase-dependent sodium/potassium pump function and is taken up by both thyroid and parathyroid tissue, whereas $^{99m}Tc$ is taken up by the thyroid alone. Using a computer, it is possible to subtract a $^{99m}Tc$ image of the patient's neck from one obtained with $^{201}$Tl, and identify parathyroid activity. Visualization depends upon the size of the gland. In general, one would expect to visualize glands larger than 500 mg. A normal parathyroid (20 mg) gland will not be visualized by this technique.

It is important to appreciate the normal anatomical position of parathyroid glands, the possible site of ectopic adenomas, and to be aware that supernumerary parathyroid glands may occur.

| | |
|---|---|
| Parathyroids in usual anatomical site | 75% |
| Ectopic parathyroid glands | 25% |
| Supernumerary (ie >4) parathyroid glands | 5% |

## CHAPTER CONTENTS

# 2.1 ANATOMY/PHYSIOLOGY

## 2.1.1 Thyroid

An understanding of the basic physiology of the thyroid and its control mechanisms is essential for the correct interpretation of thyroid scans. Figure 2.1 shows how the thyroid produces $T_4$, $T_3$ and $rT_3$, and how $T_4$ controls its own production via a negative feedback system. The eventual levels of thyroid hormone in the blood are dependent on factors other than thyroid function alone. Figure 2.2 diagrammatically illustrates the uptake of iodine (and radioiodine), incorporation into the thyroid hormone and release of thyroid hormones into the blood under TSH stimulation.

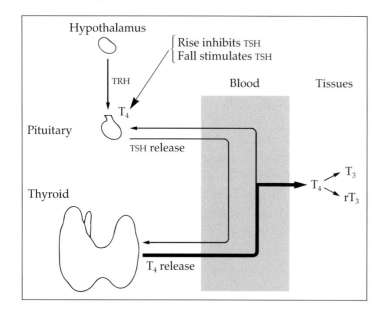

*Fig. 2.1*

*Production of $T_4$, $T_3$ and $rT_3$ in the thyroid.*

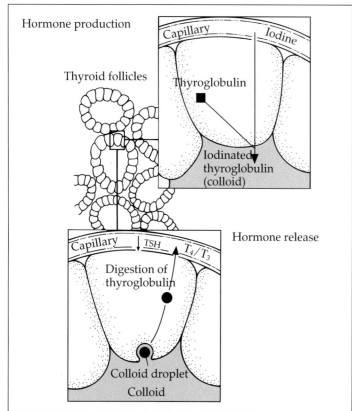

*Fig. 2.2*

*Uptake of iodine (and radioiodine), incorporation into the thyroid hormone and release of thyroid hormones into the blood under TSH stimulation.*

## 2.1.2 Adrenal gland

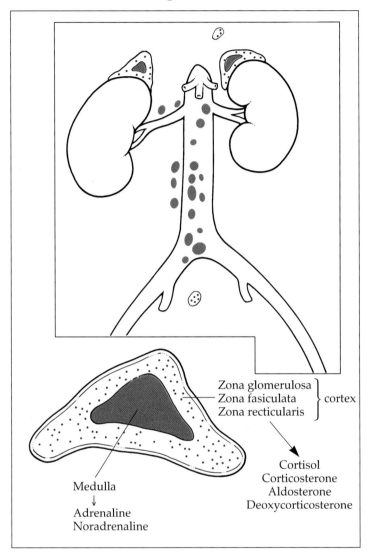

Zona glomerulosa
Zona fasiculata } cortex
Zona recticularis

Cortisol
Corticosterone
Aldosterone
Deoxycorticosterone

Medulla
↓
Adrenaline
Noradrenaline

*Fig. 2.3*

*Diagrammatic representation of the adrenal glands.*
*▒ Adrenocortical tissue: ▓ Adrenomedullary tissue.*
*Note possible extra-adrenal sites of cortical and medullary tissue.*

## 2.1.3 Parathyroid

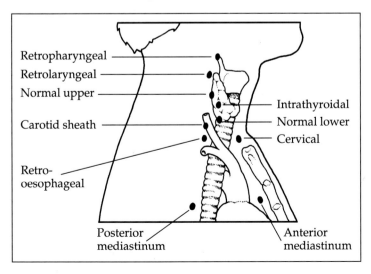

Retropharyngeal
Retrolaryngeal
Normal upper
Carotid sheath
Retro-oesophageal
Intrathyroidal
Normal lower
Cervical
Posterior mediastinum
Anterior mediastinum

*Fig. 2.4*

*While the great majority of cases of primary hyperparathyroidism are due to a single parathyroid adenoma, parathyroid hyperplasia and, more rarely, multiple parathyroid adenomas or parathyroid carcinoma may be present.*
*Parathyroid adenoma     83%*
*Parathyroid hyperplasia    15%*
*Parathyroid carcinoma     2%*

# 2.2 RADIOPHARMACEUTICALS

## 2.2.1 Thyroid imaging

*Table 2.1 Radiopharmaceuticals in thyroid imaging*

| | Production source | Decay $T_{1/2}$ | Energy (keV) | Use | Comment |
|---|---|---|---|---|---|
| $^{99m}$Tc | Generator | 6 hours | 140 | Thyroid imaging | Routine radionuclide; cheap; low radiation dose |
| $^{123}$I | Cyclotron | 13.3 hours | 159 28 | Thyroid imaging | Possibly best imaging agent; expensive and poor availability |
| $^{131}$I | Reactor | 8.1 days | 364 | Cancer imaging Uptake studies Therapy | High radiation dose due to β emission |

### $^{99m}TcO_4$ and radioiodine

It is important to appreciate the difference between the use of $^{99m}$TcO$_4$ and radioiodine ($^{131}$I, $^{123}$I, $^{132}$I, $^{125}$I) for investigation of the thyroid. Figure 2.5 shows this diagrammatically.

Very often $^{99m}$TcO$_4$ and radioiodine scans are identical. However, $^{99m}$TcO$_4$ is trapped but not bound, while radioiodines are trapped and bound. The consequences of this are as follows:

- Occasional differences in images will occur between $^{99m}$TcO$_4$ and radioiodine.
- Radioiodine needs to be used for discharge tests with perchlorate (see page 139).
- Some cancers may trap but not bind radioiodine, ie could appear 'hot' on $^{99m}$TcO$_4$ scans but 'cold' with radioiodine.
- The overall uptake of tracer by the thyroid will be higher and later with radioiodine as it is progressively incorporated into the gland—typically 30% at 24 hours compared with a peak uptake of about 4% at 20 minutes with $^{99m}$TcO$_4$.

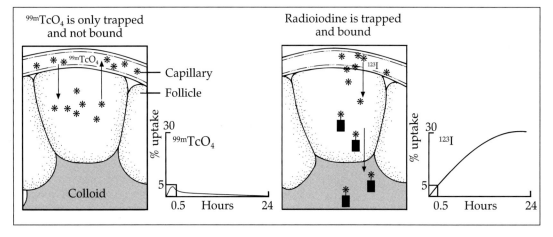

*Fig. 2.5*

*Comparison of $^{99m}TcO_4$ and radioiodine ($^{131}I$, $^{123}I$, $^{132}I$, $^{125}I$) in the investigation of the thyroid.*

## 2.2.2 Adrenal imaging

*Table 2.2 Radiopharmaceuticals for adrenal imaging*

| Organ | Hormone | Radiopharmaceutical |
|---|---|---|
| Adrenal cortex | Cortisol Aldosterone | $^{131}$I iodocholesterol $^{75}$Se selenocholesterol |
| Adrenal medulla | Catecholamines | $^{131}$I MIBG $^{123}$I MIBG |

## 2.2.3 Parathyroid imaging

*Table 2.3 Radiopharmaceuticals for parathyroid imaging*

| | Production source | Decay $T_{1/2}$ | Energy (keV) |
|---|---|---|---|
| $^{99m}$Tc | Generator | 6 hours | 140 |
| $^{201}$Tl | Cyclotron | 78 hours | 80 |

# 2.3 NORMAL SCANS WITH VARIANTS AND ARTEFACTS

## 2.3.1 Normal thyroid scan

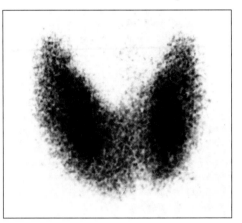 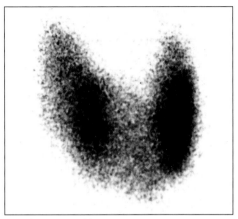 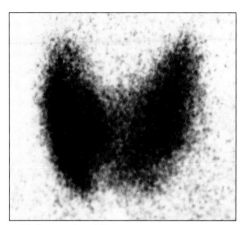

*a Anterior*              *b Left anterior oblique*              *c Right anterior oblique*

**Fig. 2.6**

*(a–c) The normal thyroid scan ($^{99m}TcO_4$).*

### Quantitation of $^{99m}TcO_4$ thyroid study

Quantitation of $^{99m}TcO_4$ uptake by the thyroid gland is simply performed. The activity in the syringe is measured under the gamma camera prior to injection. Following injection of the tracer, a 20-minute image of the thyroid is obtained. Using a computer-generated region of interest around the thyroid image, the percentage of injected activity present in the thyroid at 20 minutes can be calculated. The normal range is 0.4–4.0%.

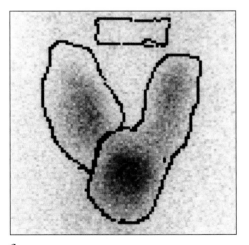

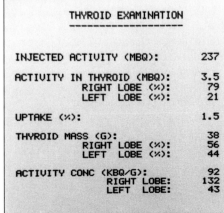

```
            THYROID EXAMINATION
            -------------------

INJECTED ACTIVITY (MBQ):           237

ACTIVITY IN THYROID (MBQ):         3.5
           RIGHT LOBE (%):          79
           LEFT  LOBE (%):          21

UPTAKE (%):                        1.5

THYROID MASS (G):                   38
           RIGHT LOBE (%):          56
           LEFT  LOBE (%):          44

ACTIVITY CONC (KBQ/G):              92
           RIGHT LOBE:             132
           LEFT  LOBE:             43
```

*a*              *b*

**Fig. 2.7**

*(a, b) Quantitation of $^{99m}TcO_4$ uptake by the thyroid gland.*

# NORMAL SCANS WITH VARIANTS AND ARTEFACTS

## Variants of normal thyroid scans

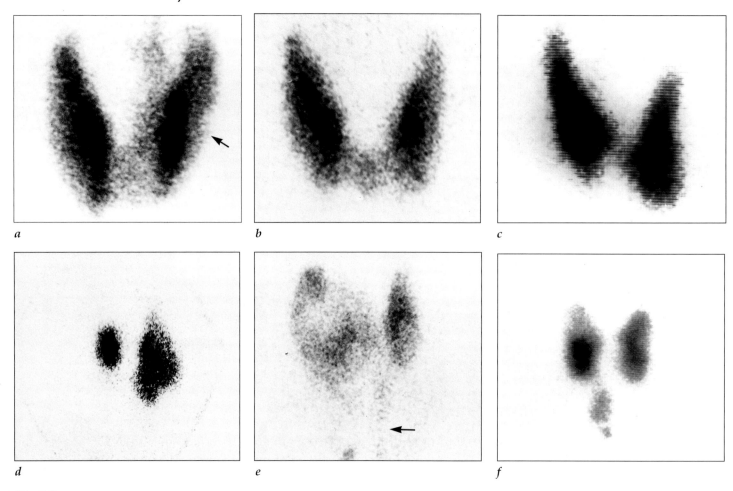

*a*      *b*      *c*

*d*      *e*      *f*

**Fig. 2.8**

*There are many variants of the normal thyroid scan. A pyramidal lobe may be seen normally, and there may be some scalloping of the edges simulating a nodule (a) (arrow). More often, the pyramidal lobe is absent (b). It is common to see some asymmetry in the size and position of thyroid lobes (c). The thyroid may appear irregular with no isthmus (d). Such appearances are most often seen after subtotal thyroidectomy, as in this case, but occasionally may be a normal variant. If the thyroid uptake is low, imaging time could be sufficiently long to allow accumulation of tracer in the oesophagus (e) (arrow). This can usually be differentiated from true extension of the thyroid tissue (f). If necessary, a repeat image after a drink of water will assist by clearing oesophageal activity.*

## 2.3.2 Adrenomedullary $^{131}$I MIBG imaging

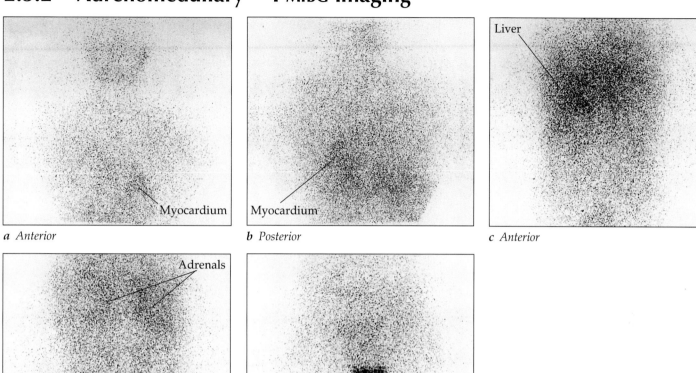

*a Anterior*    *b Posterior*    *c Anterior*

*d Posterior*    *e Anterior*

**Fig. 2.9**

Series of 24-hour images with $^{131}$I MIBG: *(a,b)* chest views; *(c)* view of abdomen; *(d)* view of abdomen and pelvis; *(e)* view of pelvis and upper femora.

Note that the myocardium is normally seen, and adrenals may also be visualized. Adrenal uptake is more commonly seen with $^{123}$I MIBG.

## 2.3.3   Normal adrenocortical scan

Initially a renal scan is obtained with $^{99m}$Tc dimercapto-succinic acid (DMSA). Using either radioactive or small lead markers, the upper poles of each kidney are identified and marks made on the patient's back with indelible ink for further reference. The radiopharmaceutical for adrenal imaging is then injected. Subsequent quantitation of adrenal uptake tracer may be of value in differentiating hyperplastic glands from normal.

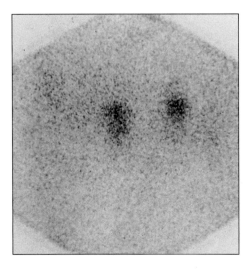

*Fig. 2.10*

*Renal DMSA scan 5 days after injection of 200 μCi $^{75}$Se selenocholesterol, showing normal adrenal images.*

- The right adrenal normally appears higher than the left.
- The right adrenal appears more active than the left because of its more posterior position.
- The normal adrenal uptake is less than, or equal to, 0.2% of the injected dose.

## 2.3.4   Normal parathyroid scan

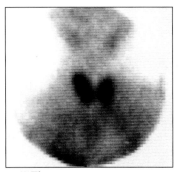 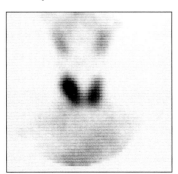 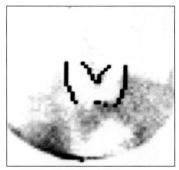 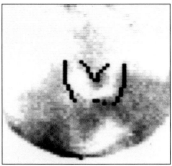

*a* $^{201}Tl$        *b* $^{99m}TcO_4$        *c* $^{201}Tl - ^{99m}TcO_4$, 100%        *d* $^{201}Tl - ^{99m}TcO_4$, 80%

*Fig. 2.11*

*Neck views: (a) $^{201}Tl$ image; (b) $^{99m}TcO_4$ image; (c) 100% $^{201}Tl$ image with $^{99m}TcO_4$ image subtracted; (d) 80% $^{201}Tl$ image with $^{99m}TcO_4$ image subtracted.*

**Normal parathyroid glands and 50% of hyperplastic glands are not visualized by this technique.**

# 2.4 CLINICAL APPLICATIONS

The clinical applications of endocrine scanning are listed below, and examples of the various clinical problems are given on subsequent pages.

**2.4.1 Clinical indications for thyroid scanning**
Assessment of thyroid nodules
Diagnosis of cause of thyrotoxicosis
Assessment of goitre
Evaluation of ectopic thyroid
Assessment of thyroid cancer

**2.4.2 Clinical indications for adrenal scanning**
Investigation of Cushing's syndrome
Investigation of Conn's syndrome (hyperaldosteronism)
Investigation of phaeochromocytoma

**2.4.3 Clinical indications for parathyroid scanning**
Parathyroid adenoma
Multiple parathyroid adenomas
Parathyroid carcinoma
Secondary hyperparathyroidism
Problems in parathyroid localization

# 2.4.1 Clinical indications for thyroid scanning

## *Assessment of thyroid nodules*

A clinically solitary thyroid nodule is one of the commonest presentations of thyroid disease. The main purpose of thyroid imaging is to detect and treat malignancy. Table 2.4 shows the common causes of thyroid nodules and their scan findings. Figure 2.12 shows one systematic approach to investigation using the thyroid scan. Other approaches would rely more heavily on ultrasound and use aspiration cytology.

*Table 2.4   Causes of thyroid nodules*

|  | Isotope scan finding | Ultrasound finding |
|---|---|---|
| Functioning adenoma | Increased uptake | Echogenic (solid) |
| Multinodular goitre | Multifocal | Multiple nodules and cysts |
| Non-functioning adenoma | Decreased uptake | Echogenic (solid) |
| Colloid nodule | Decreased uptake | Echogenic (solid) |
| Cyst | Decreased uptake | Echo-free |
| Haemorrhagic cyst | Decreased uptake | Mixed |
| Malignant tumour | Decreased uptake | Echogenic (solid) |
| Local thyroiditis | Increased or decreased uptake | Echogenic (solid) or no discrete lesion |

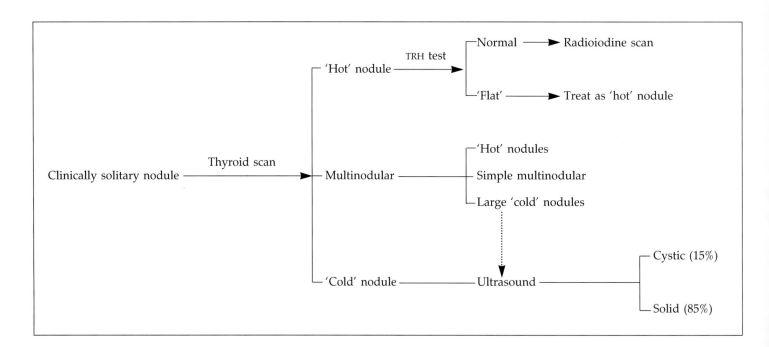

*Fig. 2.12*

*'Flow channel' for investigation of solitary thyroid nodule.*

## CLINICAL APPLICATIONS

### *Thyroid nodules: ultrasound solid*

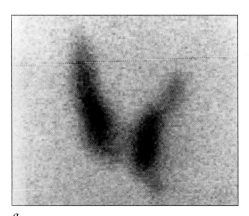

*a*

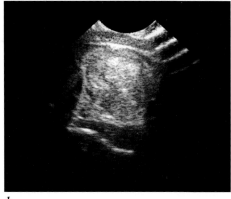

*b*

**Fig. 2.13**

*Mass in the left lobe of thyroid, which on the isotope scan (a) is seen to be non-functioning. The ultrasound scan (b) identifies a solid discrete mass. Fine-needle aspiration should be used to evaluate solid lesions.*

### *Thyroid nodules: ultrasound cystic*

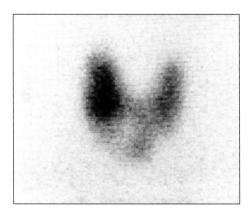

*a*

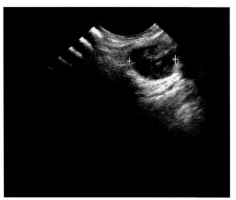

*b*

**Fig. 2.14**

*Mass in the lower pole of the right lobe of the thyroid, which on the isotope scan (a) is seen to be non-functioning and on the ultrasound (b) predominantly cystic. Fine-needle aspiration identified a colloid cyst.*

### *Thyroid nodules: use of markers*

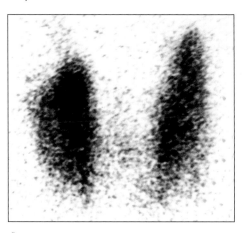

*a*

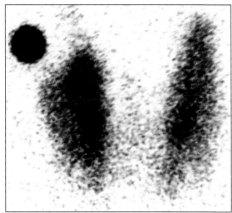

*b Marker*

**Fig. 2.15**

*Sometimes the presence of a nodule is not entirely clear, and a carefully placed radioactive marker will confirm that the palpated nodule is seen on the scan (a,b). Some care must be taken when using a pinhole collimator because of the distortion that this instrument introduces.*

- **There is no reliable method of distinguishing a solid from a cystic lesion using an isotope scan alone.**
- **Fine-needle aspiration should be used to evaluate non-functioning solid thyroid lesions.**

## Multinodular goitre

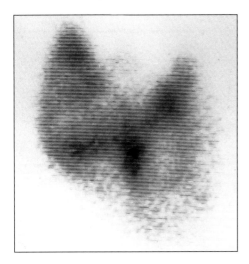

**Fig. 2.16**

$^{99m}Tc$ thyroid scan in a 63-year-old woman with a 10-year history of goitre. There is an enlarged thyroid, with non-homogeneous uptake in both lobes.

## The oblique view

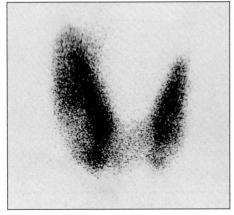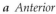  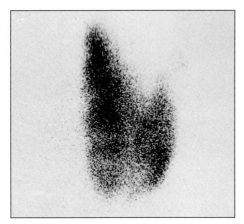  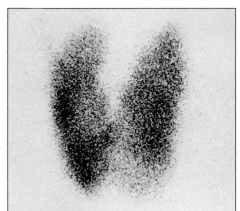

*a Anterior*                      *b Right anterior oblique*                      *c Left anterior oblique*

**Fig. 2.17**

*(a–c) Thyroid scans.*

*There is a clear-cut area of decreased tracer uptake seen in the lower pole of the right lobe, and, on the evidence of the anterior view alone, it might be concluded that there is a solitary non-functioning nodule. However, on the oblique views multiple small areas of decreased tracer uptake are seen in both lobes. The scan appearances are those of multinodular goitre, and the study emphasizes the contribution that oblique views can occasionally make.*

## CLINICAL APPLICATIONS

## The importance of 'markers'

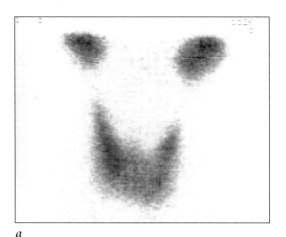

*a*

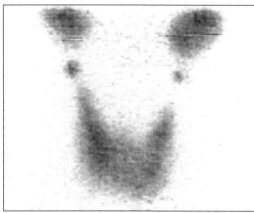

*b*

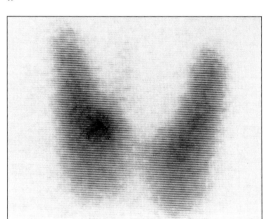

*c*

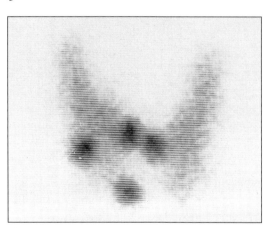

*d*

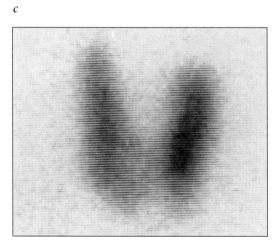

*e*

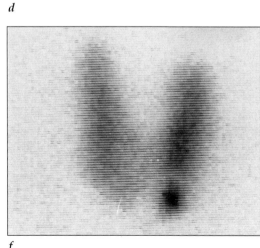

*f*

*Fig. 2.18*

*Three almost normal scans where a report could have been misleading.*

**Case 1** *The thyroid scan (a) appears relatively normal. The markers (b) indicate that the large palpable midline nodule lies above the thyroid and is due to a thyroglossal cyst.*

**Case 2** *A further example of a patient with a palpable midline thyroid nodule. The initial scan (c) appears essentially normal, but it is clear with careful marker placement (d) that the midline nodule is non-functional.*

**Case 3** *The initial thyroid scan (e) is unremarkable, although there is a small area of relatively decreased tracer uptake at the lower pole of the left lobe which corresponds to the palpable nodule. (f) Thyroid scan with nodule marker. The nodule was surgically removed, and histological examination revealed Hashimoto's thyroiditis.*

**Whenever there is a palpable nodule, it is important to correlate clinical findings with scan appearances, and careful placing of markers may be necessary.**

## CLINICAL APPLICATIONS

## Changes in cysts with time

Figures 2.19, 2.20 and 2.21 show examples of partial and complete resolution of changes following haemorrhage into a thyroid cyst. Sequential scans are often invaluable in the assessment and management of thyroid nodules.

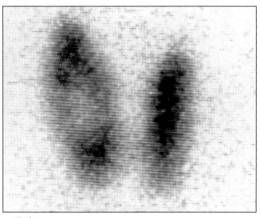

*a Before*

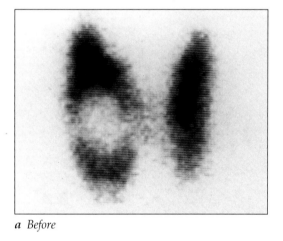

*a Before*

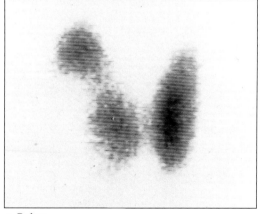

*a Before*

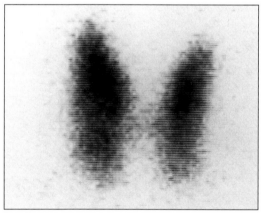

*b After*

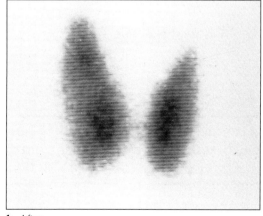

*b After*

**Fig. 2.19**

*Thyroid scan (a) before and (b) following resolution of a cyst.*

**Fig. 2.20**

*Thyroid scan (a) before and (b) following resolution of a cyst.*

**Fig. 2.21**

*Thyroid scan (a) before and (b) following aspiration of a cyst.*

## Thyroid nodule: malignant
### Papillary carcinoma

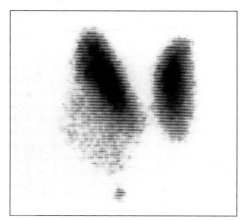

**Fig. 2.22**

*A non-functioning nodule at the lower pole of the right lobe of the thyroid. Papillary carcinoma was discovered at operation.*

There are no reliable ways of distinguishing a benign thyroid nodule from a malignant thyroid nodule on a thyroid scan. The appearance of tissue displacement should raise the suspicion of cancer, however.

### Follicular carcinoma

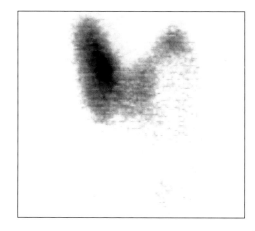

**Fig. 2.23**

*A mass in the left lobe of the thyroid in a 23-year-old woman . A non-functioning nodule is seen on the ⁹⁹ᵐTc scan which was solid on ultrasound. A follicular carcinoma was removed at operation.*

### Anaplastic carcinoma

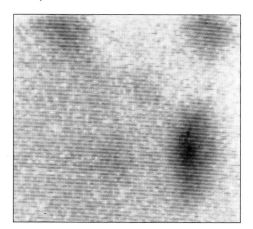

*a Patient 1*

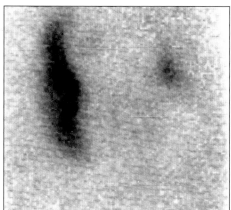

*b Patient 2*

**Fig. 2.24**

*Two examples of anaplastic carcinoma of the thyroid.*

*In the first example (a) the left lobe of the thyroid appears normal but is displaced to the left. The right lobe is replaced by a large non-functioning mass which was subsequently shown to be anaplastic carcinoma of the thyroid.*

*In the second example (b) the left lobe of the thyroid and isthmus are almost completely replaced, with the exception of a small area in the upper pole of the left lobe.*

## CLINICAL APPLICATIONS

### Thyroid nodules: functioning

Functioning nodules are almost never malignant but are important because they may cause thyrotoxicosis.

**Table 2.5 Summary of types and stages of functional nodules**

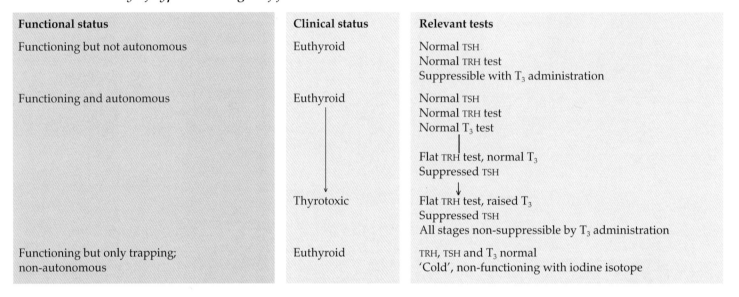

| Functional status | Clinical status | Relevant tests |
|---|---|---|
| Functioning but not autonomous | Euthyroid | Normal TSH<br>Normal TRH test<br>Suppressible with $T_3$ administration |
| Functioning and autonomous | Euthyroid<br>↓<br><br><br><br><br>Thyrotoxic | Normal TSH<br>Normal TRH test<br>Normal $T_3$ test<br><br>Flat TRH test, normal $T_3$<br>Suppressed TSH<br>↓<br>Flat TRH test, raised $T_3$<br>Suppressed TSH<br>All stages non-suppressible by $T_3$ administration |
| Functioning but only trapping; non-autonomous | Euthyroid | TRH, TSH and $T_3$ normal<br>'Cold', non-functioning with iodine isotope |

### Autonomous non-toxic nodule

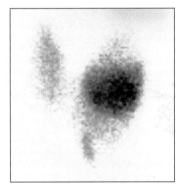

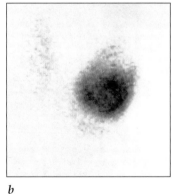

*a*

*b*

**Fig. 2.25**

*An initial thyroid scan (**a**) shows a non-toxic autonomously functioning thyroid nodule in the left lobe of the thyroid, with partial suppression of the surrounding thyroid tissue. The $T_3$ suppression test (**b**) shows no suppression of the functioning nodule.*

### Stages in the development of an autonomous toxic nodule

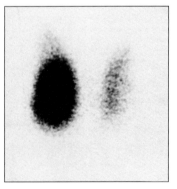

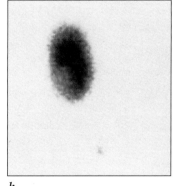

*a*

*b*

**Fig. 2.26**

*On the initial study (**a**) there is a solitary, non-toxic autonomous nodule with partial suppression of the remaining thyroid tissue. The patient subsequently became thyrotoxic, and the repeat scan (**b**) shows complete suppression of the rest of the gland. Thus there has been progression from a non-toxic autonomous nodule to a toxic autonomous nodule.*

## Misleading cases of functioning nodules

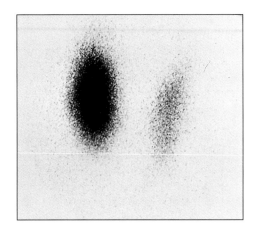

**Fig. 2.27**

**Case 1** *The initial study suggested a non-toxic autonomous nodule. However, 6 months later, while the scan appearances were essentially unchanged, the patient had developed typical clinical and biochemical features of hypothyroidism due to Hashimoto's thyroiditis. Thus, on rare occasions, patients with Hashimoto's disease may have residual nodules of tissue capable of trapping $^{99m}TcO_4$, even when, as in this case, the patient was hypothyroid.*

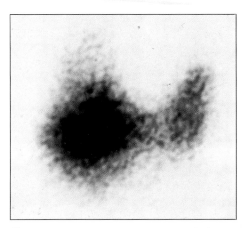
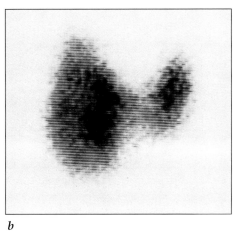

*a*     *b*

**Case 2** *A further example of the rare situation where a thyroid tumour trapped tracer. The patient presented with a lump in the right side of the neck. On $^{99m}Tc$ study (a) tracer uptake is seen at the site of the nodule, but the $^{123}I$ scan (b) does not confirm increased uptake at this site.*

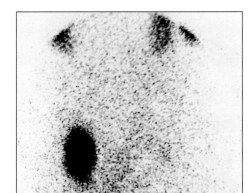

**Case 3** *There is an apparent 'hot' nodule on the right. However, this patient had a large, firm, irregular left-sided thyroid mass: the right lobe of the thyroid is in fact normal and its prominence is exaggerated because of replacement of the left lobe by tumour.*

## Diagnosis of cause of thyrotoxicosis

The thyroid scan is essential for the correct diagnosis and management of thyrotoxicosis. The common causes of hyperthyroidism with the relevant scan findings are shown in Table 2.6.

**Table 2.6  Causes of thyrotoxicosis**

| Cause | Scan finding | Comment |
|---|---|---|
| Diffuse toxic goitre (Graves' disease) | Diffuse high uptake of tracer | |
| Graves' disease developing in multinodular goitre | Diffuse irregular high uptake | TSH stimulation and thyroid stimulating antibody (TSab) measurement may be necessary to distinguish these two |
| Acute Hashimoto's disease | Diffuse high uptake | |
| Multiple toxic nodules | Irregular focal uptake | |
| Toxic nodule | Focal uptake with suppression of normal tissue | |
| Thyroiditis, painful and non-painful types | | |
| Thyrotoxicosis factitia | Low or absent uptake | |
| Iodine-induced thyrotoxicosis | | |
| Ectopic source of thyrotoxicosis | | |

## Diffuse toxicity: Graves' disease

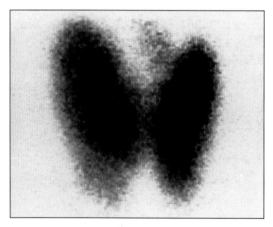

**Fig. 2.28**

*The thyroid scan shows the thyroid to be markedly enlarged, with a high uptake of tracer throughout. A pyramidal lobe is present. Quantitation of 20-minute $^{99m}Tc$ uptake confirmed a markedly increased uptake of tracer at 32% (normal 0.4–4%). The scan appearances are typically those of diffuse toxic goitre (Graves' disease).*

## Graves' disease developing in a multinodular gland

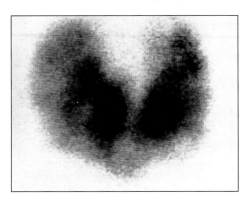

***Fig. 2.29***

*The thyroid is markedly enlarged. There is non-homogeneity of tracer uptake throughout, but the overall tracer uptake is high. These are the appearances of a diffuse toxic goitre (Graves' disease) associated with multinodular gland.*

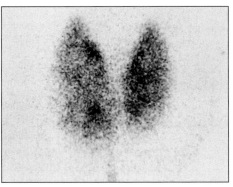

*a 0 months*

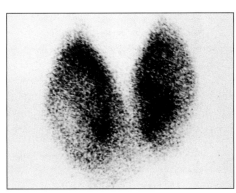

*b 2 years*

***Fig. 2.30***

*On the original study (a) the thyroid is slightly enlarged, with irregular distribution of tracer throughout. There are no clear-cut hyper- or hypofunctional nodules, and the scan appearances are those of simple non-toxic multinodular goitre. On the subsequent study (b) both lobes of the thyroid are enlarged, with irregular high uptake of tracer. There has been the development of diffuse toxic goitre superimposed on a multinodular gland.*

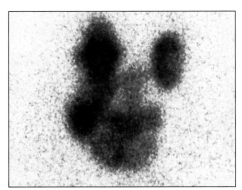

*a Before TSH*

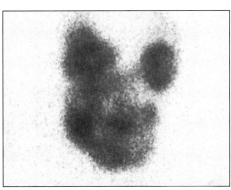

*b After TSH*

***Fig. 2.31***

*When Graves' disease develops in a multinodular gland, only the functional areas are stimulated by thyroid stimulating antibody (TSab). This can be shown by using TSH to stimulate the gland of a patient with Graves' disease. (a,b) and (c,d) demonstrate that further stimulation does not recruit any more tissue because it is already fully stimulated.*

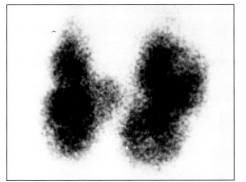

*c Before TSH*

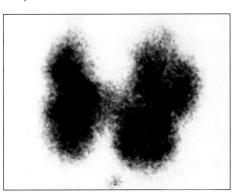

*d After TSH*

### Graves' disease in a single lobe of thyroid

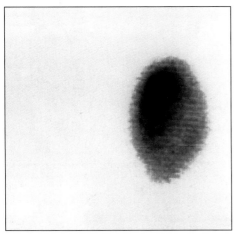

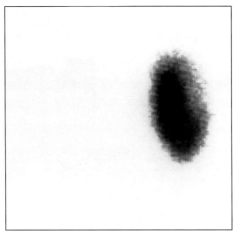

*a* 2 months, uptake 10.8%

*b* 6 months, uptake 1.7%

*Fig. 2.32*

*On the original study (a) the right lobe of the thyroid is not visualized, while the left is enlarged. Thyroid uptake is high at 10.8%. It was initially thought that there was a toxic nodule present, with suppression of the remainder of the gland. However, 6 months later, following [131]I therapy (b), the left lobe is smaller and uptake is normal (1.7%), but no functioning tissue is visualized on the right. The TSab levels were elevated. This patient had congenital absence of the right lobe of the thyroid, with Graves' disease developing in the left lobe.*

### Recurrence of Graves' thyrotoxicosis after previous thyroid surgery

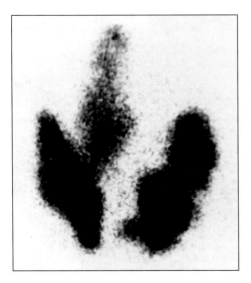

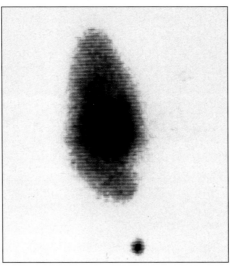

*Fig. 2.33*

*A patient with recurrence of Graves' disease following previous subtotal thyroidectomy. This is the operation that is usually performed for Graves' disease.*

*Fig. 2.34*

*Recurrence of Graves' disease in the right lobe of the thyroid following previous hemithyroidectomy.*

**Appearances of diffuse toxic goitre (Graves' disease) after thyroid-ectomy may be misleading. The isthmus is almost always removed at thyroid surgery. There may be an active pyramidal lobe or ectopic areas of function outside the immediate thyroid area. The uptake is usually high, but, because of the smaller volume of tissue, may be in the normal range. The cases in Figs 2.33 and 2.34 illustrate the differences between hemithyroid-ectomy and subtotal thyroidectomy. When the scan appearances are 'unusual', the possibility of previous surgery should be considered.**

### Thyrotoxicosis due to multiple toxic nodules

Usually a diagnosis of thyrotoxicosis due to multiple toxic nodules is made quite easily, as shown in Fig. 2.35. The features are well-demarcated nodules, evidence of suppressed perinodular thyroid tissue and an overall uptake that is often within the normal range and generally lower than is seen with Graves' disease. The normal suppressed tissue is not taking up the tracer because the high $T_4$ production by the nodules has stopped TSH production; without circulating TSH, there is practically no function of the thyroid follicular cells. This situation is the reverse to that found in Graves' disease, when the whole gland is uniformly stimulated by TSab. The demonstration of suppressed tissue may be diagnostically important and can be shown in three ways:

- Repeating the scan after im TSH injections
- Repeating the scan after antithyroid drug therapy in a dose sufficient to cause a rise in TSH (endogenous TSH stimulation)
- Repeating the scan after [131]I therapy, when the functional nodules will have reduced function and TSH will have risen to cause stimulation of previously suppressed tissue

### Multiple toxic nodular thyrotoxicosis

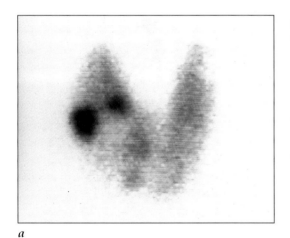

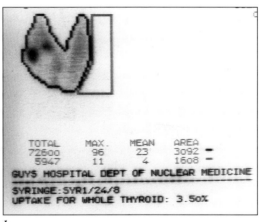

a

b

**Fig. 2.35**

**(a)** *Thyroid scan in a 40-year-old woman who presented with a goitre and thyrotoxicosis.* **(b)** *The $^{99m}Tc$ uptake of 3.50% is within the normal range.*

*Three cases illustrating recruitment of suppressed tissue using each of the three methods of increasing TSH levels*

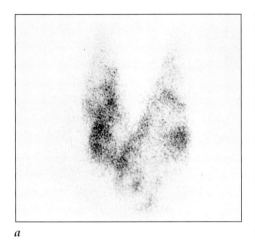

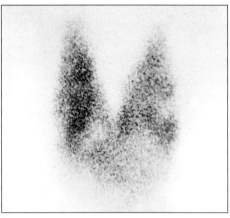

*a*

*b*

*Fig. 2.36*

**Case 1** *Thyrotoxicosis due to multiple toxic nodules. The initial study (a) shows the thyroid to be enlarged, with multiple areas of functioning tissue which, in the clinical context of thyrotoxicosis, are presumably functioning autonomously. The repeat study (b), obtained following three im injections of TSH, shows clear recruitment of perinodular thyroid tissue. This is therefore strong evidence supporting the presence of multiple toxic nodules.*

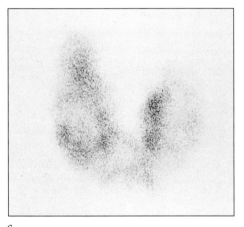

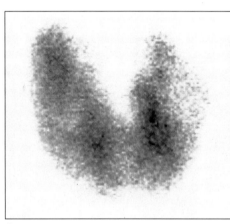

*c*

*d*

**Case 2** *Initial thyroid scan (c) and repeat scan (d) obtained following treatment with an antithyroid drug (carbimazole) at a time when the patient was biochemically hypothyroid. In comparison with the original study, the repeat scan shows more uniform distribution of tracer throughout both lobes of the thyroid and isthmus due to endogenous TSH stimulation.*

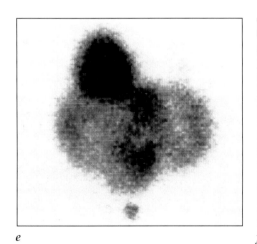

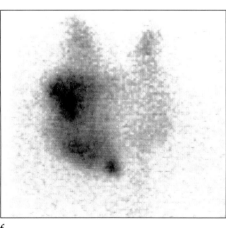

*e*

*f*

**Case 3** *On the original study (e) there is irregular uptake of tracer, with focal areas of markedly increased uptake, most notably at the upper pole of the right lobe. On the repeat study (f), obtained following definitive treatment of thyrotoxicosis with radioiodine, previously noted hyperfunctioning areas are no longer functional and there is recruitment of previously suppressed tissue, particularly in the lower pole of the right lobe and the upper pole of the left lobe. The scan findings are those of resolution of the toxic nodules following radioiodine, with recovery of suppressed tissue.*

## CLINICAL APPLICATIONS

*Radioiodine treatment for toxic nodular goitre*

There are two situations when a follow-up scan after radioiodine ($^{131}$I) therapy is clinically useful:

• By clearly establishing a diagnosis of toxic nodules and not toxic diffuse goitre, long-term follow-up is affected by the knowledge that hypothyroidism is very rare in this group of patients.

• By showing that the toxic nodules have resolved, the clinician can be confident that a recurrence of thyrotoxicosis is very unlikely.

These two points are illustrated in the two cases in Fig. 2.37. In the first there was doubt about the diagnosis; in the second there was no doubt, but the post-$^{131}$I scan shows good resolution of nodules.

*Multiple toxic nodules*

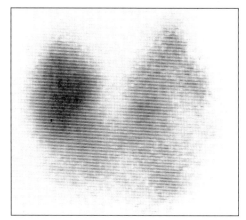

*a  0 months*

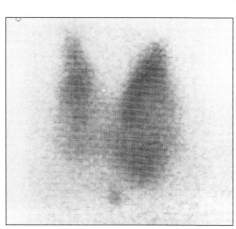

*b  9 months*

**Fig. 2.37**

**Case 1** *In the clinical context of thyrotoxicosis it is not possible from the original scan (a) to differentiate between Graves' disease superimposed on a multinodular goitre and the presence of toxic nodules. On the repeat scan (b), obtained following radioiodine therapy, the large focal area of increased tracer uptake at the upper pole of the right lobe is no longer visualized and there is relatively increased uptake throughout the left lobe of the thyroid. The sequence of scans indicates resolution of toxic nodules, with recruitment of previously suppressed thyroid tissue, following successful treatment with radioiodine.*

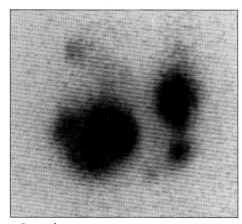

*c  0 months*

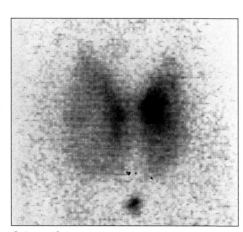

*d  6 months*

**Case 2** *The original study (c) shows the presence of multiple toxic nodules. The repeat scan (d), obtained following radioiodine therapy, shows that there has been marked resolution of 'hot' nodules, with clear visualization of previously suppressed thyroid tissue.*

*Solitary toxic nodule*

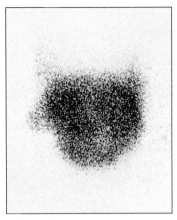

*a* 0 *months*

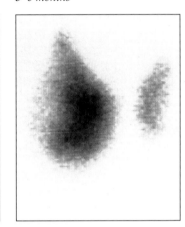

*b* 6 *months*

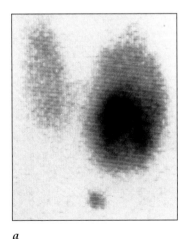

*c* 0 *months*

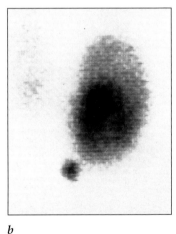

*d* 6 *months*

**Fig. 2.38**

*These two cases illustrate partial and complete resolution of the toxic nodule. If resolution is only partial there is some return of previously suppressed tissue, but the patient remains liable to relapse and may require further radioiodine therapy.*

**Case 1** *On the original study (**a**) there is a large focal area of increased tracer uptake in the midline. The right and left lobes of the thyroid are faintly visualized and the scan appearances are those of a large toxic nodule, with suppression of the remainder of the gland. The repeat scan (**b**), obtained following successful treatment with radioiodine, shows that there has been complete resolution of the nodule, with return to normal function in the rest of the gland.*

**Case 2** *On the original study (**c**) there is a single toxic nodule, with total suppression of the remainder of the gland. On the repeat scan (**d**), obtained following radioiodine therapy, the nodule is still visualized, although there has been some return of function throughout the rest of the gland. This series of scans represents partial resolution of a toxic nodule.*

**Fig. 2.39**

*Thyroid scans obtained (**a**) while receiving an antithyroid drug (carbimazole) and (**b**) 6 weeks after therapy was discontinued. It can be seen that when antithyroid therapy was discontinued, the scan appearances were those of a solitary toxic nodule, with suppression of the remainder of the gland. However, while the patient was receiving the drug, there was clearly uptake of tracer into the right lobe of the thyroid (due to endogenous TSH stimulation). If radioiodine had been given at that time, there would have been a significant risk of the patient subsequently developing hypothyroidism.*

*a*     *b*

**If a patient with a toxic nodule is treated with 131I while taking antithyroid drugs, there will be some 131I uptake into suppressed tissue (see Fig. 2.39) and the incidence of subsequent hypothyroidism rises from nearly zero to 20–30%. Thyroid scanning before 131I treatment is therefore advisable.**

## CLINICAL APPLICATIONS

*Palpable 'nodule' in hyperthyroidism*

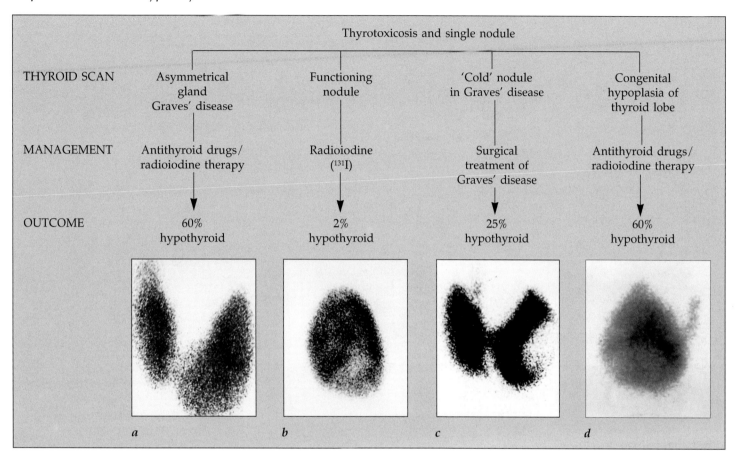

|  | | | | |
|---|---|---|---|---|
| | Thyrotoxicosis and single nodule | | | |
| THYROID SCAN | Asymmetrical gland Graves' disease | Functioning nodule | 'Cold' nodule in Graves' disease | Congenital hypoplasia of thyroid lobe |
| MANAGEMENT | Antithyroid drugs/ radioiodine therapy | Radioiodine ($^{131}$I) | Surgical treatment of Graves' disease | Antithyroid drugs/ radioiodine therapy |
| OUTCOME | 60% hypothyroid | 2% hypothyroid | 25% hypothyroid | 60% hypothyroid |
| | *a* | *b* | *c* | *d* |

### Fig. 2.40

*(a–d) There are four main reasons why a patient with hyperthyroidism could have a 'nodule'. The commonest is a functioning toxic nodule. The other three—'cold' nodule in diffuse toxic goitre (Graves' disease), an asymmetrical gland and congenital hypoplasia of thyroid lobe—are often forgotten clinically and only discovered on a scan. This has clinical importance.*

## CLINICAL APPLICATIONS

*Low uptake of tracer in the presence of clinical hyperthyroidism*

Absent thyroid uptake of tracer in a patient with thyrotoxicosis is usually a surprise finding on the scan. After checking that the tracer has been given, several causes should be considered, as illustrated in Fig. 2.41.

*Table 2.7  Causes and mechanisms of low tracer uptake in thyrotoxicosis*

| Cause | Mechanism |
|---|---|
| Subacute (De Quervain's thyroiditis) | Damage to the thyroid cell<br>Suppression of TSH by released $T_4$ |
| Thyrotoxicosis associated with high iodine ingestion including health food preparations and amiodarone. | Swamping of the body's iodine pool so that the radioactive tracer is diluted in a much larger volume and therefore proportionally less is taken up by the gland<br>Pharmacological inhibitory effect of iodine |
| Excess thyroid hormone administration<br>Ectopic thyroid hormone production (eg struma ovarii) | Suppression of TSH<br>Suppression of TSH |

*Subacute viral thyroiditis: De Quervain's thyroiditis*

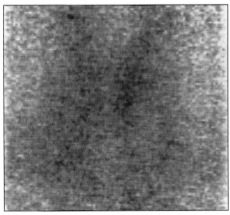

*a  0 months*

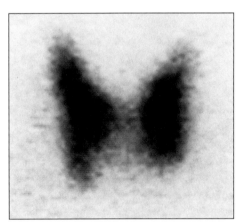

*b  4 months*

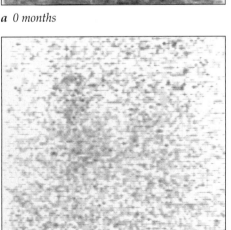

*c  0 months*

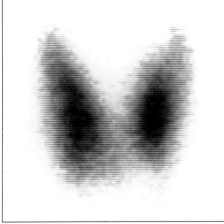

*d  12 months*

**Fig. 2.41**

***Case 1*** *On the original scan **(a)**, no significant tracer uptake is visible in the neck. Three months later the thyroid scan **(b)** is essentially normal, confirming the clinical diagnosis of resolving subacute (De Quervain's) thyroiditis.*

***Case 2*** *Thyroid scan in a 22-year-old woman with a short history of painful swelling of the thyroid. The initial scan **(c)** shows minimal uptake of traces in the thyroid region. The repeat scan **(d)** 1 year later, following resolution of symptoms, is normal.*

## CLINICAL APPLICATIONS

### High iodine uptake

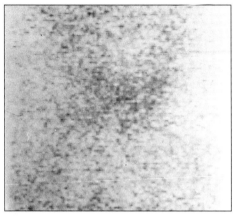

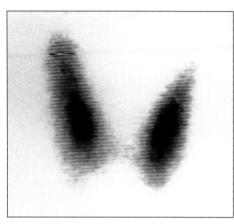

*Case 3* Thyroid scans in a 50-year-old man presenting with a goitre following ingestion of large quantities of kelp tablets. Thyroxine levels were slightly raised and the initial scan *(e)* showed no uptake. Three months later, having discontinued kelp, the scan *(f)* and the thyroid function tests returned to normal.

*e 0 months*

*f 3 months*

### Amiodarone-induced thyrotoxicosis

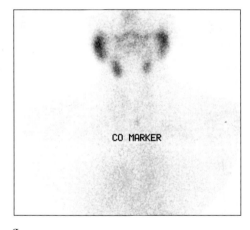

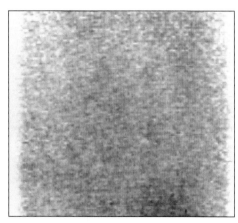

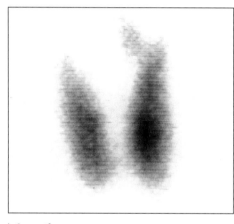

*g*

*h 0 months*

*i 8 months*

*Case 4 (g)* Thyroid scan in an 81-year-old woman who had become biochemically toxic while taking amiodarone. There is no uptake in the thyroid region, consistent with high iodine ingestion associated with amiodarone. Note the normal distribution of $^{99m}TcO_4$ in the salivary glands.

*Case 5* Thyroid scans in a 49-year-old man who developed thyrotoxicosis while taking amiodarone. *(h)* $^{99m}Tc$ scan acquired while the patient was taking amiodarone shows no uptake in the region of the thyroid. *(i)* $^{99m}Tc$ scan performed 8 months later when the patient had discontinued amiodarone but was still thyrotoxic shows uptake in the thyroid, with visualization of the pyramidal lobe.

- The high iodine content of amiodarone may induce thyrotoxicosis.
- Thyrotoxicosis may persist after amiodarone is discontinued.

## Assessment of goitre

*Table 2.8 Role of the thyroid scan in the assessment of goitre*

| Scan findings | Cause | Comment |
|---|---|---|
| Diffuse, normal uptake of tracer | Diffuse non-toxic (simple) goitre | |
| Diffuse, with high uptake of tracer | Diffuse toxic goitre (Graves' disease) | May be first indication of hyperthyroidism |
| | Lymphocytic thyroiditis (Hashimoto's disease) | Occurs in early disease |
| | Iodine deficiency | |
| | Organification defects (inherited or goitrogens) | May be difficult to distinguish |
| Diffuse, low uptake of tracer | Subacute thyroiditis (De Quervain's) | |
| | Iodine-induced goitre | May be indistinguishable on the |
| | Hashimoto's disease | scan but presentation is entirely different |
| | Lymphoma | |
| Multifocal irregularity | Simple multinodular goitre | Detection of autonomous nodule is important |
| Normal uptake of tracer | Hashimoto's disease | Diagnosis by antibodies |
| Irregular replacement of thyroid tissue | Diffuse cancer | Usually clinically apparent, but may be confused with multinodular goitre |

*Euthyroid goitre*

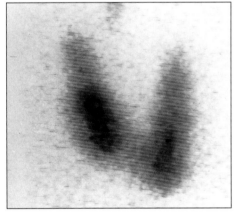

### Fig. 2.42

*Thyroid scan in a 23-year-old woman, who presented with a goitre and normal thyroid function tests, showing slight enlargement of the thyroid.*

*Graves' disease*

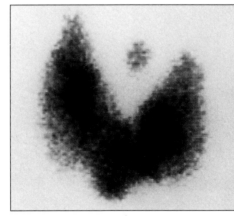 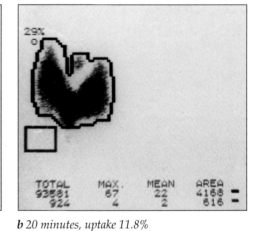

*a*                                                  *b 20 minutes, uptake 11.8%*

### Fig. 2.43

*On the thyroid scan (a) the thyroid is enlarged and shows diffusely increased uptake of tracer throughout. There is a discrete focus of activity lying above the thyroid just to the left of the midline. The scan appearances are typically those of diffuse toxic hyperplasia (Graves' disease). The small focus of activity lying above the thyroid reflects either a pyramidal lobe or else ectopic thyroid tissue. Quantitation of 20-minute $^{99m}$Tc uptake confirms that thyroid uptake is elevated at 11.8% (normal 0.4–4%).*

## CLINICAL APPLICATIONS

### Perchlorate discharge test

The perchlorate discharge test to detect inadequate organification forms part of the investigation procedure for goitre as illustrated in the following cases. The perchlorate ion $ClO_4^-$ is like the pertechnetate ion $^{99m}TcO_4^-$ and competes with iodine. An oral dose of potassium perchlorate ($KClO_4$) or an intravenous dose of sodium perchlorate ($NaClO_4$) will block further uptake of iodine and will displace and release any free unbound iodine in the follicular cell.

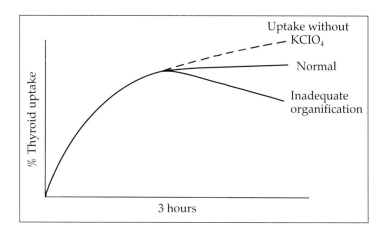

**Fig. 2.44**

*Diagrammatic representation of perchlorate discharge test.*

### Hashimoto's thyroiditis

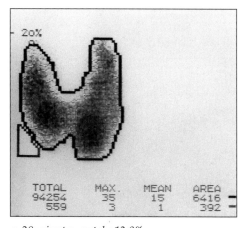

*a 20 minutes, uptake 12.9%*

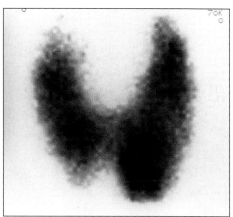

*b*

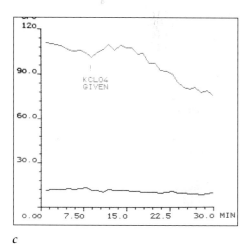

*c*

**Fig. 2.45**

*(a) 20-minute $^{99m}Tc$ quantitation. (b) Repeat scan with $^{123}I$. (c) Perchlorate discharge test.*
*    The $^{99m}Tc$ scan (a) shows the thyroid to be significantly enlarged, with diffusely increased uptake of tracer. These appearances suggest Graves' disease. However, the patient had biochemical evidence of hypothyroidism with positive thyroid antibodies. The perchlorate discharge test (c) is strongly positive, indicating that, while tracer is being trapped, a binding defect is present. This patient had Hashimoto's thyroiditis, and this pattern of results is seen occasionally when there is still increased trapping by the thyroid prior to decompensation.*

## Iodine-deficiency goitre

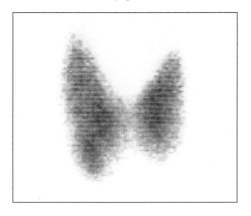

a

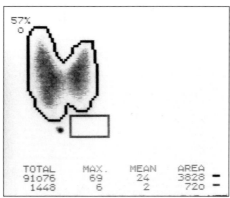

b

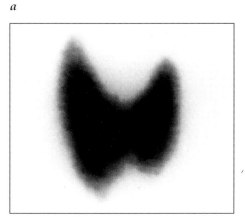

c

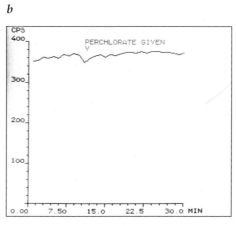

d

*Fig. 2.46*

*(a) $^{99m}$Tc thyroid scan. (b) 20-minute quantitation of tracer uptake. (c) Repeat scan with $^{123}$I. (d) Perchlorate discharge test.*

*The original scan shows the thyroid to be enlarged, with increased avidity for tracer. The perchlorate discharge test (d) is negative, indicating that there is no binding defect present. This patient had a goitre due to iodine deficiency.*

## Dyshormonogenesis

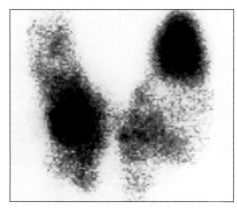

a

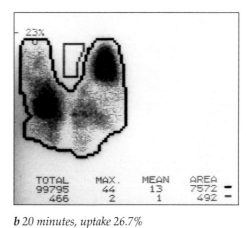

*b 20 minutes, uptake 26.7%*

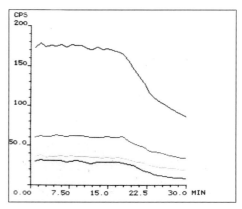

c

*Fig. 2.47*

*(a) Thyroid scan. (b) 20-minute quantitation of tracer uptake. (c) Perchlorate discharge test.*
*The original scan (a) shows the thyroid to be markedly enlarged, with non-homogeneity of tracer uptake; there are more focal areas of relatively reduced and increased uptake. Quantitation (b) shows that the thyroid uptake is significantly elevated at 26.7%. The perchlorate discharge test (c) is strongly positive. This patient had a goitre since childhood due to dyshormonogenesis.*

## CLINICAL APPLICATIONS

### Multinodular goitre

A simple non-toxic multinodular goitre will appear enlarged on the scan with irregular, usually poorly defined areas of decreased and increased tracer accumulation, corresponding to areas of fibrosis, degeneration and functional regeneration. The overall tracer uptake will be within the normal range. The following points need attention:

- An x-ray examination is necesary for confirmation of tracheal deviation.
- There is a possibility that toxic nodules will

eventually develop in all multinodular goitres and may subsequently cause thyrotoxicosis. A TRH test may be necessary for evaluation.
- If there is one non-functioning mass that is larger and different to the others, which could represent a malignancy, especially if it corresponds to a distinct palpable mass, a histological examination may be necessary for further evaluation.
- If there is any suggestion of retrosternal extension, an x-ray examination and radioiodine scan may be necessary for further evaluation.

### Simple non-toxic nodule

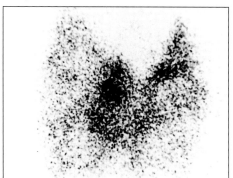

a

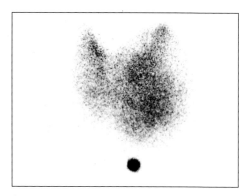

b

*Fig. 2.48*

*(a,b) Two cases of simple non-toxic multinodular goitre.*

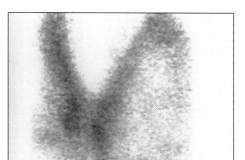

*Fig. 2.49*

*While the scan appearances are of multinodular goitre, there is a 'dominant' non-functioning nodule in the left lobe of the thyroid. This corresponded to a large palpable nodule. Such cases should be managed as a single, non-functioning nodule.*

**Ultrasensitive TSH estimation should be used to assess the significance of a functioning nodule or nodules scan on a multinodular goitre. Suppression of ultrasensitive TSH will confirm autonomous function.**

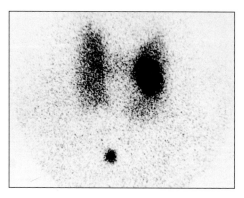

a

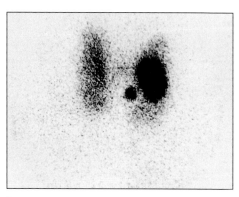

b

*Fig. 2.50*

*The original thyroid scan (a) shows a discrete focus of increased tracer uptake in the mid-zone of the left lobe. In addition, there is a photon-deficient area in the region of the isthmus and the marker on (b) indicates that this corresponds to a palpable midline nodule. The scan appearances are those of a multinodular goitre, with both hyper- and hypofunctioning nodules.*

## Evolution of a toxic nodule

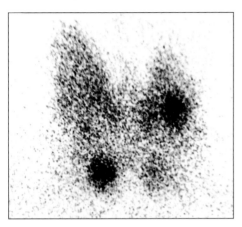 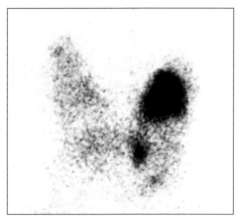 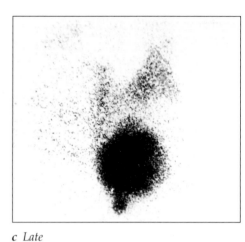

*a Early*        *b Intermediate*        *c Late*

**Fig. 2.51**

*Three examples of simple multinodular goitres with functioning nodules in various stages of evolution. (a) Early: small focal areas of increased tracer uptake with no suppression of normal tissue. Typically the TRH test would be normal, with normal thyroid function tests. (b) Intermediate: focal areas of increased uptake, with a large, more prominent nodule and some suppression of normal tissue. Typically the TRH test would be flat, with a normal $T_3$ level. (c) Late: a larger nodule is present, with more suppression of normal tissue. Typically the TRH test would be flat, with some elevation of $T_3$. This patient is developing thyrotoxicosis.*

## Suppression and stimulation tests

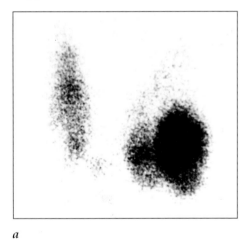 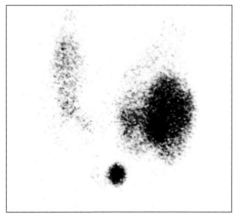 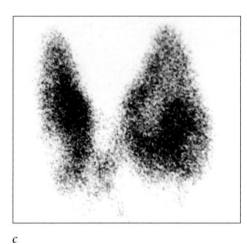

*a*        *b*        *c*

**Fig. 2.52**

*Suppression and stimulation tests combined with thyroid scanning can demonstrate a degree of autonomy and suppression of the thyroid gland. (a) A scan obtained in the resting state showing a multinodular goitre with functioning nodules and some suppression of normal thyroid tissue. (b) A scan obtained after 1 week of 80 μg $T_3$ daily showing some further suppression of non-autonomous tissue. (c) A scan obtained after three doses of 10 IU TSH (given im daily before the scan) showing that the suppressed tissue is capable of responding to further stimulation. Such a patient is not yet thyrotoxic, but is liable to develop this condition. If treatment with radioiodine ($^{131}$I) were to be given at this stage, there would be a significant risk of the patient becoming hypothyroid because of the uptake in normal tissue.*

## CLINICAL APPLICATIONS

*Retrosternal goitre*

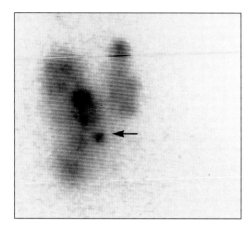

***Fig. 2.53***

*A thyroid scan obtained with $^{123}$I, showing a multinodular goitre with clear evidence of retrosternal extension on the right. A marker is present on the suprasternal notch (arrow).*

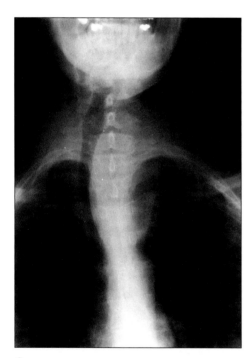

*a*

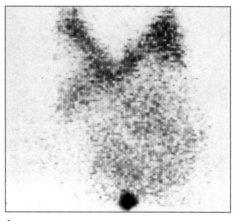

*b*

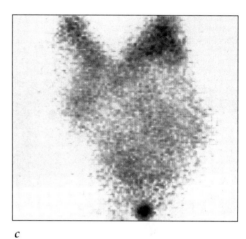

*c*

***Fig. 2.54***

*Very frequently, $^{99m}$TcO$_4$ and radioiodine scans will show an identical pattern of tracer uptake. In this case, the patient was noted to have tracheal deviation on a chest x-ray (a), and a thyroid mass was discovered. A scan was performed to ascertain whether retrosternal extension was present. (b) $^{99m}$Tc and (c) $^{123}$I scans both show a multinodular goitre with no evidence of retrosternal extension. Note, however, that there is a large non-functioning nodule occupying much of the left lobe, and the possibility of carcinoma cannot be excluded.*

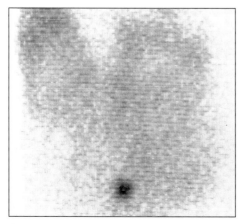

*a*

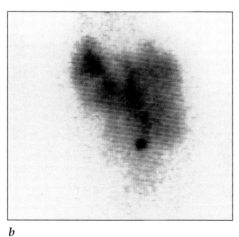

*b*

***Fig. 2.55***

*A large multinodular goitre with generally poor uptake of tracer is seen on the $^{99m}$Tc scan (a). A marker is present on the suprasternal notch and there is evidence of retrosternal extension. The $^{123}$I study (b) demonstrates a higher uptake of tracer by the gland, with clearer delineation of the borders.*

## CLINICAL APPLICATIONS

The following points should be noted in the evaluation of a retrosternal goitre:

- An isotope of iodine ($^{131}$I or $^{123}$I) is better than $^{99m}$Tc for demonstrating retrosternal extension because
  (a) there is higher uptake in the gland
  (b) there is better tissue to background ratio
  (c) there is less bone absorption by the sternum when using $^{131}$I
- The isotope $^{123}$I gives a lower radiation dose but is more expensive than $^{131}$I

- An iodine isotope is indicated when
  (a) retrosternal extension is the prime question to be answered
  (b) uptake with $^{99m}$Tc is particularly low
  (c) the lower border of the gland on a $^{99m}$Tc scan is irregular
- This technique will only demonstrate functioning retrosternal thyroid, and non-functioning may be present.

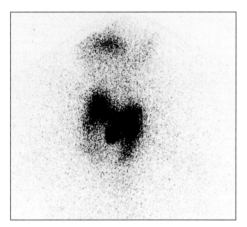

a

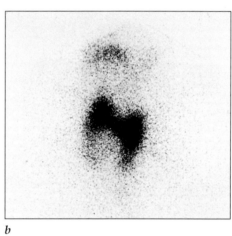

b

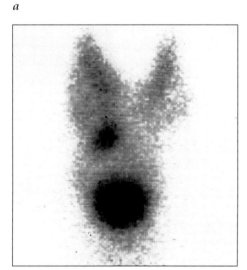

c

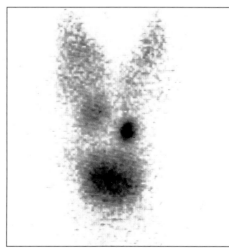

d

*Fig. 2.56*

*Functioning and non-functioning masses may be present in retrosternal goitres.*

**Case 1** *Thyroid scans obtained with $^{123}$I (a) and with a marker on the suprasternal notch (b), showing a multinodular goitre with retrosternal extension. There is a large non-functioning nodule in the lower pole of the right lobe, extending across the midline.*

**Case 2** *Thyroid scans obtained with $^{123}$I (c) and with a marker on the suprasternal notch (d) showing a multinodular goitre with striking retrosternal extension. In addition, there are two focal areas of relatively increased tracer uptake, one at the lower pole of the right lobe and the other, much larger, lying retrosternally. The scan appearances are suggestive of autonomously functioning nodules, but there is no evidence of suppression of the remaining thyroid tissue.*

**CLINICAL APPLICATIONS**

## Goitre associated with low uptake of tracer on scan
## Thyroiditis

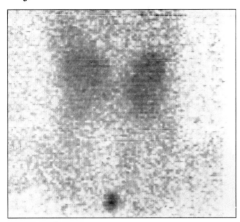

*a  0 months*

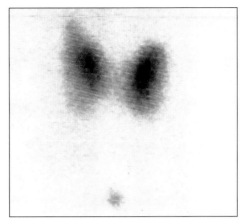

*b  5 months*

*Fig. 2.57*

*A patient who presented with biochemical and clinical evidence of hyperthyroidism together with tenderness in the neck. A thyroid scan at the time (a) showed low uptake of tracer by the gland. A repeat scan (b), obtained when thyroiditis had resolved, was normal.*

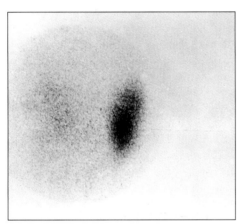

*a  0 months*

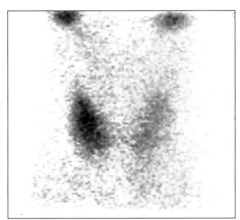

*b  3 weeks, uptake 0.41%*

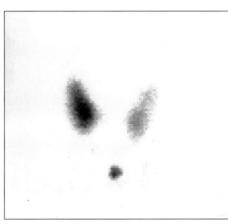

*c  7 weeks, uptake 2.06%*

*Fig. 2.58*

*A male patient who presented with a tender, firm swelling in the right side of his neck. On the original scan (a) the left lobe of the thyroid appears relatively normal, but there is essentially no uptake on the right. The scan findings raise the possibility of replacement of the right lobe of the thyroid, and carcinoma cannot be excluded. An operation was recommended, but when the patient was seen for review 3 weeks later the right-sided symptoms had resolved, and he was complaining of pain in the left side of his neck. A repeat scan was obtained (b) which shows clear improvement in the right lobe of the thyroid, with low uptake on the left. One month later, the patient was asymptomatic. A further scan (c) shows overall improvement, although there is still slight reduction of tracer uptake by the left lobe of the thyroid. This patient represents an unusual case of thyroiditis, initially involving one lobe of the thyroid and subsequently the other.*

*Thyroxine*

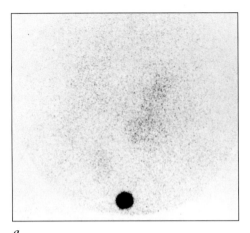

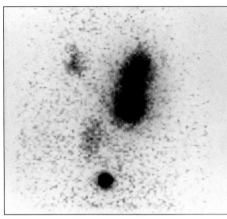

a

b

**Fig. 2.59**

*A patient with a past history of thyroid surgery for a multinodular goitre who was subsequently placed on a suppressive dose of thyroxine. The initial scan (**a**), obtained while the patient was receiving thyroxine, shows extremely low uptake of tracer. A repeat study for reassessment of the gland (**b**) was obtained one month after discontinuation of thyroxine. The scan appearances in this case represent a combination of multinodular change and previous thyroid surgery.*

*A case of Hashimoto's thyroiditis and lymphoma*

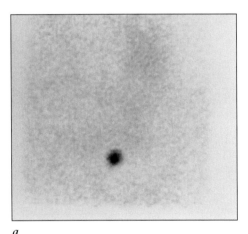

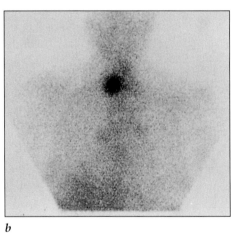

a

b

**Fig. 2.60**

*The thyroid scan (**a**) shows extremely poor uptake of tracer throughout the thyroid, in keeping with the clinical picture of hypothyroidism due to Hashimoto's thyroiditis. The gallium-67 ($^{67}$Ga) scan (**b**) of the neck and thorax shows intensely increased tracer accumulation in the region of the thyroid, with much less striking but nevertheless abnormal hilar activity. This patient had thyroid lymphoma, which has a known association with Hashimoto's thyroiditis. In addition, there is evidence of active lymphoma in the hilar regions.*

**Gallium-67 can be used diagnostically in a patient with Hashimoto's thyroiditis who develops further swelling in the neck while taking T$_4$ replacement therapy, when a routine thyroid scan cannot be employed.**

## Evaluation of ectopic thyroid

### Thyroid development and possible clinical outcome

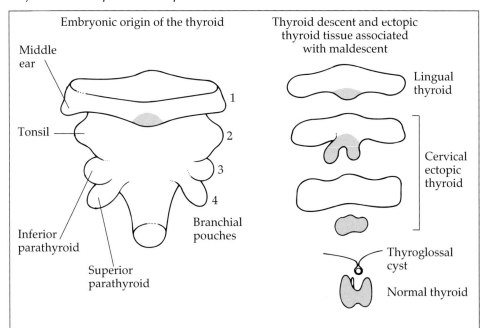

**Fig. 2.61**

*Thyroid development.*

### Table 2.9 Scan appearances for evaluation of ectopic thyroid

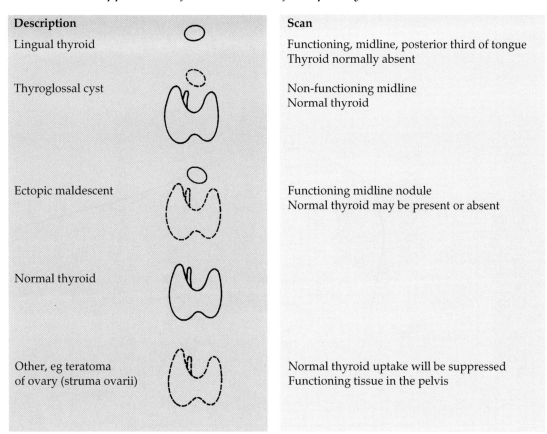

| Description | | Scan |
|---|---|---|
| Lingual thyroid | | Functioning, midline, posterior third of tongue<br>Thyroid normally absent |
| Thyroglossal cyst | | Non-functioning midline<br>Normal thyroid |
| Ectopic maldescent | | Functioning midline nodule<br>Normal thyroid may be present or absent |
| Normal thyroid | | |
| Other, eg teratoma<br>of ovary (struma ovarii) | | Normal thyroid uptake will be suppressed<br>Functioning tissue in the pelvis |

## Ectopic thyroid

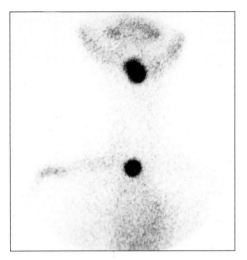

**Fig. 2.62**

*A thyroid scan showing no functioning thyroid tissue in the neck, but an area of avid tracer accumulation lying in the midline which corresponds to the posterior part of the tongue (lingual thyroid).*

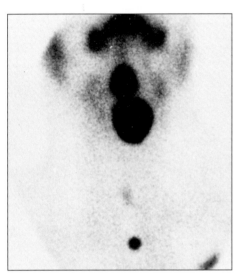

**Fig. 2.63**

*Thyroid scan showing two sites of functioning thyroid tissue: the smaller, at the posterior end of the tongue, represents lingual thyroid; the larger, in the upper neck in the midline, corresponds to a palpable mass. There is very little functioning thyroid tissue in the normal position. There are thus two sites of ectopic thyroid tissue: lingual and midline. It is highly probable that this patient would become hypothyroid if the midline mass were to be removed, with the additional possibility of considerable enlargement of the lingual thyroid. Note that this is not the appearance of a thyroglossal cyst, which is non-functioning on a thyroid scan.*

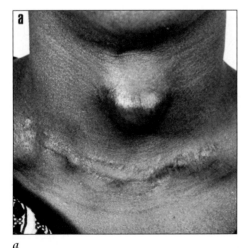 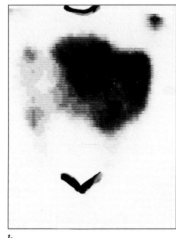 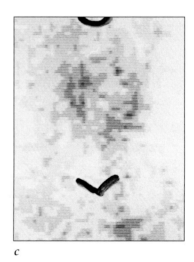

*a*        *b*        *c*

**Fig. 2.64**

*(a) A patient who developed a midline swelling following subtotal thyroidectomy. The scans show functioning (b) and, after T³, suppressible (c) ectopic thyroid tissue.*

## Thyroglossal cyst

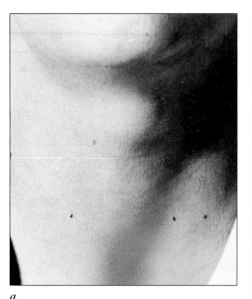

*a*

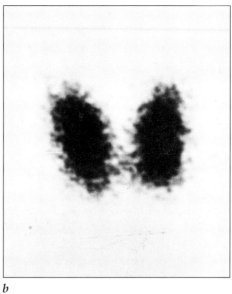

*b*

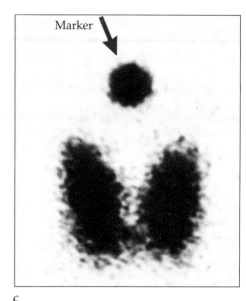

Marker

*c*

**Fig. 2.65**

*(a)* *A patient with a midline swelling. The thyroid scan* *(b,c)* *is normal, with no tracer uptake at the site of the swelling (marker). These are the typical findings with a thyroglossal cyst.*

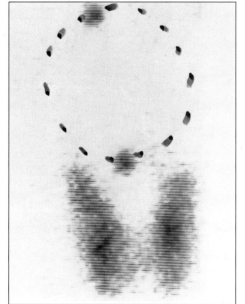

**Fig. 2.66**

*A woman with a large midline swelling. The thyroid scan demonstrates a normal thyroid with no tracer uptake in the large swelling, consistent with a thyroglossal cyst.*

## CLINICAL APPLICATIONS

### Assessment of thyroid cancer

Radionuclide thyroid scanning is used in the management of thyroid cancer at several stages:

(1) In diagnosis (see the sections on cold nodules and goitre)
(2) To assess the presence of normal thyroid tissue left behind after surgery for thyroid cancer
(3) To assess the presence of residual functioning thyroid tumour
(4) To assess the metastatic spread of functioning thyroid cancer
(5) To assess the suitability of the thyroid tumour for radioiodine ($^{131}$I) therapy.

It is essential to have a working knowledge of the behaviour of thyroid tumours in respect of their ability to accumulate tracer (Table 2.10).

**Table 2.10 Comparison of thyroid tumours based on ability to accumulate tracer**

| Histology | Comment |
|---|---|
| Pure papillary with no colloid formation | Rarely take up significant $^{131}$I |
| Papillary with follicular elements producing colloid | May take up significant amounts of $^{131}$I |
| Follicular | Usually take up $^{131}$I |
| Anaplastic | Never take up $^{131}$I |
| Medullary | Never take up $^{131}$I |
| Lymphoma | Never take up $^{131}$I |

### Thyroid cancer

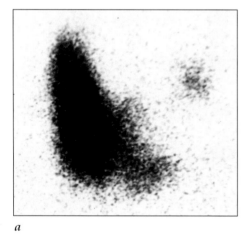
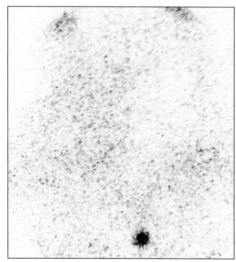
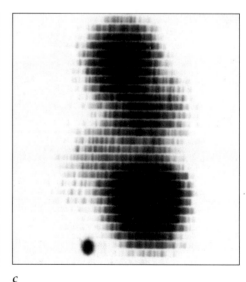

a

b

c

**Fig. 2.67**

*A case illustrating the commonest presentation of thyroid cancer. The patient presented with a left-sided thyroid nodule which was non-functioning and solitary on the thyroid scan (a). The likelihood of cancer was therefore about 10%. The nodule was removed and found to be a follicular carcinoma, and total thyroidectomy was then performed. The postoperative thyroid scan at four days (b) showed no remaining functioning tissue. T₄ replacement was not given, and the patient was rescanned with $^{131}$I at 4 weeks postoperatively (at which time the TSH level was greater than 40 mU/litre and serum T₄ was low, 15 mmol/litre). Functioning thyroid tissue is clearly visible (c), which could be either tumour or residual normal tissue.*

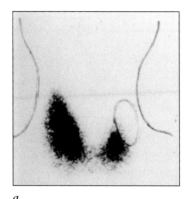
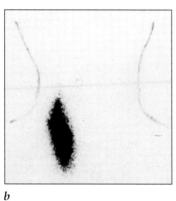
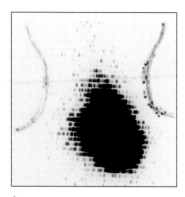

*a*      *b*      *c*

*Fig. 2.68*

*In contrast with Fig. 2.67, a case presented in a similar way with a non-functioning 'cold' nodule in the upper pole of the left lobe of the thyroid (**a**). A total left and subtotal right hemithyroidectomy was performed confirming follicular carcinoma. The postoperative scan (**b**) shows residual functional thyroid tissue on the right. The patient received an ablative dose of ¹³¹I and was rescanned 3 months later with ¹³¹I (**c**). The normal right-sided tissue has been destroyed and the residual tumour tissue on the left is now accumulating ¹³¹I in response to the higher levels of TSH.*

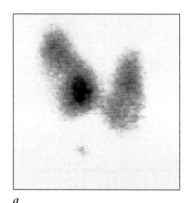
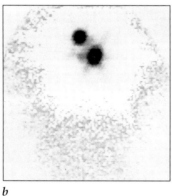
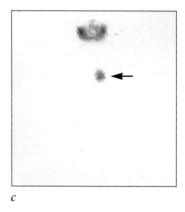

*a*      *b*      *c*

*Fig. 2.69*

*A thyroid scan (**a**) revealed a 'cold' nodule in the right mid-lobe of the thyroid. At surgery, a follicular carcinoma was discovered. Following total thyroidectomy, a ¹³¹I scan (**b**) revealed two foci of avid tracer uptake in the thyroid surgical bed. A 3000 MBq (81 mCi) therapeutic dose of ¹³¹I was given. Nine months later, a repeat ¹³¹I scan (**c**) showed a small focus of activity in the neck (arrow). There has been clear improvement following therapy, but there is persistent residual tissue (tumour), and further ¹³¹I therapy will be required.*

- Solitary 'cold' nodules have a probability of malignancy of about 10%.
- Differentiated thyroid cancer does not accumulate ¹³¹I at normal TSH stimulation.
- Levels greater than 30 mU/litre of TSH must be shown to be certain that a potentially functioning tumour is not missed.
- ¹³¹I is the optimal isotope for demonstrating small amounts of residual tissue.
- At the time of the first scan after surgery, it is not possible to distinguish normal from malignant thyroid tissue.
- After a therapeutic dose of ¹³¹I, any residual uptake after more than six months is likely to represent residual cancer.

## CLINICAL APPLICATIONS

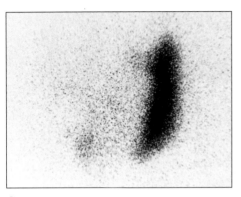
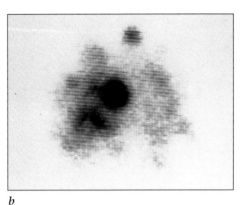

*a*                                    *b*

• **Replacement rather than displacement is a feature of thyroid cancer.**

• **Thyroid tumours do not take up tracer until after ablation of the thyroid gland, when the TSH has risen.**

• **Microscopic lung metastases are often seen with ¹³¹I when the chest x-ray is clear; they will respond well to ¹³¹I therapy.**

*Fig. 2.70*

*A patient with a history of having received external radiotherapy some 20 years earlier who presented with a right-sided thyroid mass. The thyroid scan (a) shows the typical features of cancer: non-function and replacement rather than displacement of normal tissue. A histological examination revealed a follicular carcinoma, and a total thyroidectomy was performed. The ¹³¹I scan performed 4 weeks postoperatively (b) showed some residual functioning thyroid cancer in the surgical bed and wide-spread lung metastases, at a time when the chest x-ray was normal.*

## Whole-body radioiodine (¹³¹I) scan

Whole-body scans using ¹³¹I are undertaken to assess residual thyroid cancer and metastases. The normal sites of radioiodine uptake, however, need to be known so that a correct interpretation can be made.

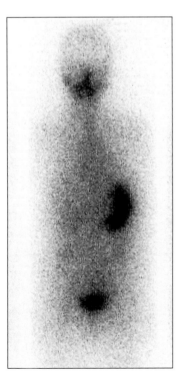
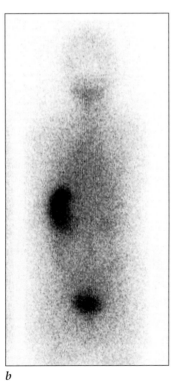

*a*                    *b*

*Fig. 2.71*

*(a,b) Normal whole-body scan in a patient following total thyroidectomy for papillary carcinoma of the thyroid. The normal biodistribution of iodine in the salivary glands, stomach and bladder can be seen.*

## CLINICAL APPLICATIONS

*Whole-body scans showing resolution of metastases*

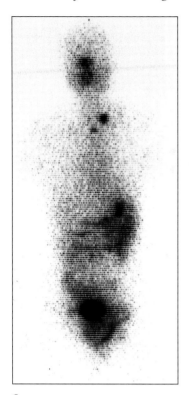

a                                    b

### Fig. 2.72

*(a) An anterior view of a patient scanned 72 hours after an oral dose of [131]I. Apart from the normal sites of uptake, tracer is seen in the tumour in the surgical bed. (b) A repeat scan obtained 6 months later following a therapeutic dose of [131]I to destroy the tumour. This is now a normal scan.*

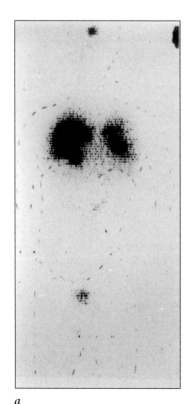
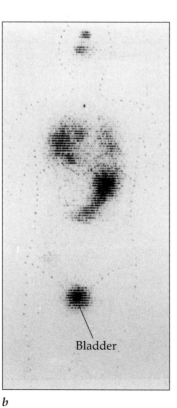

Bladder

a                           b                           c

### Fig. 2.73

*A follicular carcinoma of the thyroid in a patient with metastases to lung and skull, as shown on the first whole-body [131]I scan (a). The patient was treated on two occasions with [131]I, and the follow-up scans (b) and (c) obtained 6 months after each [131]I therapy show progressive resolution of the metastases.*

## CLINICAL APPLICATIONS

*Post-therapy ¹³¹I whole-body scan*

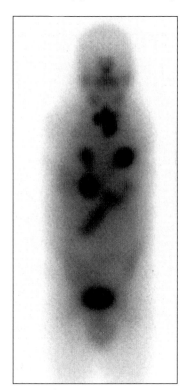 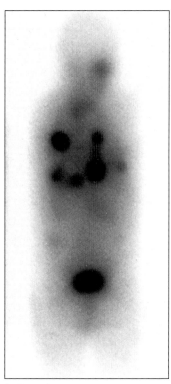

*a Anterior*          *b Posterior*

***Fig. 2.74***

*(a,b) Post-therapy whole-body ¹³¹I scan in a patient with recurrent follicular carcinoma. Images show multiple tumour sites in the neck and lung fields.*

*Discrepancy between scanning and therapeutic dose of radioiodine*

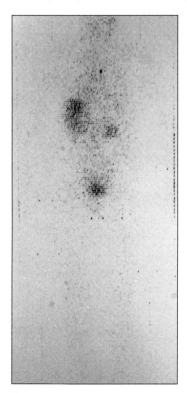 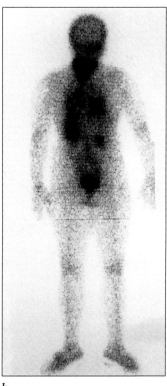

*a*          *b*

***Fig. 2.75***

*(a) A posterior view of a patient with a follicular carcinoma. Lung metastases were not detected, but a repeat scan (b) after a 150 mCi (5550 MBq) therapeutic dose of radioiodine clearly shows functioning lung metastases. This is unusual, but illustrates that when there is doubt about metastases a repeat scan after the therapeutic dose is worthwhile.*

**CLINICAL APPLICATIONS**

*$^{201}$Tl uptake in thyroid cancer*

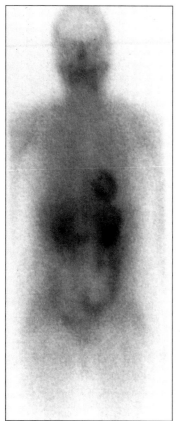

*a Anterior*

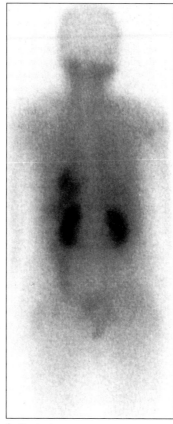

*b Posterior*

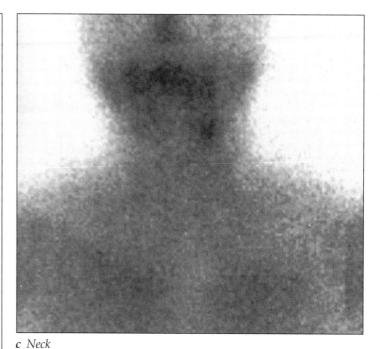

*c Neck*

**Fig. 2.76**

*(a–c) Whole body $^{201}$Tl scan with local view demonstrating $^{201}$Tl uptake in the left side of the neck at the site of a nodule. The scan shows normal distribution of $^{201}$Tl in the rest of the body.*

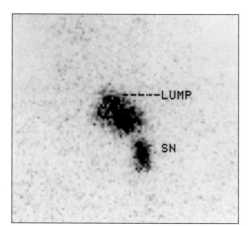

**Fig. 2.77**

*A scan showing the anterior neck and chest view 30 minutes after the injection of $^{201}$Tl. There is a marker on the suprasternal notch. The patient had a total thyroidectomy for papillary thyroid cancer and was on thyroxine. The positive $^{201}$Tl uptake indicated local recurrence which was confirmed histologically.*

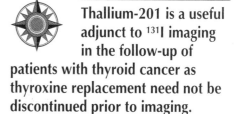

**Thallium-201 is a useful adjunct to $^{131}$I imaging in the follow-up of patients with thyroid cancer as thyroxine replacement need not be discontinued prior to imaging.**

## Medullary carcinoma of the thyroid (MTC)

### $^{99m}Tc$ scan appearance in MTC

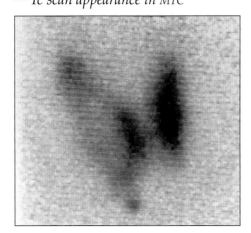

**Fig. 2.78**

*Thyroid scan from a 68-year-old man who presented with bone metastases and was subsequently found to have a thyroid nodule in the right lobe. This was found to be MTC at operation.*

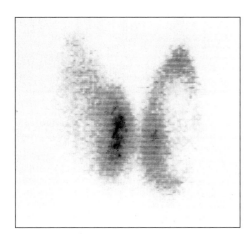

**Fig. 2.79**

*A thyroid scan from the daughter of the patient in Fig. 2.78, discovered on routine screening of the family. She was found to have a multinodular goitre on palpation, and the scan confirmed this. Note that the scan appearances indicate dominant 'cold' nodules in each lobe. A thyroidectomy was performed which confirmed medullary carcinoma.*

- **Large, dominant 'cold' nodules in a multinodular gland may be malignant.**
- **Medullary carcinoma may be familial.**
- **Medullary carcinoma of the thyroid may be bilateral, and multifocal.**

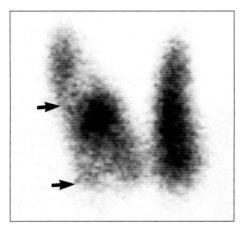

**Fig. 2.80**

*Thyroid scan from a 64-year-old woman who presented with a mass in the right side of the thyroid, showing two areas of reduced uptake (arrows) which were found to be MTC at surgery.*

## CLINICAL APPLICATIONS

$^{99m}Tc(V)$ DMSA *appearances in* MTC

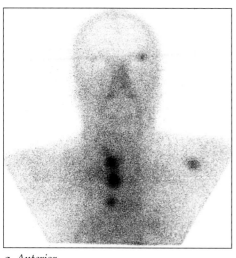
*a* Anterior

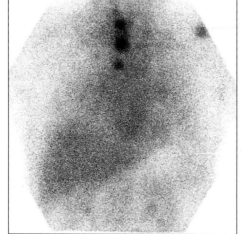
*b* Anterior

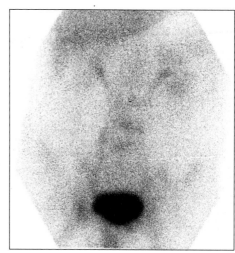
*c* Anterior

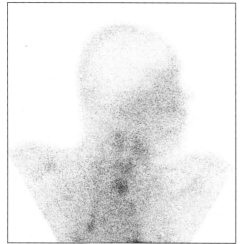
*d* Posterior

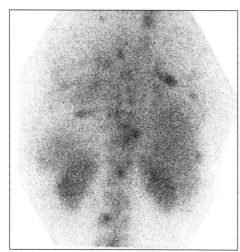
*e* Posterior

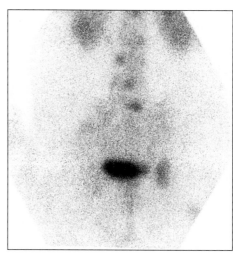
*f* Posterior

**Fig. 2.81**

$^{99m}Tc(V)$ DMSA *scan in a 54-year-old man with a past history of surgery to the thyroid for* MTC *who presented with neck masses and bone pain. There are focal areas of abnormality in the right side of the neck (a–c) and throughout the skeleton (d–f).*

$^{99m}Tc(V)$ DMSA **is a cheap, available radiopharmaceutical for investigating patients with** MTC.

### $^{131}I$ MIBG appearances in MTC

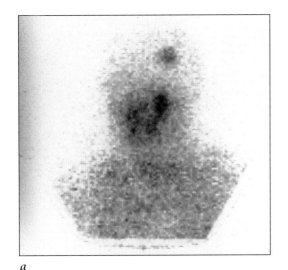

a

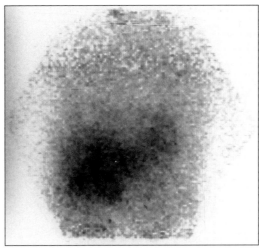

b

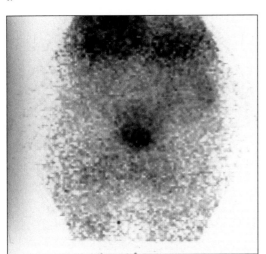

c

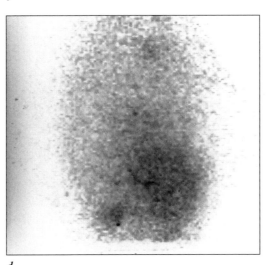

d

**Fig. 2.82**

$^{131}I$ MIBG scan from a 64-year-old man with MIBG uptake in **(a)** skull metastases, **(c)** left iliac crest and **(d)** right paralumbar region. **(b)** No uptake was seen in the chest. The patient was subsequently treated with a therapeutic dose of $^{131}I$ MIBG with a good palliative response.

**Due to the low sensitivity of MIBG imaging in patients with MTC (about 30%), MIBG imaging should only be used to assess its potential for therapy in patients with known recurrent disease.**

# 2.4.2 Clinical indications for adrenal scanning

## Investigation of Cushing's syndrome

*Table 2.11 Scan appearances in Cushing's syndrome*

| Cause | Scan appearance |
|---|---|
| Bilateral hyperplasia (caused by pituitary adenoma or ectopic ACTH) | Bilateral increased uptake |
| Adenoma | Unilateral uptake with suppression of the contralateral side |
| Carcinoma | Variable, depending on the metabolic activity of the tumour. Most often there is no uptake, but there may be faint or even high uptake. There is suppression of the contralateral side |

## Adrenal hyperplasia

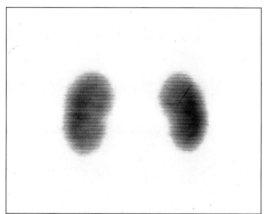

*a* DMSA

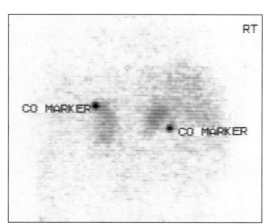

*b* DMSA *with markers*

### Fig. 2.83

*(a,b)* DMSA *scan acquired initially to identify upper poles of kidneys.* [75]Se *selenocholesterol images acquired at (c) 7 and (d) 9 days post-injection confirm bilateral symmetrical uptake in the adrenal glands consistent with adrenal hyperplasia.*

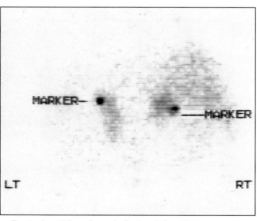

*c Posterior,* [75]Se *selenocholesterol day 7*

*d Posterior,* [75]Se *selenocholesterol day 9*

## CLINICAL APPLICATIONS

## Adrenal adenoma

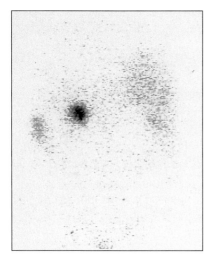

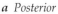

*a* Posterior

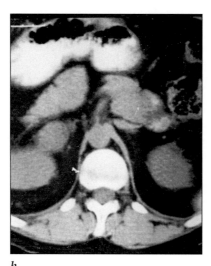

*b*

### Fig. 2.84

*(a) View of abdomen 3 days after injection of $^{75}$Se selenocholesterol. (b) CT scan of abdomen.*

*The selenocholesterol scan shows increased tracer uptake in the left adrenal. The CT scan shows the left-sided adrenal adenoma. Note that there is suppression of the right adrenal because of autonomous production of cortisol from the adenoma.*

## Adrenal carcinoma

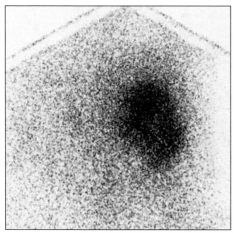

Posterior

### Fig. 2.85

*View of abdomen 4 days after iv injection of $^{75}$Se selenocholesterol. The adrenal scan shows high uptake into a right-sided, large, irregular mass. There is suppression of the normal left adrenal, which is not visualized. Scan appearances were due to an adrenal carcinoma.*

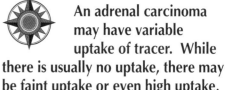

**An adrenal carcinoma may have variable uptake of tracer. While there is usually no uptake, there may be faint uptake or even high uptake, as in the case shown in Fig. 2.85.**

## Investigation of Conn's syndrome (hyperaldosteronism)

*Table 2.12 Scan appearances in Conn's syndrome*

| Cause | Scan appearance |
|---|---|
| Adenoma | (a) Asymmetric early tracer uptake without dexamethasone suppression |
| | (b) Unilateral uptake with dexamethasone suppression of the contralateral gland |
| Bilateral hyperplasia | Bilateral early uptake with and without dexamethasone suppression |

## *Adrenal adenoma*

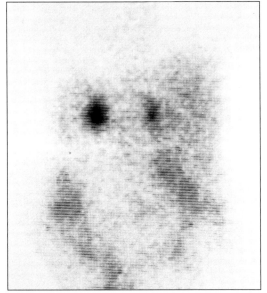

*a Posterior*

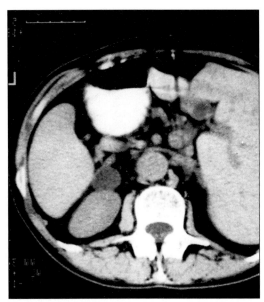

*b*

**Fig. 2.86**

*(a) View of abdomen 3 days after injection of [75]Se selenocholesterol. (b) CT scan of abdomen.*

*The patient was a 60-year-old woman who presented with hypertension and hypokalaemia, and was subsequently found to have a Conn's tumour. The adrenal scan shows increased uptake of tracer into the left adrenal gland. Note that the normal right adrenal is clearly visualized. The CT scan confirms the left adrenal tumour.*

• The typical scan appearance in Conn's syndrome is one adrenal gland showing moderately increased tracer uptake, the other being normal.
• The CT scan may be less helpful in Conn's syndrome than with other adrenal tumours, since the adenoma is often small (less than 2 cm).

## CLINICAL APPLICATIONS

### Dexamethasone suppression test

Dexamethasone is a potent synthetic glucocorticoid which normally causes adrenal suppression. Because of the low dosage used, it does not significantly interfere with steroid measurements in the blood or urine and is therefore used to help establish the cause of Cushing's syndrome. In the context of Conn's syndrome, one expects to visualize both adrenals but, if dexamethasone is given, an autonomously functioning adenoma will still be visualized but there will be suppression of the normal contralateral gland. When bilateral hyperplasia is present, both glands will still be visualized with low doses of dexamethasone, although there may be suppression when higher doses are used.

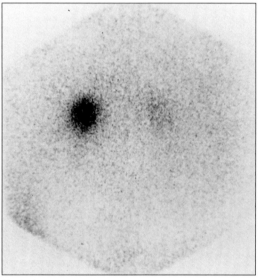

Posterior

**Fig. 2.87**

*View of abdomen 5 days after injection of $^{75}$Se selenocholesterol (while receiving dexamethasone).*

*In this case of Conn's syndrome there is unilateral left-sided uptake into the tumour. There is very poor tracer uptake into the normal right adrenal gland, because of dexamethasone suppression. (Courtesy of Dr K Britton, London, UK.)*

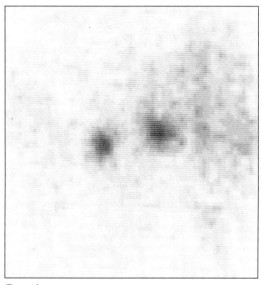

Posterior

**Fig. 2.88**

*View of abdomen 4 days after injection of dexamethasone.*

*The common cause of Conn's syndrome is a benign adrenal adenoma. However, on occasion, hyperaldosteronism may be due to bilateral hyperplasia. In this case, bilateral adrenal uptake of tracer is seen during a dexamethasone suppression test.*

## Investigation of phaeochromocytoma

While phaeochromocytomas are usually intra-adrenal (80%), and unilateral (90%), it is nevertheless important to detect those at extramedullary sites, which may occur anywhere from the base of the skull to the bladder. Ten per cent of tumours are malignant, and metastases may take up $^{131}$I MIBG.

*Preoperative*

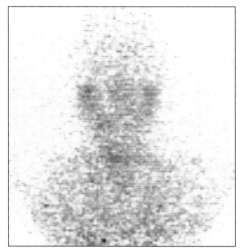

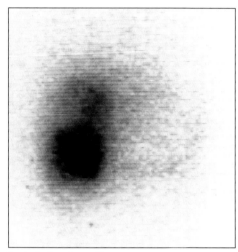

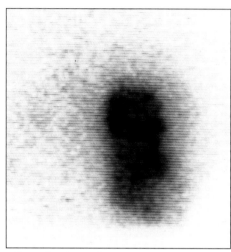

*a Anterior, 0 months*        *b Anterior, 0 months*        *c Posterior, 0 months*

*Postoperative*

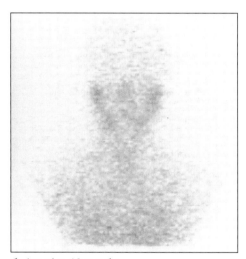

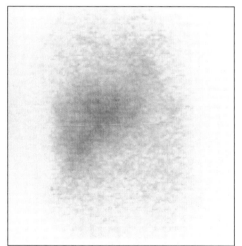

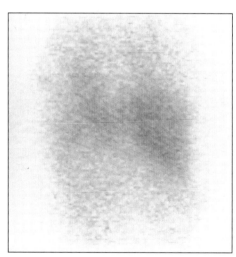

*d Anterior, 18 months*       *e Anterior, 18 months*       *f Posterior, 18 months*

**Fig. 2.89**

*(a–f)* $^{131}$I MIBG *scan in a 41-year-old woman with symptoms of phaeochromocytoma and raised urinary VMA levels.*

*There is intense tracer uptake **(b,c)** in the region of the right adrenal gland. At surgery, a large mass was removed which had invaded the kidney. A follow-up study was performed at 18 months **(d–f)** at which no abnormal uptake was seen and the VMA level was normal.*

## CLINICAL APPLICATIONS

### Malignant phaeochromocytoma

Malignant phaeochromocytomas are rare but, when they metastasize, the deposits will usually accumulate MIBG in the same way as the primary or benign phaeochromocytomas (see page 163). Apart from identifying the sites of spread of the tumour, the scan permits an assessment of the potential for treating these tumours with therapeutic doses of $^{131}$I MIBG.

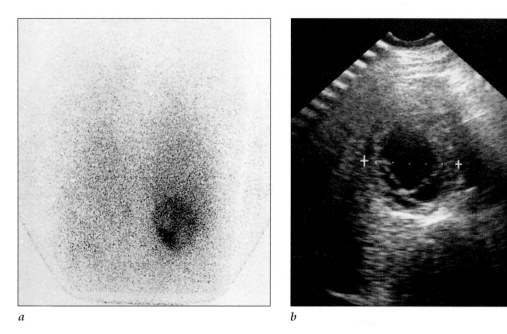

a                                        b

**Fig. 2.90**

*A 73-year-old woman who presented with high blood pressure and anxiety attacks. Serum noradrenaline levels were grossly elevated and the $^{123}$I MIBG scan (a) shows uptake in the region of the right adrenal gland. The uptake is non-homogeneous and the ultrasound (b) identifies a septated lesions. A malignant phaeochromocytoma was removed at surgery.*

## 2.4.3  Clinical indications for parathyroid scanning

### *Parathyroid adenoma*

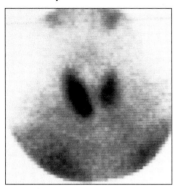 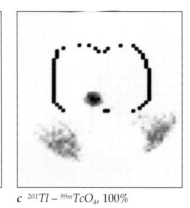 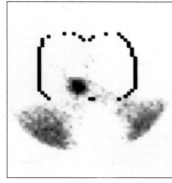

*a* $^{201}Tl$      *b* $^{99m}TcO_4$      *c* $^{201}Tl - {}^{99m}TcO_4$, 100%      *d* $^{201}Tl - {}^{99m}TcO_4$, 80%

**Fig. 2.91**

*(a) $^{201}Tl$ image. (b) $^{99m}TcO_4$ image. (c) Subtraction image, 100%. (d) Subtraction image, 80%.*
   *The patient was a 70-year-old man with primary hyperparathyroidism. Subtraction identifies the discrete focus of $^{201}Tl$ avidity at this site, indicating parathyroid adenoma. This finding was confirmed at surgery.*

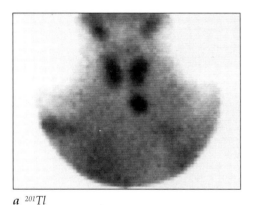 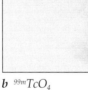 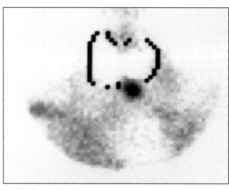

*a* $^{201}Tl$      *b* $^{99m}TcO_4$      *c* $^{201}Tl - {}^{99m}TcO_4$

**Fig. 2.92**

*(a) $^{201}Tl$ image. (b) $^{99m}TcO_4$ image. (c) Subtraction image.*
   *The patient was a 59-year-old woman with primary hyperparathyroidism. There is a single moderately enlarged area present below the lower pole of the left lobe of the thyroid gland which shows uptake of $^{201}Tl$ but without corresponding uptake of $^{99m}TcO_4$. The scan findings are those of parathyroid adenoma at the left lower lobe of the thyroid. This finding was confirmed at surgery.*

- **The majority of parathyroid adenomas are associated with the lower aspect of the thyroid lobes.**
- **The majority of parathyroid adenomas will be apparent from subjective evaluation of the $^{201}Tl$ and $^{99m}TcO_4$ images.**
- **Combined $^{201}Tl/^{99m}TcO_4$ imaging has approximately 70% sensitivity for a parathyroid adenoma.**

## Multiple parathyroid adenomas

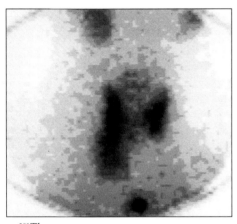 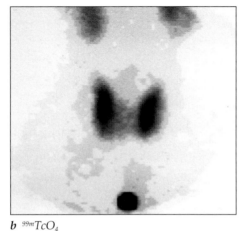 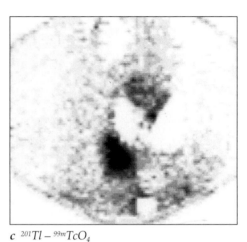

*a* $^{201}Tl$                    *b* $^{99m}TcO_4$                    *c* $^{201}Tl - {}^{99m}TcO_4$

**Fig. 2.93**

*(a)* $^{201}Tl$ *image.* *(b)* $^{99m}TcO_4$ *image.* *(c)* *Subtraction image.*

*This study from a patient with primary hyperparathyroidism shows a clear focus of increased tracer uptake at the lower aspect of the right lobe of the thyroid but with a further focus at the upper pole. At surgery, two parathyroid adenomas were found. This is an extremely uncommon finding.*

## Parathyroid carcinoma

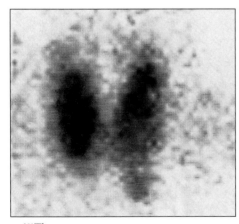 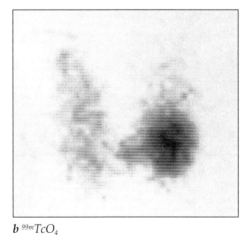 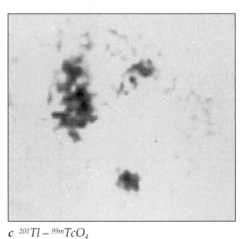

*a* $^{201}Tl$                    *b* $^{99m}TcO_4$                    *c* $^{201}Tl - {}^{99m}TcO_4$

**Fig. 2.94**

*(a)* $^{201}Tl$ *image.* *(b)* $^{99m}TcO_4$ *image.* *(c)* *Subtraction image.*

*In this case the thyroid pertechnetate scan appearances suggest an autonomously functioning nodule at the lower pole of the left lobe of the thyroid, with suppression of the remainder of normal thyroid tissue. However, it is apparent that on the $^{201}Tl$ scan there is a focus of increased tracer uptake at the lower pole of the left lobe of the thyroid, which is confirmed on the subtraction image. There is some further mismatch over the thyroid area, but this is misleading in the presence of an autonomously functioning thyroid nodule. At surgery, parathyroid carcinoma was found, corresponding to the focus at the lower aspect of the left lobe of the thyroid.*

 **The majority of para-thyroid carcinomas are functional, but non-functioning tumours may occasionally be found.**

## CLINICAL APPLICATIONS

# *Secondary hyperparathyroidism*

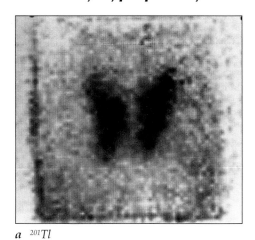

*a* $^{201}Tl$

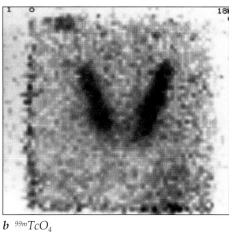

*b* $^{99m}TcO_4$

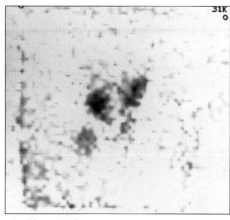

*c* $^{201}Tl - ^{99m}TcO_4$

**Fig. 2.95**

*(a) $^{201}Tl$ image. (b) $^{99m}TcO_4$ image. (c) Subtraction image.*

*This patient had chronic renal failure with severe secondary hyperparathyroidism and bone disease. Combined $^{201}Tl/^{99m}TcO_4$ parathyroid imaging revealed three large, discrete foci of activity in the right upper, lower and left upper poles of the thyroid. Further, there is a probable fourth small focus of activity at the lower pole of the left lobe of the thyroid. The scan findings were due to severe parathyroid hyperplasia.*

**In the more typical cases of secondary hyperparathyroidism approximately 50% of hyperplastic glands will not be visualized. The case illustrated in Fig. 2.95 is unusual, and scanning seldom reveals such striking changes.**

## *Problems in parathyroid localization*

The main difficulty associated with parathyroid imaging occurs when there is an associated thyroid problem. The following cases illustrate some of these difficulties.

### *Thyroid nodule*

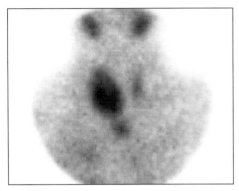 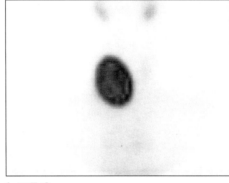 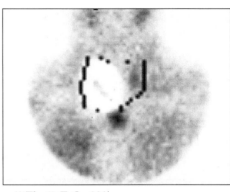

*a* $^{201}Tl$        *b* $^{99m}TcO_4$        *c* $^{201}Tl - {}^{99m}TcO_4$, 80%

**Fig. 2.96**

*(a)* $^{201}Tl$ *image.* *(b)* $^{99m}TcO_4$ *image.* *(c) Subtraction image.*

   *This study shows an autonomous nodule in the right lobe of the thyroid with suppression of the left lobe seen on the $^{99m}Tc$ scan* ***(b)***. *The subtraction scan* ***(c)*** *shows two areas of* $^{201}Tl$ *uptake: one at the lower pole of the right lobe at the site of the parathyroid adenoma, and one in the region of the suppressed left thyroid lobe.*

 **False positive parathyroid scans may be obtained when the thyroid contains a non-functioning or autonomously functioning nodule.**

### *Multinodular goitre*

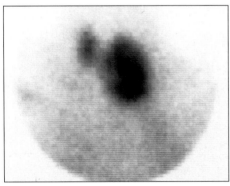 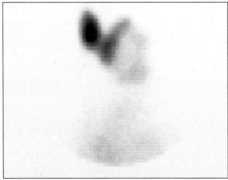 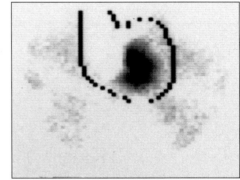

*a* $^{201}Tl$        *b* $^{99m}TcO_4$        *c* $^{201}Tl - {}^{99m}TcO_4$, 80%

**Fig. 2.97**

*(a)* $^{201}Tl$ *image.* *(b)* $^{99m}TcO_4$ *image.* *(c) Subtraction image.*

   *The $^{99m}TcO_4$ scan shows a multinodular gland with more marked enlargement of the left lobe of the thyroid than the right. There is some mismatching between $^{201}Tl$ and $^{99m}TcO_4$, with a large area of $^{201}Tl$ uptake in the lower pole of the left lobe* ***(c)*** *not matched by similar $^{99m}TcO_4$ uptake. The scan findings are due to a large multinodular goitre. An adenoma would have to be massive to account for these changes, and this is extremely unlikely.*

 **Extreme caution must be exercised when interpreting a parathyroid study in the presence of thyroid disease. When extensive multinodular change is present, the study may be uninterpretable, as illustrated by the cases in Fig. 2.97.**

# CHAPTER 3

# RENAL

Renal imaging with technetium-99m ($^{99m}$Tc) labelled isotopes is widely performed and provides both anatomical and functional information relating to the urinary tract. However, the great strength of these studies, as is so often the case in nuclear medicine, is the functional data that is generated, since anatomical definition cannot approach the fine detail obtained with radiographic and ultrasonic investigations. In general, two types of investigation are commonly performed: static and dynamic imaging.

## Static imaging

Renal images are usually obtained some 3 hours following intravenous injection of $^{99m}$Tc dimercaptosuccinic acid (DMSA). DMSA is taken up by the proximal tubules and fixed there. Since rapid loss of tracer does not occur, several views of the kidneys can be obtained. This is of particular relevance in paediatrics, where it may be important to identify sites of cortical scarring (eg in children with recurrent urinary tract infection or reflux), which, on occasion, are best seen on the oblique views. The static renal images obtained provide good definition of the cortical outline and, in addition, show the relative distribution of functional tissue. The ratio of tracer uptake between kidneys provides a measure of divided renal function. By selecting regions of interest within an individual kidney, it is also possible to measure the relative function at these sites; this may be of particular relevance when a duplex system is present.

## Dynamic imaging

Dynamic imaging is performed most often with $^{99m}$Tc diethylenetriamine pentaacetic acid (DTPA), which is a true chelate and is excreted by the kidney purely by glomerular filtration. In contrast to DMSA, the tracer is rapidly excreted, and thus rapid sequential renal imaging must be performed. The images that are obtained provide information relating to renal vascularity, renal function and excretion. Following an intravenous bolus of $^{99m}$Tc DTPA, an image is obtained for the first 30 seconds which provides a 'vascular image', with the major blood vessels and perfusion to both kidneys, liver and spleen being visualized. The amount of activity at each site reflects the relative vascularity. Renal function is assessed at 2 minutes after injection, when there is good renal visualization and an image will show the relative distribution of function between the kidneys. Thereafter, cortical activity rapidly diminishes as the tracer is excreted by glomerular filtration. By 5 minutes, activity is normally seen in the collecting systems, and serial images are obtained up to 30 minutes which show progressive excretion of tracer. If there is any suggestion of obstruction, it is important to mobilize the patient and obtain a subsequent image to ensure that there is no functional hold-up caused by patient positioning. If the question of obstruction has not been resolved, the study will need to be extended and further images obtained following diuretic administration. $^{99m}$Tc MAG3 is now becoming widely used as an alternative dynamic renal imaging agent. The extraction efficiency of MAG3 is 2.5 times that of DTPA, leading to better image quality with a lower absorbed radiation dose.

## CHAPTER CONTENTS

# 3.1 ANATOMY/PHYSIOLOGY

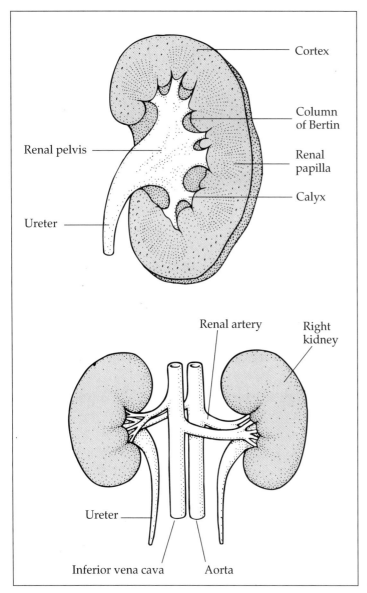

**Fig. 3.1**

*Anatomy of the kidney.*

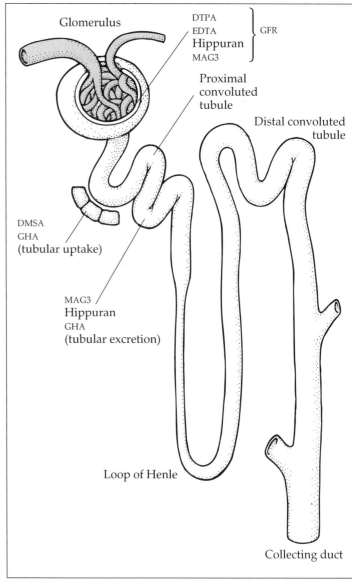

**Fig. 3.2**

*Renal physiology.*

# 3.2  RADIOPHARMACEUTICALS

*Table 3.1  Radionuclides in renal disease*

| Method | Radiopharmaceutical | Site of excretion | Function measured |
|---|---|---|---|
| Glomerular filtration rate (GFR) Effective renal plasma flow (ERPF) | $^{51}$Cr ethylenediaminetetraacetic acid (EDTA) $^{125}$I iothalamate $^{131}$I/$^{125}$I hippuran | Glomerular filtration  Glomerular filtration and tubular excretion | Total renal function and plasma flow |
| Static imaging | $^{99m}$Tc DMSA $^{99m}$Tc glucoheptonate (GHA) | Proximal tubular accumulation 10–20% excretion | Divided renal function Distribution of intrarenal function Ectopic sites of renal tissue |
| Dynamic imaging | $^{99m}$Tc DTPA $^{123}$I hippuran $^{99m}$Tc MAG3 | Glomerular filtration Glomerular filtration and tubular excretion | Renal perfusion Total renal function Divided renal function Outflow tract damage |
| Radionuclide cystogram | $^{99m}$Tc DTPA | Glomerular filtration | Vesicoureteric reflux Residual urine volume |

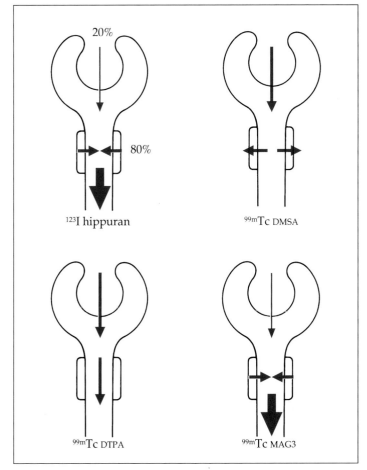

### Fig. 3.3

*Mechanisms of radiopharmaceutical clearance.*

# 3.3 NORMAL SCANS WITH VARIANTS AND ARTEFACTS

## 3.3.1 Normal static $^{99m}$Tc DMSA images

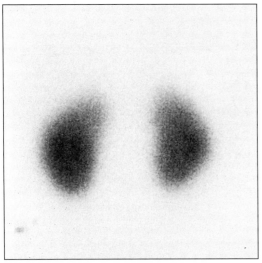

*a* Posterior

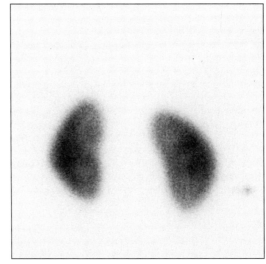

*b* Anterior

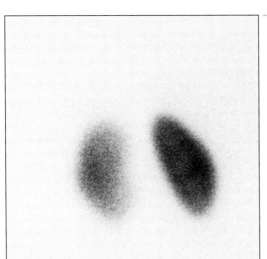

*c* Right posterior oblique

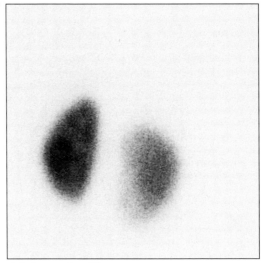

*d* Left posterior oblique

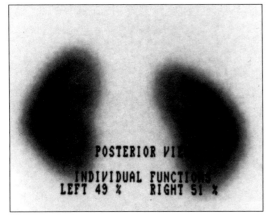

*e* Quantitation

*Fig. 3.4*

*(a–d)* Normal static $^{99m}$Tc DMSA analogue images obtained 3 hours after injection. *(e)* Quantitation image. As the radionuclide is taken up in the proximal tubules, the images represent functioning cortical tissue.

Occasionally more detail can be identified in the renal parenchyma.

When divided renal function is required, anterior and posterior views are adequate. However, if areas of cortical scarring are to be identified, eg in children with recurrent urinary tract infection or reflux, then oblique views are necessary to provide good definition of cortical outline.

## 3.3.2 Quantitation of DMSA study

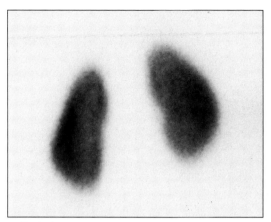

*a Posterior*

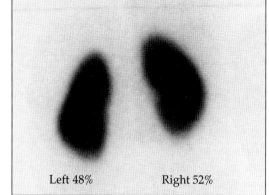

Left 48%   Right 52%

*b Posterior*

Fig. 3.5

*Quantitation study on a normal static ⁹⁹ᵐTc DMSA renal scan. (a) Posterior view. (b) Relative kidney contribution to renal function.*

• Approximately 60% of injected DMSA is taken up by the kidneys, but it should be remembered that 10–15% is excreted. If the bladder is not emptied before imaging and is included in the field of view, it will be clearly visualized. However, on occasion, when the kidney is damaged, there may be increased excretion of DMSA with bladder visualization.

• Percentage of divided function should be calculated from anterior and posterior images using the geometric mean.

## 3.3.3 Normal SPECT DMSA scans

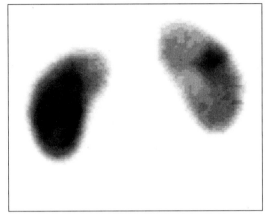

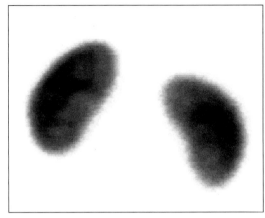
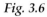

*Fig. 3.6*

*(a,b)* DMSA *scan planar views.*

*a* Anterior

*b* Posterior

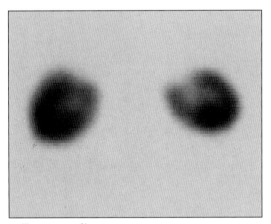
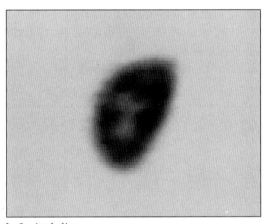

*Fig. 3.7*

*(a)* Transaxial, *(b)* sagittal and *(c)* coronal sections of normal DMSA scan.

*a* Transverse slice

*b* Sagittal slice

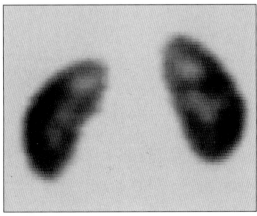

SPECT **imaging permits the visualization of smaller lesions and scars by visualizing the entire renal parenchyma with no overlying tissue.**

*c* Coronal slice

## 3.3.4   Normal DMSA variants

### *Duplex kidneys*

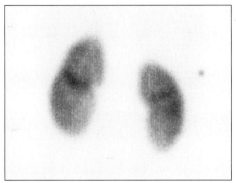

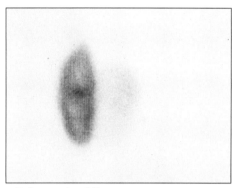

*a  Posterior*

*b  Anterior*

*c  Left posterior oblique*

***Fig. 3.8***

*(a–c)* DMSA *scan. The transverse bands seen on both kidneys, particularly on the left, identify a duplex collecting system.*

### *Uncomplicated horseshoe kidney*

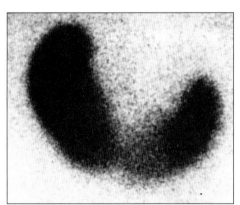

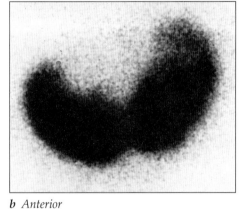

***Fig. 3.9***

*(a–d) Two typical examples of uncomplicated horseshoe kidney where fusion occurs between the lower poles. The connecting bridge may function normally or act as a fibrous bridge. The axes of the kidney will incline towards the midline.*

*a  Posterior*

*b  Anterior*

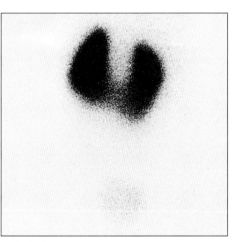

**Always image anteriorly as well as posteriorly to assess the function of the fused bridge adequately.**

*c  Posterior*

*d  Anterior*

## NORMAL SCANS WITH VARIANTS AND ARTEFACTS

### *Crossed renal ectopia*

The malrotated kidney is usually fused anteriorly to the lower pole of a kidney in the normal position.

*Case 1*

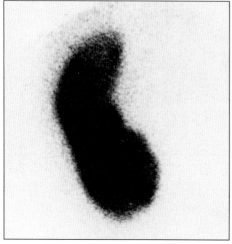

*a  Anterior*

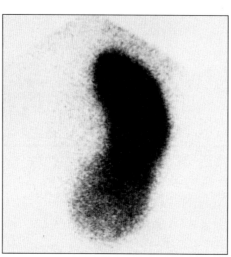

*b  Posterior*

*Case 2*

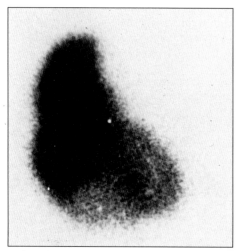

*c  Anterior*

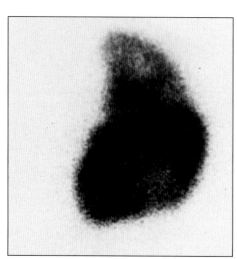

*d  Posterior*

**Fig. 3.10**

*(a, b) Case 1; (c, d) case 2: two DMSA scans of two patients showing the typical appearances of crossed renal ectopia. The anterior abdomen must always be imaged to assess the function of the ectopic kidney.*

## NORMAL SCANS WITH VARIANTS AND ARTEFACTS

## Complete failure of ascent (pancake kidney)

When there is no ascent from the original sacral position, the two kidneys are fused in the midline of the pelvis.

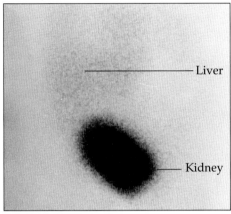

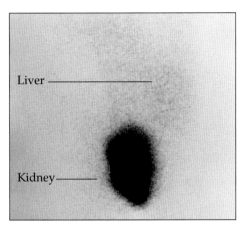

*a* Anterior

*b* Posterior

*Fig. 3.11*

*(a, b)* DMSA *scan. Pancake kidney.*

## Pelvic kidney

More frequently, one kidney only fails to ascend normally. This is often associated with decreased function and obstruction.

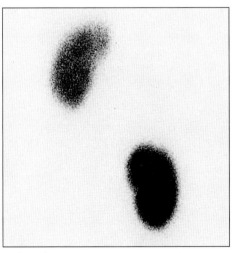

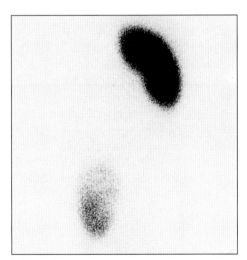

*a* Anterior

*b* Posterior

*Fig. 3.12*

*(a, b)* DMSA *scan. The right kidney is normal. The left kidney is lying in the pelvis.*

## 3.3.5 Normal dynamic ⁹⁹ᵐTc DTPA images

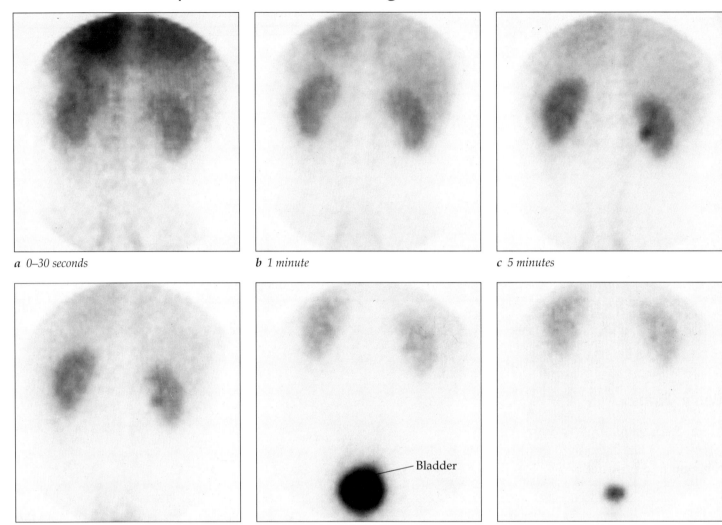

*a 0–30 seconds*  *b 1 minute*  *c 5 minutes*

*d 10 minutes*  *e 20 minutes*  *f Post-micturition*

**Fig. 3.13**

*Normal dynamic ⁹⁹ᵐTc DTPA renal scan images.* **(a)** *First 30 seconds (first pass), showing renal perfusion and vascular structures.* **(b)** *Image at 1 minute, showing the distribution of renal function, with uptake in each kidney reflecting the relative contribution to the total GFR.* **(c, d)** *Images at 5 and 10 minutes after injection, showing excretion into the collecting system. Note that the ureters are usually not seen.* **(e)** *Image 20 minutes after injection, showing the bladder. There should be little activity in the kidneys at this time.* **(f)** *Post-micturition image.*

## 3.3.6   Normal DTPA quantitation

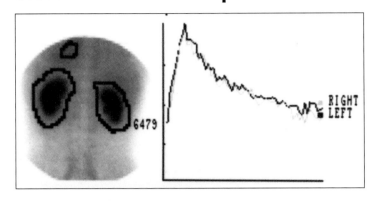

**Fig. 3.14**

*Time–activity (T/A) curve from normal DTPA renal scan. The renogram curve consists of several separate segments. The initial steep upward rise is the tracer appearance and represents renal blood flow. The more gradually rising second segment is the accumulation phase and reflects filtration of the tracer and entry into the renal tubules, with the point of maximum accumulation at the peak of the curve. The downward sloping segment is the excretory curve and reflects the loss of radioactivity as the tracer leaves the kidney to be excreted into the bladder. The individual GFR is measured from background-subtracted images of the kidneys between 80 and 180 seconds after injection. In this case differential GFR was equal.*

### Lasix washout

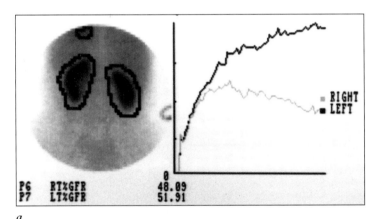

*a*

### Reflux study

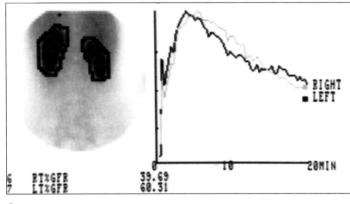

*a*

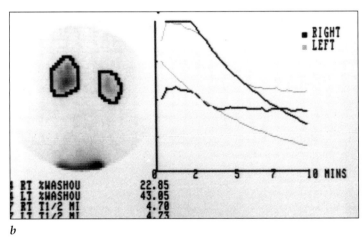

*b*

**Fig. 3.15**

**(a)** *A renogram showing abnormal phase three of curve due to dilatation of left-sided collecting system.* **(b)** *Following Lasix administration, good washout curves are obtained from both sides.*

*b*

**Fig. 3.16**

**(a, b)** *Following the initial phase of the study, the patient is asked to micturate and data acquisition is performed during micturation. Regions of interest are placed around the bladder and kidneys. The curve (1) demonstrates the high initial counts in the bladder area falling with micturition, but no rise is seen in the curves from the renal regions of interest (2, 3). This is a negative reflux study.*

# NORMAL SCANS WITH VARIANTS AND ARTEFACTS

## 3.3.7 Normal ⁹⁹ᵐTc MAG3 study

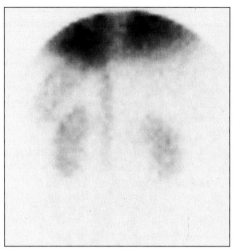

*a* 0–20 seconds

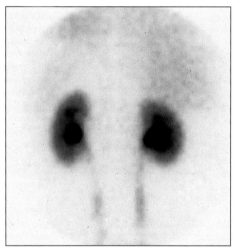
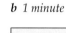

*c* 5 minutes

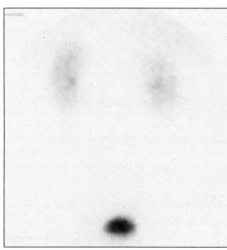

*e* Post-micturition

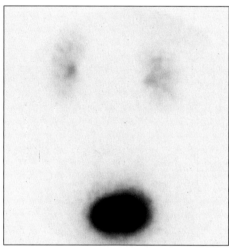

*b* 1 minute

*d* 20 minutes

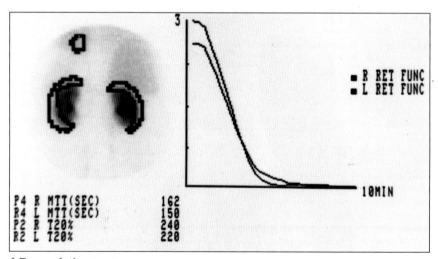

| | | |
|---|---|---|
| P4 R MTT(SEC) | | 162 |
| R4 L MTT(SEC) | | 150 |
| P2 R T20% | | 240 |
| R2 L T20% | | 220 |

*f* Deconvolution curve

**Fig. 3.17**

*(a–f) Normal dynamic ⁹⁹ᵐTc MAG3 study with symmetrical pattern of perfusion, uptake and excretion. Due to the higher extraction of ⁹⁹ᵐTc MAG3 (2.5 times that of DTPA), the activity levels passing through the kidneys are higher (for an equivalent administered dose) than for DTPA. Visualization of the ureters (c) is a normal feature on a ⁹⁹ᵐTc MAG3 study. (f) demonstrates the deconvolution curve from which the mean transit time for each kidney can be determined.*

# 3.3.8 Normal DTPA variants

## Extrarenal pelvis

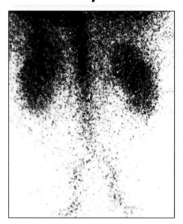 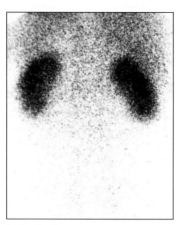 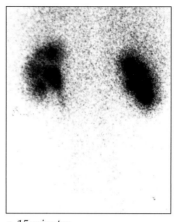 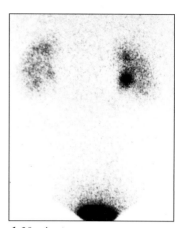

*a* 30 seconds     *b* 2 minutes     *c* 15 minutes     *d* 30 minutes

**Fig. 3.18**

*(a–d) In this example of a normal dynamic $^{99m}$Tc DTPA renal scan study activity is seen in the right renal pelvis (on the 30-minute image), reflecting an extrarenal pelvis, and there is also some pooling in the upper pole calyx. These are normal variants.*

## Renal nephroptosis

Positioning of a patient can affect the position of the kidney, as illustrated in Fig. 3.19.

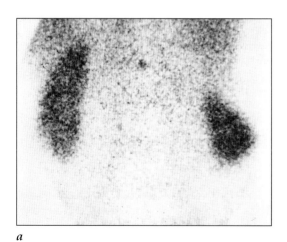 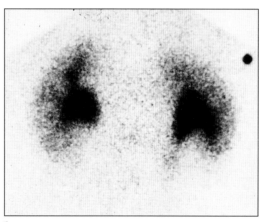

*a*     *b*

**Fig. 3.19**

*(a) 2-minute image, sitting.*
*(b) 20-minute image, lying.*

**Downward displacement of the kidney (nephroptosis) may cause significant errors of quantitation. Patients should be imaged in the supine position to reduce this source of error.**

## NORMAL SCANS WITH VARIANTS AND ARTEFACTS

## Delayed emptying of renal pelvis

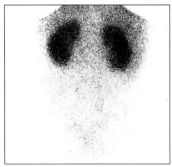

*a* 2 minutes

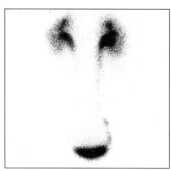

*b* 20 minutes

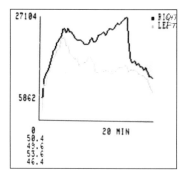

*c*

### Fig. 3.20

*(a,b)* A normal variant of a dynamic renal scan, showing progressive accumulation of tracer in the pelvis of the right kidney until the pelvis contracts and releases the tracer. The transient visualization of the ureter is not abnormal, but continuous visualization of the ureter indicates a dilated ureter. The T/A curve *(c)* clearly shows initial emptying of the pelvis followed by progressive filling before rapid emptying occurs.

## Increased urine flow rate

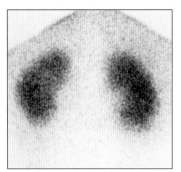

*a* 2 minutes

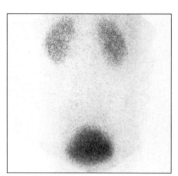

*b* 20 minutes

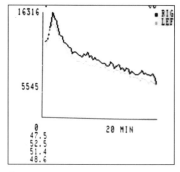

*c*

### Fig. 3.21

*(a,b)* Repeat study (of the same patient as in Fig. 3.20) with increased diuresis. *(c)* T/A curve, showing rapid continuous clearance and emptying of tracer from the collecting system. When a patient is given a diuretic before the $^{99m}$Tc DTPA injection, there is very rapid transit with no hold up at all, thus excluding obstruction.

The case in Figure 3.21 illustrates the marked differences that can occur simply as the result of physiological alterations, in this instance differences in urine flow.

## Crossed renal ectopia

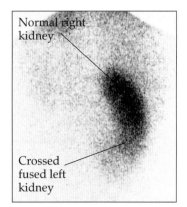

*a* 1–2 minutes

Normal right kidney

Crossed fused left kidney

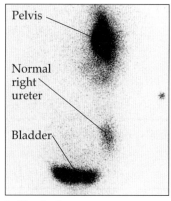

*b* 10 minutes

Pelvis

Normal right ureter

Bladder

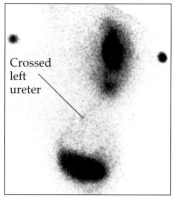

*c* 20 minutes

Crossed left ureter

### Fig. 3.22

*(a–c)* Crossed ectopia, dynamic study. A 30-year-old patient who was referred with right loin pain and had a previously diagnosed absent left kidney. Posterior view DTPA scan.

The DTPA scan shows the classic appearances of crossed renal ectopia, with both ureters inserting into the bladder normally, but crossing to the lower pole of the renal mass.

# 3.4 CLINICAL APPLICATIONS

The clinical applications of renal imaging are listed below, and examples of the various clinical problems are given on subsequent pages.

**3.4.1 Renal function**
Renal function in urinary tract infection
Renal tubular dysfunction
Renal function with calculi
Assessment of function after percutaneous renal stone removal

**3.4.2 Obstruction**
Indications for radionuclide scans
Appearance of obstruction: DMSA scan
Appearance of obstruction: DTPA scan
Assessment of obstruction
Renal scan with diuretic washout
DMSA scans in obstruction
Difficulties in assessing obstruction

**3.4.3 Reflux nephropathy**
Role of radionuclide studies in reflux nephropathy
Advantages of radionuclude studies over micturating cystography
Demonstration of cortical scarring
Renal scarring: DMSA and DTPA scans
Demonstration of reflux

**3.4.4 Trauma**
Bullet injuries to the kidney
Shrapnel injuries causing urinary leaks
Assessment of kidneys following abdominal trauma
Vascular study to assess trauma

**3.4.5 Renal failure**
Indications for renal scanning in acute renal failure
Diagnosis of pre-renal failure
Diagnosis of ATN
Monitoring changes in the anuric patient
Diagnosis of complications
Assessment of probable prognosis

**3.4.6 Space-occupying lesions**
Indications for radionuclide scans
Causes of space-occupying lesions
Pseudotumour
Tumour
Renal cyst
Renal calculus

**3.4.7 Congenital and ectopic abnormalities**
Congenital abnormalities
Reduplication
Cystic disease
Abnormalities of fusion
Abnormalities of ascent

**3.4.8 Vascular disorders and hypertension**
Indications for assessment of renal blood supply with radionuclides
Indications for investigation of hypertension with radionuclides
Renal artery stenosis (RAS)
Renal infarct
Preoperative assessment of aortic aneurysm
Follow-up after surgery or angioplasty
Functional assessment of angioplasty
Postoperative assessment

**3.4.9 Renal transplant**
Renal transplant complications
Normal renal transplant
Acute rejection
Chronic rejection
Two cases of cortical scarring in renal transplants demonstrated on DMSA scans
Transplant ATN
Vascular complications
Urinary complications
Biopsy complications

## CLINICAL APPLICATIONS

# 3.4.1 Renal function

Radionuclide renal imaging with quantitation provides the only non-invasive accurate method of measuring the contribution of an individual kidney to overall renal function. In addition, the technique can be used to assess the regional distribution of function within an individual kidney. For most purposes, a static imaging agent (DMSA) is the pharmaceutical of choice because:

- It closely reflects the total parenchymal function
- The distribution and uptake change only very slowly with time—unlike the dynamic agents (DTPA, MAG3)
- The background is low, with a very high target/background ratio
- Multiple views can be obtained
- Exact timing after injection is not critical.

## *Renal function in urinary tract infection*

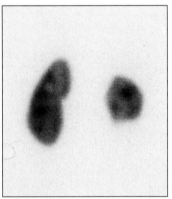 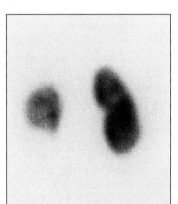 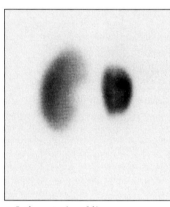

*a Posterior*  *b Anterior*  *c Left posterior oblique*

*Fig. 3.23*

*(a–c)* DMSA *scan in a 19-year-old woman with a history of recurrent urinary tract infections, showing a small irregular right kidney contributing only 29% to overall GFR.*

## *Renal tubular dysfunction*

*Poor DMSA uptake by kidneys*

 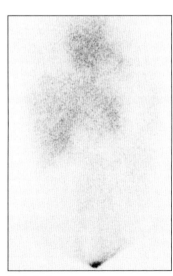

*a Posterior*  *b Anterior*

*Fig. 3.24*

*(a, b)* DMSA *scan. A 12-year-old girl with only mild renal impairment.*

*The scan shows almost no uptake into the kidneys, with tracer seen in blood pools of the liver, spleen and heart. In this case there is a clear discrepancy between the degree of renal impairment and the impairment of DMSA uptake. This is due to renal tubular dysfunction.*

 **In some cases of renal tubular dysfunction, such as renal tubular acidosis, there may be very poor uptake of DMSA by the kidneys** which may result, on rare occasions, in misleading information about renal function.

## CLINICAL APPLICATIONS

## *Renal function with calculi*

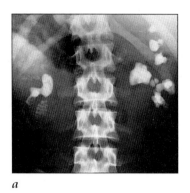

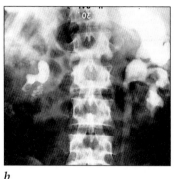

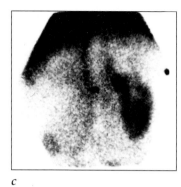

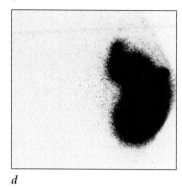

*a*  *b*  *c*  *d*

**Fig. 3.25**

*(a) Control film and (b) intravenous urogram (IVU) from a patient with renal stones. Divided renal function cannot be accurately assessed from the IVU, but can readily be obtained from the functional phase of the DTPA scan (c) or the DMSA scan (d). Both the scans show absent function on the left.*

**The IVU often gives unreliable information about renal function and the distribution of function within a kidney.**

## *Assessment of function after percutaneous renal stone removal*

### *Using DTPA*

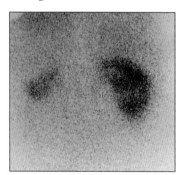

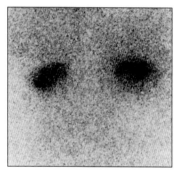

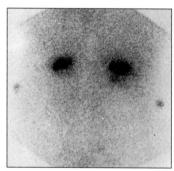

*a 2 minutes, before*  *b 20 minutes, before*  *c 2 minutes, after*  *d 20 minutes, after*

**Fig. 3.26**

*DTPA images (a, b) before and (c, d) after removal of a right-sided renal stone. The postoperative study shows loss of function of the lower half of the right kidney, attributable to vascular injury during attempted pyelolithotomy.*

### *Using DMSA*

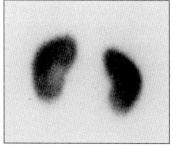

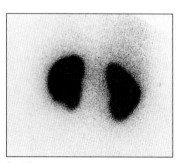

*a Before*  *b After*

**Fig. 3.27**

*The first DMSA scan (a) only shows the decreased function associated with the pelvic stone in the left kidney. The post-lithotomy scan (b) shows a focal loss of function at the lower pole which is due to damage by the track.*

## 3.4.2 Obstruction

### *Indications for radionuclide scans*

- Measurement of renal function in known obstruction
- Assessment of equivocal obstruction after IVU or ultrasound
- Baseline during a period of observation
- Preoperative evaluation
- Postoperative comparison.

### *Appearance of obstruction: DMSA scan*

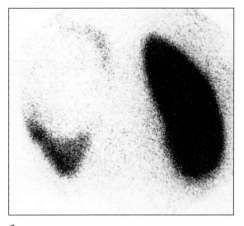

a

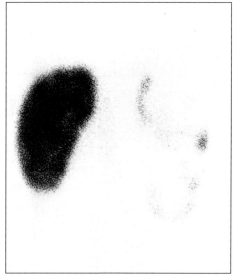

b

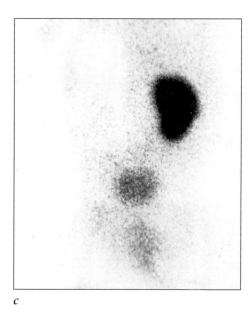

c

*Fig. 3.28*

*DMSA study. Three separate cases of obstruction showing the spectrum of significant renal impairment progressing to a non-functioning kidney. (**a**) Left-sided obstruction with one single photon-deficient area. (**b**) Obstruction of the right kidney with gross calyceal dilatation and some residual functioning tissue between the calyces. (**c**) Loss of function in the left kidney with a photon-deficient space representing the obstructed non-functioning kidney.*

- **When a kidney contributes less than 15% to the total renal function, there will usually be no improvement after relief of obstruction.**
- **Radionuclides are not used to investigate the site or cause of obstruction and should not be used to exclude obstruction as a cause of acute renal failure.**

## *Appearance of obstruction: DTPA scan*

### Pelviureteric junction obstruction

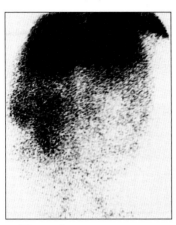 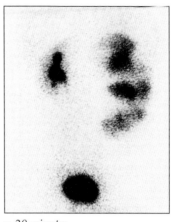 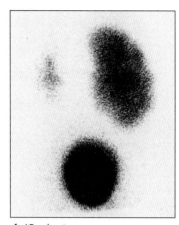

*a 30 seconds*   *b 2 minutes*   *c 20 minutes*   *d 45 minutes*

**Fig. 3.29**

DTPA *scan. A patient with right-sided pelviureteric junction (PUJ) obstruction. (a) 30-second image, showing normal renal blood flow on the left but no definite renal blood flow on the right. (b) 2-minute image, showing a rim of functioning tissue around the photon-deficient calyces. (c) 20-minute image, showing gradual filling of the calyces. (d) 45-minute image, showing that drainage is complete from the left side but a large volume system is full of tracer on the right.*

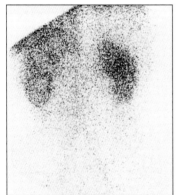 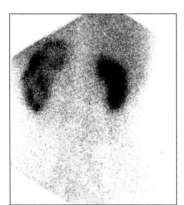 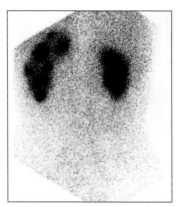 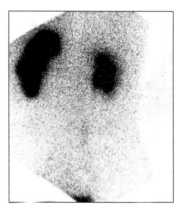

*a 30 seconds*   *b 2 minutes*   *c 15 minutes*   *d 30 minutes*

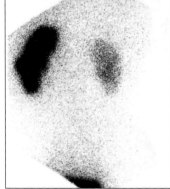

**Fig. 3.30**

*(a–e)* DTPA *study. A further case of* PUJ *obstruction.*

*The appearance of multiple hot spots in obstruction, as seen in the 15-minute image, is common before the collecting system is full, and is an indication of obstruction and slow transit, not of dilatation. Increasing the urine flow rate with diuretic will help to distinguish between obstruction and dilatation. In this case there is dilatation of the right collecting system, which clears following diuretic, but there is no change in the appearances of the left kidney, which is obstructed.*

*e 10 minutes, post-diuretic*

## CLINICAL APPLICATIONS

### Obstruction of the upper pole calyx

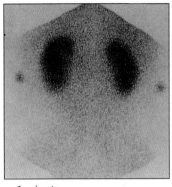
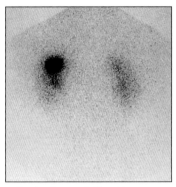
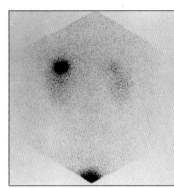

*a 1 minute*      *b 20 minutes*      *c 2 minutes, post-diuretic*      *d 10 minutes, post-diuretic*

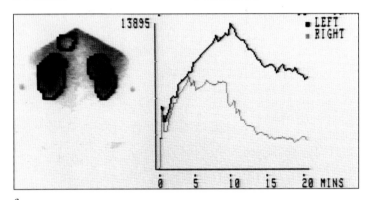

*e*

**Fig. 3.31**

**(a–d)** DTPA scan. **(e)** Renogram curve.

   This study shows dilatation of the left upper pole calyx which drains incompletely, even following diuretic administration. In this case there is obstruction of the upper pole calyx. Note that renogram curves do not indicate obstruction and can be misleading in cases such as this where there is focal pathology.

### Obstructed moiety of a duplex kidney

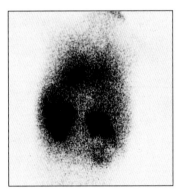
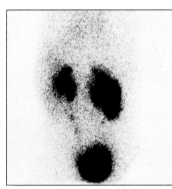
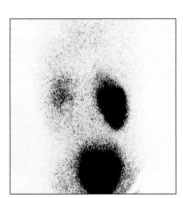

*a 2 minutes*      *b 10 minutes*      *c 30 minutes*      *d 10 minutes, post-diuretic*

**Fig. 3.32**

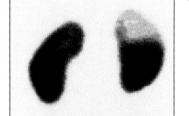

*e Posterior,* DMSA

DTPA *scans.* **(a)** *2-minute image, showing poor function of the lower moiety of the right duplex kidney.* **(b)** *10-minute image, showing some excretion into the obstructed lower moiety.* **(c)** *30-minute image, showing activity in the collecting system.* **(d)** *10 minutes after diuretic administration, showing washout of tracer from all except the obstructed lower moiety.* **(e)** DMSA *scan, showing the appearance of an obstructed upper moiety of a right duplex kidney.*

## CLINICAL APPLICATIONS

## Assessment of obstruction

As functional information is being generated with DTPA studies, measurements can provide the following information, which may be of value in the assessment of obstruction:

• Divided renal function
• Diuretic washout rates
• Deconvolution measurements for retention function and transit times.

### Divided renal function

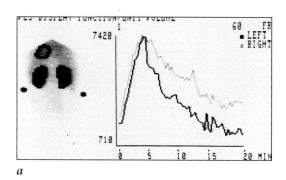

*a*

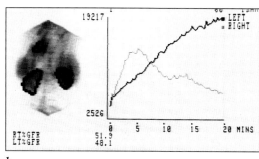

*b*

**Fig. 3.33**

**(a)** *Normal T/A curve compared with* **(b)** *T/A curve from a case of left-sided obstruction. Note the normal divided function in the obstructed kidney before significant damage has occurred.*

### Diuretic washout rate

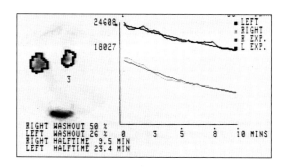

**Fig. 3.34**

*T/A curve from the obstructed case following administration of diuretic. Note the slow washout on the obstructed left side — only 26% is washed out, with a slow (23-minute) $T_{1/2}$.*

### Deconvolution studies

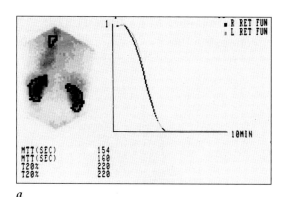

*a*

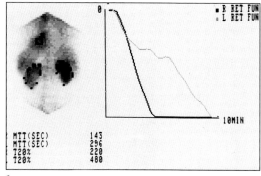

*b*

**Fig. 3.35**

**(a)** *Normal.* **(b)** *Abnormal. Note the delayed renal parenchymal transit time of the obstructed left kidney.*

## Renal scan with diuretic washout

### Dynamic DTPA

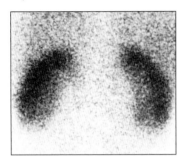

*a* 2 minutes

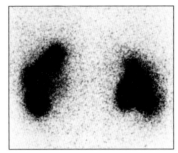

*b* 10 minutes

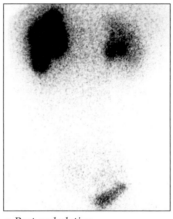

*c* Post-ambulation

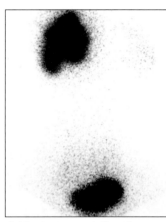

*d* 10 minutes, post-diuretic

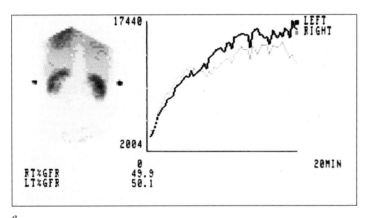

*e*

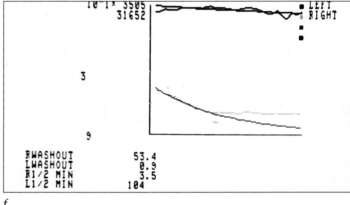

*f*

**Fig. 3.36**

*An 18-year-old woman who had a history of recurrent loin pain after drinking fluids. An IVU showed probable left-sided PUJ obstruction, and the questions that needed resolution were (1) the degree of obstruction, and (2) the degree of functional impairment secondary to the obstruction.*

*The 2-minute dynamic DTPA image (a) shows good selective uptake of tracer in both kidneys, with equal divided function. The 10-minute image (b) shows approximately equal dilatation of both collecting systems. Following bladder emptying and the effect of gravity (ambulation) (c), there is almost complete drainage from the right kidney, but none at all from the left. The image taken 10 minutes after diuretic administration (d) shows that there is no washout from the left side, but complete washout from the right. The T/A curve for 0–20 minutes (e) shows a steady rise in both renal areas. The GFR is equally divided between the two kidneys. The T/A curve following diuretic (f) shows that there is no washout from the left side, but the right side is normal.*

*This study therefore confirmed significant left-sided PUJ obstruction which, so far, had not led to any loss of renal function.*

- A fall in the T/A curve before 20 minutes virtually excludes obstruction, but a rising curve, while suggestive, does not prove the presence of obstruction.
- The effect of gravity in causing emptying of the collecting systems excludes obstruction, but failure to do so does not confirm the presence of obstruction.
- The combination of failure to drain following ambulation together with failure to washout with diuresis confirms PUJ obstruction.

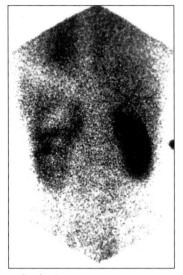

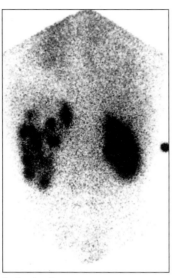

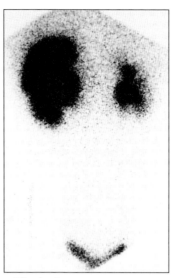

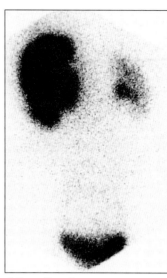

*a* 2 minutes          *b* 5 minutes          *c* 20 minutes          *d* Post-diuretic

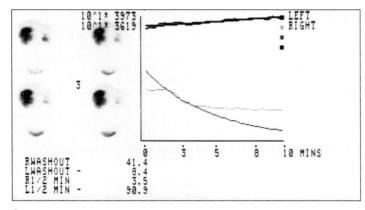

*e*

```
RWASHOUT        41.4
LWASHOUT -       8.4
R1/2 MIN -       3.5
L1/2 MIN -      90.9
```

*Fig. 3.37*

*A 19-year-old woman with recurrent left-sided loin pain and hydronephrosis. A dynamic DTPA renal scan with diuretic (frusemide) washout was obtained as a baseline functional study prior to pyeloplasty.*

*The 2-minute functional study (**a**) shows dilatation of the left kidney, with decreased function (32% of the total GFR). The 5-minute image (**b**) shows dilated calyces on the left. The 20-minute image (**c**) shows marked dilatation of the left collecting system, with delay in excretion. There is also some dilatation, but much less marked, of the right collecting system. The image taken following diuretic (**d**) shows that instead of washout there has been further accumulation of the tracer. This is reflected by the negative value for washout on the computer-generated curves (**e**). This finding is only seen in the more severe cases of obstruction.*

Accurate measurement of residual renal function may be difficult when there is a grossly enlarged collecting system present. Function must be measured before filling of the system occurs. For example, in the case in Fig. 3.37, if function was measured at 20 minutes, it would be grossly overestimated. However, on the functional image it can, on occasion, be difficult to define the cortical outline accurately and also to select appropriate sites for background subtraction.

## CLINICAL APPLICATIONS

*Importance of postural drainage*

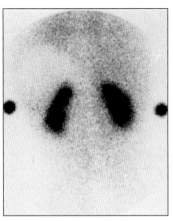 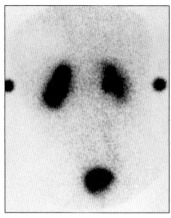 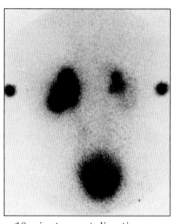 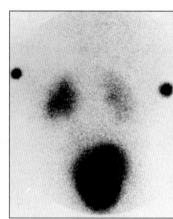

*a* 5 minutes      *b* 20 minutes      *c* 10 minutes, post-diuretic      *d* Post-posture change

**Fig. 3.38**

*(a–d) Dynamic $^{99m}Tc$ DTPA renal scan. A 2-year-old child who was being reassessed 2 months following left pyeloplasty for PUJ obstruction.*

*It is apparent that there are bilaterally dilated collecting systems, more marked on the left, with no drainage on the left before diuretic administration. Following diuretic, there is significant washout on the right, with some pooling in upper pole calyx. On the left there is incomplete emptying. With change in posture there is marked washout on the left, with further emptying on the right. This patient therefore has a dilated collecting system on the left, which is not obstructed.*

*Note that, in this case, diuretic study alone would have been misleading and was only performed prior to change in posture/mobilization because the patient had been sedated, and there was concern that he would wake up with change in posture.*

 • Functional studies in such cases provide the necessary confirmation for surgical treatment, and also provide a baseline functional measurement for subsequent follow-up to assess the future growth of the kidney and the effect of surgical intervention.

• When there is markedly decreased renal function, an impaired diuretic response may be obtained; thus false positives for obstruction can occur in the presence of dilatation. A doubling of the dose of diuretic is therefore recommended in this situation.

**CLINICAL APPLICATIONS**

## DMSA *scans in obstruction*

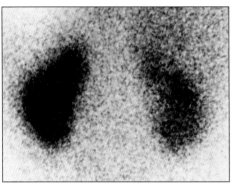
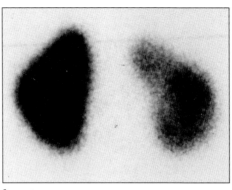

*a* DTPA

*b* DMSA

### Fig. 3.39

*A 3-year-old child with right-sided PUJ obstruction.*

*The functional DTPA image (a) shows a normal left kidney and impaired function of the right which contributes 27% to the total GFR. The DMSA study (b) provides similar information, although scarring in the right kidney is more apparent. The measured contribution of the right kidney to the total GFR is 30%.*

*In this case DMSA and DTPA studies correlate reasonably well. However, if DMSA is not performed carefully, it may overestimate function in the presence of obstruction.*

*A case illustrating how DMSA scans may be misleading in the assessment of function when the kidney is obstructed*

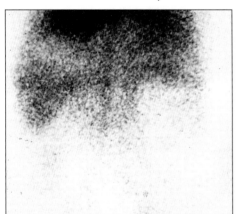
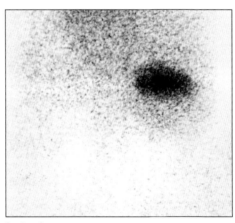

*a* 30 seconds, DTPA

*b* 2 minutes, DTPA

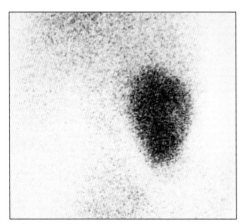
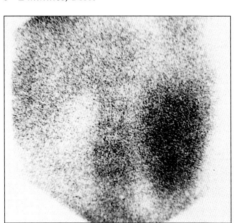

*c* 30 minutes, DTPA

*d* 3 hours, post-DMSA

### Fig. 3.40

*(a–c) DTPA renal scan. (d) 3-hour image post-DMSA.*

*The DTPA study shows markedly impaired perfusion of the right kidney, with only a small area of functioning renal tissue at the upper pole. The 30-minute image shows the dilated collecting system. The similarity between the DMSA scan and the 30-minute DTPA image is striking. Taken in isolation, the DMSA study would indicate reasonable function in the right kidney. However, there is almost complete obstruction, and when the DMSA study was obtained, all of the tracer normally excreted by the kidney was retained in the renal area. This case therefore illustrates well how DMSA may overestimate renal function in the presence of obstruction.*

## Difficulties in assessing obstruction

False positive diagnosis of obstruction may occur:

- When the patient is dehydrated
- If collecting systems are grossly dilated, as washout is partially volume-dependent
- In neonates, because the GFR and hence the diuretic response to frusemide is less
- In the elderly, since the GFR may be decreased
- With chronic renal failure

- If the diuretic is not given intravenously, ie is extravasated at the injection site
- Too soon after operation for PUJ obstruction
- In the presence of gross reflux.

False negative diagnosis rarely occurs, but may do so:

- If the obstruction is in the lower tract and measurements are taken from the upper tract
- The obstruction is intermittent.

### Newborn infant: investigation of obstruction

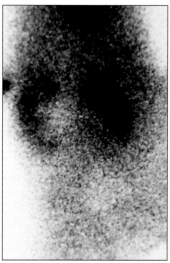

*a 2 minutes*

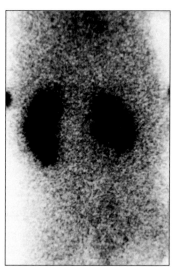

*b 10 minutes*

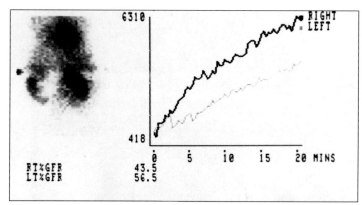

*c*

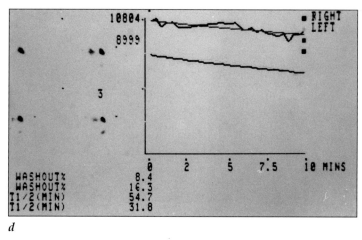

*d*

**Fig. 3.41**

Dynamic $^{99m}$Tc DTPA study in a 6-week-old baby who had been shown to have dilated, possibly obstructed, collecting systems in utero by ultrasound.

The 2-minute image **(a)** shows approximately symmetrical function with a photon-deficient area in the renal pelvis on the left. The 10-minute image **(b)** shows dilatation of both collecting systems. The T/A curve **(c)** shows progressive accumulation in the dilated systems. The T/A curve following diuretic **(d)** shows poor washout from the collecting systems. The DTPA study confirms the dilatation and probably indicates bilateral obstruction.

The GFR in infants is low, and the response to diuretic is less compared with older children, therefore false positives may occur; this must be taken into account when investigating newborn infants. A study showing lack of obstruction is of more significance than one such as this, showing possible obstruction.

## Renal impairment and bilateral PUJ obstruction

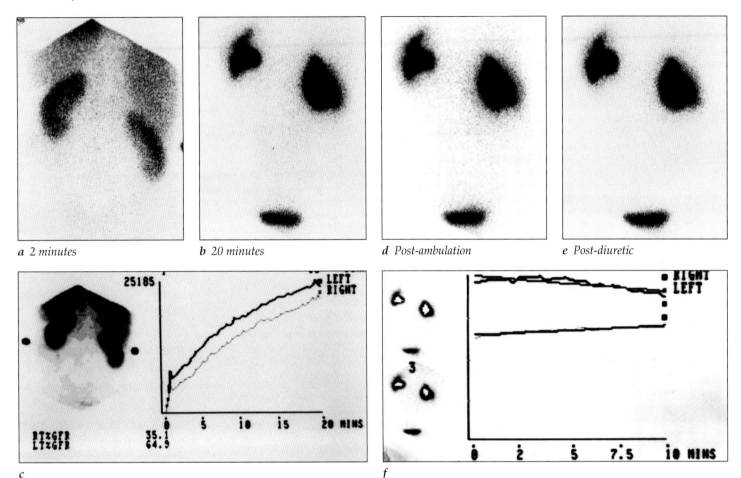

*a* 2 minutes      *b* 20 minutes      *d* Post-ambulation      *e* Post-diuretic

*c*                               *f*

**Fig. 3.42**

DTPA *renal scan in a 62-year-old woman with an incidental finding of dilated collecting systems when she was having ultrasound for an abdominal mass. She was asymptomatic with the exception of intermittent backache. The clinical issues were to document function in the two kidneys, and assess the degree of obstruction.*

*The 2-minute image* **(a)** *shows good selective excretion of* DTPA, *with some impaired function on the right (35% of the total* GFR*). The 20-minute image* **(b)** *shows good rapid excretion into dilated collecting systems bilaterally. The T/A curve* **(c)** *shows progressive filling of both collecting systems. The image taken after bladder emptying and ambulation* **(d)** *shows that there is no significant emptying of the collecting systems. Immediately prior to administration of diuretic both systems are dilated and full, the right more than the left. Following diuretic* **(e)**, *there is no significant washout of the tracer. The T/A curve following diuretic* **(f)** *confirms the lack of washout from either kidney.*

*The* DTPA *scan has shown that there is some decreased function of the right kidney. There are bilaterally dilated collecting systems which do not wash out following diuretic, thus suggesting bilateral obstruction which is more marked on the right than on the left. This patient had chronic renal impairment and, because of the poor function, the diuretic study overestimated the degree of obstruction.*

**With deteriorating renal function, the diagnosis of obstruction using diuretic renography becomes increasingly unreliable.**

## Lower urinary tract obstruction

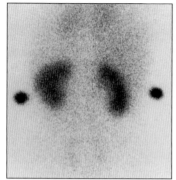

*a 2 minutes*

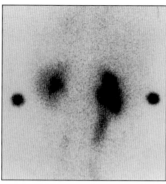

*b 10 minutes*

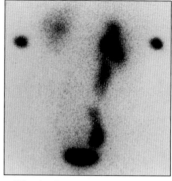

*c 20 minutes*

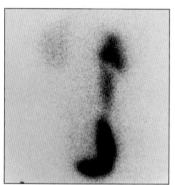

*d Pre-diuretic*

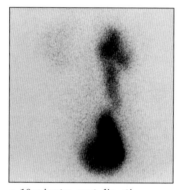

*e 10 minutes, post-diuretic*

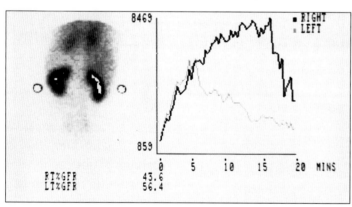

*f*

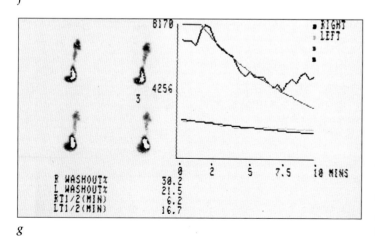

*g*

### Fig. 3.43

*(a–g)* DTPA *renal scan with diuretic washout. Normal renal washout in the presence of lower urinary tract obstruction.*

*The 2-minute functional image (a) shows good and relatively symmetrical function, with the left kidney contributing 55% to the total* GFR. *The 10-minute image (b) shows normal tracer passage through the left kidney and dilatation of the right collecting system and ureter. The 20-minute image (c) shows further dilatation of the right collecting system and ureter. The pre-diuretic image (d) shows drainage from the upper tract, but further accumulation in the lower half of the ureter. The image taken 10 minutes after diuretic (e) shows further drainage from the upper tract, with pooling in the lower ureter. The T/A curve (f) demonstrates a progressive rise of the tracer on the right, but there is a dramatic fall following diuretic. Quantitative analysis (g) shows 30% washout on the right, with $T_{1/2}$ of 6 minutes, which is normal.*

*The* DTPA *study confirms lower tract dilatation, but the washout from the renal pelvis is within normal limits. This case was subsequently shown to have obstruction at the level of the vesicoureteric junction.*

**It is important to be aware that with lower urinary tract obstruction there may be washout from the upper tract into a grossly dilated lower tract. Thus if only the renal area is measured, false negative results for obstruction may be obtained.**

## Urethral valves

### Bilateral vesicoureteric obstruction

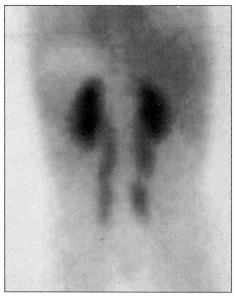

*a  5 minutes*

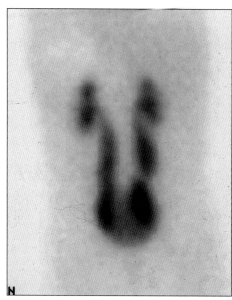

*b  10 minutes*

*c  20 minutes*

### Postoperative vesicoureteric obstruction

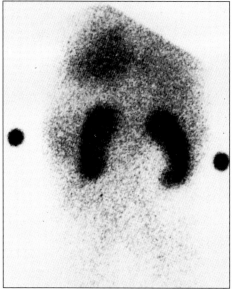

*d  2 minutes*

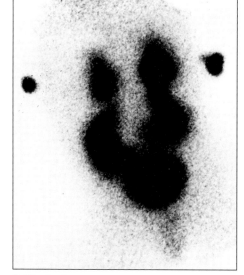

*e  10 minutes*

*f  20 minutes*

**Fig. 3.44**

*Two further cases scanned with DTPA illustrating some of the difficulties in assessing obstruction in the lower urinary tract. These are both cases of urethral valves. In the first (a–c) there is bilateral vesicoureteric obstruction. The second case (d–f) is that of a 2-year-old child being reassessed following an operation for urethral valves. The scan demonstrates persisting hold-up at the vesicoureteric junction level.*

**A post-micturition film may be useful to exclude obstruction at the lower end of the ureter as a full bladder may obscure the obstructed ureter.**

## Intermittent obstruction
### Aged 1 month

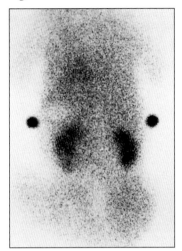 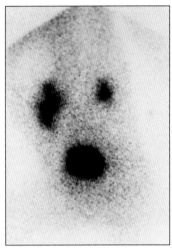 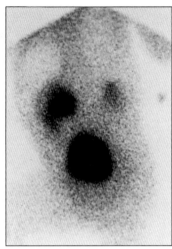

*a  1 minute*  *b  Pre-diuretic*  *c  Post-diuretic*

### Aged 2 months

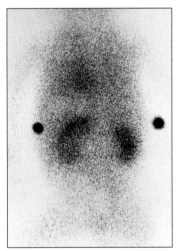 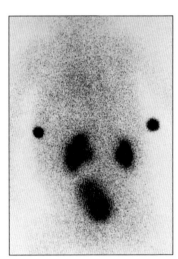 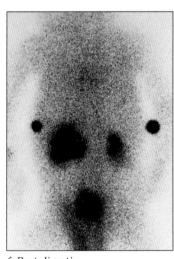

*d  1 minute*  *e  Pre-diuretic*  *f  Post-diuretic*

**Fig. 3.45**

*A 1-month-old infant with intrauterine diagnosis of hydronephrosis. The series of four DTPA studies shows intermittent obstruction with sudden loss of renal function.*

***Study 1 (a)** 1-minute functional phase: L, 58%; R, 42% of GFR. **(b)** Pre- and **(c)** post-diuretic, showing partial hold-up at the left PUJ.*

***Study 2 (d)** 1-minute functional phase: L, 46%; R, 54% of GFR. **(e)** Pre- and **(f)** post-diuretic, showing left-sided obstruction.*

### Aged 3 months

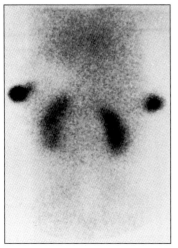

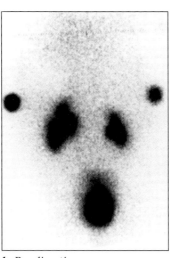

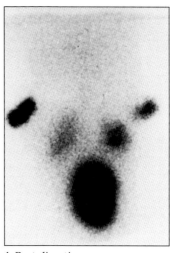

*g* 1 minute

*h* Pre-diuretic

*i* Post-diuretic

***Study 3 (g)*** *1-minute functional phase: L, 45%; R, 55% of* GFR. ***(h)*** *Pre- and* ***(i)*** *post-diuretic, showing normal washout with no obstruction.*

### Aged 15 months

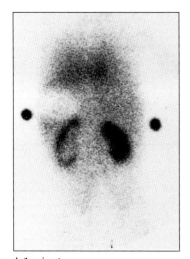

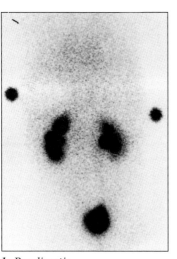

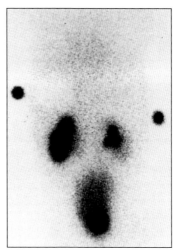

*j* 1 minute

*k* Pre-diuretic

*l* Post-diuretic

***Study 4 (j)*** *1-minute functional phase: L, 25%; R, 75% of* GFR. ***(k)*** *Pre- and* ***(l)*** *post-diuretic, showing definite obstruction.*

*This series dramatically illustrates that obstruction may be intermittent. Over a period of 14 months the studies indicated partial obstruction, complete obstruction and normal washout on the left. However, a final study once again indicated obstruction, which was associated with a significant loss of function.*

- Obstruction may be intermittent.
- A prominent photon-deficient area is frequently seen on infant studies and is due to milk in the stomach after a recent feed, given to assist sedation.

## *PUJ obstruction: postoperative follow-up*

### *Preoperative study*  *Postoperative study*

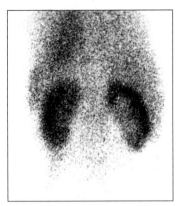

*a 2 minutes*

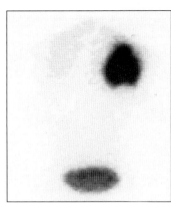

*d Post-diuretic*

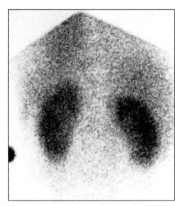

*f 2 minutes*

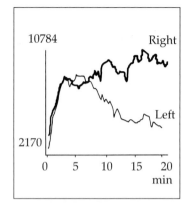

*h T/A curve*

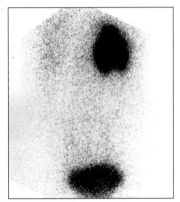

*b 10 minutes*

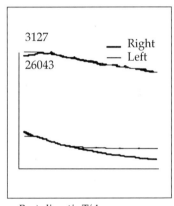

*e Post-diuretic T/A curve*

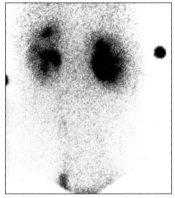

*g 10 minutes*

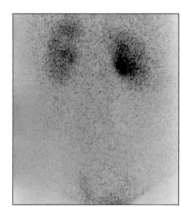

*i After ambulation*

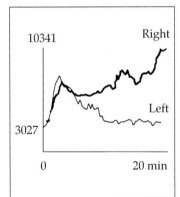

*c TA curve*

**Fig. 3.46**

*A 24-year-old woman with right-sided hydronephrosis. The initial study was performed to assess the renal function and as baseline for the follow-up.*

*Preoperative views: (a) 2-minute DTPA image; (b) 10-minute DTPA image; (c) T/A curve; (d) effect of diuretic; (e) T/A curve following diuretic. Postoperative views: (f) 2-minute DTPA image; (g)10-minute DTPA image; (h) T/A curve; (i) effect of gravity.*

*The initial study shows well-functioning kidneys, with a dilated right collecting system, which failed to wash out with gravity and diuretic. However, following pyeloplasty, it is seen that there is improved function. Furthermore, while there is still a dilated collecting system, and the initial T/A curves are identical, this drains rapidly with gravity alone.*

## CLINICAL APPLICATIONS

### The importance of diuretic in excluding obstruction

*Preoperative study*

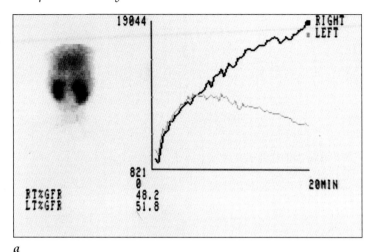
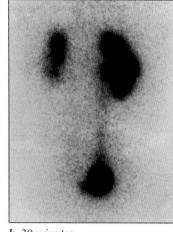
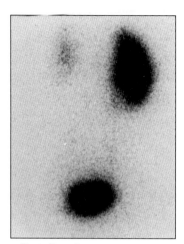

*a*                              *b* 30 minutes           *c* Post-diuretic

### Postoperative study

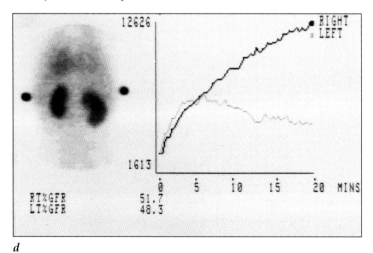
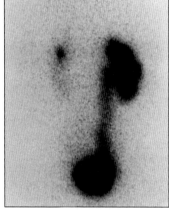
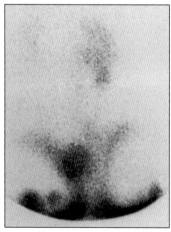

*d*                              *e* 30 minutes           *f* Post-diuretic

**Fig. 3.47**

A 2-year-old child with recurrent urinary tract infection and a diagnosis of PUJ obstruction on the right side. DTPA studies were performed before and after surgery for PUJ obstruction.

Preoperative views: **(a)** T/A curve; **(b)** 30-minute image; **(c)** image following diuretic. Postoperative views: **(d)** T/A curve; **(e)** 30-minute image; **(f)** image following diuretic.

The T/A curves are identical, indicating the difficulty in differentiation between dilatation alone and dilatation with obstruction. The difference is clearly seen when diuretic is used: before surgery there is no washout, while after surgery the washout is essentially complete.

Following a pyeloplasty operation, a DTPA study may appear to show persistent obstruction. Following diuretic and delayed imaging, washout will be observed if the operation was successful.

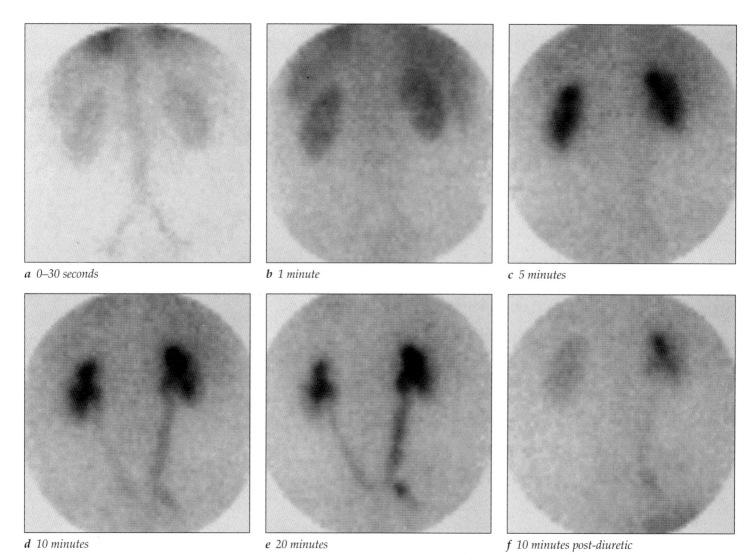

*a 0–30 seconds*          *b 1 minute*          *c 5 minutes*

*d 10 minutes*          *e 20 minutes*          *f 10 minutes post-diuretic*

### Fig. 3.48

*Possible ureteric obstruction in a 63-year-old man with an ileal conduit urinary diversion following cystectomy for carcinoma of the bladder. Bilateral ureteric dilatation was noted on ultrasound.*

*(a–f)* A DTPA *study was performed to assess the presence of an obstruction. At 10 minutes* ***(d)*** *the ureters are visualized, confirming dilatation, and at 20 minutes* ***(e)*** *there is significant activity remaining in the collecting systems and ureters. Following diuretic administration* ***(f)****, there is washout of activity, and activity is seen in the small bowel.*

## CLINICAL APPLICATIONS

# 3.4.3 Reflux nephropathy

## *Role of radionuclide studies in reflux nephropathy*

- Determination of presence or absence of renal scars
- Measurement of individual kidney function
- Identification of presence or absence of reflux.

*Table 3.2   Grades of vesicoureteric reflux*

| Grade | MCUG | Radionuclide studies |
|---|---|---|
| I | Reflux into the ureter only | Direct[a] method will detect. Indirect[b] method may not |
| II | Reflux into ureter and upper collecting system with no dilatation | |
| III<br>IV<br>V | As II, with progressive degrees of dilatation | Both radionuclide methods will detect all grades but will not reliably distinguish them |
| Intrarenal | Reflux into the collecting tubules | |

[a]Direct, instillation of tracer directly into bladder.
[b]Indirect, utilizes the tracer excreted into the bladder following a routine DTPA scan.

## *Advantages of radionuclide studies over micturating cystography*

- Lower radiation doses
- No catheterization
- Simultaneous assessment of renal function.

## *Demonstration of cortical scarring*

### Cortical scarring

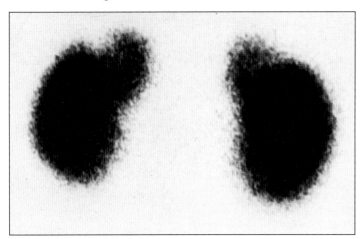

*Posterior*

**Fig. 3.49**

*Bilateral upper pole scarring is a typical and common finding, as demonstrated on this DMSA scan.*

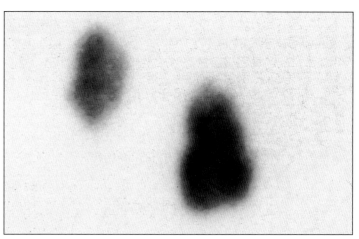

*Posterior*

**Fig. 3.50**

*Bilateral renal reflux. The posterior view DMSA scan alone shows scarring of both kidneys, particularly the left.*

### SPECT *to show cortical scarring*

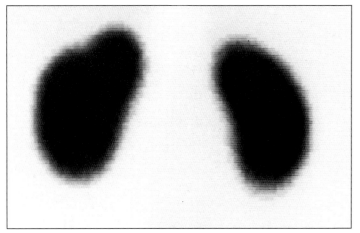

*a  Posterior planar*

**Fig. 3.51**

*Upper pole scarring demonstrated with a SPECT DMSA scan. (a) Posterior DMSA planar renal scan. Scarring of the upper pole of the left kidney is clearly visualized on a coronal SPECT section (b). Note how the SPECT study shows the relationship between the scar and the underlying calyces much more clearly than the DMSA planar renal scan.*

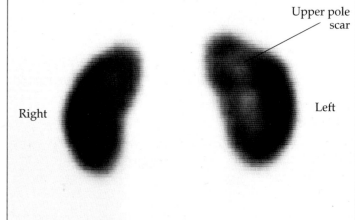

*b  Coronal SPECT*

- DMSA is the radiopharmaceutical of choice to show cortical scarring.
- Multiple views are necessary to show scars optimally.
- DMSA is the radiopharmaceutical of choice for assessment of divided function.

## CLINICAL APPLICATIONS

## Further examples of scarring

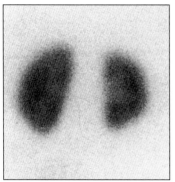
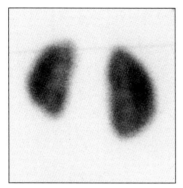

*a Anterior*    *b Posterior*

**Fig. 3.52**

**(a, b)** DMSA scans.
There are scars in both the upper and lower poles on the left. The left kidney is slightly smaller than the right and contributes 42% to the total GFR. Dilatation of the calyces is noted in both kidneys. These changes are attributable to bilateral reflux, with evidence of scarring and some loss of function in the right kidney.

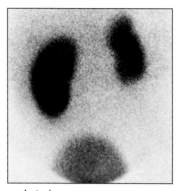
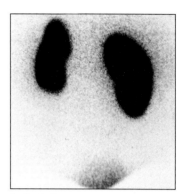

*a Anterior*    *b Posterior*

**Fig. 3.53**

**(a, b)** DMSA scans.
The right kidney is normal, but the left kidney is contracted and scarred. The left kidney contributes 28% to the total GFR. Note that the bladder is in the field of view and has not been emptied prior to imaging.

## Resolution of DMSA changes

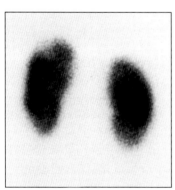
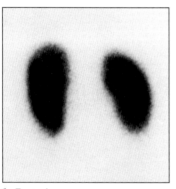

*a Posterior*    *b Posterior*

**Fig. 3.54**

A 6-year-old child with a urinary tract infection.
Posterior view DMSA scans show **(a)** irregularity of the left upper pole and **(b)** almost complete resolution 1 month later.

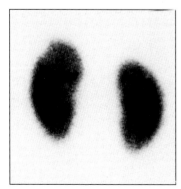
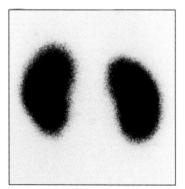

*a Posterior, 0 months*    *b Posterior, 4 months*

**Fig. 3.55**

A 5-year-old child with reflux and infection.
**(a)** Posterior view DMSA scan showing upper pole irregularity.
**(b)** Four months later this has resolved.

DMSA **abnormalities seen within 3 months of an acute infection may resolve. A follow-up study should therefore be performed to differentiate transient change due to pyelonephritis from persistent renal scarring.**

*An unusual case demonstrating the combination of obstruction and reflux*

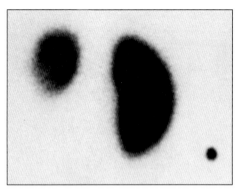

*a* *Posterior,* DMSA

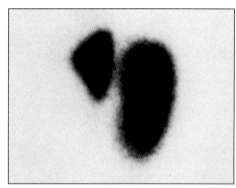

*b* *Left posterior oblique,* DMSA

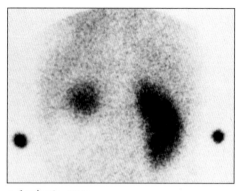

*c* *1 minute,* DTPA

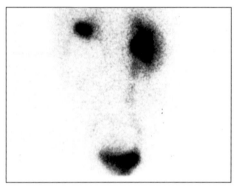

*d* *10 minutes,* DTPA

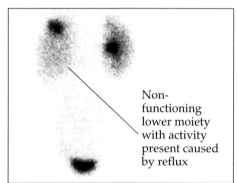

Non-functioning lower moiety with activity present caused by reflux

*e* *Post-micturition,* DTPA

**Fig. 3.56**

*An 8-year-old girl who presented with enuresis.*

*(**a, b**) The* DMSA *scans show a normal right kidney and functioning tissue only in the upper moiety of the duplex left kidney.*
*(**c, d**) The* DTPA *scans show a photon-deficient lower left moiety caused by obstruction. However, after micturition (**e**) this obstructed moiety 'fills in' as a result of vesico-ureteric reflux, which was subsequently confirmed on a micturating cystogram.*

---

*A duplex kidney with reflux*

Normal upper moiety

Damaged lower moiety

Scarring of lower pole

**Fig. 3.57**

DMSA *scan. There is loss of function of the left lower moiety of a duplex kidney and scarring of the lower pole of the right kidney. However, divided renal function is approximately equal (R, 52%).*

*Renal contraction*

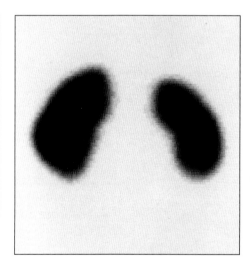

**Fig. 3.58**

DMSA *scan. A further case of reflux showing generalized diminution in the functioning mass of the right kidney, which contributes 40% to the total* GFR. *However, there are no discrete cortical scars present.*

• **Reflux most commonly occurs into the lower moiety of a duplex kidney. Obstruction most commonly affects the upper moiety.**
• **Generalized renal contraction without clear-cut scars may be a consequence of reflux.**

## *Renal scarring:* DMSA *and* DTPA *scans*

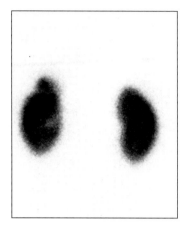 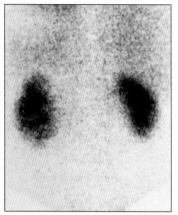 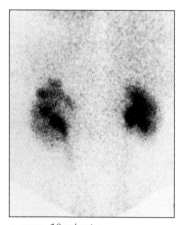 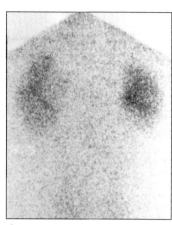

*a* DMSA      *b* DTPA, *2 minutes*      *c* DTPA, *10 minutes*      *d* DTPA, *20 minutes*

**Fig. 3.59**

*The posterior* DMSA *study (a) clearly shows upper moiety scarring. The* DTPA *scan (b) also shows this, but less well, and the dilated calyces close to the surface are well identified (c). These drain normally, showing that there is no obstruction (d).*

- DTPA **will not demonstrate scars as well as** DMSA**.**
- **Calyceal dilatation without obstruction is a feature of previous reflux.**

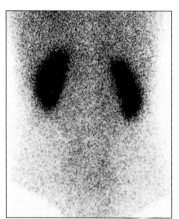 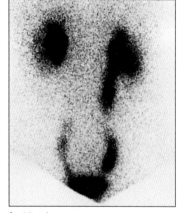 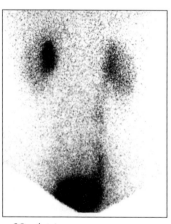 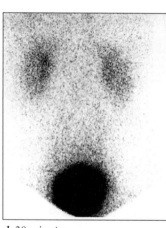

*a 2 minutes*      *b 10 minutes*      *c 20 minutes*      *d 30 minutes*

**Fig. 3.60**

*(a–d) A further case showing features of previous reflux. The* DTPA *scan shows marked bilateral collecting system dilatation with rapid drainage.*

**Some features of reflux, including scarring, dilatation of calyces and visualization of the ureter, may be residual effects of previous reflux, and do not indicate that reflux is still occurring.**

## CLINICAL APPLICATIONS

## *Demonstration of reflux*

Renal scars and pelvicalyceal dilatation show that reflux has occurred in the past. Other methods are required to show that reflux is continuing. Reflux may be demonstrated as the bladder is filling (filling phase reflux) or during micturition (emptying phase reflux). The gold standard is the micturating cystogram, but radionuclide methods are valuable adjuncts, especially for follow-up.

*Table 3.3   Comparison of direct and indirect radionuclide methods*

| Method | Advantages | Disadvantages |
|---|---|---|
| Direct | All age groups<br>Low radiation dose<br>Detects grade I reflux | Requires catheterization |
| Indirect | No catheterization<br>Provides individual renal function information | Only suitable over 3 years of age<br>Only detects grades II–IV reflux |

### *Filling phase reflux*
Excretory phase of a dynamic study with DTPA or MAG3

### *Vesicoureteric reflux*

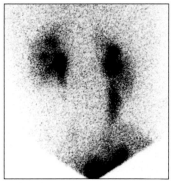

*a  15 minutes*

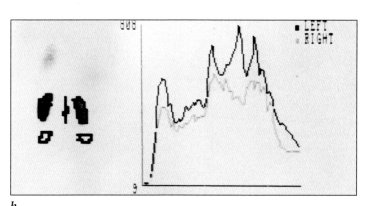

*b*

**Fig. 3.61**

*The DTPA scan (a) shows dilatation of both collecting systems. The T/A curve (b) demonstrates the intermittent spikes caused by urine refluxing into the collecting systems.*

## CLINICAL APPLICATIONS

*Ureteric reflux associated with cortical scarring*

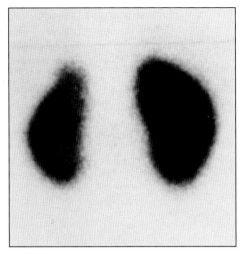

*a* DMSA

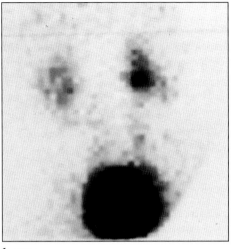

*b* DTPA

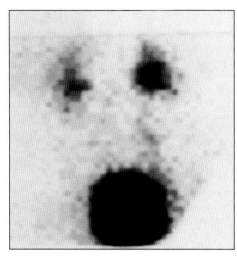

*c* DTPA

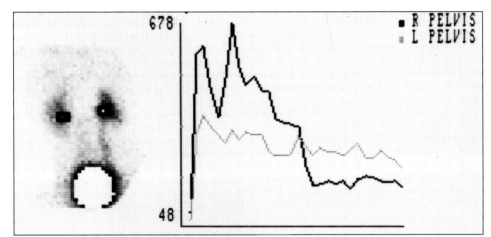

*d*

**Fig. 3.62**

*A 9-year-old child with recurrent urinary infection.*

*The DMSA scan (a) shows a normal right kidney with a scarred left kidney and impaired function. The DTPA study (b, c) shows reflux occurring into both kidneys before bladder emptying commences. Note that there is more reflux into the normal right kidney than the left kidney. (d) The T/A curve shows 'spiking' caused by reflux.*

• All phases of the DTPA study may provide information about vexicoureteric reflux. In the particular case shown in Fig. 3.62, there is evidence of reflux occurring while the bladder is full before micturition commences.

• Reflux is not always associated with scarring or damage of the kidney.

## CLINICAL APPLICATIONS

### Emptying phase reflux

Emptying phase reflux can be performed in one of two ways: the indirect method or the direct method. In the indirect method intravenously injected radionuclide is allowed to accumulate in the bladder, whereas in the direct method the radionuclide is instilled directly into the bladder.

Indirect micturating reflux studies are difficult to perform, and are subject to errors. The following points should be noted:

- The collecting systems must be allowed to drain as much as possible before commencing the investigation
- There should be no patient movement, since false positives may occur
- The presence of reflux should be confirmed on the images

- After significant reflux, the bladder will refill as the kidney empties
- It is important to obtain a stable baseline for a few minutes before micturition
- In order to detect minor reflux, regions of interest (ROI) should be drawn around the collecting system and not the whole kidney
- T/A curves generated from renal ROI should be displayed without the bladder to detect minor reflux.

### Bladder and renal T/A curves

Bladder and renal T/A curves will increase the accuracy of detecting reflux. A typical reflux T/A curve is shown in Fig. 3.63.

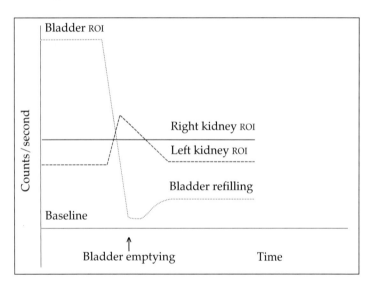

**Fig. 3.63**

*Typical reflux T/A curve with normal right kidney and refluxing left kidney (ROI = regions of interest).*

### Demonstration of vesicoureteric reflux during micturition

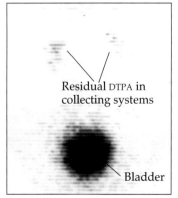

*a Before micturition*

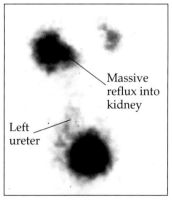

*b During micturition*

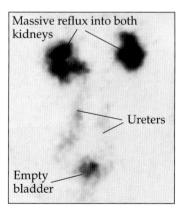

*c After micturition*

**Fig. 3.64**

*After a routine DTPA scan, when most of the tracer is in the bladder, demonstration of vesicoureteric reflux is possible. Continuous imaging before (a), during (b) and after micturition (c) shows DTPA refluxing up into the pelvicalyceal system.*

*Indirect DTPA reflux study: follow-up*

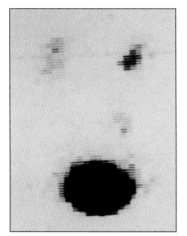

*a* Before micturition

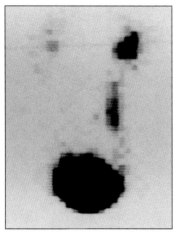

*b* Before micturition

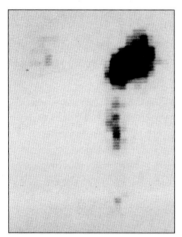

*c* During micturition

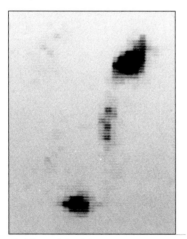

*d* After micturition

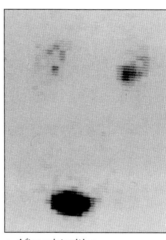

*e* After micturition

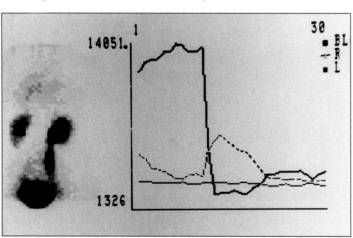

*f*

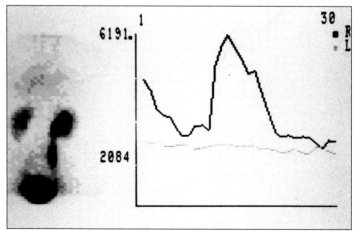

*g*

### Fig. 3.65

*A 5-year-old child with known vesicoureteric reflux and a past history of recurrent urinary tract infection.*

*At the initiation of micturition (a, b) there is reflux into the right kidney and ureter. At the completion of micturition (c) massive reflux has occurred, which then drains back into the bladder as pressure diminishes (d, e). The T/A curve (f) demonstrates rapid bladder emptying, with right-sided reflux and subsequent drainage. The T/A curve, (g) using the full scale, shows the right-sided reflux more clearly.*

*The DTPA reflux study is useful for follow-up. In this particular case the child was previously shown to have bilateral vesicoureteric reflux, and the present study demonstrated that left-sided reflux had resolved, but right-sided reflux remained moderately severe.*

## CLINICAL APPLICATIONS

### Reflux and chronic renal failure

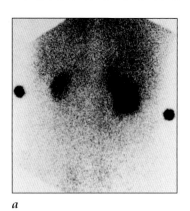

*a*

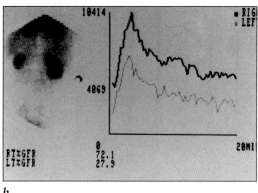

*b*

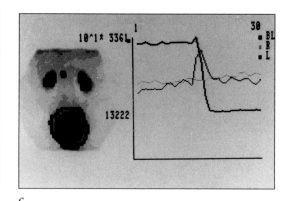

*c*

**Fig. 3.66**

*Chronic renal failure due to bilateral reflux. A 30-year-old patient with chronic renal failure. The DTPA scan (a, b) shows bilateral impaired function with extensive scarring. The indirect reflux study (c) confirms reflux into the left kidney.*

### Reflux into a non-functioning kidney

**Fig. 3.67**

*(a–c) Dynamic DTPA scan. Gross reflux into a non-functioning kidney in a 38-year-old woman with multiple previous operations on both ureters for strictures. (d, e) DTPA images and (f) T/A curve post-diuretic. There is dilatation of the left collecting system and upper ureter which clears completely following diuretic, but there is gross reflux into the non-functioning right kidney. Note the rising curve on the T/A study following diuretic due to reflux.*

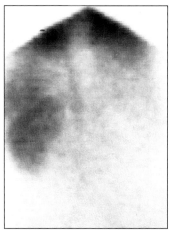

*a 30 seconds*

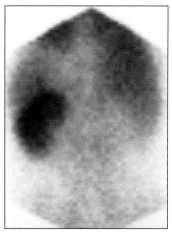

*b 2 minutes*

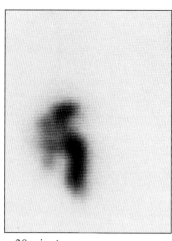

*c 20 minutes*

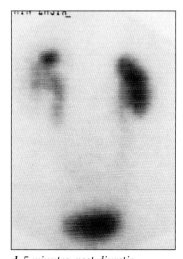

*d 5 minutes, post-diuretic*

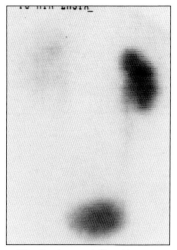

*e 10 minutes, post-diuretic*

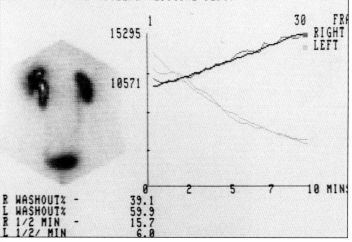

*f*

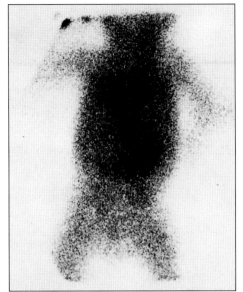

*a* 2 minutes

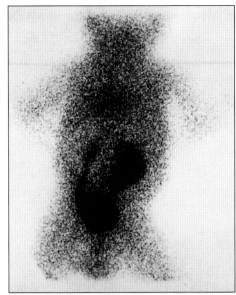

*b* 15 minutes

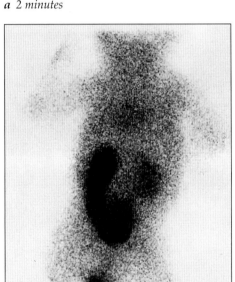

*c* 5 minutes, post-diuretic

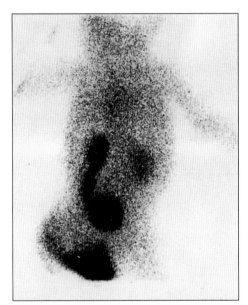

*d* 15 minutes, post-diuretic

*Fig. 3.68*

*Reflux into a non-functioning kidney. On the 2- and 15-minute DTPA images (**a, b**) the left kidney seems to be non-functional. The right kidney is somewhat dilated, and there is reflux into the left ureter. On the 5-minute image following diuretic (**c**) the right collecting system is clear, but there is massive reflux into the non-functioning kidney. On the 15-minute image following diuretic (**d**) reflux is still apparent, but there has been some emptying into the bladder.*

**Reflux into a kidney can cause confusion and may result in either an overestimate of function if the measurement is made after the parenchymal phase, or a misdiagnosis of obstruction.**

## 3.4.4 Trauma

*Table 3.4 Classification and consequences of trauma*

| *Mild trauma:* | *Consequence* | *Moderate trauma:* | *Consequence* |
|---|---|---|---|
| Parenchymal contusion | Focal loss of function | Renal laceration | Haemorrhage |
| Haematomas: | | Ruptured kidney | Haemorrhage |
| intrarenal | Infection | Collecting system damage | Urinary leaks |
| perinephric | Infection | *Severe trauma:* | |
| Minor lacerations | Haemorrhage | Shattered kidney | Haemorrhage |
| | | Renal artery thrombosis | Renal infarction |
| | | Renal artery avulsion | Renal infarction |

## *Bullet injuries to the kidney*

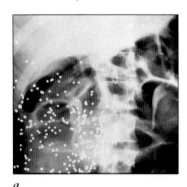 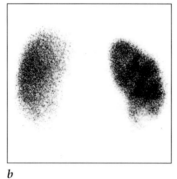

*a*        *b*

**Fig. 3.69**

*The IVU (a) shows the result of a shotgun injury. The DMSA scan, oblique view (b) shows loss of function of the lower pole of the right kidney caused by direct injury. Note the multiple focal areas of decreased activity caused by absorption by lead shot.*

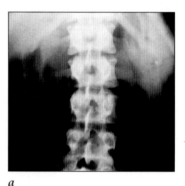 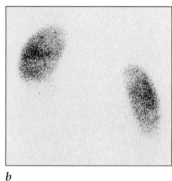

*a*        *b*

**Fig. 3.70**

*Penetrating bullet injury to the left flank. The IVU (a) shows damage to the left transverse process of L3. The DMSA scan (b) shows loss of function of the lower pole of the left kidney.*

## *Shrapnel injuries causing urinary leaks*

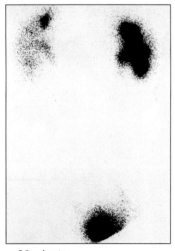 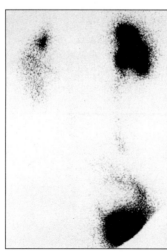

*a 20 minutes*        *b 40 minutes*

**Fig. 3.71**

*Injury to abdomen from shrapnel, causing a urinary leak. The 20-minute DTPA image (a) shows dilatation of the right collecting system only. At 40 minutes (b) the urinary leak from the lower end of the right ureter becomes apparent.*

 **It is essential to obtain delayed images of the abdomen to detect urinary leaks.**

## Assessment of kidneys following abdominal trauma

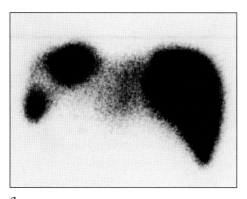

*a*

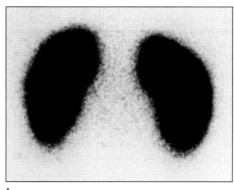

*b*

*Fig. 3.72*

*A 13-year-old boy who was admitted following a road traffic accident with pain and guarding in the left side of the abdomen, but with no other features present. The clinical issue was whether this boy had sustained significant splenic or renal trauma. The colloid liver/spleen scan (a) clearly demonstrates the presence of haematoma in the spleen. In this case the DMSA scan (b) was normal. While only the posterior view is shown here, it is important to obtain anterior, posterior and oblique views in such cases. This study confirmed that there was no renal haematoma or renal tear.*

**Radionuclide studies are probably the investigations of choice for rapid assessment of upper abdominal trauma.**

## Vascular study to assess trauma

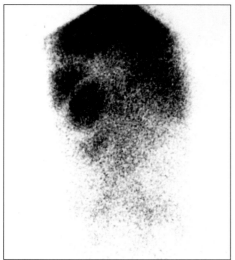

*a  Posterior, 30 seconds*

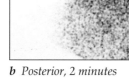

*b  Posterior, 2 minutes*

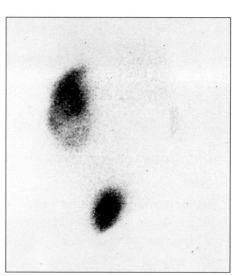

*c  Posterior, 3½ hours*

*Fig. 3.73*

*(a–c) Renal scan (GHA). Ruptured right kidney following abdominal trauma. A 5-year-old boy with a non-functioning right kidney and a ruptured left kidney following abdominal trauma.*

*On the vascular study (a) there is reduced flow to the lower pole of the left kidney, with a distinct area of absent activity also seen on the functional image (b). On the delayed image (c) there is confirmation of reduced function in the lower pole and probable upper calyceal dilatation. No right-sided renal function is noted. The scan findings were attributable to a ruptured left kidney at the lower pole.*

# 3.4.5   Renal failure

*Table 3.6   Classification of renal failure in relation to dynamic renal scan findings*

| Cause of acute renal failure | Scan features |
|---|---|
| Obstruction | Variable blood flow<br>Dilated calyces |
| Pre-renal, eg haemorrhage, hypotension, diarrhoea | Normal blood flow<br>Good uptake<br>Delayed intrarenal transit<br>Minimal excretion |
| Acute tubular necrosis (ATN), eg secondary to pre-renal causes, tissue damage (trauma etc), nephrotoxins | Almost normal blood flow<br>Absent or poor uptake<br>No excretion |
| Parenchymal disease, eg glomerulonephritis | Severely impaired blood flow<br>Poor uptake<br>Poor or absent excretion<br>Delayed intrarenal transit |
| Vascular (arterial or venous obstruction) | Severely impaired blood flow<br>Poor or absent uptake<br>No excretion |
| Chronic renal failure | Small kidneys<br>Poor blood flow<br>Little or no uptake or excretion |

## *Indications for renal scanning in acute renal failure*

- To diagnose pre-renal failure
- To diagnose acute tubular necrosis (ATN)
- To monitor changes in the anuric patient
- To diagnose complications
- To assess the probable prognosis.

## CLINICAL APPLICATIONS

# *Diagnosis of pre-renal failure*

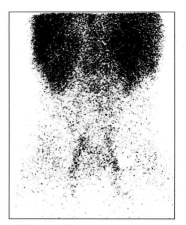 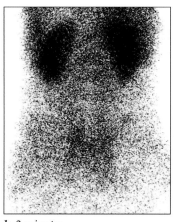 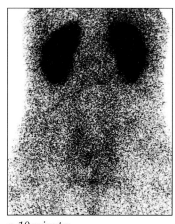 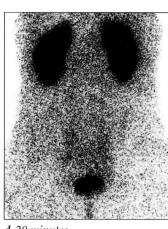

*a* 30 seconds    *b* 2 minutes    *c* 10 minutes    *d* 20 minutes

*Fig. 3.74*

*A 16-year-old male with nephrotic syndrome who presented with acute oliguria. DTPA scan: (a) 30-second image, showing almost normal blood flow; (b) 2-minute image showing symmetrical good uptake; (c, d) progressive accumulation of DTPA at 10 and 20 minutes after injection.*

*The DTPA scan shows some diminution of blood flow to both kidneys, but with moderately good filtration. Thereafter there is progressive concentration of tracer, with delayed transit.*

 **These are the appearances of acute pre-renal hypovolaemic failure, and are not typical of acute tubular necrosis. The management implication is that such a patient may respond to rehydration and plasma expanders.**

*Fig. 3.75*

*Typical time–activity curve of pre-renal failure.*

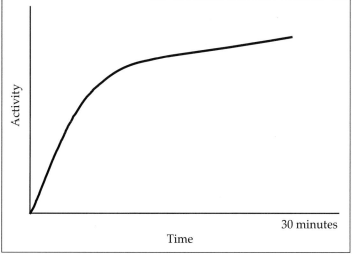

30 minutes

Time

 **In the presence of renal failure radionuclide imaging cannot be used to *exclude* obstruction; this is the role of ultrasound.**

## *Diagnosis of* ATN

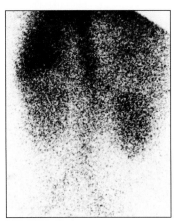

*a 0 minutes*

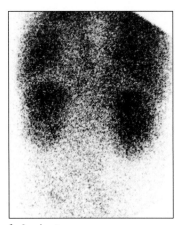

*b 2 minutes*

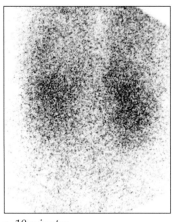

*c 10 minutes*

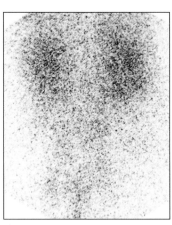

*d 20 minutes*

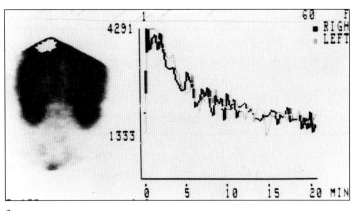

*e*

### Fig. 3.76

*(a–d) Dynamic* DTPA *image and (e) T/A curve in a 68-year-old woman who presented with acute renal failure following diarrhoea and vomiting. The likely clinical diagnosis was* ATN, *but in order that appropriate management could be undertaken, this diagnosis had to be confirmed rapidly with no associated morbidity. The* DTPA *scan does this, and provides the characteristic appearances shown here.*

*An ultrasound examination should also be performed to exclude obstruction which is not identified by* DTPA *in the presence of acute renal failure.*

## ATN *in an infant*

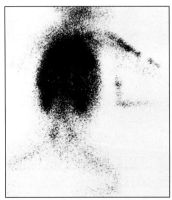

*a 30 seconds*

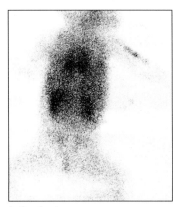

*b 2 minutes*

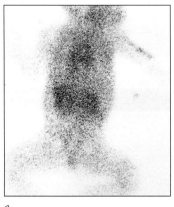

*c*

### Fig. 3.77

DTPA *scan: (a) 30-second image showing good renal blood flow; (b) 2-minute image showing a blood pool image only, with no selective uptake; (c) the blood pool image fades, with no excretion.*

• **For the evaluation of acute renal failure in children a combination of** DTPA **renal scan and ultrasound is usually sufficient and avoids the risks associated with contrast media.**

• **Note that the resolution of images in children is often poor in comparison with those obtained in adults.**

## Comparison of ATN and parenchymal disease

**Table 3.7**  *DTPA scan results in ATN and parenchymal disease*

| DTPA scan | ATN | Parenchymal disease |
|---|---|---|
| Blood flow | Good | Poor |
| 2-minute uptake | Blood pool only | Poor |
| Excretion | Nil | Poor to nil |

### ATN

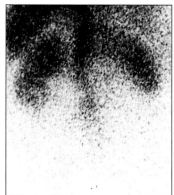 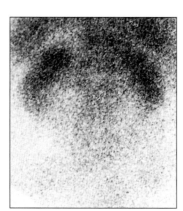 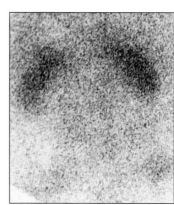

*a  30 seconds*

*b  2 minutes*

*c  20 minutes*

**Fig. 3.78**

*(a–c)* DTPA *scan in a patient with* ATN, *showing well perfused non-functioning kidneys.*

### Glomerulonephritis

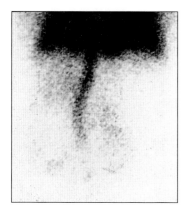 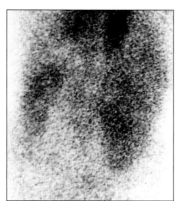 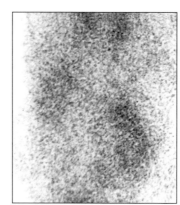

*a  30 seconds*

*b  2 minutes*

*c  30 minutes*

**Fig. 3.79**

*(a–c)* DTPA *scan in a patient with glomerulonephritis, showing poor perfusion and minimal tracer accumulation and excretion.*

 The DTPA scan provides a positive diagnosis of ATN; most other causes of acute renal failure will differ, but they are usually individually indistinguishable from each other.

## CLINICAL APPLICATIONS

## *Monitoring changes in the anuric patient*

In the absence of urine output, the radionuclide scan is the only simple non-invasive way to monitor the progress of renal failure.

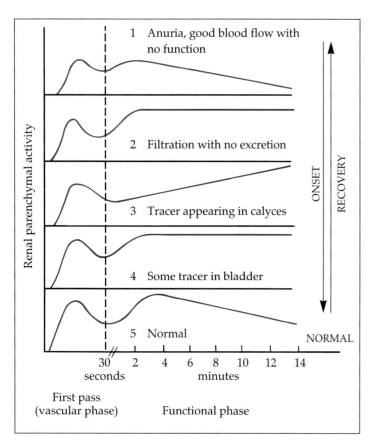

**Fig. 3.80**

*The phases through which the renal T/A curves change during onset and recovery of ATN. Initially (1), the blood flow is slightly diminished and there is a blood pool only, with no filtration at 2 minutes; this fades as the tracer leaves the blood compartment to diffuse into the larger extracellular fluid space. As recovery occurs (2, 3, 4), there is a gradual improvement in blood flow and more tracer is filtered, which increases the uptake at 2 minutes; however, with poor tubular flow, the tracer progressively concentrates in the kidney (3). Finally (5), there is the normal picture of good blood flow with rapid filtration and rapid clearance from the parenchyma into the collecting system. Note that the appearances during recovery are the same as those seen when classic ATN develops from pre-renal failure (except in reverse order).*

## CLINICAL APPLICATIONS

## Normal recovery from ATN

### Acute phase

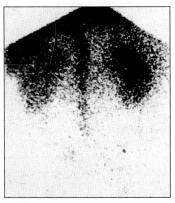
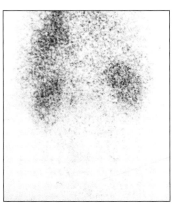

*a  30 seconds*　　*b  2 minutes*　　*c  30 minutes*

### Recovery phase

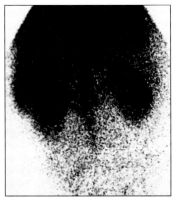
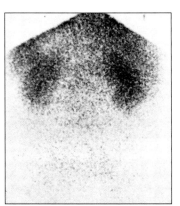
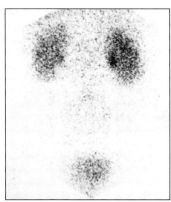

*d  30 seconds*　　*e  2 minutes*　　*f  30 minutes*

**Fig. 3.81**

*(a–c) DTPA scan. The classic appearance of ATN — well-maintained blood flow with blood pool only at 2 minutes; this fades with no excretion. (d–f) During recovery the blood flow increases and the 2-minute image represents filtered tracer as well as blood pool. The tracer is retained in the kidney and some is excreted.*

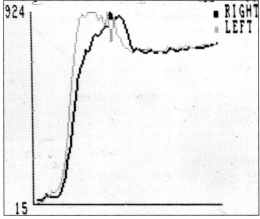
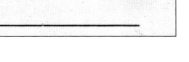

*a*

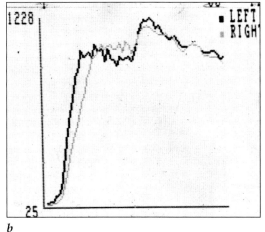

*b*

**Fig. 3.82**

*T/A curves during recovery from ATN. The intermediate T/A curve (a) shows that there is very little tracer filtered, but it is retained in the renal parenchyma, resulting in a horizontal third phase. On recovery, the T/A curve (b) shows that there is more tracer filtered and, with increasing tubular urine flow, the third phase falls as tracer leaves the kidney and enters the bladder.*

- **Recovery time will vary from a few days to a few months.**
- **Retention of tracer in the kidney from 2 minutes to 30 minutes is the first sign of recovery.**

## Deterioration of function during treatment

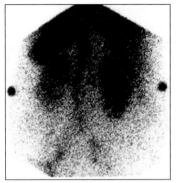
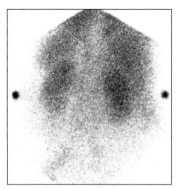
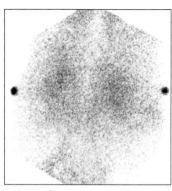

*a* 0 months, 30 seconds     *b* 0 months, 2 minutes     *c* 0 months, 20 minutes

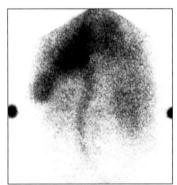
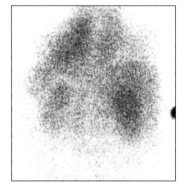
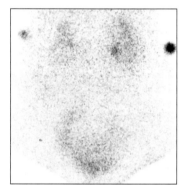

*d* 2 months, 30 seconds     *e* 2 months, 2 minutes     *f* 2 months, 20 minutes

### Fig. 3.83

*A patient with acute faecal peritonitis following perforation who developed acute renal failure.*

*The initial DTPA study (a–c) shows the typical appearances of ATN. However, the second scan 2 months later (d–f) shows gross deterioration of blood flow to both kidneys, with no recovery of function. This study illustrates well the value of the DTPA scan in following a patient with renal failure.*

## Diagnosis of complications

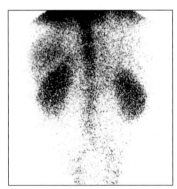
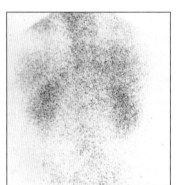

*a* 0 months, 30 seconds     *b* 0 months, 2 minutes     *c* 0 months, 20 minutes

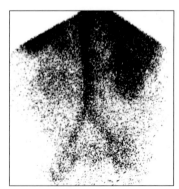
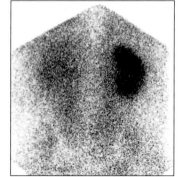
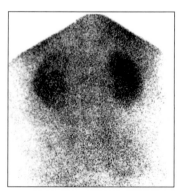

*d* Repeat, 30 seconds     *e* Repeat, 2 minutes     *f* Repeat, 20 minutes

### Fig. 3.84

*A 63-year-old man who presented with acute renal failure.*

*The original DTPA study (a–c) shows the typical features of ATN. The patient gradually made a good recovery, but subsequently had a second episode of oliguria. The repeat DTPA study (d–f) shows improved perfusion and function of the right kidney, but there has been striking deterioration in the perfusion of the left kidney. This patient was shown to have superimposed left renal vein thrombosis.*

## CLINICAL APPLICATIONS

# Assessment of probable prognosis

## Haemolytic uraemic syndrome

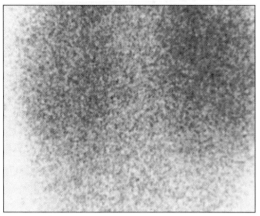

*a  0 months*

*b  0 months*

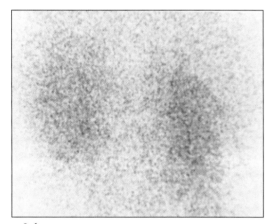

*c  3 days*

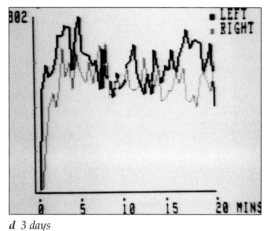

*d  3 days*

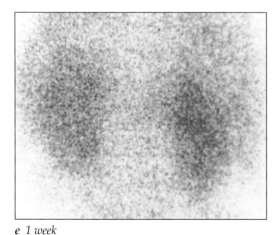

*e  1 week*

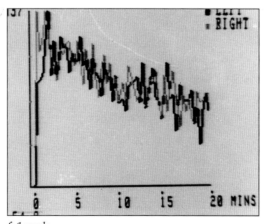

*f  1 week*

*Fig. 3.85*

*(a, b) A 2-minute DTPA image with T/A curve, which shows almost absent blood flow and function typical of haemolytic uraemic syndrome. The repeat study (c, d) 3 days later shows that there has been some recovery of blood flow. The subsequent study (e, f) 1 week after the onset of renal failure shows that the blood flow has improved further, but with superimposed ATN.*

The appearances of a dynamic renal scan are a good guide to prognosis in acute vascular disease, but may be misleading in other conditions, most notably haemolytic uraemic syndrome in children, when there may be virtually absent blood flow with subsequent complete recovery.

## CLINICAL APPLICATIONS

### Post-surgical aneurysm

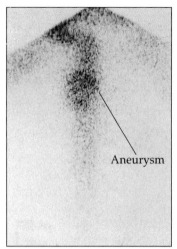
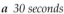

*a 30 seconds*

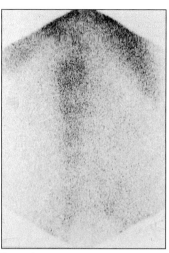

*b 2 minutes*

*c 20 minutes*

**Fig. 3.86**

*A 72-year-old man who had an emergency renal scan performed following abdominal surgery for an aortic aneurysm.*

*The dynamic DTPA 30-second image (a) shows an aortic aneurysm, with absent renal blood flow. The 2-minute image (b) shows a dilated aorta, but with no renal blood pool. On the 20-minute image (c) there is no excretion of tracer seen.*

*This patient had developed acute renal failure, and the differential diagnosis lay between ATN and absent blood flow caused by a ligated renal artery. This study clearly demonstrates the latter diagnosis, and this information was important for subsequent management.*

### Renal failure caused by loss of blood supply

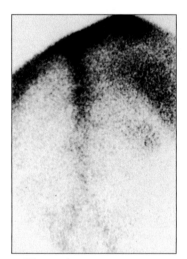

*a 30 seconds*

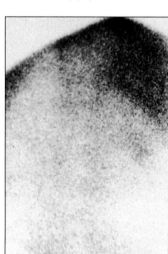

*b 2 minutes*

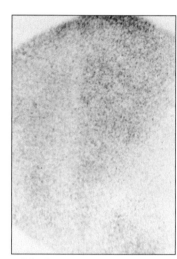

*c 20 minutes*

**Fig. 3.87**

*(a–c) DTPA scan.*

*The scan shows severe impairment of blood flow and associated ATN of the right kidney caused by an embolus following cardiac surgery. (The left kidney was non-functional.)*

## CLINICAL APPLICATIONS

### Bilateral renal artery stenosis: DTPA

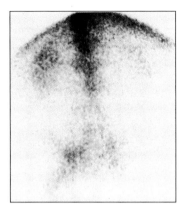 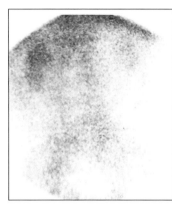

*a  30 seconds*  *b  2 minutes*  *c  20 minutes*

**Fig. 3.88**

**(a–c)** DTPA *scan. Severe bilateral renal artery stenosis.*
*The scan shows blood flow to the left kidney, but with* ATN. *There is no blood flow to the right kidney.*

### Renal artery stenosis: MAG3

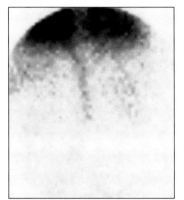 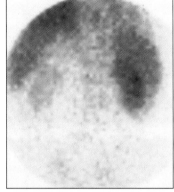 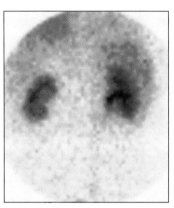 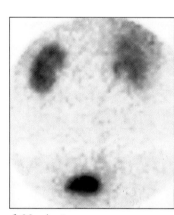

*a  0–30 seconds*  *b  1 minute*  *c  10 minutes*  *d  20 minutes*

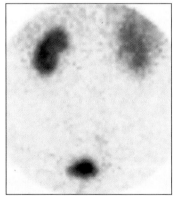 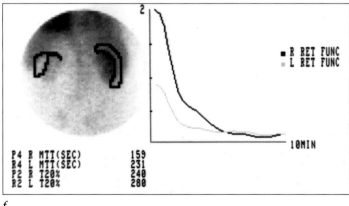

*e  Post-micturition*  *f*

| | | |
|---|---|---|
| P4 R MTT(SEC) | 159 | ■ R RET FUNC |
| R4 L MTT(SEC) | 231 | ⊡ L RET FUNC |
| P2 R T20% | 240 | |
| R2 L T20% | 280 | |

**Fig. 3.89**

MAG3 *study in a 72-year-old man with a history of hypertension, showing* **(a)** *reduced perfusion of left kidney, slow uptake of tracer at 1 minute* **(b)**, *and prolonged parenchymal transit at 10 minutes* **(c)**, *20 minutes* **(d)** *and post-micturition* **(e)**, *confirming left renal artery stenosis.* **(f)** *Curves of parenchymal transit confirm prolonged transit on left.*

### Chronic renal impairment: DTPA

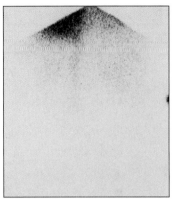 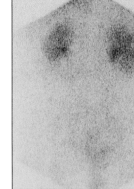 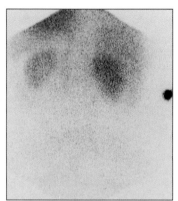

*a 30 seconds*          *b 2 minutes*          *c 20 minutes*

- DTPA scans will only rarely contribute to the management of patients with contracted kidneys who are in chronic renal failure.
- A DTPA study cannot exclude the presence of obstruction in such cases.

*Fig. 3.90*

*A 71-year-old woman with known previous hypertension and ischaemic heart disease who developed acute on chronic renal failure.*

*The dynamic image (a) shows bilateral poorly perfused kidneys. The 2-minute image (b) shows very poor selective accumulation on both sides, the right kidney contributing 57% to the total GFR. On the 20-minute image (c) there is very slow transit of a small amount of tracer.*

*The DTPA scan showed the non-specific appearances of chronic renal failure, with some decreased size in the kidneys, generalized decrease in perfusion and function with relatively slow transit of tracer.*

### Chronic renal impairment: MAG3

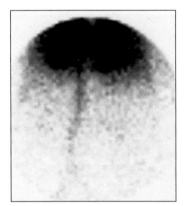 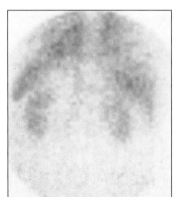 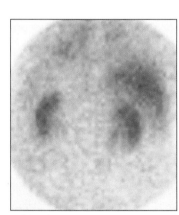

*a 0–30 seconds*          *b 1 minute*          *c 20 minutes*

MAG3 is the agent of choice in patients with renal failure, since the better renal extraction improves visualization.

*Fig. 3.91*

*A 74-year-old woman with a long history of diabetes, hypertension and gradually rising creatinine.*

*The MAG3 study (a–c) confirms symmetrical poor uptake and prolonged transit in bilaterally small kidneys.*

# 3.4.6 Space-occupying lesions

Radionuclide scanning has a limited use in investigating renal masses because other investigations (such as ultrasound, IVU, CT and arteriography) provide the information necessary for the diagnosis and management of these patients.

### Indications for radionuclide scans

- To investigate a possible pseudotumour
- To assess the blood flow of a lesion if arteriography is contraindicated.

### Causes of space-occupying lesions

- Pseudotumour
- Tumour
- Cyst
- Calculus
- Abscess.

### Pseudotumour

#### Definition

Unusually shaped masses of normal renal tissue resembling pathological masses.

#### Causes

- Dromedary hump (lateral margin, left kidney)
- Exaggerated Column of Bertin
- Focal compensatory hypertrophy (regenerating nodules).

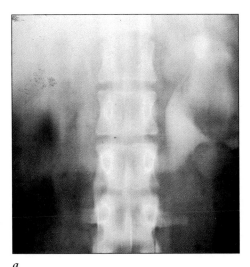

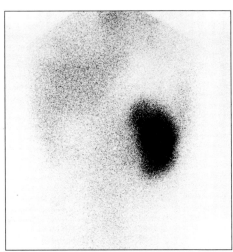

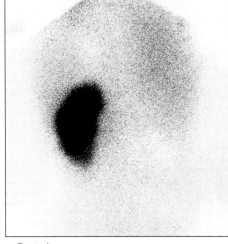

*a*  *b Anterior*  *c Posterior*

*Fig. 3.92*

*A 19-year-old woman who had a previous right nephrectomy because of chronic reflux presented with a mass in her left kidney.*

*A large, space-occupying lesion is seen on the IVU (a). However, the DMSA scan — anterior (b), posterior (c) — indicates that the space-occupying lesion represents functional renal tissue, thus confirming the presence of a pseudotumour.*

**Pseudotumours are capable of accumulating and excreting radiopharmaceuticals — unlike true tumours.**

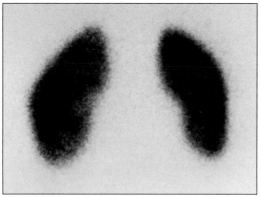

*a Posterior*

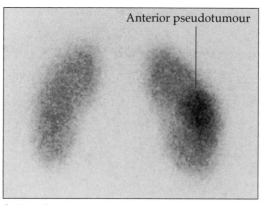

Anterior pseudotumour

*b Anterior*

**Investigating a pseudotumour:**
- **Multiple views using DMSA are necessary**
- **Careful correlation with IVU or ultrasound is essential.**

### Fig. 3.93

*In this case a mass had been identified on ultrasound and confirmed by an IVU. A DMSA scan was performed to assess whether the mass represented functional renal tissue. On the posterior (a) and anterior (b) views there is no space-occupying lesion seen, and the anterior view shows a functioning swelling at the site of the mass. This study therefore confirmed the presence of a pseudotumour, which requires no further investigation or treatment.*

## Tumour

### Hypernephroma

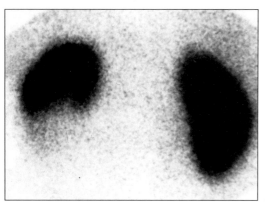

*a*

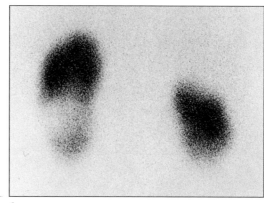

*b*

### Fig. 3.94

*(a–d) Four cases of hypernephroma, showing a variety of appearances on posterior DMSA imaging.*

*There are no specific features to suggest malignant tumour rather than other causes of space-occupying renal masses.*

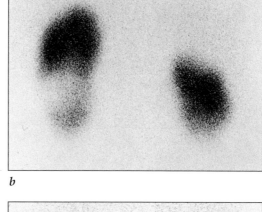

*c*

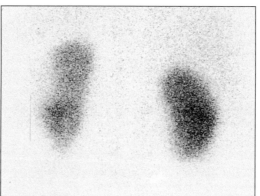

*d*

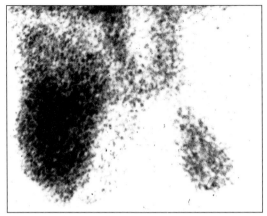

*a  30 seconds, blood flow*

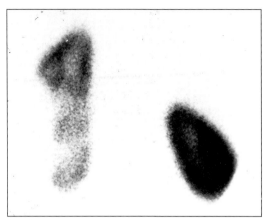

*b  3 hours*

### Fig. 3.95

*(a, b)* DMSA *scan. Hyper-nephroma of the left kidney.*

*The markedly increased blood flow to the tumour corresponds to the area of absent function shown on the scan.*

## Renal cyst

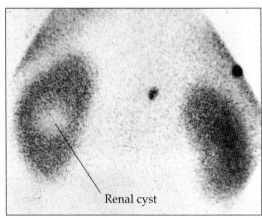

Renal cyst

*a*

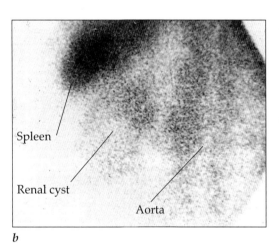

Spleen

Renal cyst

Aorta

*b*

### Fig. 3.96

*The photon-deficient area on the* DMSA *scan (a) corresponds to a similar photon-deficient area on the* $^{99m}$*Tc red blood cell scan (b). Absent blood flow makes a hypernephroma unlikely.*

 **The early 30-second images of the** DMSA **scan can be used to assess renal perfusion of a lesion.**

## Renal calculus

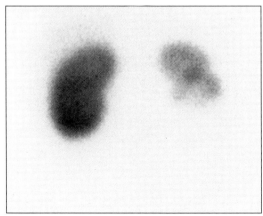

*a  Anterior*

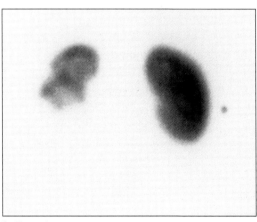

*b  Posterior*

### Fig. 3.97

*A 52-year-old woman with a left-sided staghorn calculus scan on* IVU.

*The* DMSA *scan (a,b) confirms impaired function on the left side (23% of* GFR) *and identifies that the lower pole of the left kidney is non-functioning.*

## 3.4.7    Congenital and ectopic abnormalities

### Congenital abnormalities

- Reduplication
- Cystic disease:
  - (a)  Infantile
  - (b)  Adult
  - (c)  Polycystic
  - (d)  Solitary cysts
  - (e)  Medullary sponge kidney

- Abnormalities of fusion:
  - (a)  Horseshoe kidney
  - (b)  Crossed renal ectopia
- Abnormalities of ascent:
  - (a)  Pancake kidney
  - (b)  Pelvic kidney.

### Reduplication

*Duplex kidney*

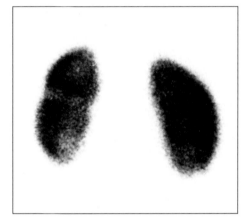
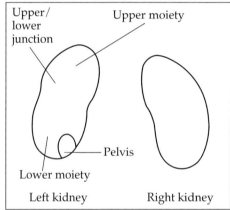

*Fig. 3.98*

*Posterior DMSA scan of a typical duplex kidney on the left side.*

- A duplex system is suspected if there is scan evidence of:
  - (a) elongated kidney
  - (b) lateral mid-zone impression
  - (c) unusual position of collecting system.
- The reduplicated ureters from a duplex kidney may:
  - (a) join soon after leaving the upper or lower moiety
  - (b) join anywhere between the kidney and the bladder
  - (c) enter the bladder separately.
- A duplex system is associated with reflux, which occurs most often in the lower moiety.
- The upper moiety may become obstructed.

**CLINICAL APPLICATIONS**

## *Cystic disease*

### *Polycystic kidneys*

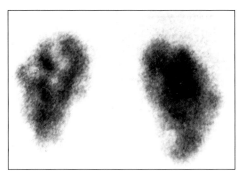

*a* Case 1, Posterior

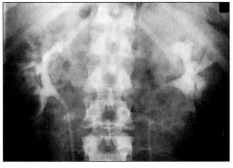

*b* Case 1, IVU

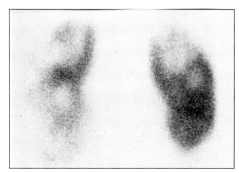

*c* Case 2, Posterior

**Fig. 3.99**

**Case 1 (a)** *Posterior* DMSA *scan, showing multiple photon-deficient areas in both kidneys.*
**(b)** *An* IVU *of the same patient.*
**Case 2: (c)** *Posterior* DMSA, *showing large cysts in both kidneys.*
    *In both cases multiple space-occupying lesions are present on* DMSA *studies, in keeping with known polycystic disease.*

### *Solitary cyst*

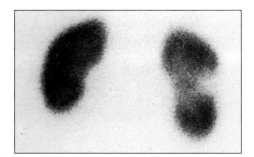

*a* Posterior

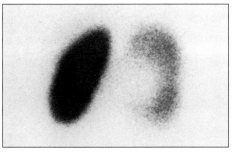

*b* Left posterior

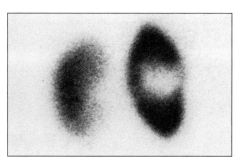

*c* Right posterior, oblique

**Fig. 3.100**

*(a–c)* DMSA *scan in a 64-year-old man who presented with left-sided renal colic and symptoms of prostatic enlargement.*
    *A large non-functioning focal lesion is seen in the mid-zone of the right kidney. This right renal cyst, which was confirmed on ultrasound, was an incidental finding. The left kidney is seen to be normal.*

### *Medullary sponge kidney*

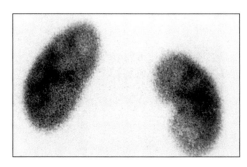

**Fig. 3.101**

*On the* DMSA *study patchy distribution of the tracer is seen throughout the parenchyma of both kidneys, which have prominent calyces.*

## Abnormalities of fusion

### Horseshoe kidney

Fusion occurs between the lower poles. The connecting bridge may function normally or act as a fibrous bridge. The axes of the kidney will incline towards the midline. Obstruction, stone, and infection are common complications.

### Horseshoe kidney with impaired function

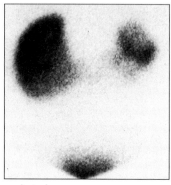 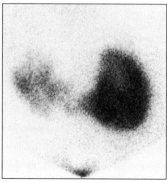

*a* Anterior     *b* Posterior

**Fig. 3.102**

*(a, b)* DMSA scan.
   *The decreased left-sided function in this case is caused by infection.*

### Horseshoe kidney and obstruction

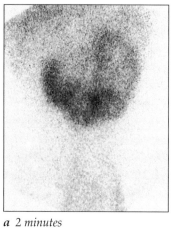 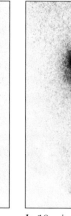 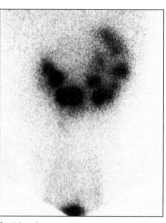  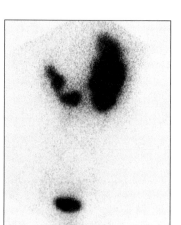 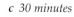 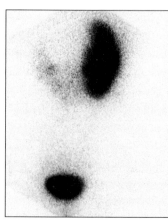

*a* 2 minutes     *b* 10 minutes     *c* 30 minutes     *d* 15 minutes

**Fig. 3.103**

*A 15-year-old male with horseshoe kidney who developed left hydronephrosis. Anterior view DTPA study: (a) 2-minute image; (b) 10-minute image; (c) 30-minute image after micturition, (d) 15-minute image after iv diuretic and (e) T/A curve after diuretic.*
   *The DTPA study shows a dilated left collecting system, which fails to wash out with diuretic. Measurements show only 18% washout with a $T_{1/2}$ of 148 minutes.*

*e*

## *Abnormalities of ascent*

### *Pelvic kidney*

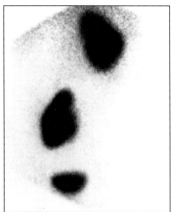

*a Anterior*

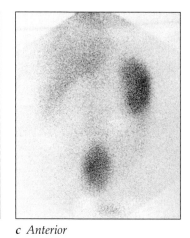

*b Anterior*

*c Anterior*

**Fig. 3.104**

Three cases of pelvic kidney imaged with DMSA anteriorly. Usually the kidney is well separated from the bladder **(a)**, but confusion with the bladder and the possibility of overlooking the pelvic kidney may occur if the kidney is superimposed on the bladder **(b)**, or when there is chronic renal failure **(c)**.

• If an ectopic kidney is suspected, or only one kidney is seen on the posterior view, always obtain anterior views which include the pelvis.
• Be sure that the 'bladder' is not a pelvic kidney.
• If necessary, re-image after micturition.

### *Pancake kidney*

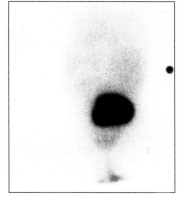

*a Posterior*

*b Anterior*

**Fig. 3.105**

**(a, b)** DMSA scan in a 2-year-old child with a solitary midline kidney or pancake kidney.

### *Cross-fused renal ectopia*

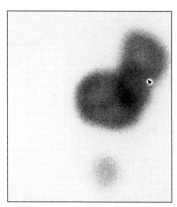

*a Anterior*

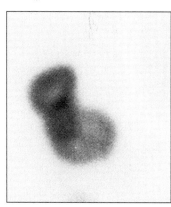

*b Posterior*

**Fig. 3.106**

**(a, b)** DMSA scan in a 5-year-old child with spina bifida, demonstrating cross-fused renal ectopia.

## Obstructed pelvic kidney

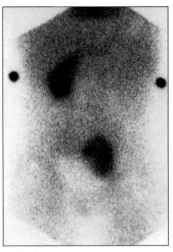

*a* 1 minute

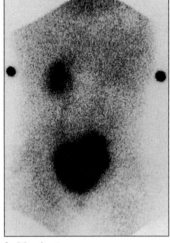

*b* 20 minutes

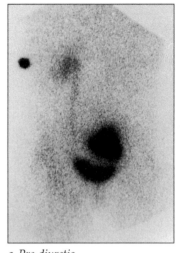

*c* Pre-diuretic

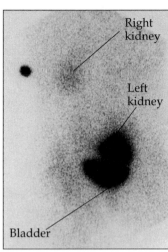

Right
kidney

Left
kidney

Bladder

*d* Post-diuretic

**Fig. 3.107**

DTPA *scan. An 8-year-old child with known spina bifida and a pelvic kidney.*

*The child had been troubled with recent recurrent urinary tract infections, and stones were noted in the pelvic kidney on an* IVU. *The function was difficult to assess on the* IVU, *and a* DTPA *study was requested to assess function in the pelvic kidney and the degree of obstruction. The 1-minute image (a) shows a pelvic kidney and a photon-deficient bladder. The 20-minute image (b) shows filling of the bladder with a dilated collecting system in the pelvic kidney. The images before (c) and after (d) diuretic show poor drainage from the partially obstructed pelvic kidney.*

*The* DTPA *study clearly shows that both kidneys are of approximately equal function, calculated at 48% of the total* GFR *in the left pelvic kidney. It is also apparent that there is gross dilatation of the collecting system, with some obstruction of outflow from the pelvic kidney.*

**A pelvic kidney may be confused with bladder activity in a neonate.**

## Pelvic kidney with dilatation

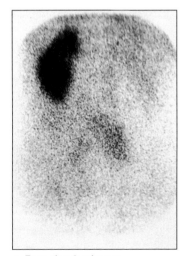

*a* Posterior, 2 minutes

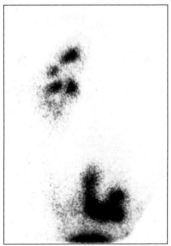

*b* Posterior, 20 minutes

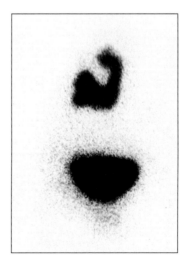

*c* Anterior, 30 minutes

**Fig. 3.108**

*(a–d)* DTPA *renal scan.*

*This scan shows how poorly the pelvic kidney may be visualized from the posterior aspect in the early phases. Note that dilatation without obstruction is frequently seen in a pelvic kidney because there is failure of full development as well as failure of ascent.*

# 3.4.8   Vascular disorders and hypertension

## Indications for assessment of renal blood supply with radionuclides

* When diminished renal blood supply is suspected:
  (a) Hypertension, due to renal artery stenosis
  (b) Renal infarction
     (i)  Whole kidney
     (ii) Focal, eg embolus
* Pre- and post-intervention follow-up:
  (a) Before surgery for aortic aneurysm
  (b) Before surgery for renal artery stenosis
  (c) Before angioplasty.

## Indications for investigation of hypertension with radionuclides

* Patient under 40 years with severe hypertension
* IVU suggests features of renal artery stenosis
* Renal bruit
* Hypertension associated with known arterial disease, eg Takayasu's disease
* Hypertension poorly controlled with antihypertensives
* Deteriorating renal function.

## Renal artery stenosis (RAS)

### Choice of radiopharmaceutical

* $^{99m}$Tc DMSA is rapid, reliable and cheap as a screening test. Significant RAS results in lower DMSA uptake. A difference of greater than ±5% should be investigated further.

* $^{123}$I hippuran measures renal plasma flow. RAS causes decreased uptake and delayed intrarenal transit time.
* $^{99m}$Tc MAG3 is now a cheaper and more available alternative to $^{123}$I hippuran.

### $^{123}$I hippuran

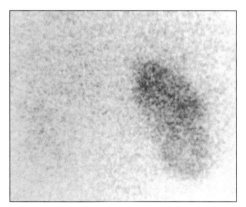

a 1 minute

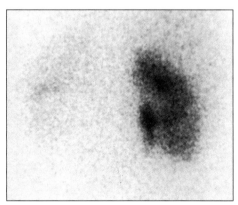

b 5 minutes

c 10 minutes

d

```
                              8858          ■ RIGHT
                                            ▪ LEFT



                              1489

    PEAK(SEC)        260
    PEAK(SEC)        40.0
    RIGHT %GFR       76.0
    LEFT  %GFR       23.0
```

**Fig. 3.109**

**(a–c)** *Hippuran scan in a patient who presented with hypertension.* **(d)** *T/A curve.*

*The study shows the delayed accumulation of $^{123}$I hippuran in a normal-sized left kidney typical of RAS.*

## CLINICAL APPLICATIONS

$^{99m}Tc$ MAG3

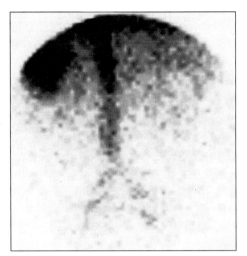 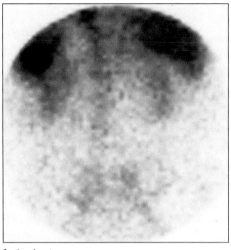 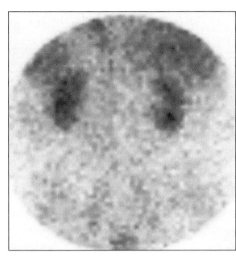

*a 0–30 seconds*  *b 1 minute*  *c 20 minutes*

### Fig. 3.110

*(a–c)* MAG3 *scan in a 52-year-old man with a history of peripheral vascular disease and hypertension.*

*Bruit heard over the abdomen together with the scan demonstrate poorly perfused, small kidneys with prolonged transit. An arteriogram confirmed severe aortic and renal artery stenosis.*

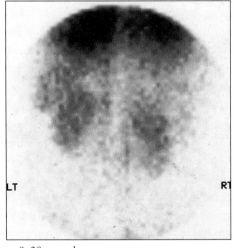 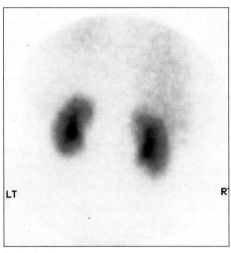 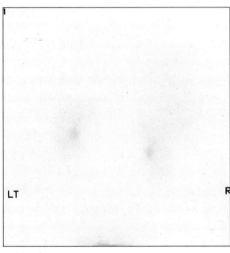

*a 0–30 seconds*  *b 1 minute*  *c 20 minutes*

### Fig. 3.111

*A 29-year-old woman with a history of renal artery stenosis was treated surgically.*

*The postoperative $^{99m}Tc$ MAG3 study (a–c) demonstrates good symmetrical perfusion and function, confirming resolution of the renal artery stenosis.*

 MAG3 or hippuran, because of their closer dependence on renal plasma flow, are more sensitive than DTPA for detecting impaired renal blood flow. Quantitation of uptake, retention and transit times will add information to the visual inspection of images.

## CLINICAL APPLICATIONS

*DTPA*

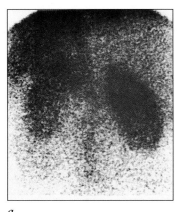 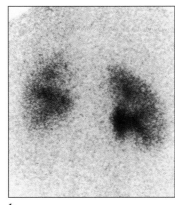

*a*        *b*

**Fig. 3.112**

*(a, b) A DTPA scan performed on the same patient as in Fig. 3.109 shows some diminution of blood flow and function, but the changes are less marked.*

*DMSA and* $^{123}I$ *hippuran*

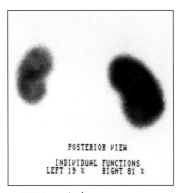 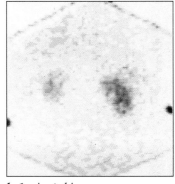 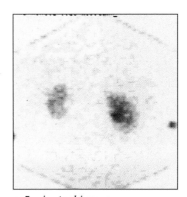 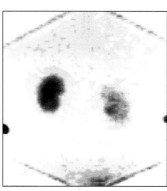

*a* DMSA, *posterior*     *b* 1 minute hippuran     *c* 5 minutes hippuran     *d* 20 minutes hippuran

**Fig. 3.113**

*A 70-year-old man who was being investigated for uncontrolled hypertension. (a) Posterior DMSA scan. (b–d)* $^{123}I$ *hippuran scan at 1 minute (b), 5 minutes (c) and 20 minutes (d) after injection.*

*The initial screening study with DMSA shows decreased function of the left kidney. Because of the discrepancy between the two kidneys, a* $^{123}I$ *hippuran scan was performed; this showed the typical feature of delayed tracer transit through the left renal parenchyma.*

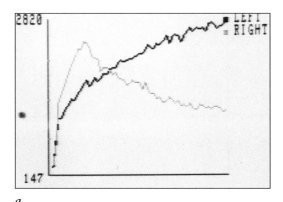 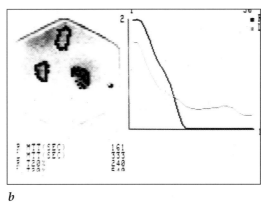

*a*        *b*

**Fig. 3.114**

*The T/A curve (a) from both kidneys in the same patient as in Fig. 3.113 shows the delayed accumulation in the left kidney. The parenchymal transit times and retention functions (b) confirm the delayed parenchymal transit line.*

## Segmental RAS

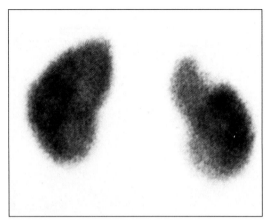

a  Posterior, DMSA

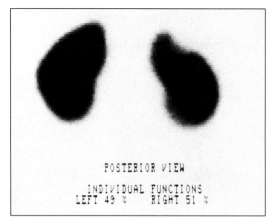

POSTERIOR VIEW

INDIVIDUAL FUNCTIONS
LEFT 49 %    RIGHT 51 %

b Quantitation

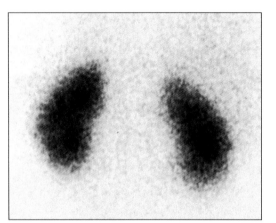

c  2 minutes, hippuran

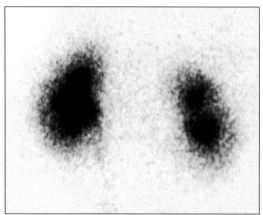

d  15 minutes, hippuran

### Fig. 3.115

A 16 year old female who presented with malignant hypertension. Previous investigations, including IVU, ultrasound and arteriogram, were all normal.

The posterior DMSA scan (a) shows a large clear-cut defect at the upper pole of the right kidney. Quantitation (b) shows no overall difference in function. On the 2-minute hippuran study (c) the lesion is undetectable, but the 15-minute hippuran scan (d) shows prolonged retention at the site of the lesion which is partly due to delayed transit caused by 'segmental artery stenosis'. A subsequent selective arteriogram confirmed an arterial lesion at that site, and partial nephrectomy cured the hypertension.

- DMSA is very sensitive for segmental RAS.
- DMSA and hippuran together may provide the best evaluation of suspected renal hypertension.
- DMSA and hippuran scans can be performed on the same hospital visit.

## Bilateral RAS

### Pre-angiogram

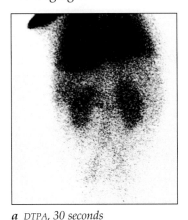

*a* DTPA, 30 seconds

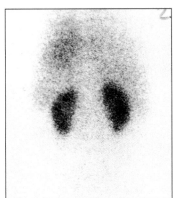

*b* DTPA, 2 minutes

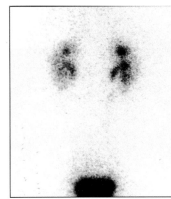

*c* DTPA, 20 minutes

### Fig. 3.116

*A 15-year-old male who presented with hypertension. (a–c)* DTPA *renal scan. (d, e) arteriogram showing multiple stenoses. (f)* DMSA *scan.*

*The initial* DTPA *and* DMSA *scans were normal, in spite of bilateral* RAS.

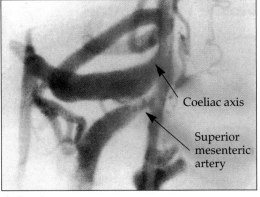
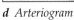

*d* Arteriogram

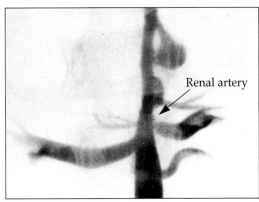

*e* Arteriogram

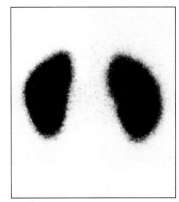

*f* DMSA

### Post-angiogram

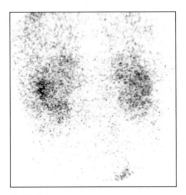

*a* DMSA

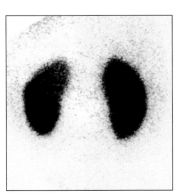

*b* DMSA

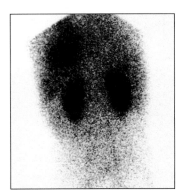

*c* DTPA

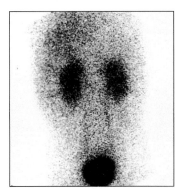

*d* DTPA

### Fig. 3.117

*Same case as in Fig. 3.116.* DMSA *scan: (a) following arteriogram; (b) 2 weeks later.* DTPA *scan: (c) 1-minute image; (d) 20-minute image (both also 2 weeks later).*

*Following the arteriogram, there was an episode of acute renal failure, and the* DMSA *scan shows no uptake. After recovery the* DMSA *scan shows a focal defect at the upper pole of the left kidney, and the* DTPA *scan now shows delayed parenchymal transit time.*

- **Radionuclide investigations depend on asymmetry, and therefore symmetrical RAS may be missed, but prolonged transit times may be measurable.**
- **When RAS is critical, contrast agents for x-ray procedures may cause renal failure.**

## Renal infarct

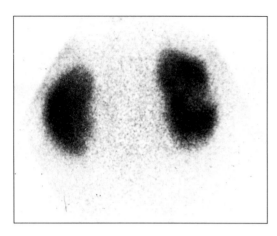

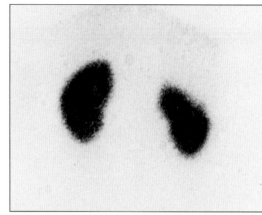

**Fig. 3.118**

*A 63-year-old man who was admitted with a 12-hour history of right loin pain. He was known to be sensitive to contrast media. The DMSA scan shows a focal lesion in the right kidney attributable to a renal infarct.*

**Fig. 3.119**

*A 60-year-old man with mitral valve disease and atrial fibrillation who developed loin pain. The DMSA scan shows focal loss of renal tissue in the upper pole, attributable to renal infarction.*

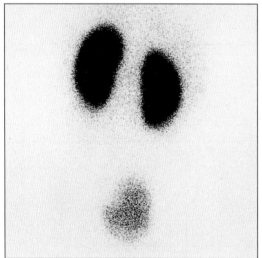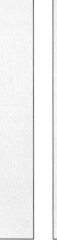

*a 0 months*

*b 7 months*

**Fig. 3.120**

*A 14-year-old boy with neurofibromatosis. Renal scan (DMSA): **(a)** initial study; **(b)** repeat study 7 months later.*

*This patient was known to have neurofibromatosis and presented with hypertension. The possibility of renal artery stenosis was considered and a DMSA study was obtained as part of the initial work-up. This was normal. However, the repeat study 7 months later showed no function on the right. The patient had undergone an autonephrectomy.*

## *Preoperative assessment of aortic aneurysm*

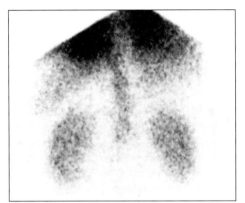

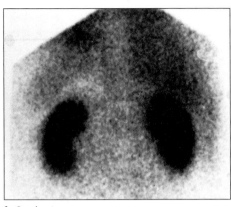

*a 30 seconds*

*b 2 minutes*

**Fig. 3.121**

*(a, b)* DTPA scan. A patient with a stenosis of the descending aorta.

   The arteriogram and IVU suggested loss of perfusion to the left kidney. A DTPA scan was performed to assess the perfusion and function preoperatively. The kidneys can be seen to be well perfused with symmetrical function. The level of aortic narrowing can be easily seen.

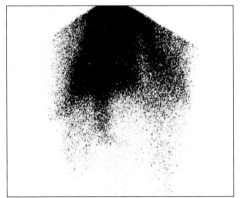

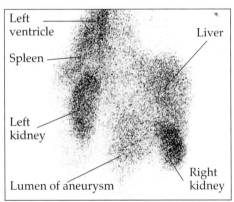

Left ventricle

Liver

Spleen

Left kidney

Lumen of aneurysm

Right kidney

*a 30 seconds*

*b 2 minutes*

**Fig. 3.122**

*(a, b)* DTPA scan. A 74-year-old man with an aortic aneurysm.

   Radionuclide investigation was performed to assess the preoperative blood flow of both kidneys. The DTPA scan shows good blood flow to both kidneys symmetrically, with normal aortic lumen to the level of the renal arteries. The 2-minute image shows a dilated aortic lumen below the aortic artery.

- Nuclear medicine studies are not diagnostic of an aneurysm — only the lumen is identified.
- All patients should have a renal blood flow study preoperatively as a baseline.

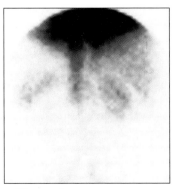

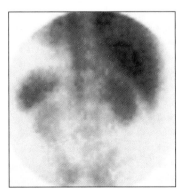

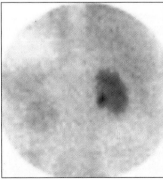

*a 30 seconds*

*b 2 minutes*

*c 20 minutes*

**Fig. 3.123**

*(a–c)* DTPA scan in a 69-year-old man, showing severely impaired perfusion following aortic dissection. The left kidney is extremely poorly perfused and is not functioning; the right kidney is poorly perfused and is functioning poorly. Non-visualization of the lower aorta is noted.

## CLINICAL APPLICATIONS

### *Follow-up after surgery or angioplasty*

*Preoperative*

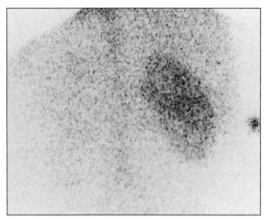

*a  30 seconds*

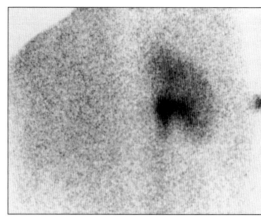

*b  10 minutes*

**Fig. 3.124**

*The preoperative DTPA scan images at 30 seconds (**a**) and 10 minutes (**b**) show poor blood flow and function on the left. The corresponding DTPA scan images postoperatively (**c, d**) show loss of perfusion and function of the left kidney. These last two scan images also show a large haematoma on the left side caused by bleeding, and associated induced ATN of the right kidney.*

*Postoperative*

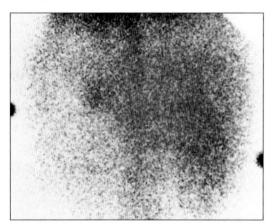

*c  30 seconds*

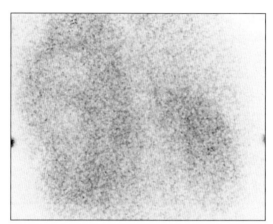

*d  10 minutes*

## Functional assessment of angioplasty

*Features of RAS affected by angioplasty*

- Decreased renal blood flow
- Decreased GFR
- Delayed excretion
- Prolonged mean parenchymal transit time.

*Pre-angioplasty*

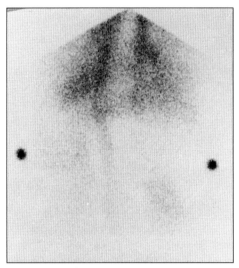

*a 0–30 seconds*

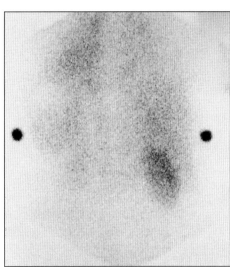

*b 1–2 minutes*

### Fig. 3.125

A 61-year-old woman with known bilateral RAS and malignant hypertension. Pre- and post-angioplasty. Renal scan (dynamic DTPA): **(a)** perfusion view (0–30 seconds); **(b)** parenchymal function (1–2 minutes); **(c)** perfusion view (0–30 seconds); **(d)** parenchymal function (1–2 minutes).

On the original study **(a, b)** both kidneys show impaired blood flow and impaired function, the left kidney being more severely affected than the right. Following angioplasty of the right renal artery, there has been marked improvement in the perfusion and function of the right kidney **(c, d)**.

*Post-angioplasty*

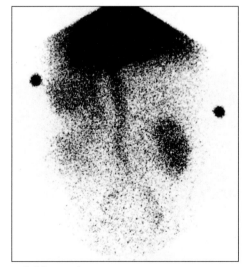

*c 0–30 seconds*

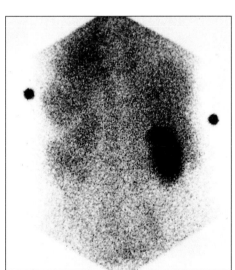

*d 1–2 minutes*

## Pre-angioplasty

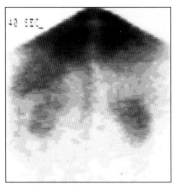

*a* 0–30 seconds

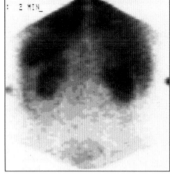

*b* 2 minutes

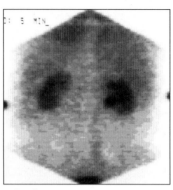

*c* 5 minutes

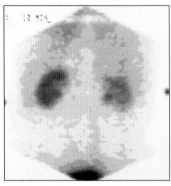

*d* 10 minutes

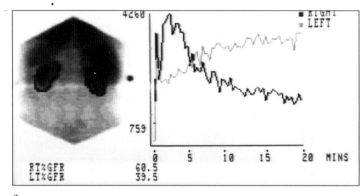

RT%GFR   60.5
LT%GFR   39.5

*e*

## Post-angioplasty

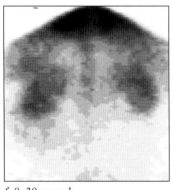

*f* 0–30 seconds

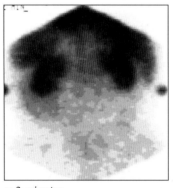

*g* 2 minutes

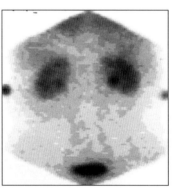

*h* 5 minutes

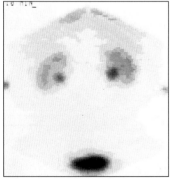
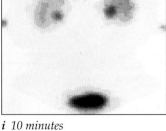

RT%GFR   49.9
LT%GFR   50.1

*i* 10 minutes

*j*

### *Fig. 3.126*

*Renal artery stenosis.* DTPA *scans, (a–d) pre- and (f–i) post-angioplasty.*

*Vascular phase: (a) pre-angioplasty; (f) post-angioplasty. Note the decreased blood flow in the left kidney, which improves after angioplasty.*

*2-minute image: (b) pre-angioplasty; (g) post-angioplasty. Note the decreased uptake (38%) in the left kidney increasing after angioplasty to 50% of the total* GFR.

*5-minute image: (c) pre-angioplasty; (h) post-angioplasty. Note the delay in excretion of tracer from the left side becoming equal after angioplasty.*

*10-minute image: (d) pre-angioplasty; (i) post-angioplasty. Note again the relative increase in tracer uptake on the left side becoming equal after angioplasty; this reflects an improved mean transit time on the left side.*

*T/A curves (e) and (j): note the delayed accumulation and decreased* GFR *before angioplasty, which improves after treatment.*

**Functional follow-up with tracers is the optimal method for investigating the effect of angioplasty, ie the effect of the stenoses is more important than the appearance.**

## *Postoperative assessment*

*Preoperative*

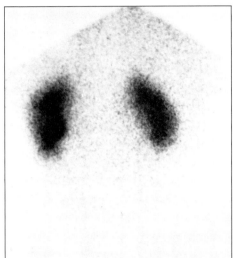

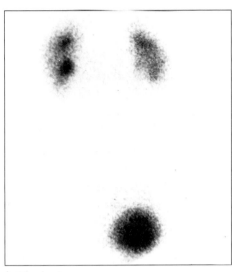

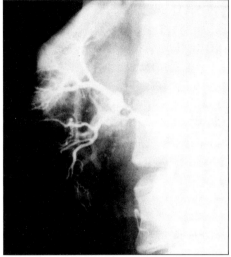

*a 5 minutes*

*b 20 minutes*

*c*

*Postoperative*

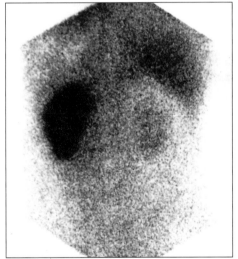

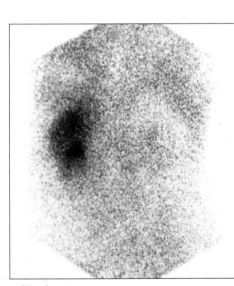

*d 5 minutes*

*e 20 minutes*

### Fig. 3.127

*A 25-year-old patient with hypertension caused by right renal artery stenosis. (**a, b**) Initial DTPA scan. (**c**) Arteriogram, showing tight right RAS. (**d, e**) Postoperative DTPA scan.*

*The initial DTPA scan shows relatively normal blood flow, but with slightly decreased function and prolonged transit of the right kidney. The immediately postoperative follow-up scan for assessment shows gross loss of function, with a surrounding 'halo' caused by a perirenal haematoma, which was subsequently evacuated.*

## 3.4.9   Renal transplant

### *Renal transplant complications*

- Rejection:
  - (a) Hyperacute (irreversible)
  - (b) Acute (reversible)
  - (c) Chronic
- ATN
- Drugs — cyclosporin
- Vascular complications:
  - (a) Renal artery occlusion
- (b) Renal artery stenosis
- (c) Renal venothrombosis
- (d) Renal infarct
- Urinary complications:
  - (a) Leaks
  - (b) Lymphocoele
  - (c) Obstruction
- Biopsy complications.

### *Normal renal transplant*

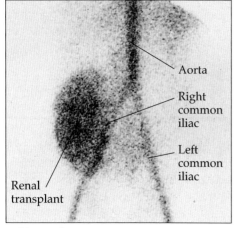 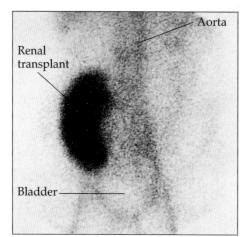 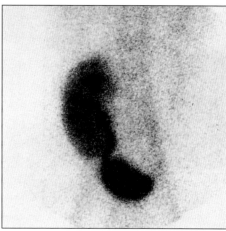

*a  30 seconds*

*b  2 minutes*

*c  30 minutes*

**Fig. 3.128**

*Dynamic (DTPA) renal scan of a normal renal transplant.*

## CLINICAL APPLICATIONS

### Quantitation

Quantitative information can be obtained from a dynamic renal scan in transplant patients, which may be of considerable value in the serial assessment of these patients. The two main parameters which are measured are (1) flow index which is derived from the first 30 seconds of the study and reflects renal blood flow; and (2) uptake index which is derived from the image at 1–2 minutes and reflects parenchymal function.

$$(1)\ \frac{\text{Flow}}{\text{index}} = \frac{\text{Iliac area to peak}}{\text{Renal area to peak}} \times 100$$

$$(2)\ \text{Uptake} = \frac{\text{Renal counts/pixel}}{\text{Background counts/pixel}} \times 100$$

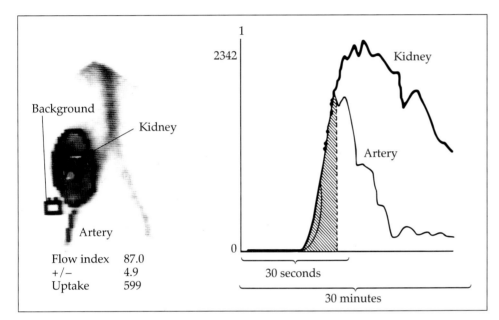

Flow index 87.0
+/− 4.9
Uptake 599

**Fig. 3.129**

*Quantitation in a renal transplant patient*

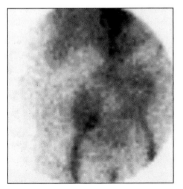

*a  0–30 seconds*  *b  5 minutes*  *c*

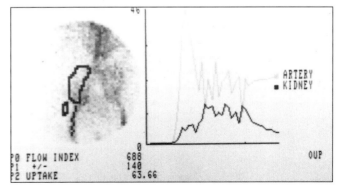

**Fig. 3.130**

*Quantitation in a poorly perfused, poorly functioning transplant. (a, b) Dynamic DTPA scan. (c) Transplant renogram curve with flow index and uptake index.*

This 42-year-old woman had a renal transplant performed which functioning well initially. Two weeks after transplant the urine output fell. The scan shows a poorly perfused, poorly functioning transplant with a high flow index indicating poor perfusion and a low uptake index indicating poor function.

## Variants

### End-to-side anastomosis

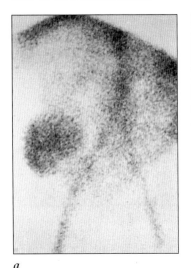
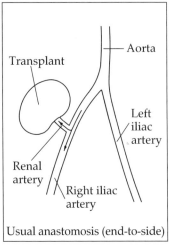

*a*

### End-to-end anastomosis

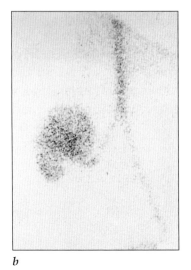
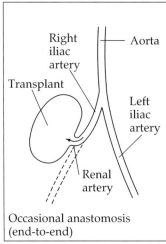

*b*

**Fig. 3.131**

30-second DTPA *images.*

*The most common anastomosis in renal transplant surgery is an end-to-side anastomosis **(a)**, usually employing a patch of iliac artery from the donor. Occasionally, an end-to-end anastomosis **(b)** is necessary because of the lack of arterial tissue. This is much more likely to result in renal artery stenosis, and obviously the distal iliac artery cannot be used as an area of interest to compare with renal blood flow.*

### Renal transplant in pregnancy

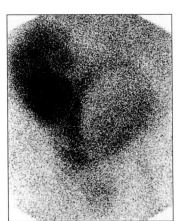

5 minutes

**Fig. 3.132**

DTPA *renal scan of a pregnant renal transplant patient, showing the uterus and placenta.*

### Renal transplant with renal polycystic disease

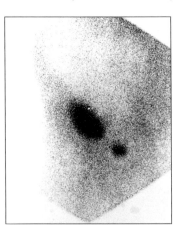

**Fig. 3.133**

DTPA *renal scan of a patient with massive polycystic kidneys and a renal transplant, showing a large photon-deficient area attributable to polycystic renal mass.*

## CLINICAL APPLICATIONS

### *Acute rejection*

*Features of acute rejection*

- Decreased blood flow
- Decreased uptake
- Prolonged intrarenal transit time

- Decreased excretion
- Ureteric dilatation
- Increased renal size.

*Day 1 post-transplant*

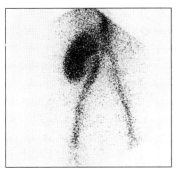 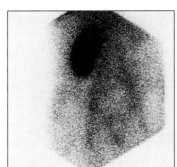

*a  30 seconds*    *b  2 minutes*

*Day 4 post-transplant*

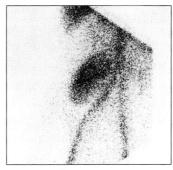 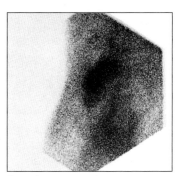

*e  30 seconds*    *f  2 minutes*

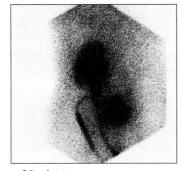

*c  20 minutes*

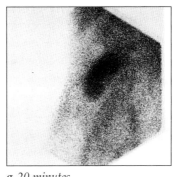

*g  20 minutes*

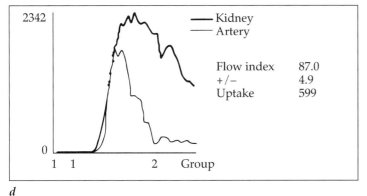

| | |
|---|---|
| Flow index | 87.0 |
| +/− | 4.9 |
| Uptake | 599 |

*d*

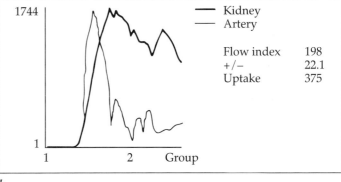

| | |
|---|---|
| Flow index | 198 |
| +/− | 22.1 |
| Uptake | 375 |

*h*

### Fig. 3.134

*The common DTPA scan appearances of acute rejection, showing decreased blood flow and function. Day 1 post-transplant: (**a**) 30 seconds, good blood flow; (**b**) 2 minutes, good uptake; (**c**) 20 minutes, good excretion (note catheter); (**d**) T/A curves, with flow indices and uptake. Day 4 post-transplant: (**e**) 30 seconds, decreased blood flow; (**f**) 2 minutes, decreased uptake; (**g**) 20 minutes, no excretion; (**h**) T/A curves, with flow indices and uptake.*

**On the DTPA scan alone rejection and cyclosporin toxicity are indistinguishable; both may cause decreased perfusion and decreased GFR.**

## *Severe acute rejection*

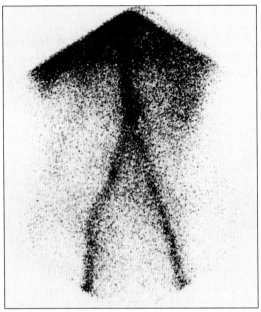

*a 30 seconds*

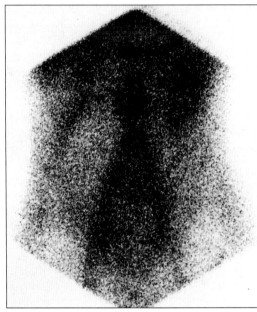

*b 2 minutes*

### *Fig. 3.135*

*(a, b) DTPA images. Same case as in Fig. 3.134.*

*Despite antirejection therapy, this episode progressed to an avascular irreversible graft.*

*Note the photon-deficient area at the site of the kidney and the vascular rim around the rejected graft caused by a hyperaemic inflammatory response.*

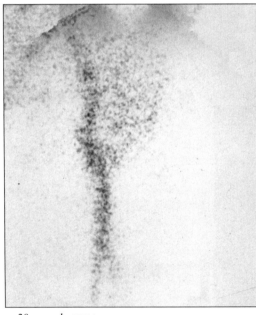

*a 30 seconds, DTPA*

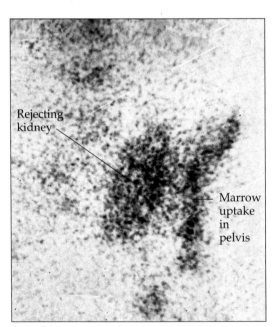

Rejecting kidney

Marrow uptake in pelvis

*b Colloid*

### *Fig. 3.136*

*A further case of acute rejection.*

*The 30-second DTPA image (a) shows poor blood flow. The sulphur colloid scan (b) shows high uptake of tracer in the rejecting kidney.*

*In addition to sulphur colloid, other agents such as indium-labelled white cells or platelets have been advocated for the detection of acute rejection. However, these agents are relatively insensitive.*

## *Chronic rejection*

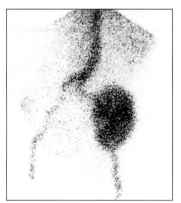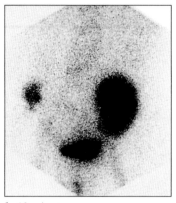

*a 30 seconds*          *b 10 minutes*

### Fig. 3.137

*A 49-year-old man with a well-functioning, left-sided renal transplant, together with a previous right-sided transplant which shows the end stages of a chronically rejected graft.*

*On the vascular DTPA image (a) the left-sided transplant is seen to be well perfused, but there is markedly impaired perfusion to the right kidney. The 10-minute image (b) shows the left kidney to be normal in size with good function. However, the right kidney is small, shows irregular cortical outline and has poor function.*

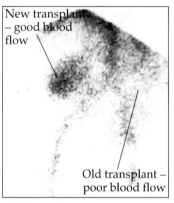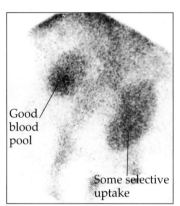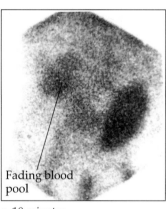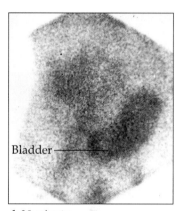

New transplant – good blood flow

Old transplant – poor blood flow

Good blood pool

Some selective uptake

Fading blood pool

Bladder

*a 30 seconds*   *b 2 minutes*   *c 10 minutes*   *d 30 minutes*

### Fig. 3.138

*(a–d) A patient with a chronically rejected left-sided renal transplant, together with a new right-sided transplant which shows the features of ATN.*

*This series of DTPA images illustrates well the different features of ATN and chronic rejection.*

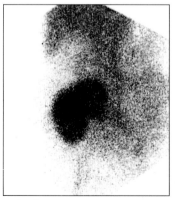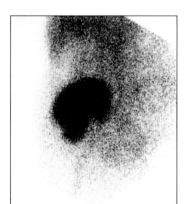

*a 2 minutes*          *b 2 minutes*

### Fig. 3.139

*Renal scarring in chronic rejection. DTPA images of a renal transplant at 2 minutes: (a) soon after the graft had been inserted and (b) several months later, showing the development of a lower pole scar.*

 **Progressive renal scarring is frequently seen in a chronic deteriorating transplant.**

## *Two cases of cortical scarring in renal transplants demonstrated on DMSA scans*

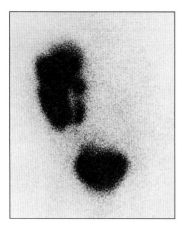

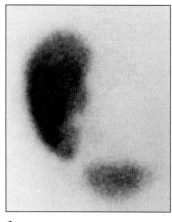

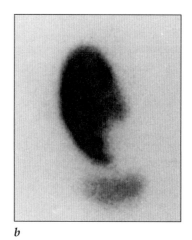

*a*

*b*

**Fig. 3.140**

*In this case, the renal outline is markedly irregular, indicating extensive cortical scarring.*

**Fig. 3.141**

*In this case there was deterioration of function of the renal transplant. A DTPA scan raised the possibility of thinning of the lower pole. The DMSA scan (a) confirmed a lower pole scar, but note that this is best demonstrated on the oblique view (b).*

## *Transplant ATN*

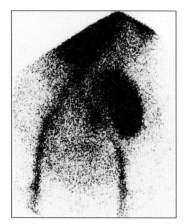

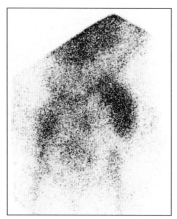

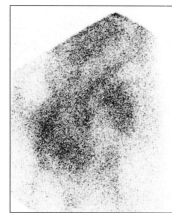

*a  30 seconds*

*b  2 minutes*

*c  20 minutes*

**Fig. 3.142**

*Typical ATN.*
*The DTPA 30-second image (a) shows excellent blood flow. The 2-minute image (b) shows a blood pool only, with no selective filtration. The 20-minute image (c) shows loss of the blood pool image as the tracer diffuses to the extracellular space. No excretion is seen.*

• ATN is a common finding postoperatively with non-related donor kidneys. The value of the DTPA scan is in monitoring the blood flow until function returns, which may take several weeks.

## *Vascular complications*

### *Acute vascular occlusion*

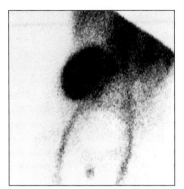

*a  30 seconds*

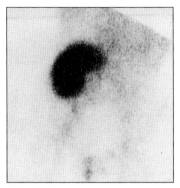

*b  2 minutes*

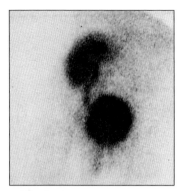

*c  10 minutes*

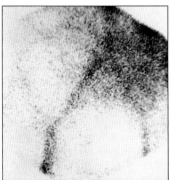

*d  30 seconds*

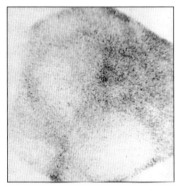

*e  2 minutes*

**Fig. 3.143**

*(a–c) Initial* DTPA *series of a normally functioning transplant. (d, e)* DTPA *images following acute renal artery occlusion causing graft infarction.*

### *Avascular graft*

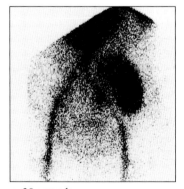

*a  30 seconds*

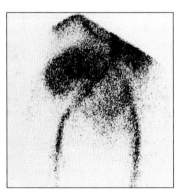

*b  30 seconds*

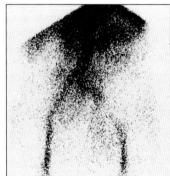

*c  30 seconds*

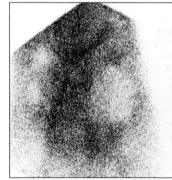

*d  2 minutes*

**Fig. 3.144**

*The initial 30-second* DTPA *scan (a) shows good perfusion of left renal transplant. Acute rejection then caused an avascular graft and a new transplant was inserted in the right iliac fossa, shown by the second* DTPA *scan (b); this subsequently became avascular as a result of renal artery thrombosis.*

*The final 30-second* DTPA *scan shows loss of perfusion of both transplants (c) with an avascular space in the 2-minute image (d).*

**Avascular graft may be due to:**
- **Arterial thrombosis**
- **End stage rejection**
- **Hyperacute rejection**
- **Venous occlusion.**

**These are indistinguishable on the scan.**

## CLINICAL APPLICATIONS

*Renal artery aneurysm*

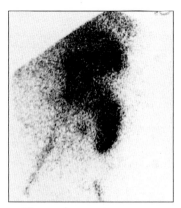
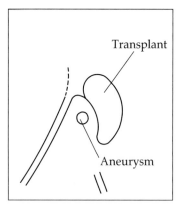
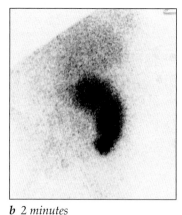
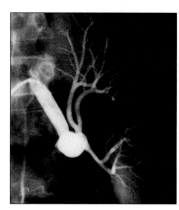

*a  30 seconds*                    *b  2 minutes*                    *c*

**Fig. 3.145**

*(a, b)* DTPA *dynamic phase. (c) Arteriogram. A renal transplant patient who developed an aneurysm at the renal artery anastomosis. The common iliac artery had been tied at the time of surgery. Absence of this vessel is seen on the* DTPA *scan.*

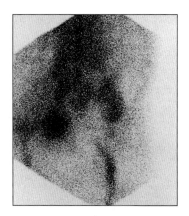
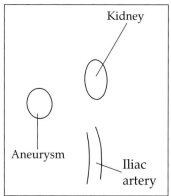

**Fig. 3.146**

*Internal iliac artery aneurysm. $^{99m}Tc$* DTPA *image of anterior pelvis, 1 minute after injection.*

*On the transplant study an aneurysm was noted arising from the right internal iliac artery. This patient died from an acute haemorrhage from the aneurysm before surgery could be performed.*

**CLINICAL APPLICATIONS**

## *Urinary complications*

### *Ureteric leaks*

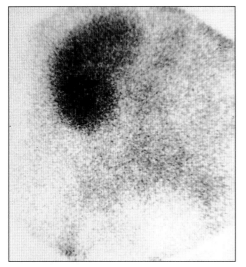 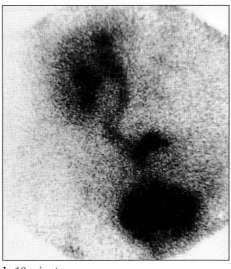 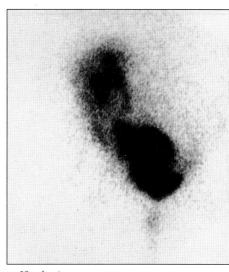

*a* 2 minutes     *b* 10 minutes     *c* 60 minutes

**Fig. 3.147**

*(a–c)* DTPA *scan series, showing a well-functioning transplant with a urine leak at the lower end of the ureter. The 60-minute image shows how the leak and the bladder may fuse and mask the finding of the leak.*

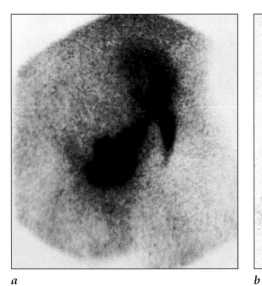 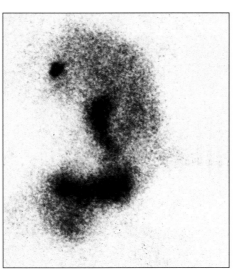 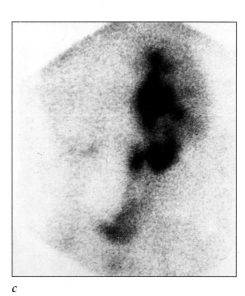

*a*     *b*     *c*

**Fig. 3.148**

*(a–c) Three further examples of the appearances of a urinary leak on the* DTPA *scan.*

- A functioning transplant is necessary to detect a leak.
- Delayed views and views after micturition may be necessary to detect the leak.
- Leaks are usually, but not always, painful.

## Lymphocoele

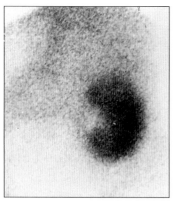 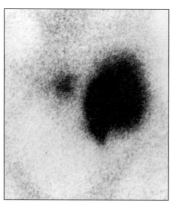

*a 5 minutes*  *b 30 minutes*

**Fig. 3.149**

*(a, b)* DTPA *scan of postoperative transplant lymphocoele in common position between the bladder and the kidney, causing pressure on the ureter and consequently obstruction.*

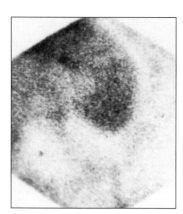

**Fig. 3.150**

DTPA *scan of transplant lymphocoele surrounding the kidney. There is distortion of the bladder but no obstruction.*

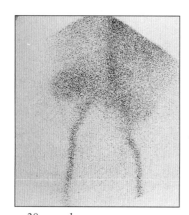 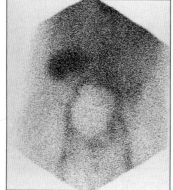 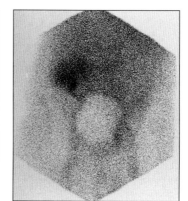 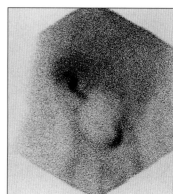

*a 30 seconds*  *b 1 minute*  *c 5 minutes*  *d 10 minutes*

**Fig. 3.151**

*(a–d)* Dynamic DTPA *phase image. A 4-week-old renal transplant with good perfusion and function.*
*The large pelvic lymphocele could be mistaken for a full bladder. Note the tracer collecting in the distorted bladder on the 10-minute image.*

## Obstruction

### Obstruction due to lymphocoele

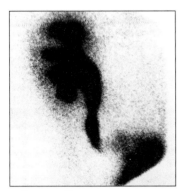

*a* Preoperative

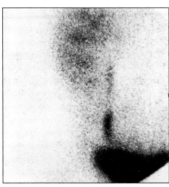

*b* Postoperative

**Fig. 3.152**

*The preoperative scan (a) shows a lymphocoele causing distortion of the bladder with ureteric partial obstruction. The postoperative scan (b) shows no distortion and free drainage.*

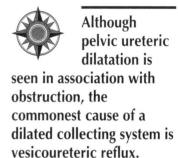

**Although pelvic ureteric dilatation is seen in association with obstruction, the commonest cause of a dilated collecting system is vesicoureteric reflux.**

### Obstruction due to blood clot

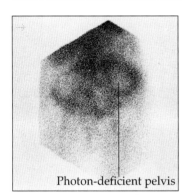

Photon-deficient pelvis

**Fig. 3.153**

*Obstruction with anuria. Obstruction may be a problem in a graft with primary non-function, and may be a cause for failure of the graft to recover from ATN or cyclosporin. The only clue may be, as here, a photon-deficient area centrally. In this case it was due to a blood clot in the renal pelvis.*

**Failure of recovery of function from ATN should be investigated with ultrasound to exclude obstruction.**

## *Biopsy complications*

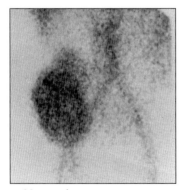

*a* 30 seconds

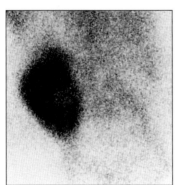

*b* 2 minutes

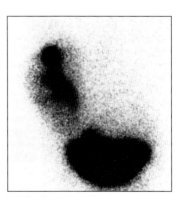

*c* 20 minutes

**Fig. 3.154**

*(a–c) DTPA scan, showing decreased perfusion at the upper pole, with an associated dilated calyx. This was due to a scar occurring after a renal biopsy.*

# CHAPTER 4

# TUMOUR

Nuclear medicine has a significant role to play in the management of oncology patients, contributing to both diagnosis and follow-up. In addition to diagnostic imaging, nuclear medicine techniques are also used in the treatment of malignancy.

Nuclear medicine investigations may be non-specific. Non-specific investigations are investigations that demonstrate tumour sites (usually secondary sites) but are not specific for malignancy. Non-specific techniques include technetium-99m ($^{99m}$Tc) liver/spleen colloid imaging for liver metastases, $^{99m}$Tc diphosphonate bone imaging for bone metastases, and thyroid imaging with $^{99m}$Tc pertechnetate ($^{99m}$TcO$_4$) and $^{99m}$Tc(V) dimercaptosuccinic acid ($^{99m}$Tc(V) DMSA) for primary medullary thyroid carcinomas. Thallium-201 ($^{201}$Tl) is also a radiopharmaceutical that, in addition to its established use in myocardial imaging, may be used to image tumours. Gallium-67 ($^{67}$Ga) citrate may be used to image a variety of tumours as well as sites of infection and inflammation. Lastly, $^{99m}$Tc nanocolloid may be used to visualize tumour deposits within bone

marrow and $^{99m}$Tc diethylenetriamine pentaacetic acid (DTPA), the dynamic renal imaging agent, has also been used to image neurofibromas.

Tumour imaging may also be undertaken with radiopharmaceuticals that are specific for tumours, such as iodine-123/131 *meta*-iodobenzylguanidine ($^{123/131}$I MIBG), which is specific for neuroendocrine tumours. Iodine-131 ($^{131}$I) is specific for follicular thyroid carcinomas, and indium-111 ($^{111}$In) octreotide is specific for tumours expressing somatostatin receptors.

Tumour-associated monoclonal antibodies labelled with $^{111}$In, $^{123}$I/$^{131}$I or $^{99m}$Tc have also been developed for tumour imaging. While many of these are still under evaluation, a few are now commercially available.

Tumour imaging studies contribute to the diagnosis, staging and follow-up of neoplastic disease. If significant tumour uptake is seen on the diagnostic study, some radiopharmaceuticals such as $^{131}$I and $^{131}$I MIBG may be used in therapeutic doses to treat the malignancy.

## CHAPTER CONTENTS

# 4.1   RADIOPHARMACEUTICALS

*Table 4.1   Radiopharmaceuticals for tumour imaging*

| Radiopharmaceutical | Tumour demonstrated |
|---|---|
| *Non-specific* | |
| $^{99m}$Tc liver/spleen colloid | Liver metastases |
| $^{99m}$Tc diphosphonate | Primary bone tumours<br>Bone metastases |
| $^{99m}$TcO$_4$ | Thyroid tumours |
| $^{201}$Tl | Medullary thyroid carcinoma |
| $^{99m}$Tc(V) DMSA | Medullary thyroid carcinoma |
| $^{67}$Ga | Lymphoma<br>Hepatoma<br>Bronchial carcinoma |
| $^{99m}$Tc nanocolloid | Bone marrow tumour deposits |
| $^{99m}$Tc DTPA | Neurofibromata |
| *Specific* | |
| $^{131}$I | Follicular thyroid carcinoma |
| $^{123/131}$I MIBG | Neuroendocrine NG |
| $^{111}$In octreotide | Somatostatin-receptor receptor-positive tumours |
| $^{111}$In/$^{123/131}$I/$^{99m}$Tc monoclonal antibodies | Specific antigen-positive tumours |

*Table 4.2   Mechanisms of tumour localization for tumour-specific agents*

| Site of localization | Mechanism |
|---|---|
| Intracellular | Metabolic, eg $^{131}$I, $^{131}$I MIBG |
| Tumour cell membrane | Receptor binding, eg $^{111}$In octreotide, $^{111}$In monoclonal antibodies |
| Surrounding normal tissue | Uptake into normal tissue adjacent to tumour site, eg liver/colloid uptake in normal Kupffer's cells adjacent to liver metastases |

# 4.2 NORMAL SCANS WITH VARIANTS AND ARTEFACTS

## 4.2.1 ⁹⁹ᵐTc liver/spleen colloid

⁹⁹ᵐTc colloid has a role in liver/spleen imaging by nature of its uptake in reticuloendothelial cells within these organs. Replacement of liver tissue by tumour cells can be visualized as photon-deficient areas.

**Fig. 4.1**

*(a–d) Normal ⁹⁹ᵐTc liver/spleen scan, showing uniform colloid uptake within the Kupffer's cells of the liver and the reticuloendothelial cells of the spleen. Uniform uptake is normal. Multiple views are required, however, to confirm the absence of photon-deficient lesions in all areas of the liver and spleen.*

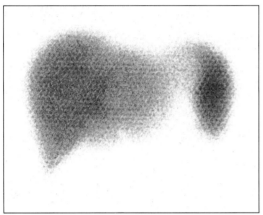

*a Anterior*

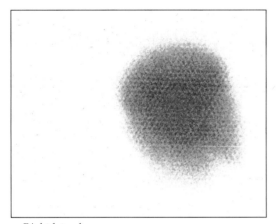

*b Posterior*

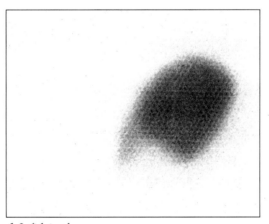

*c Right lateral*

*d Left lateral*

## 4.2.2 ⁹⁹ᵐTc diphosphonate

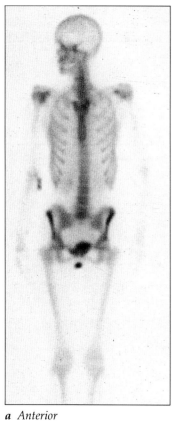 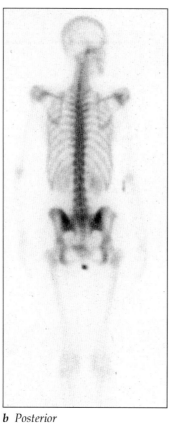

*a* Anterior      *b* Posterior

⁹⁹ᵐTc diphosphonate is taken up by the osteoblasts that are normally active throughout the skeleton. In the normal skeleton there is uniform, symmetrical distribution of tracer.

*Fig. 4.2*

*(a, b) Normal whole-body bone scan, demonstrating uniform, symmetrical distribution of tracer.*

## 4.2.3 ⁹⁹ᵐTcO₄

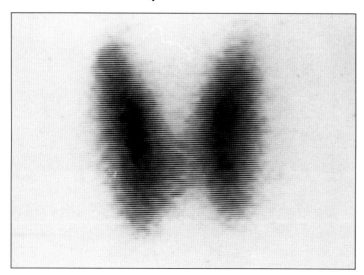

⁹⁹ᵐTcO₄ is trapped by thyroid follicular cells that are uniformly distributed throughout the gland in the normal thyroid.

*Fig. 4.3*

*⁹⁹ᵐTcO₄ scan, demonstrating the typical appearance of a normal thyroid gland.*

## NORMAL SCANS WITH VARIANTS AND ARTEFACTS

# 4.2.4   ⁶⁷Ga

*Table 4.3   Normal distribution of ⁶⁷Ga*

| Always | Variable |
|---|---|
| Bone marrow | Spleen |
| Liver | Salivary glands |
| Gut | Lacrimal glands |
| Nasal sinuses | Sweat |
| | Kidneys (first 24 hours only) |
| | Breast (lactation or prolactin-releasing drugs) |

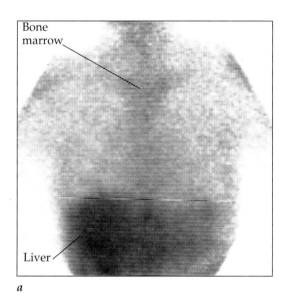

*a*

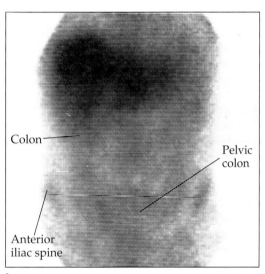

*b*

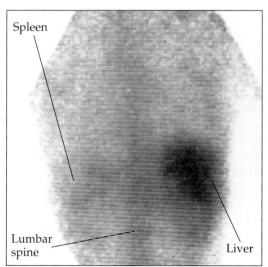

*c*

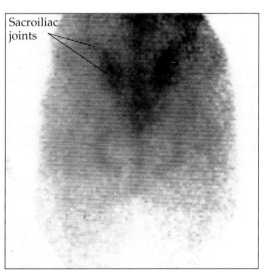

*d*

*Fig. 4.4*

*(a–d) ⁶⁷Ga scan of neck, chest, abdomen and pelvis 48 hours after injection, showing the normal distribution. Head and limb views are obtained in addition when clinically indicated.*

## NORMAL SCANS WITH VARIANTS AND ARTEFACTS

### *Pitfalls*

*Problem of bowel activity*

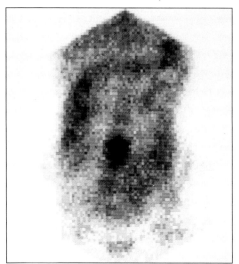
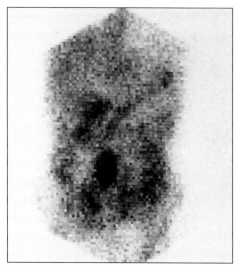

*a* Anterior

*b* Anterior

**Fig. 4.5**

*(a)* $^{67}$*Ga scan of the abdomen (48 hours), showing central massive tracer uptake and widespread bowel uptake. (b)* $^{67}$*Ga scan (72 hours).*

*The central uptake has remained, while the bowel uptake has changed significantly in distribution. Central uptake was due to a mass of lymphomatous nodes around the iliac bifurcation.*

**When tracer uptake is seen in the abdomen on the first $^{67}$Ga scan (usually 48 hours), the study should be repeated at 72 hours, and even 96 hours if necessary, to distinguish normal bowel from focal disease.**

*Post-radiation sialitis*

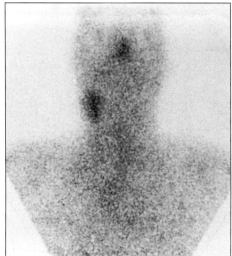
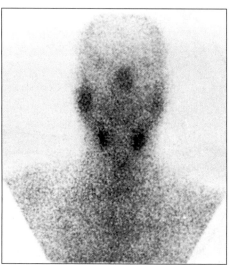

*a* Anterior

*b* Anterior

**Fig. 4.6**

*(a) Anterior view of neck and chest, showing uptake in Hodgkin's lymphoma involving right cervical lymph node. (b) Same view obtained following radiotherapy.*

*This study shows resolution of disease, but there is striking uptake of tracer in the salivary glands. This was due to radiation sialitis, and this study was initially reported as indicating recurrent disease.*

**Radiation sialitis, especially involving the submandibular glands, commonly occurs after upper mantle radiation therapy. Radiation sialitis accumulates $^{67}$Ga.**

# NORMAL SCANS WITH VARIANTS AND ARTEFACTS

## *Variants*

### *Breast uptake of ⁶⁷Ga*

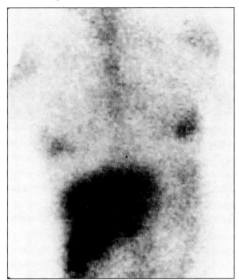

*Anterior*

**Fig. 4.7**

*Anterior view of thorax and abdomen. ⁶⁷Ga uptake is seen in both breasts.*
  *The commonest cause of breast uptake is drug administration, usually an antiemetic, which causes prolactin release.*

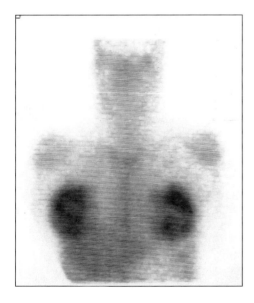

**Fig. 4.8**

*A 23–year old woman with marked ⁶⁷Ga accumulation in the breasts. The patient was subsequently discovered to have a prolactin secreting pituitary adenoma causing galactorrhea.*

In ⁶⁷Ga studies:
- **Faint salivary gland uptake may be normal**
- **Slight axillary uptake may be caused by ⁶⁷Ga being excreted in sweat.**

## 4.2.5 $^{201}$Tl

$^{201}$Tl not only has a normal distribution in the myocardium, but also in the liver, lungs, thyroid and skeletal muscle. The normal pattern of uptake must be understood if tumour imaging is to be undertaken.

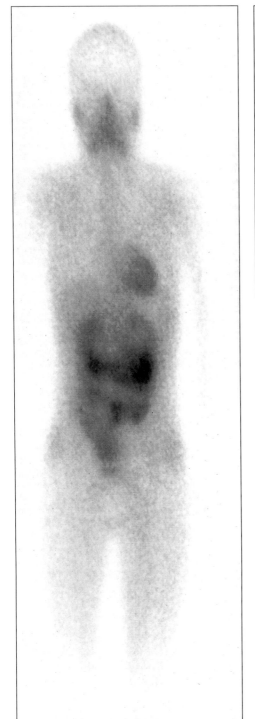

*a Anterior*

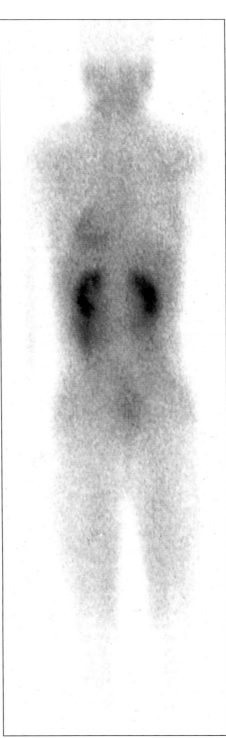

*b Posterior*

### Fig. 4.9

*(a, b) Whole-body $^{201}$Tl scan, showing normal distribution.*

## NORMAL SCANS WITH VARIANTS AND ARTEFACTS

## 4.2.6 $^{99m}$Tc(V) DMSA

$^{99m}$Tc(V) DMSA has little non-specific uptake. Uptake is faintly visualized in the axial skeleton, kidneys and bladder. At the usual imaging time of 2 hours, significant blood pool activity is identified in the region of the heart and great vessels, liver and testes. Breast visualization may be a normal feature in women and appears unrelated to the menstrual cycle or pregnancy. Uptake in the region of the pituitary is noted in some patients.

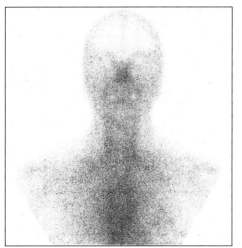

*a Anterior*

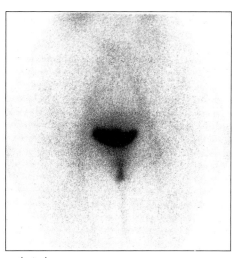

*c Anterior*

**Fig. 4.10**

*Normal whole body $^{99m}$Tc(V) DMSA scan in a female: (a) anterior view of head and neck; (b) anterior view of chest and abdomen; (c) anterior view of pelvis; (d) posterior view of thorax; (e) posterior view of pelvis.*

*b Anterior*

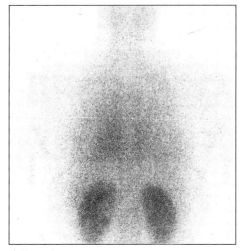

*d Posterior*

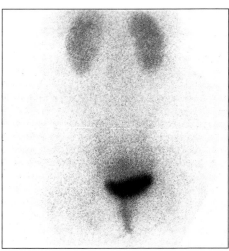

*e Posterior*

## 4.2.7 Miscellaneous non-specific techniques

### $^{99m}$Tc nanocolloid

$^{99m}$Tc nanocolloid is taken up into the reticuloendothelial cells of the body, with significant bone marrow uptake. In childhood the active marrow occupies much of the skeleton, but in adults the active marrow is normally located in the axial skeleton and proximal long bones only. The distribution is symmetrical.

### $^{99m}$Tc DTPA

$^{99m}$Tc DTPA is generally used as a dynamic renal imaging agent. It is rapidly cleared from the bloodstream by the kidneys and is excreted into the bladder. There is little non-specific uptake.

## NORMAL SCANS WITH VARIANTS AND ARTEFACTS

# 4.2.8    $^{123/131}$I MIBG

## Normal distribution

MIBG labelled with $^{123}$I or $^{131}$I is taken up into tissues containing chromoffin tissue and tissues with a rich sympathetic and parasympathetic nerve supply. Normal tissues visualized include salivary glands, myocardium, liver and adrenal glands. MIBG is excreted via the kidneys into the bladder.

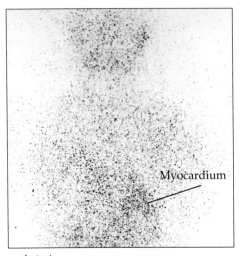

a Anterior

b Posterior

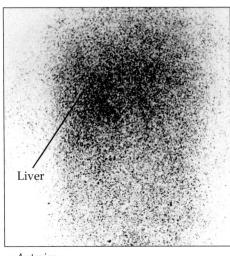

c Anterior

### Fig. 4.11

Series of 24-hour images with $^{131}$I MIBG:
(a) anterior view of chest; (b) posterior view of chest; (c) anterior view of abdomen; (d) posterior view of abdomen and pelvis; (e) anterior view of pelvis and upper femora.

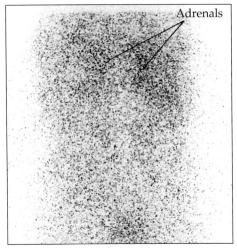

d Posterior

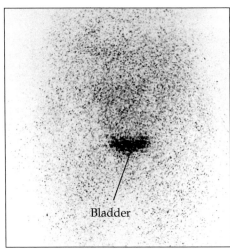

e Anterior

## NORMAL SCANS WITH VARIANTS AND ARTEFACTS

# 4.2.9   $^{111}$In octreotide

$^{111}$In octreotide (pentetreotide) is an octapeptide that has a similar biodistribution to somatostatin and therefore enables somatostatin receptor-positive tumours to be imaged.

*3-hour scan*

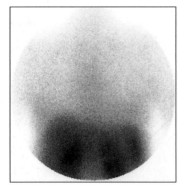 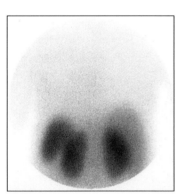 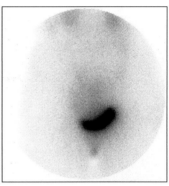 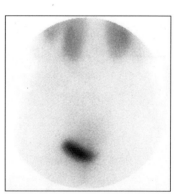

*a  Anterior chest*       *b  Posterior chest*       *c  Anterior abdomen*       *d  Posterior abdomen*

*24-hour scan*

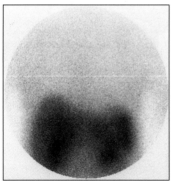 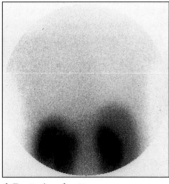 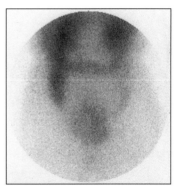 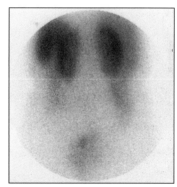

*e  Anterior chest*       *f  Posterior chest*       *g  Anterior abdomen*       *h  Posterior abdomen*

**Fig. 4.12**

Normal $^{111}$In octreotide scan. The normal biodistribution is seen at 3 hours **(a–d)**, with faint activity in the blood pool and activity in the liver, spleen, kidney and bladder. At 24 hours **(e–f)** non-specific gut activity is also visualized and activity in the spleen has increased.

## 4.2.10 Monoclonal antibodies

Monoclonal antibodies are IgG class molecules that are theoretically specific for a single tumour antigen. They can be used whole or as fragments.

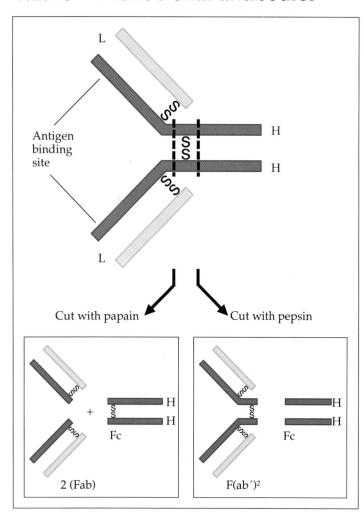

**Fig. 4.13**

*Diagrammatic representation of the IgG molecule: L, light chain; H, heavy chain; SS, disulphide band; Fab, variable portion of IgG molecule; Fc, constant portion of IgG molecule.*

*Table 4.4   Monoclonal antibodies for tumour imaging*

| Antigen | Tumour |
|---|---|
| *Non-specific: dedifferentiation antigens* | |
| Anti-CEA antibody | Colorectal |
| | Ovary |
| *Specific* | |
| HMFG 1 | |
| HMFG 2 | Ovary |
| B72.3 | Ovary |
| | Colorectal |
| PR1 A3 | Colorectal |
| PLAP | Seminoma |
| P97 | Melanoma |

*Table 4.5   Radionuclides for antibody imaging*

| Radionuclide | Advantages | Disadvantages |
|---|---|---|
| $^{131}I$ | Cheap<br>Long half-life | Poor image quality |
| $^{123}I$ | Good image quality | Relatively short half-life<br>Expensive |
| $^{111}In$ | Long half-life<br>Moderate image quality | Expensive<br>DTPA chelate increases uptake in bone marrow |
| $^{99m}Tc$ | Cheap<br>Available | Short half-life may be inappropriate for tumours with low vascularity or low antibody affinity |

# 4.3 CLINICAL APPLICATIONS

The clinical applications of tumour imaging are listed below, and examples of the various clinical problems are given on subsequent pages.

**4.3.1** $^{99m}$**Tc liver/spleen colloid**
Diagnosis of metastases
Staging of malignancy
Follow-up

**4.3.2** $^{99m}$**Tc diphosphonate**
Diagnosis of metastases
Staging
Follow-up
Soft tissue uptake of diphosphonate
Diagnosis of primary bone tumours
Benign bone disease in patients with malignancy

**4.3.3** $^{99m}$**TcO$_4$**
Diagnosis of primary differentiated thyroid tumours

**4.3.4** $^{99m}$**Tc nanocolloid**
Tumour infiltration
Site of biopsy for marrow aspiration
Post-radiation effects

**4.3.5** $^{99m}$**Tc DTPA**
Neurofibromatosis
$^{99m}$Tc DTPA uptake in a plexiform neurofibroma

**4.3.6** $^{67}$**Ga**
$^{67}$Ga uptake in lymphoma
$^{67}$Ga uptake in bronchial carcinoma
$^{67}$Ga uptake in hepatoma
$^{67}$Ga uptake in other tumours
Staging
$^{67}$Ga in follow-up of lymphoma

**4.3.7** $^{201}$**Tl**
$^{201}$Tl imaging in recurrent thyroid cancer

**4.3.8** $^{99m}$**Tc(V) DMSA**
Diagnosis of MTC
Staging
Follow-up
Registration of $^{99m}$Tc(V) DMSA images with MRI

**4.3.9** $^{123/131}$**I MIBG**
Malignant phaeochromocytoma
Neuroblastoma
Carcinoid syndrome

**4.3.10** $^{111}$**In octreotide**
$^{111}$In octreotide in MTC
$^{111}$In octreotide in breast cancer
$^{111}$In octreotide in carcinoid: comparison with $^{123}$I MIBG

**4.3.11** **Monoclonal antibodies**
Breast carcinoma
Melanoma
Colon carcinoma
Ovarian carcinoma

**4.3.12** **Therapy**
Role of radionuclide imaging post-therapy
$^{131}$I therapy
Samarium-135 EDTMP therapy
$^{131}$I MIBG therapy

# 4.3.1 $^{99m}$Tc liver/spleen colloid

The use of $^{99m}$Tc colloid in oncology patients has significantly declined since the refinement of liver ultrasound to detect liver metastases. $^{99m}$Tc colloid imaging is, however, particularly useful for performing serial investigations in patients with known malignancy in order to follow progression of disease or to identify response to treatment.

## Diagnosis of metastases

Liver metastases are identified as photon-deficient areas within the liver. They may be multiple or single, large or small. Miliary metastases of the liver may be suspected if the colloid scan shows the liver to be enlarged with patchily reduced uptake.

**Table 4.6  Tumours that commonly metastasize to the liver**

Colorectal
Ovary
Breast
Lymphoma
Melanoma

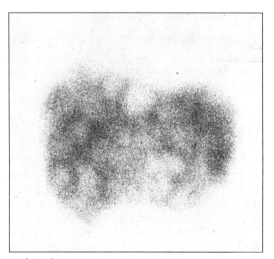

*a Anterior*

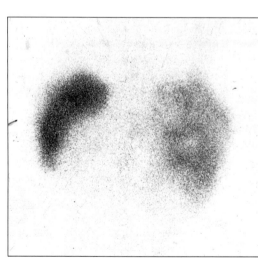

*b Posterior*

*Fig. 4.14*

*A 63–year old female with a history of rectal bleeding and sigmoid carcinoma diagnosed on a colonoscopic biopsy.*

*The $^{99m}$Tc liver/spleen colloid scan prior to surgery (**a, b**) shows multiple large defects typical of colonic metastases.*

## CLINICAL APPLICATIONS

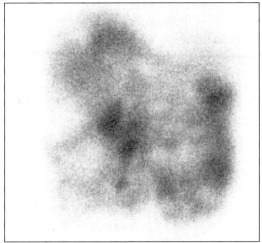
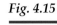

*a Anterior*

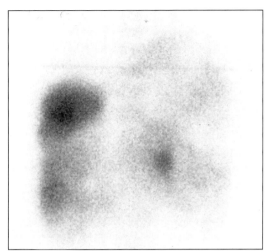

*b Posterior*

### Fig. 4.15

*An 87–year–old female who presented with an ulcerated breast cancer and jaundice.*

*The $^{99m}$Tc liver/spleen (a, b) colloid scan demonstrates widespread replacement of liver tissue by metastases.*

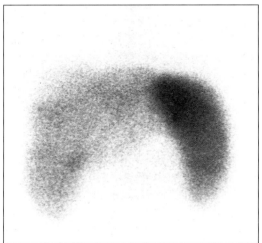

*a Anterior*

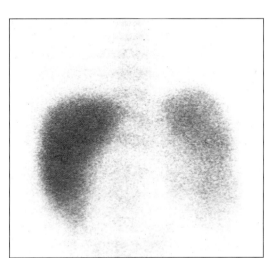

*b Posterior*

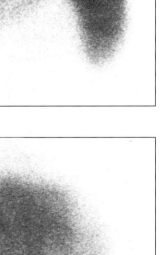

*c Right lateral*

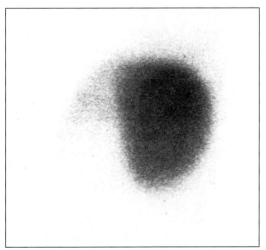

*d Left lateral*

### Fig. 4.16

*An elderly female with newly diagnosed breast cancer and abnormal liver function tests.*

*The $^{99m}$Tc liver/spleen colloid scan (a–d) shows diffusely reduced uptake of tracer in the spleen, with more focal abnormalities seen on the right lateral views (c). The scan appearances are those of miliary metastases from carcinoma of the breast, subsequently confirmed on CT.*

## CLINICAL APPLICATIONS

## Staging of malignancy

Management decisions in patients with newly diagnosed malignancy are influenced by the presence of distant metastases at the time of presentation. The accurate staging of the disease is therefore essential to plan treatment and also to determine prognosis.

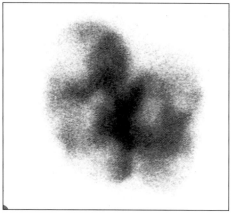

a Anterior    b Posterior

**Fig. 4.17**

*A 54–year–old patient with a breast lump diagnosed as cancer on biopsy. The liver was enlarged at the time of presentation and liver function tests were abnormal.*

*The* ⁹⁹ᵐTc *liver/spleen colloid scan (a, b) shows multiple metastases in both lobes of the liver, confirming metastases. The patient was categorized as having stage 4 disease and radical surgery to the breast was not performed.*

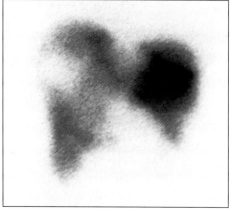

a Anterior    b Posterior

c Right lateral    d Left lateral

**Fig. 4.18**

*A 44–year–old female with known breast cancer treated by mastectomy 6 years earlier. The patient presented with right hypochondrical discomfort and raised liver function tests.*

*A* ⁹⁹ᵐTc *liver/spleen colloid scan (a–d) was performed to restage the patient prior to commencing chemotherapy.*

## Follow-up

$^{99m}$Tc liver/spleen colloid imaging enables an estimate of the number, size and distribution of metastases to be assessed. By inspection of serial studies, progression or regression of metastases can be readily assessed.

### Progression of disease

*Initial study*

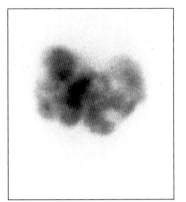
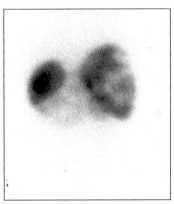
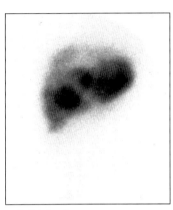
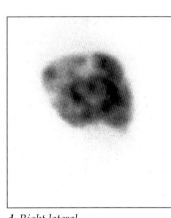

*a  Anterior*      *b  Posterior*      *c  Left lateral*      *d  Right lateral*

### 4 months later

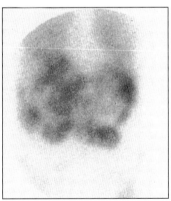
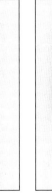
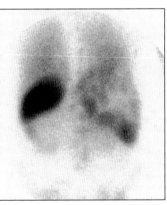
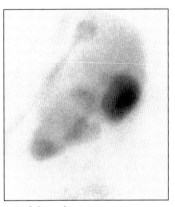
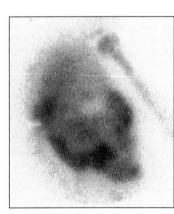

*e  Anterior*      *f  Posterior*      *g  Left lateral*      *h  Right lateral*

**Fig. 4.19**

*A 45–year–old woman with known carcinoma of the breast was shown to have multiple liver metastases on $^{99m}$Tc liver/spleen colloid imaging (a–d). Four months later she became extremely unwell and repeat imaging (e–h) demonstrated progression, with replacement of liver tissue by tumour. Lung uptake of colloid was visualized; this is a non-specific finding associated with profound debility.*

## Regression of disease

### Pre-chemotherapy

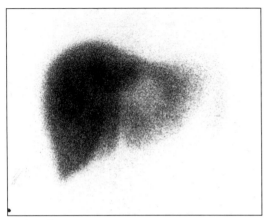

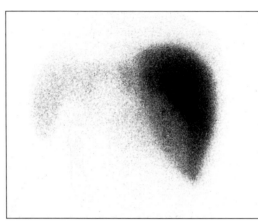

*a Anterior*

*b Posterior*

### Post-chemotherapy

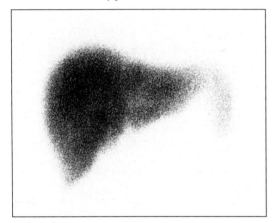

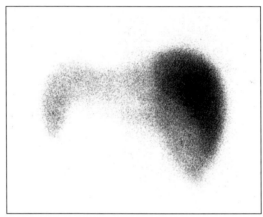

*c Anterior*

*d Posterior*

**Fig. 4.20**

**(a, b)** $^{99m}$Tc liver/spleen colloid scan in a 64–year–old male with colonic carcinoma and liver metastases. Following chemotherapy with 5-fluorouracil the liver/spleen scan **(c, d)** shows significant, though not complete, regression of disease.

## 4.3.2    $^{99m}$Tc diphosphonate

### Diagnosis of metastases

One of the main indications for bone imaging using $^{99m}$Tc diphosphonate is the diagnosis of metastases. The whole-body nature of a bone scan permits the extent of metastatic involvement to be assessed.

Since the bone scan becomes positive at a metastatic site many months before an abnormality can be detected on an x-ray, $^{99m}$Tc diphosphonate bone imaging is the investigation of choice for patients with known malignancy and clinically suspected bone metastases.

**Table 4.7    Tumours that commonly metastasize to the skeleton**

| |
|---|
| Bronchus |
| Breast |
| Prostate |
| Thyroid |
| Renal |

### Bone metastases in carcinoma of the bronchus

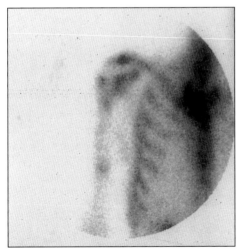
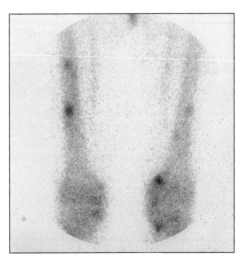

a Anterior                    b Anterior                    c Anterior

**Fig. 4.21**

A 50–year–old woman who was a known heavy smoker with a carcinoma of the bronchus developed a pain in the left shoulder.

The bone scan **(a–c)** shows uptake in the femora, right humerus, left shoulder and left 4th rib at sites of metastatic spread.

## CLINICAL APPLICATIONS

*Bone metastases in carcinoma of the prostate*

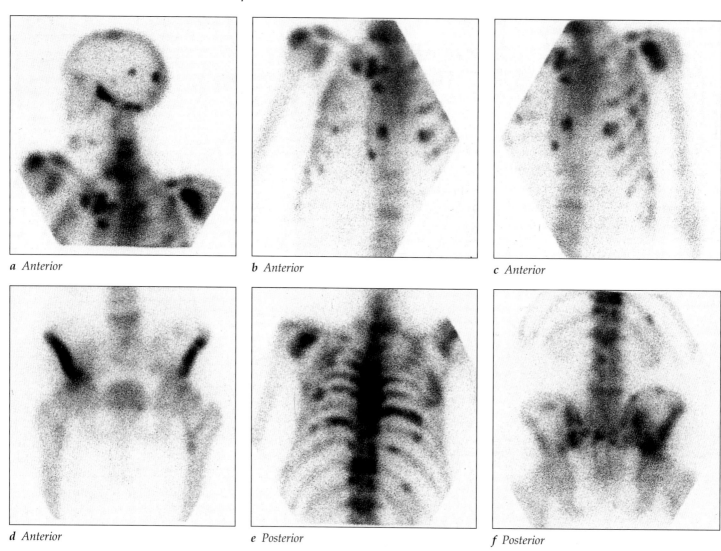

*a* Anterior       *b* Anterior       *c* Anterior

*d* Anterior       *e* Posterior       *f* Posterior

**Fig. 4.22**

*A 73–year–old man presented with prostatism and generalized bone pain.*
   *The bone scan **(a–f)** demonstrates multiple areas of intense uptake throughout the skeleton, diagnostic of multiple metastases from carcinoma of the prostate.*

## Bone metastases in carcinoma of the breast

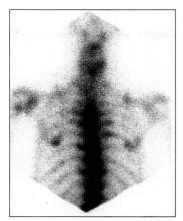 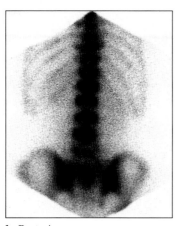 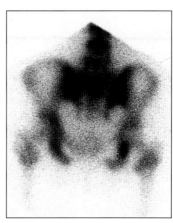

*a* Posterior                *b* Posterior                *c* Posterior

**Fig. 4.23**

*A 60-year-old woman with known breast cancer and bone metastases. The patient developed anaemia and a bone scan (a–c) demonstrated diffusely increased uptake throughout the axial skeleton and poor visualization of the kidneys consistent with a superscan of malignancy. Note that bladder activity is faintly visualized, confirming that this patient has functioning kidneys that are not visualized due to intense uptake in the skeleton.*

## Bone metastases in carcinoma of the thyroid

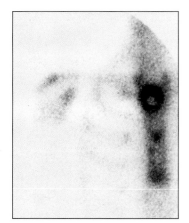 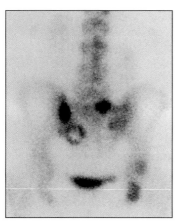

*a* Anterior              *b* Posterior

**Fig. 4.24**

*An 80-year-old woman with a large, craggy thyroid nodule and a pulsatile mass over the sternum.*

*The bone scan (a,b) shows lytic lesions in the sternum and sacrum, with increased uptake seen in the sacroiliac regions and right ischium, and the lower sternum. At surgery a follicular thyroid carcinoma was removed.*

 **Bone metastases from thyroid carcinoma are occasionally lytic.**

## Bone metastases in carcinoma of the kidney

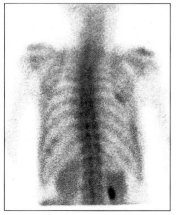 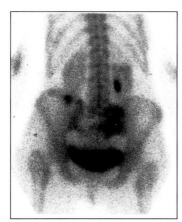

*a* Posterior              *b* Posterior

**Fig. 4.25**

*An 84-year-old woman with a hypernephroma of the right kidney. A bone scan (a,b) was performed to investigate a rising calcium level which demonstrated a photon-deficient area at the upper pole of the right kidney and bone lesions in the left iliac crest, right sacroiliac joint and ribs bilaterally at sites of metastatic spread.*

## CLINICAL APPLICATIONS

### *Staging*

Management decisions, such as whether to embark on radical surgery following the initial diagnosis, are significantly influenced by an accurate assessment of the extent of disease at presentation. The $^{99m}$Tc diphosphonate bone scan provides an extremely sensitive technique for identifying the presence of metastases.

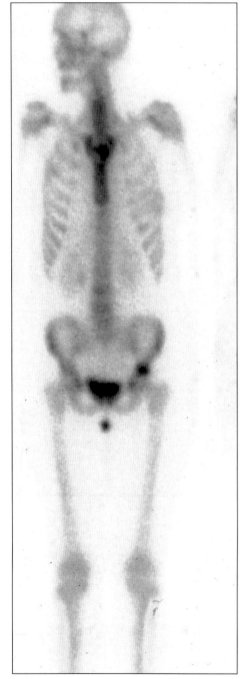

*a  Anterior*

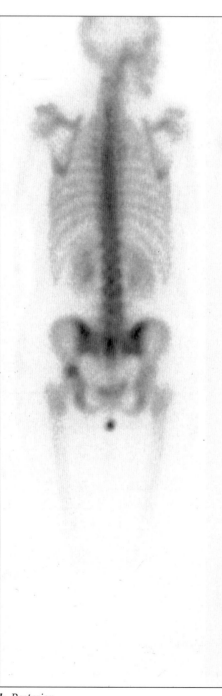

*b  Posterior*

**Fig. 4.26**

*A 53-year-old woman with newly diagnosed breast cancer and palpable axillary nodes.*

*The whole-body scan (a,b) shows uptake in the manubrium sternum and left superior acetabulum. The scan findings are those of metastases of breast carcinoma, confirming stage 4 disease.*

## CLINICAL APPLICATIONS

## Follow-up

Since the bone scan can accurately define the presence and extent of bone metastases, it can be used to monitor the patient throughout the course of the disease.

Deterioration can be detected either by an increase in uptake at the site of a known lesion, by an increase in size of a known lesion or by an increase in the number of lesions.

Regression following successful therapy may be acccompanied by a transient increase in uptake at the site of a healing metastasis. Usually, however, the uptake decreases in intensity. With time the actual number of lesions will reduce.

### Progression of disease

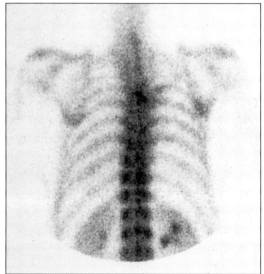

*a Posterior, 0 months*

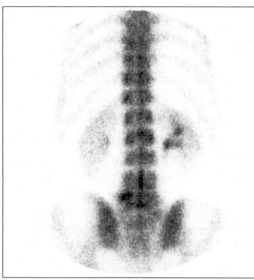

*b Posterior, 0 months*

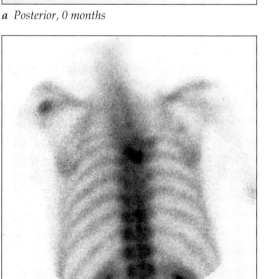

*c Posterior, 3 months*

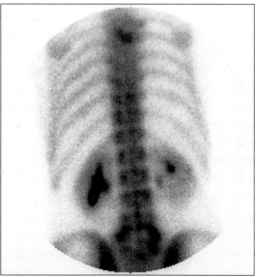

*d Posterior, 3 months*

**Fig. 4.27**

*A 33-year-old woman with known skeletal metastases.*

*A bone scan of the posterior spine (a,b) shows uptake at L5, with diffuse uptake also seen at T6 and T7.*

*A bone scan performed 3 months later when the patient developed severe mid-thoracic pain (c,d) shows more intense uptake at previously identified sites, with a new lesion seen in the upper thoracic spine.*

# CLINICAL APPLICATIONS

## Regression of disease

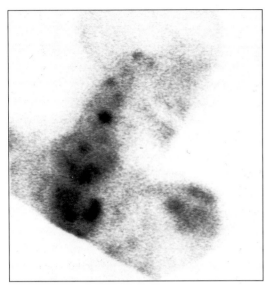

*a Anterior, 0 months*

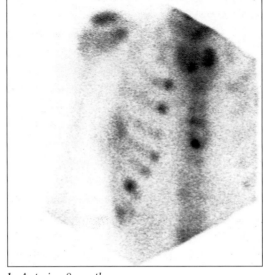

*b Anterior, 0 months*

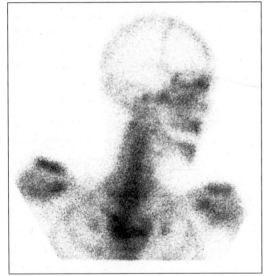

*c Anterior, 12 months*

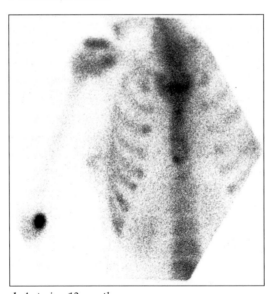

*d Anterior, 12 months*

**Fig. 4.28**

*A 40-year-old woman with recurrence of carcinoma in the right breast and bone pain.*

*The initial bone scan (a,b) shows multiple areas of intense uptake throughout the spine, ribs and sternum. The patient was treated with chemotherapy and a repeat scan one year later shows significant improvement (c,d), with less intense uptake in the sternum and ribs. There has been complete resolution of the cervical spine lesions.*

**A repeat bone scan should generally not be performed in under 6 months unless new symptoms develop in the interim.**

## CLINICAL APPLICATIONS

## *Soft tissue uptake of diphosphonate*

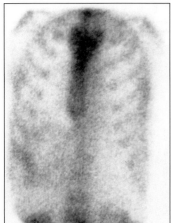

*Anterior*

### Fig. 4.29

*Anterior view of thorax and upper abdomen.*

*In this case there is marked non-homogeneous tracer uptake in an enlarged liver.*

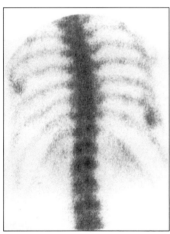

*a Posterior*

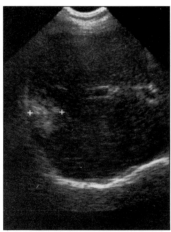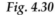

*b*

### Fig. 4.30

*(a) Posterior view of thorax and upper abdomen. (b) Ultrasound of liver.*

*In this case a discrete focus of increased tracer uptake, which is not related to bone, is seen lying clearly between the right 10th and 11th ribs. This lesion represented MDP uptake in a single metastasis, which is shown on the ultrasound of the liver.*

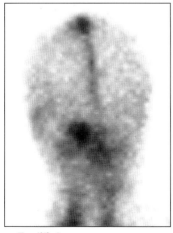

*a Equilibrium*

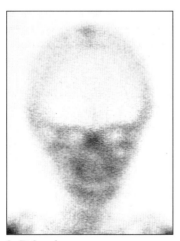

*b Delayed*

### Fig. 4.31

$^{99m}Tc$ MDP *bone scan:* (a) *anterior view of skull, blood pool image;* (b) *anterior view of skull, delayed image.*

*The equilibrium* $^{99m}Tc$ MDP *bone scan image was obtained a few minutes after injection. This shows abnormal blood pool in the region of the right orbit. The delayed image is normal. This child had a rhabdomyosarcoma of the right orbit. The study was being performed to investigate the possibility of local bony involvement and skeletal metastases. This is a further example of a non-specific agent, inasmuch as it indicates a large blood volume in the lesion, but does not reveal anything more about the pathology which is present.*

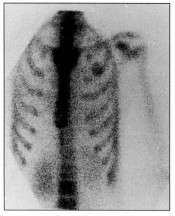

*a Anterior*

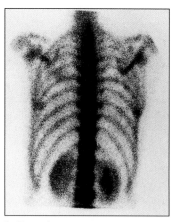

*b Posterior*

### Fig. 4.32

*(a,b) Bone scan, demonstrating uptake in a soft tissue lesion in the left upper chest. This was subsequently found to be a primary adenocarcinoma of the lung.*

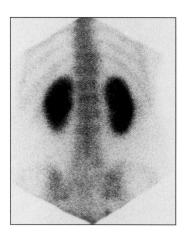

### Fig. 4.33

*Intense $^{99m}$Tc diphosphonate accumulation in the kidneys in a patient with hypercalcaemia of malignancy.*

## Diagnosis of primary bone tumours

Primary bone tumours are associated with increased uptake of $^{99m}$Tc diphosphonate at the sites of primary and secondary disease (see Chapter 1, pages 50–6).

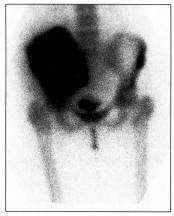

*a Anterior*

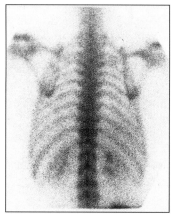

*b Posterior*

### Fig. 4.34

*A 23-year-old woman with known chondroblastic osteogenic sarcoma of the right ileum.*

*The bone scan (a) shows intense uptake in the region of the right ileum. The remainder of the scan (b) was normal.*

## *Benign bone disease in patients with malignancy*

### Degenerative disease

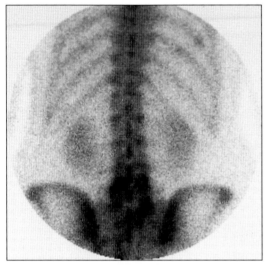

*Posterior*

**Fig. 4.35**

*Moderate uptake seen on a bone scan at the level of L5 in a patient with breast carcinoma and back pain. The scan findings are non-specific, but an x-ray of this area confirms degenerative disease at L5.*

### Osteoporotic collapse

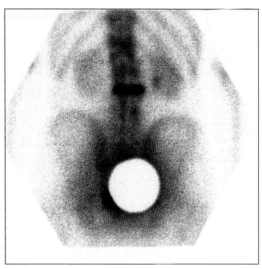

*Anterior*

**Fig. 4.36**

*Linear uptake seen at the level of L3 in a patient with prostate cancer on hormone therapy. In the absence of other lesions, the scan findings are those of osteoporotic collapse, but a repeat scan should be performed at 6 months to confirm reduction in uptake if the lesion is benign.*

### Radiation necrosis

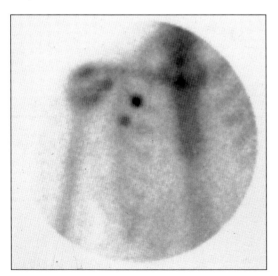

*Anterior*

**Fig. 4.37**

*A 52-year-old woman with known breast cancer.*
*The bone scan shows two foci of uptake in the right hemithorax. The patient had undergone radiotherapy to this area 12 years previously and the scan findings are those of radiation necrosis of the ribs in the field of radiotherapy.*

# 4.3.3 $^{99m}TcO_4$

Nodular change within the thyroid is not uncommon and is only due to malignancy in a small percentage of cases. The thyroid scan using $^{99m}TcO_4$ or $^{123}I$ is the only imaging technique which enables the identification of functioning or non-functioning thyroid tissue to be made. Functioning thyroid tissue at the site of a nodule virtually excludes malignancy. In 10% of cases, non-functioning nodules which are solid on ultrasound will be found to be malignant (see Chapter 2, pages 150–2).

## Diagnosis of primary differentiated thyroid tumours

### Diagnosis of follicular carcinoma

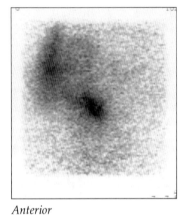

Anterior

### Diagnosis of papillary carcinoma

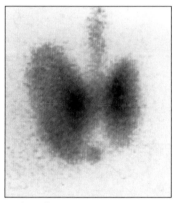 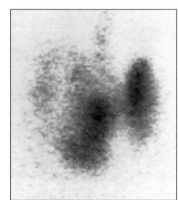

*a* Anterior      *b* Anterior

**Fig. 4.38**

*$^{99m}TcO_4$ thyroid scan of a patient with asymmetrical goitre, most marked on the left. The scan shows grossly abnormal uptake in the left lobe suggestive of thyroid replacement. The lesion was solid on ultrasound. At surgery a follicular carcinoma with significant vascular invasion was removed.*

 **The combination of an ultrasound scan and a $^{99m}TcO_4$ scan is essential for determining subsequent management in patients with solitary thyroid nodules.**

**Fig. 4.39**

*(a,b) $^{99m}TcO_4$ scan, showing the development of a discrete cold nodule in an enlarged right lobe of the thyroid over a period of 1 year. The lesion was solid on ultrasound and a papillary carcinoma was diagnosed on fine-needle aspiration.*

### $^{131}I$ imaging in thyroid cancer

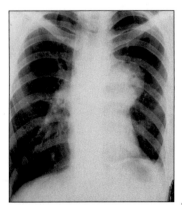 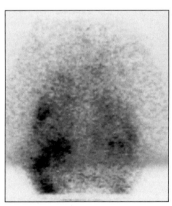 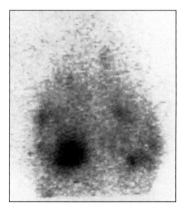

*a* X-ray      *b* Posterior, 3 months post-surgery      *c* Posterior, 6 months post-surgery

**Fig. 4.40**

*Serial $^{131}I$ study of the chest in the same patient as Fig. 4.38.*

*The chest x-ray (a) shows a large mass in the left hilum. The posterior $^{131}I$ scan of the chest (b) performed 3 months after surgery for primary tumour reveals widespread uptake in lung metastases. The posterior $^{131}I$ scan of the chest (c) performed 6 months later shows an increase of abnormality, despite intervening $^{131}I$ therapy.*

**CLINICAL APPLICATIONS**

# 4.3.4 ⁹⁹ᵐTc nanocolloid

*Table 4.8 Use of ⁹⁹ᵐTc nanocolloid for bone marrow imaging in malignancy*

Diagnosis of sites of tumour infiltration
Selection of sites for bone marrow biopsy
Assessment of post-radiotherapy effects

## *Tumour infiltration*

In patients with known malignancy, bone marrow scanning may be of value for determining suitable sites for biopsy, or for detecting metastases. Often, the marrow scan will not provide more information than other screening tests, such as the radionuclide bone scan, but on occasion dramatic results can be obtained.

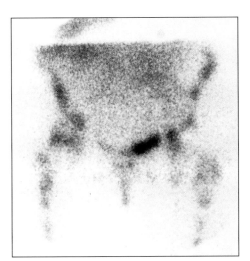

*a  Anterior, bone marrow scan*

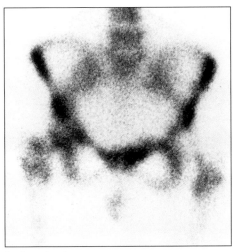
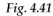

*b  Anterior, bone scan*

**Fig. 4.41**

*(a) Bone marrow scan: anterior view of pelvis and upper femora. (b) Bone scan: anterior view of pelvis and upper femora.*

*The patient was a 64-year-old woman with bronchial carcinoma and bone metastases. The bone scan shows evidence of metastases in the pelvis and upper femora. In this case the marrow study shows multiple defects, essentially matching the bone scan findings.*

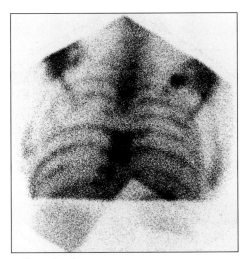

*a  Posterior, bone marrow scan*

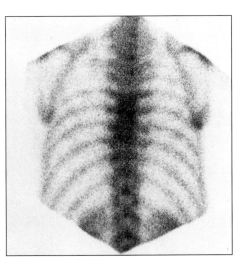

*b  Posterior, bone scan*

**Fig. 4.42**

*(a) Bone marrow scan: posterior view of thoracic spine. (b) Bone scan: posterior view of thoracic spine.*

*The patient was a 43-year-old woman with breast carcinoma and back pain. The marrow scan shows obvious marrow replacement at T-5, with left 4th and 6th ribs not visualized. The bone scan was originally thought to be normal, but the left 4th rib is not visualized. Nevertheless, it is apparent that findings on the marrow scan are more obvious, with additional lesions being seen. A subsequent biopsy confirmed metastatic involvement in the upper thoracic spine.*

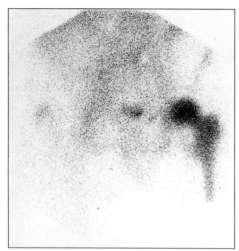

a  Anterior, bone marrow scan

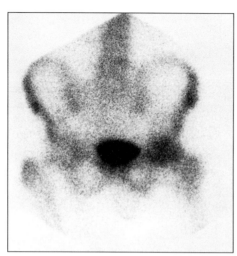

b  Anterior, bone scan

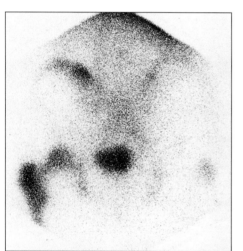

c  Posterior, bone marrow scan

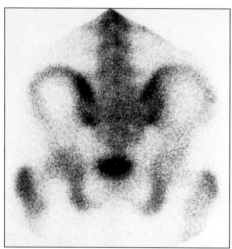

d  Posterior, bone scan

**Fig. 4.43**

*(a)* Bone marrow scan: anterior view of pelvis. *(b)* Bone scan: anterior view of pelvis. *(c)* Bone marrow scan: posterior view of pelvis. *(d)* Bone scan: posterior view of pelvis.

The patient was a 52-year-old man with carcinoma of the lung. The most striking finding on the bone scan views is increased tracer uptake in the region of the left femoral head. Findings on the marrow scan are dramatic, with strikingly increased tracer uptake in the left upper femur, extending into the shaft. However, elsewhere in the pelvis and in the right femur there is marked reduction of tracer uptake, except for a small area at the left upper posterior pelvis. There was extensive marrow replacement by tumour.

## Site of biopsy for marrow aspiration

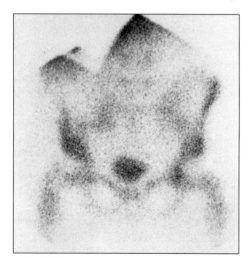

a  Anterior

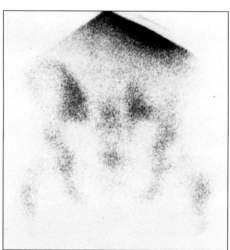

b  Posterior

**Fig. 4.44**

Bone marrow scan: *(a)* anterior view of pelvis; *(b)* posterior view of pelvis.

The patient was a 28-year-old man with recurrent Hodgkin's disease. He was previously treated with total nodular radiation, and was currently being considered for bone marrow harvest followed by very high-dose chemotherapy and marrow reinfusion. The oncologists wanted to know if there was a suitable site for marrow biopsy. It is apparent that there is reduced uptake in the right hemipelvis, but the remainder of the pelvis and both femora show slightly increased activity. The left hemipelvis was therefore chosen as a suitable site for marrow harvest.

## Post-radiation effects

The reticuloendothelial function of bone marrow is very sensitive to the effect of external radiation. The following two cases illustrate the effect of radiation.

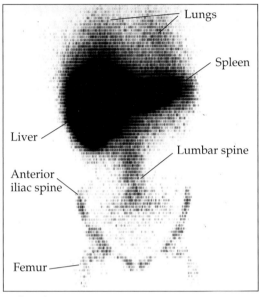

*a  Anterior*

*b  Posterior*

**Fig. 4.45**

*(a) Anterior and (b) posterior views of a marrow scan in a patient with Hodgkin's disease following upper mantle radiotherapy.*

*Note the normal marrow distribution below the diaphragm but absence of uptake in the upper axial skeleton.*

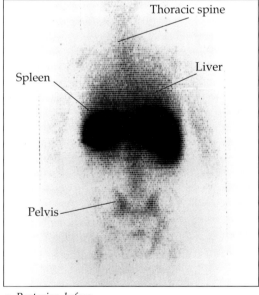

*a  Posterior, before*

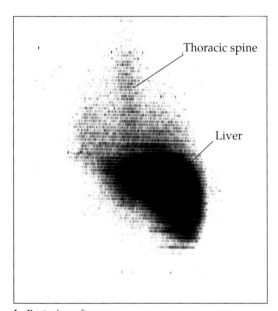

*b  Posterior, after*

**Fig. 4.46**

*Posterior views of a patient (a) before and (b) after lower abdominal radiation therapy for lymphoma.*

*Note the normal lower marrow activity before treatment, with no uptake afterwards. There has also been a splenectomy.*

## 4.3.5  $^{99m}$Tc DTPA

$^{99m}$Tc DTPA, while normally used for dynamic renal imaging, has been shown to be taken up into sites of neurofibromatosis.

### *Neurofibromatosis*

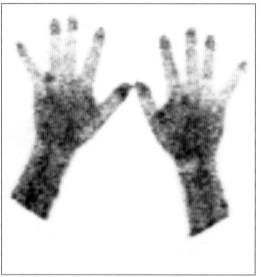

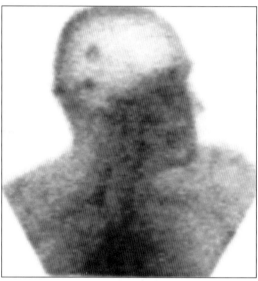

*a  1 hour*

*b  1 hour*

**Fig. 4.47**

*$^{99m}$Tc DTPA scan at 1 hour: (a) hands; (b) posterior skull.*

*The patient was a 58-year-old man with multiple neurofibromatosis. The scan images show the focal uptake in the web space between the 4th and 5th left fingers and in the right posterior skull.*

### $^{99m}$Tc DTPA *uptake in a plexiform neurofibroma*

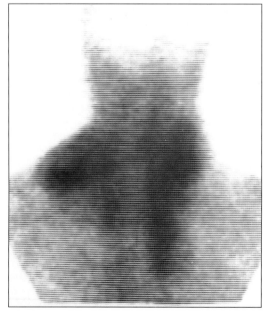

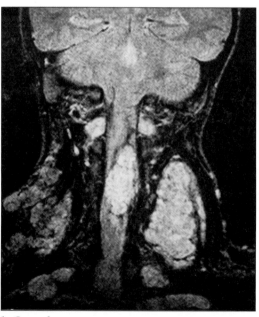

*a  Posterior*

*b  Coronal*

**Fig. 4.48**

*(a) Posterior view of neck and upper thorax, showing uptake of $^{99m}$Tc DTPA into an extensive plexiform neurofibroma. Note extension of tumour alongside the sympathetic chain. (b) Coronal MR study, showing the extensive tumour.*

*The patient was an eight-year-old boy with known plexiform neurofibroma causing brachial plexus signs and evidence of spinal cord compression. The imaging studies were undertaken as a baseline prior to surgery, which was planned to relieve the cord compression.*

# 4.3.6    $^{67}$Ga

*Table 4.6    Tumours imaged with $^{67}$Ga*

| |
|---|
| Lymphoma |
| Bronchial carcinoma |
| Hepatoma |
| Others |

## $^{67}$Ga uptake in lymphoma

### Clinical indications for $^{67}$Ga scanning in lymphoma

• As a baseline to establish that the tumour is $^{67}$Ga-avid for subsequent follow-up

• Assessment for suspected hilar pathology

• Pretreatment staging as an adjunct to other staging procedures

• Follow-up as an adjunct to other investigations

• Follow-up when there is a systemic indication, eg fever, pruritis, weight loss.

### $^{67}$Ga uptake at sites of primary lymphoma

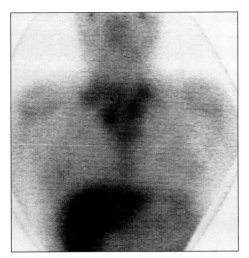

*a Anterior*

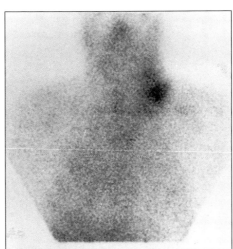

*b Anterior*

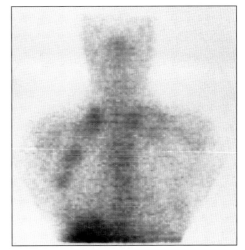

*c Anterior*

**Fig. 4.49**

*Examples of $^{67}$Ga accumulation in lymphoma. (**a**) Anterior view of chest, showing bilateral supraclavicular and upper mediastinal uptake. (**b**) Anterior view of chest, showing left supraclavicular and cervical uptake. (**c**) Anterior view of chest, showing bilateral supraclavicular uptake and right axillary disease.*

## Diagnosis of lymphoma

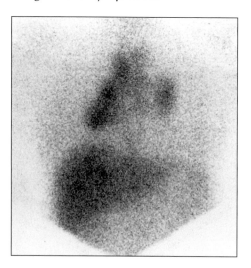

**Fig. 4.50**

*Anterior view of chest and upper abdomen.*
*This patient was being investigated for hilar gland enlargement shown on a chest x-ray. The $^{67}Ga$ study shows avid uptake in the glands bilaterally, indicating active disease. Lymphoma was subsequently confirmed in this case.*

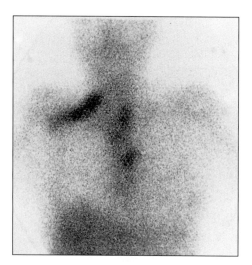

**Fig. 4.51**

*This patient presented with general malaise and had signs of brachial plexus compression. A malignancy was suspected, but initial investigations yielded negative results. A $^{67}Ga$ scan was requested, and the study shows uptake in and around nerves in the brachial plexus, together with some focal mediastinal disease. A lymphoma was diagnosed by mediastinal biopsy, and the patient responded well to chemotherapy.*

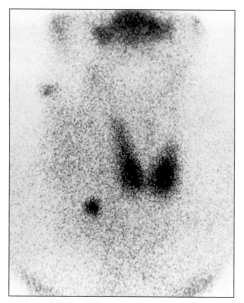

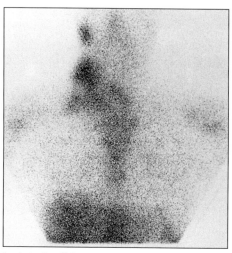

**Fig. 4.52**

*(a) $^{99m}TcO_4$ thyroid scan, anterior view of neck. Markers are placed on a palpable mass. (b) $^{67}Ga$ study, anterior view of neck and chest.*
*This patient presented with a mass in her neck, and this was initially thought to be a thyroid neoplasm. The thyroid scan, however, shows a normal thyroid, which is clearly displaced by an external mass. The $^{67}Ga$ scan shows avid uptake in the cervical glands and upper mediastinum. This patient had a lymphoma, not of thyroid origin.*

*b Anterior, $^{67}Ga$*

*a Anterior, $^{99m}TcO_4$*

## ⁶⁷Ga uptake in bronchial carcinoma

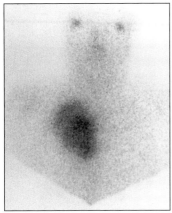

*a  Anterior, ⁶⁷Ga*

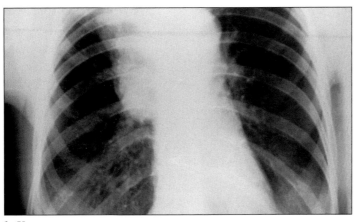

*b  X-ray*

**Fig. 4.53**

*(a) ⁶⁷Ga study, anterior view of upper thorax. (b) Chest x-ray.*

*The chest x-ray shows a mass in the right upper zone. The ⁶⁷Ga scan shows tracer uptake in this mass. The patient was subsequently shown to have a bronchial carcinoma.*

**⁶⁷Ga is a non-specific tumour seeker and has variable uptake in lung tumours. It is rarely useful in the differential diagnosis of a lung mass.**

## ⁶⁷Ga uptake in hepatoma

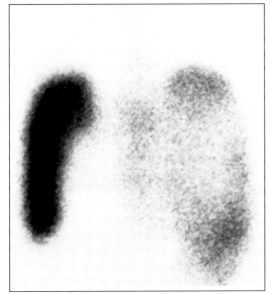

*a  Posterior, liver/spleen colloid*

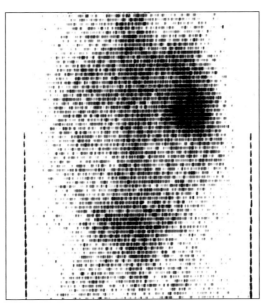

*b  Posterior, ⁶⁷Ga*

**Fig. 4.54**

*(a) Colloid liver/spleen scan, posterior view. (b) ⁶⁷Ga scan (rectilinear), posterior view.*

*This patient was an alcoholic with known cirrhosis, who presented with weight loss. The liver scan shows a space-occupying lesion, and on the ⁶⁷Ga study there is focal tracer uptake corresponding to the liver mass. This patient was found to have a hepatoma.*

## $^{67}$Ga uptake in other tumours

### $^{67}$Ga uptake in colon CA

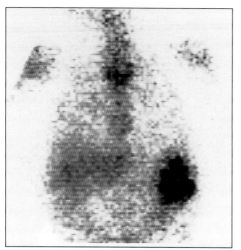

a Anterior

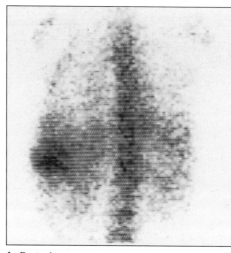

b Posterior

**Fig. 4.55**

$^{67}$Ga study: **(a)** anterior and **(b)** posterior views of thorax and upper abdomen.

This patient was being investigated for PUO. The $^{67}$Ga study shows abnormal tracer accumulation in the left hypochondrium, and this was subsequently shown to be due to a splenic flexure carcinoma of the colon.

### $^{67}$Ga uptake in lymphoplasmocytoma

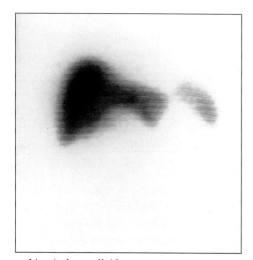

a Liver/spleen colloid

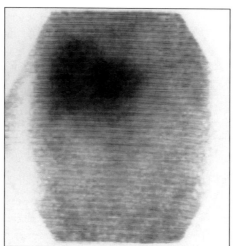

b $^{67}$Ga

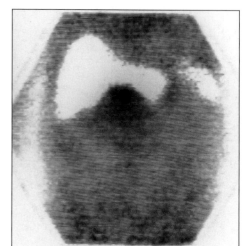

c Subtraction

**Fig. 4.56**

A 75-year-old male with a known lymphoplasmocytoma, polyarthropathy and hepatomegaly.

The $^{99m}$Tc liver/spleen colloid scan **(a)** shows a photon-deficient area in the region of the porta hepatis, which fills in on $^{67}$Ga imaging **(b)**. The subtraction image **(c)** confirms a $^{67}$Ga-avid tumour.

## CLINICAL APPLICATIONS

## *Staging*

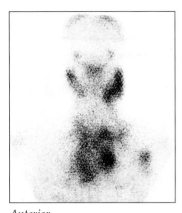

*Anterior*

**Fig. 4.57**

*This patient presented with supraclavicular lymph nodes which were biopsied and confirmed to be lymphoma.*

*The ⁶⁷Ga study shows the supraclavicular nodes but also identifies tumour in the upper mediastinum and left axilla.*

## Interpretation of ⁶⁷Ga uptake by liver

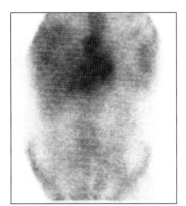

*a Anterior, ⁶⁷Ga*

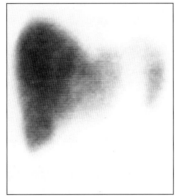

*b Anterior, liver colloid*

**Fig. 4.58**

**Case 1 (a)** *Anterior view of abdomen with ⁶⁷Ga, showing focal uptake in the epigastrium.* **(b)** *Anterior view of colloid liver scan, showing slight reduction of tracer uptake in the region of the left lobe. This appearance is due to focal disease, but may be normal when there is a 'thin' left lobe.*

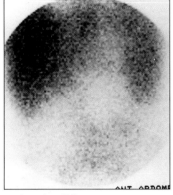

*c Anterior, ⁶⁷Ga*

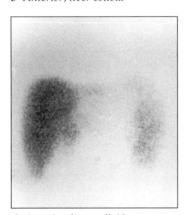

*d Anterior, liver colloid*

**Case 2 (c)** *Anterior view of abdomen with ⁶⁷Ga, showing apparent normal distribution of tracer uptake in the liver.* **(d)** *Anterior view of colloid liver scan, showing a focal defect in the left lobe.*

*In both cases the patient had lymphoma deposits in the left lobe of the liver. Since ⁶⁷Ga accumulates in both lymphoma and normal liver, disease may be 'camouflaged' against a background of tracer uptake in normal liver. In the first case the colloid scan **(b)** could not be interpreted without the ⁶⁷Ga study **(a)**, and in the second case the ⁶⁷Ga study **(c)** could not be interpreted without the colloid scan **(d)**.*

- ⁶⁷Ga uptake in the liver may be difficult to interpret.
- A colloid liver scan should always be performed following a ⁶⁷Ga study, and they should be interpreted together.

## CLINICAL APPLICATIONS

# ⁶⁷Ga in follow-up of lymphoma

## Relapse

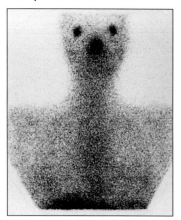 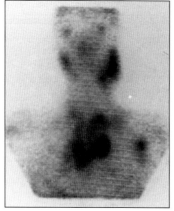

*a* Anterior, 0 months    *b* Anterior, 24 months

**Fig. 4.59**

*A 48-year-old woman with successfully treated Hodgkin's lymphoma.*

*The ⁶⁷Ga scan of the head and neck (a) shows a normal pattern of ⁶⁷Ga uptake after chemotherapy and radiotherapy. Two years later the patient represented with recurrent night sweats. A repeat ⁶⁷Ga scan (b) demonstrates widespread recurrence in the left neck, mediastinum and left axilla.*

## Resolution

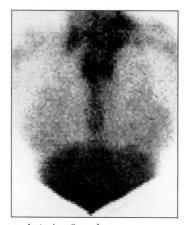 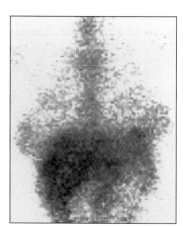

*a* Anterior, 0 weeks    *b* Anterior, 2 weeks post-therapy

**Fig. 4.60**

*(a) Anterior view of chest. (b) Repeat view 2 weeks after radiation therapy.*

*On the original study of this patient with Hodgkin's lymphoma it is apparent that there is massive tracer uptake bilaterally in the supraclavicular nodes and upper mediastinum. A repeat study was obtained because there was some doubt as to the effectiveness of radiation therapy. It is apparent that there is now no abnormal uptake.*

## Distinction of relapse from infection

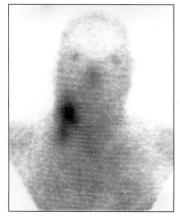 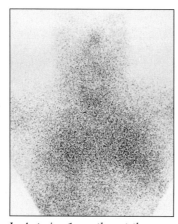

*a* Anterior, 0 months    *b* Anterior, 1 month post-therapy

**Fig. 4.61**

*(a) Anterior view of head and upper chest. (b) Repeat view 1 month after chemotherapy.*

*This patient with Hodgkin's lymphoma had a baseline staging study which showed uptake in the right cervical and supraclavicular nodes. The repeat study was performed because, following therapy, the patient had a persistent fever. It is apparent that the disease activity has resolved, but there is slight increased tracer uptake diffusely over the lung fields. This may be due to cytotoxic drug pneumonitis or superadded opportunistic infection in an immunocompromised patient.*

 **⁶⁷Ga is a good guide to the activity of disease when avid uptake has previously been demonstrated in a tumour.**

**CLINICAL APPLICATIONS**

# 4.3.7 $^{201}$Tl

Although $^{201}$Tl is primarily used as a myocardial imaging agent, it has also been used to diagnose a variety of tumours. Tumours in which $^{201}$Tl uptake has been documented are:

- Bronchus
- Thyroid
- Breast
- Lymphoma
- Brain
- Osteosarcoma
- Ewing's tumour
- Hepatoma
- Oesophagus

## $^{201}$Tl imaging in recurrent thyroid cancer

$^{201}$Tl is taken up by follicular, papillary and medullary thyroid cancers. It has a particular role in the management of patients with $^{131}$I-negative tumours such as Hurthlé cell tumours, and in patients who develop signs of local recurrence while on thyroxine and in whom $^{131}$I imaging is not possible.

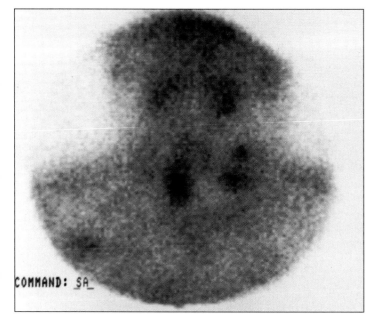

*Fig. 4.62*

$^{201}$Tl scan of the neck in an elderly female patient who had follicular carcinoma of the thyroid resected five years previously. She was maintained on thyroxine, but thyroglobulin estimations had been rising slowly despite negative $^{131}$I scans.

One month prior to the scan the patient had noticed enlarging masses in her neck. The $^{201}$Tl scan was performed with the patient on thyroxine and confirmed tumour recurrence in the midline and in the left supraclavicular region.

# 4.3.8 $^{99m}$Tc(V) DMSA

$^{99m}$Tc(V) DMSA is a non-specific tumour imaging agent taken up into a number of different and disparate tumours. Its main use clinically is in the management of medullary thyroid carcinoma (MTC). This rare tumour is characterized by its slow growing nature and patients may survive many years despite distant metastases. $^{99m}$Tc(V) DMSA is taken up at sites of both soft tissue and bone recurrence.

## Diagnosis of MTC

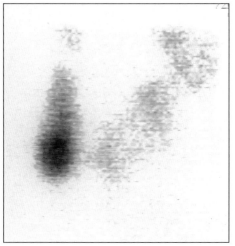

*a* Anterior

**Fig. 4.63**

*A 70-year-old patient presenting with a neck mass.*

*The $^{99m}$Tc thyroid scan (a) demonstrates a non-functioning lesion in the left lobe of the thyroid which was solid on ultrasound. In view of the patient's long history of diarrhoea, a serum calcitonin estimation was performed. While the results of this test were awaited, a $^{99m}$Tc(V) DMSA scan was performed (b–d) which demonstrates uptake of $^{99m}$Tc(V) DMSA in the region of the thyroid mass, confirming an MTC. This was also confirmed on fine-needle aspiration.*

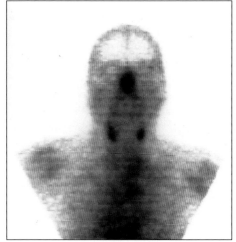

*b* Anterior

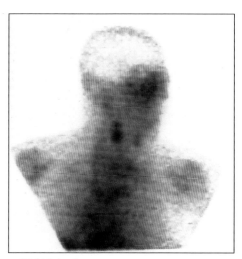

*c* Right lateral

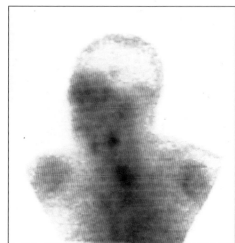

*d* Left lateral

## CLINICAL APPLICATIONS

### *Staging*

Many patients with MTC have metastases at the time of initial diagnosis. These are frequently asymptomatic, and in view of the slow growing nature of the disease, the presence of distant metastases does not contraindicate aggressive surgery in the neck and mediastinum.

**Table 4.7   Sites of spread in MTC**

Local lymph nodes
Mediastinial lymph nodes
Skeleton
Liver
Lungs

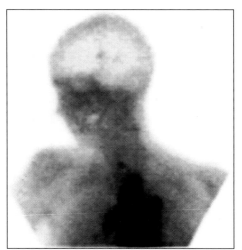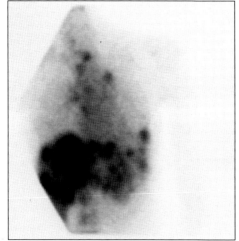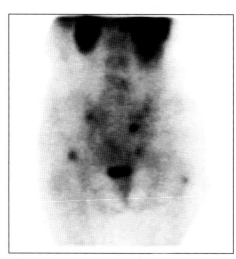

a *Anterior*                b *Anterior*                c *Posterior*

### *Fig. 4.64*

*A 67-year-old with a 15-year history of MTC and stable calcitonin levels. Six months prior to imaging the calcitonin levels started to rise and the patient developed diarrhoea and bone pain.*

*$^{99m}Tc(V)$ DMSA scan shows recurrence in the thyroid bed and mediastinum (**a**), liver and ribs (**b**), and pelvis and upper right femur (**c**).*

## CLINICAL APPLICATIONS

## Follow-up

The main therapeutic tool in MTC is surgery to all accessible lesions. $^{99m}$Tc(V) DMSA performed before and after surgery enables the success of the surgery to be determined.

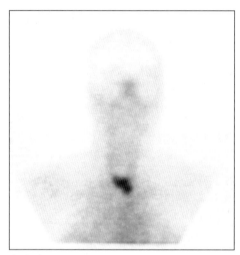

Anterior

**Fig. 4.65**

*Postoperative $^{99m}$Tc(V) DMSA scan in a patient with MTC, showing residual tumour at the site of surgery.*

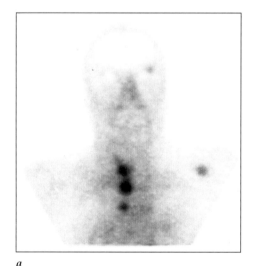

a                              b

**Fig. 4.66**

*A 67-year-old man with a 5-year history of MTC.*

*A $^{99m}$Tc(V) DMSA scan (a) was performed, since the patient represented with masses in the right side of the neck. The scan confirms recurrent tumour, but also identifies bone metastases in the left shoulder and left orbit.*

*Following further surgery a repeat scan (b) showed residual tumour in the neck. The bone metastases were unaltered.*

 **False positive uptake may be observed in patients who have recently had a sternotomy or who have benign bone disease.**

## CLINICAL APPLICATIONS

### Registration of $^{99m}Tc(V)$ DMSA images with MRI

$^{99m}Tc(V)$ DMSA provides a highly specific tool for studying patients with MTC. Its sensitivity in low-volume disease is less than 80%, however. By combining the images acquired by MRI with the $^{99m}Tc(V)$ DMSA image optimum sensitivity and specificity is obtained.

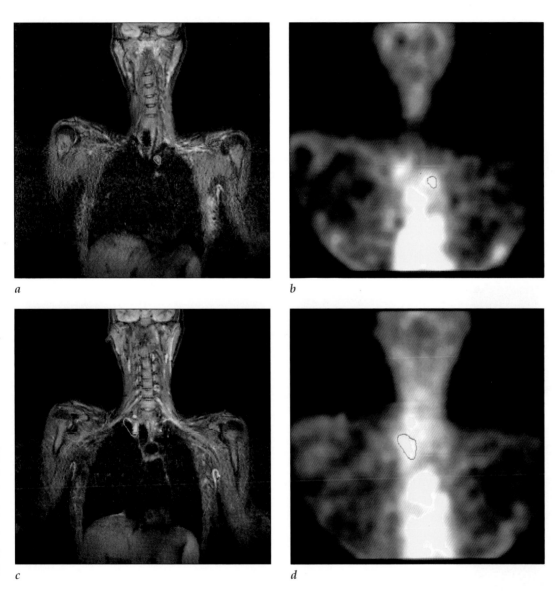

a

b

c

d

**Fig. 4.67**

*Registered coronal images, (a,c) MRI, (b,d) $^{99m}Tc(V)$ DMSA, localizing small tumour deposits on an anatomically accurate MRI scan.*

## CLINICAL APPLICATIONS

### 4.3.9 $^{123/131}$I MIBG

*Table 4.7* MIBG-*accumulating tumours*

| Tumour type | Sensitivity |
|---|---|
| Phaeochromocytoma | 85% |
| Neuroblastoma | 90% |
| Carcinoid | 40% |
| Medullary thyroid carcinoma (MTC) | 30% |
| Paraganglioma | 30% |

## Malignant phaeochromocytoma

Malignant phaeochromocytomas are rare, but, when they metastasize, the deposits will usually accumulate MIBG in the same way as the primary or benign phaeochromocytomas. Apart from identifying the sites of spread of the tumour, the scan permits an assessment of the potential for treating these tumours with therapeutic doses of $^{131}$I MIBG.

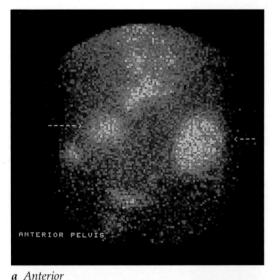

*a Anterior*

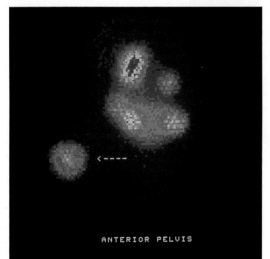

*b Anterior*

*Fig. 4.68*

*Case 1 (a)* *Anterior view of abdomen and pelvis 24 hours after* $^{131}$I MIBG *injection, showing deposits in the pelvis and abdomen (arrows).*

*Case 2 (b)* *Anterior view of abdomen and pelvis 24 hours after injection of* $^{123}$I MIBG, *showing multiple tumours in the bladder wall and in nodes above the bladder. Note also deposit in the right upper femur (arrow). (Courtesy of Professor D Ackery, Southampton, UK.)*

## Neuroblastoma

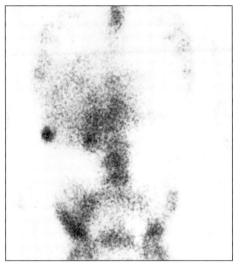

*a Anterior, bone scan*

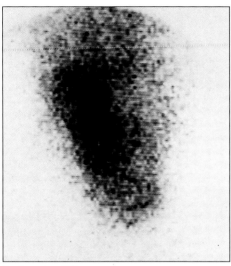

*b Anterior, ¹³¹I MIBG*

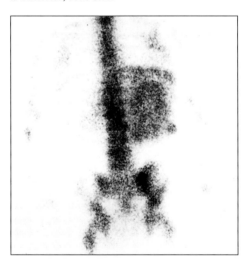

*c Posterior, bone scan*

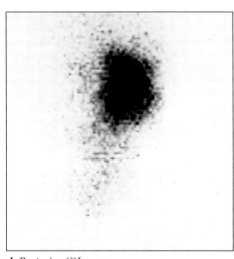

*d Posterior, ¹³¹I MIBG*

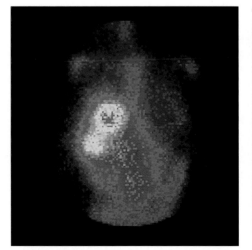

*a Anterior*

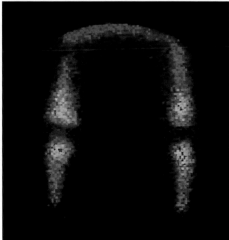

*b Anterior*

### Fig. 4.69

**(a)** *Anterior view of abdomen and pelvis of an* MDP *bone scan, showing a focus of increased tracer uptake in the right ilium. However, in addition, there is diffuse soft tissue uptake in the right hypochondrium.* **(b)** *Anterior 48-hour* MIBG *scan view of abdomen, uptake in the same site as seen with* MDP. **(c)** *Posterior* MDP *bone scan view of abdomen and pelvis, showing multiple focal abnormalities throughout the skeleton and, in addition, showing soft tissue uptake.* **(d)** *Posterior* MIBG *scan view of abdomen showing uptake in the soft tissue mass.*

*The patient was a 4-year-old boy who presented with a right-sided abdominal mass caused by neuroblastoma. Had surgery not been successful, the uptake in this case is high enough to justify undertaking treatment with a therapeutic dose of* ¹³¹I MIBG.

• The case illustrated in Fig. 4.69 provides a good example of a specific and a non-specific radiopharmaceutical. The ⁹⁹ᵐTc diphosphonate is non-specific, and does not reveal anything about pathology. The ¹³¹I MIBG is specific, indicating a tumour of neural crest origin.

### Fig. 4.70

**(a)** *Anterior view of chest and abdomen, showing a large multifocal neuroblastoma accumulating* ¹³¹I MIBG *in a child.* **(b)** *Anterior view of femora, showing* ¹³¹I MIBG *uptake in the marrow.*

Note that tracer uptake in long bones is always abnormal on a MIBG scan, since it indicates marrow involvement.

# Carcinoid syndrome

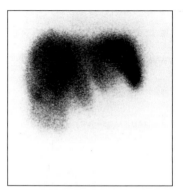

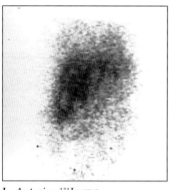

*a  Anterior, liver/spleen colloid*

*b  Anterior, ¹³¹I MIBG*

**Fig. 4.71**

*(a) Anterior view of colloid liver/spleen scan. (b) Anterior abdominal view of ¹³¹I MIBG scan.*

*This patient had carcinoid syndrome and liver metastases. The liver scan shows non-homogeneity of tracer uptake, but with the suggestion of more focal defects at the lower right lobe. MIBG uptake is seen at this site.*

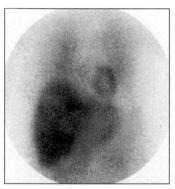

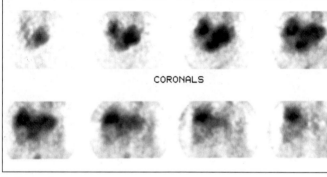

CORONALS

*a  Anterior, 1 hour*

*b  Coronal SPECT*

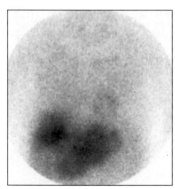

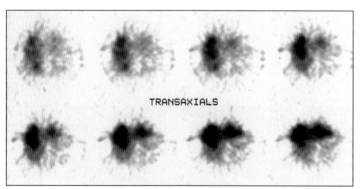

TRANSAXIALS

*c  Anterior, 24 hours*

*d  Transaxial SPECT*

**Fig. 4.72**

*Anterior ¹²³I MIBG scan (a) at 1 hour and (c) at 24 hours in a patient with carcinoid tumour.*

*The 1-hour image (a) shows relatively photon-deficient areas in the liver on the predominantly blood pool image. At 24 hours (c), the ¹²³I MIBG has accumulated in the previously photon-deficient areas. SPECT imaging (b,d) confirms focal localization within the liver metastases.*

*This patient was subsequently treated with ¹³¹I MIBG (see page 312, this chapter).*

SPECT **at 24 hours with** ¹²³I MIBG **increases the sensitivity of liver metastases detection.**

**CLINICAL APPLICATIONS**

# 4.3.10    $^{111}$In octreotide

$^{111}$In octreotide, an octapeptide analogue of somato-statin, is a newly developed tumour imaging agent whose clinical role is still being defined. As the mecha-nism of uptake relies on the presence of somatostatin receptors on the tumour membrane, a positive study indicates that the tumour may respond to somatostatin therapy. Similarly, a negative study indicates that somatostatin therapy is unlikely to be beneficial.

*Table 4.8    Tumours showing $^{111}$In octreotide uptake*

Neuroblastoma
Phaeochromocytoma
Carcinoid
Pancreatic islet cell
Glomus tumour
Medullary thyroid
Lymphoma
Breast

## $^{111}$In octreotide in MTC

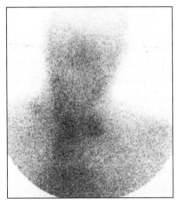

*a Anterior*

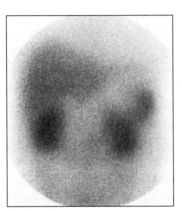

*b Anterior*

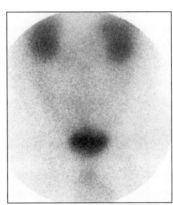

*c Anterior*

**Fig. 4.73**

$^{111}$In octreotide scan in a patient with primary medullary thyroid cancer. There is uptake at the site of the primary tumour (**a**). No other sites of disease are identified (**b,c**).

## $^{111}$In octreotide in breast cancer

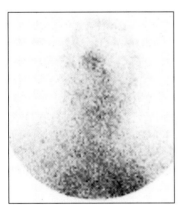

*a Anterior*

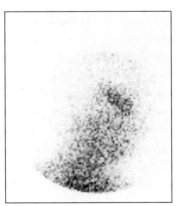

*b Right lateral*

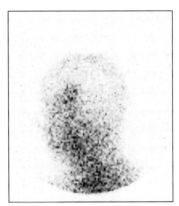

*c Left lateral*

**Fig. 4.74**

(**a–c**) $^{111}$In octreotide scan in a patient with breast cancer and a known cerebral metastasis, showing uptake in the right frontoparietal region at the site of metastasis.

**CLINICAL APPLICATIONS**

## *¹¹¹In octreotide in carcinoid: comparison with ¹²³I MIBG*

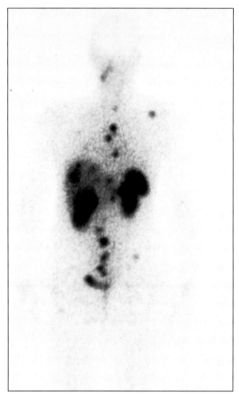

*a  Anterior,¹¹¹In octreotide*

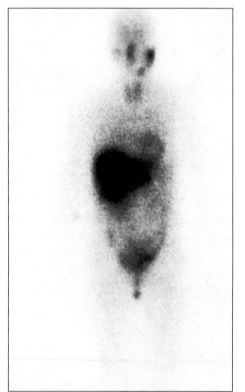

*c  Anterior, ¹²³I MIBG*

*b  Posterior, ¹¹¹In octreotide*

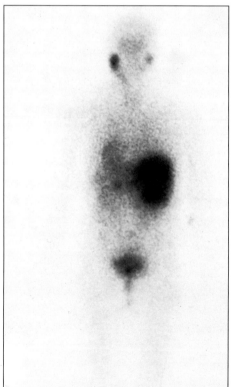

*d  Posterior, ¹²³I MIBG*

*Fig. 4.75*

*(a,b)* ¹¹¹*In octreotide scan in a patient with metastatic carcinoid, showing multiple lesions in the liver, spine and abdomen. (c,d)* ¹²³*I MIBG scan in the same patient, showing minimal MIBG accumulation in the tumour sites. (Courtesy of Prof. M. Fischer, Kassell, Germany.)*

## 4.3.11 Monoclonal antibodies

### *Breast carcinoma*

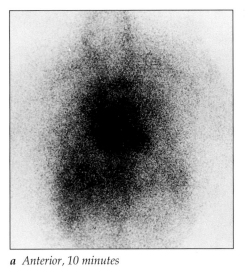 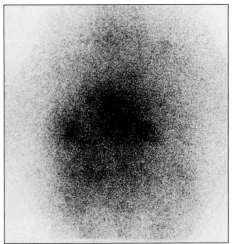 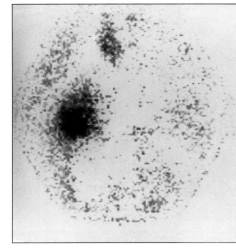

*a Anterior, 10 minutes*      *b Anterior, 24 hours*      *c Anterior, 24 hour view – 10 minute view*

### Fig. 4.76

**(a)** *Anterior view of chest and abdomen 5–10 minutes after injection of $^{131}$I-labelled anti-breast cancer antigen monoclonal antibody, showing the normal blood pool distribution of labelled protein at 10 minutes.* **(b)** *Same view at 24 hours, showing uptake in a right breast tumour.* **(c)** *Same view with 10-minute view subtracted from the 24-hour view, showing more clearly the uptake into the right breast tumour.*

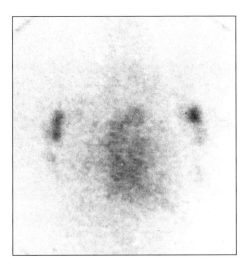

### Fig. 4.77

*$^{123}$I HMFG 2, an antibody to milk fat globule, was injected into the web spaces of both hands of a patient with a right-sided breast carcinoma.*

*At 24 hours uptake in both axillae was symmetrical despite unilateral breast disease, confirming non-specific uptake in normal lymph nodes of this antibody.*

## Melanoma

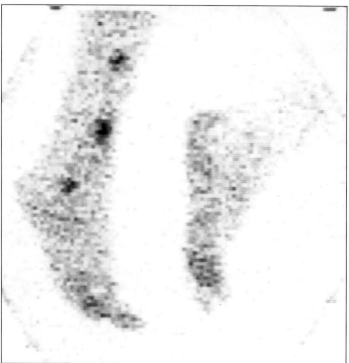

*Lateral, 24 hours*

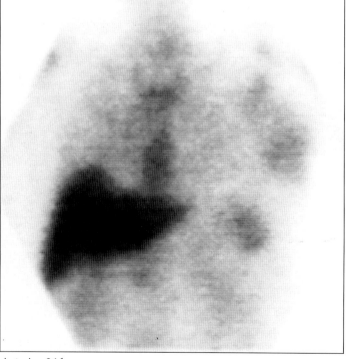

*Anterior, 24 hours*

**Fig. 4.78**

*Lateral view of right leg 24 hours after injection of $^{131}$I-labelled anti-melanoma monoclonal antibody, showing uptake into three cutaneous melanoma deposits.*

**Fig. 4.79**

*Anterior view of chest 24 hours after injection of $^{131}$I-labelled anti-melanoma monoclonal antibody, showing uptake in a left axillary melanoma metastasis.*

## Colon carcinoma

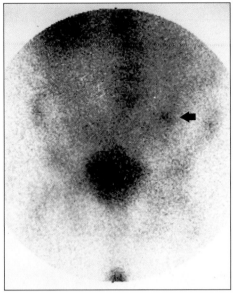

a Anterior

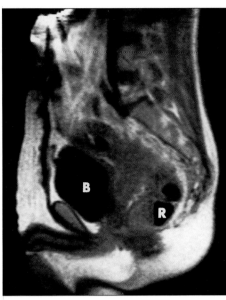

b

### Fig. 4.80

A 62-year-old male with suspected recurrence of a rectal tumour following a previous Hartman's procedure.

(a) Anterior image of the pelvic cavity 48 hours following administration of 80 MBq [111]In B72.3 antibody (Oncoscint). The image shows intense uptake of antibody centrally in the pelvis. A further site of focal uptake (arrow) can also be seen above and to the left of this mass, at the level of the iliac crest. This uptake is at the site of a colostomy and has been recognized as a normal feature of such studies. Normal distribution of activity may also be seen in the bone marrow.

(b) Sagittal T1-weighted MRI image through the pelvis of this patient demonstrating the tumour mass situated between the urinary bladder (B) and the rectum (R). (Courtesy of Drs AC Perkins and ML Wastie, Nottingham, UK.)

## Ovarian carcinoma

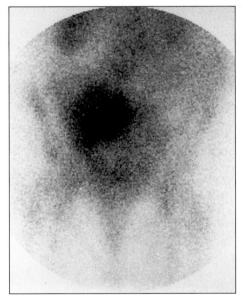

a Anterior

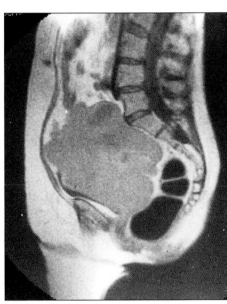

b

### Fig. 4.81

A 78-year-old woman with a suspected primary ovarian carcinoma.

(a) Anterior view of the pelvic region 48 hours following administration of 80 MBq [111]In OC 25 F(ab´)[2] antibody. Intense accumulation of activity can be seen in the right side of the pelvic cavity, consistent with a malignant tumour. Faint accumulation of activity may also be seen in the bone tumour.

(b) Sagittal SE 560/40 T1-weighted MRI image through the pelvis, demonstrating the limits of this large ovarian tumour.

Following surgery, histology confirmed an adenocarcinoma of the ovary. (Courtesy of Drs AC Perkins and ML Wastie, Nottingham, UK.)

# 4.3.12 Therapy

Although gamma (γ) ray production is not essential in a radionuclide used for therapy, a low abundance of γ photons permits imaging in the post-therapy period.

## Role of radionuclide imaging post-therapy

• Confirm uptake at known tumour sites
• Identify unknown tumour sites not visualized with low tracer doses
• Permit approximate dosimetric calculations to be undertaken
• Confirm retention at tumour site by delayed imaging.

## $^{131}I$ therapy

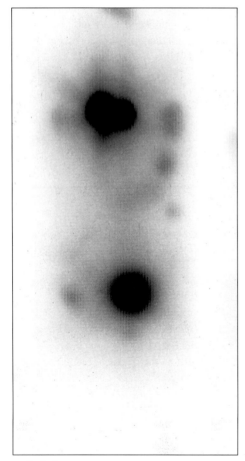

a Anterior

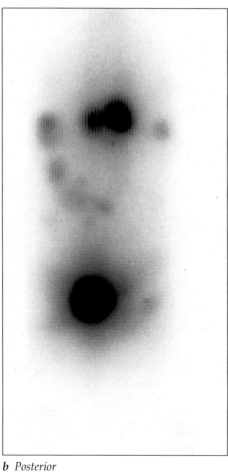

b Posterior

**Fig. 4.82**

*(a,b) Post-therapy whole-body $^{131}I$ scan confirming uptake in recurrent disease in the anterior mediastinum. A right lower rib lesion not seen on the tracer scan is also visualized, as is a lesion in the right iliac crest.*

**CLINICAL APPLICATIONS**

## Samarium-153 EDTMP therapy

*Bone scan*

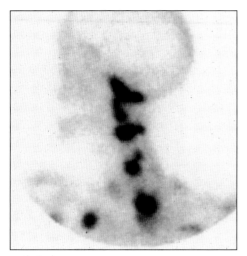

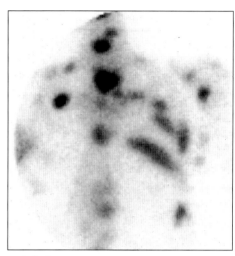

*a Anterior*    *b Anterior*    *c Anterior*

¹⁵³*Sm* EDTMP

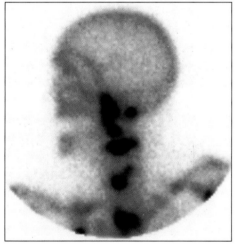

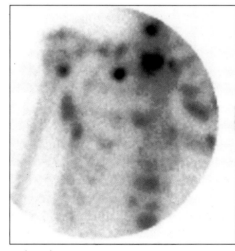

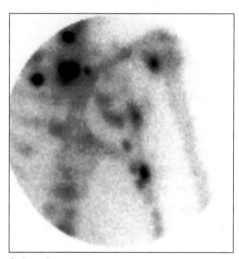

*d Anterior*    *e Anterior*    *f Anterior*

**Fig. 4.83**

**(a–c)** *Bone scan of a patient with metastases from carcinoma of the prostate.*

*The patient underwent palliative therapy for bone pain using samarium-153* EDTMP *(¹⁵³Sm* EDTMP*). The post-therapy ¹⁵³Sm* EDTMP **(d–f)** *shows uptake of the therapy dose at sites of previous ⁹⁹ᵐTc diphosphonate uptake.*

# $^{131}$I MIBG therapy

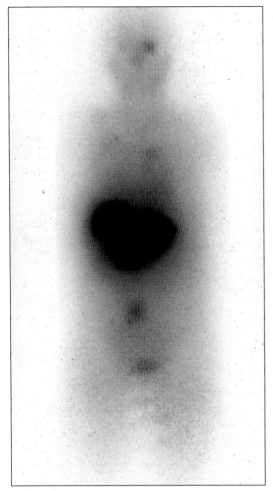

a Anterior

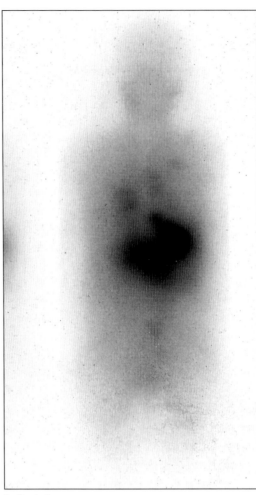

b Posterior

**Fig. 4.84**

**(a,b)** Post-therapy scan in a patient treated with $^{131}$I MIBG for carcinoid.

The scan shows good uptake in the liver, lungs, orbit and abdominal lesions.

# CHAPTER 5

# BRAIN

Radionuclide brain scans utilize three major groups of agents (see Table 5.1), each of which investigates a completely different physiological process. The blood–brain barrier (BBB) agents such as technetium-99m diethylenetriamine pentaacetic acid (⁹⁹ᵐTc DPTA) localize within the vasculature in a normal study, and are only seen in the brain in regions when there has been breakdown of the blood–brain barrier or the formation of new 'leaky' capillaries. Planar imaging with these agents is usually performed, although single photon emission computed tomography (SPECT) may aid lesion localization.

The cerebral perfusion agents such as technetium-99m (⁹⁹ᵐTc) HMPAO or iodine-123 (¹²³I) IMP are taken up into the brain in proportion to the regional cerebral blood flow. A normal study with these agents will therefore show radiotracer within the brain, with abnormalities usually being indicated by areas of relatively decreased activity. In order to accurately define regional cerebral perfusion, SPECT imaging is usually vital. These radiotracers are gradually supplanting the BBB agents for many conditions such as the investigation of stroke, dementia and epilepsy because of their increased sensitivity and specificity. However, BBB agents still have clinical utility, and may sometimes be the agents of choice. Static imaging with either BBB or cerebral perfusion tracers may be preceded by a dynamic blood flow study, which may provide valuable information about the extracranial vessels and major cerebral vasculature. Some lesions such as arterio-venous malformations will be best seen during the dynamic study. Repeated imaging in a BBB study over several hours can give useful information, since tumours in particular can show differences in the rates of accumulation of tracers with different tumour histologies. Tumours may also be investigated using thallium-201 (²⁰¹Tl).

The third group of agents used in brain scanning are those used to investigate CSF dynamics. These are injected into the subarachnoid space. An example is indium-111 (¹¹¹In) DPTA. Planar imaging is usually performed.

Computed tomography (CT) or magnetic resonance (MRI) scanning, when available, will usually be the primary investigation of choice in many neurological conditions. Radionuclide brain scans may be used as a screening method for patients, decreasing the number who will then require CT scans. In some conditions the ability of these studies to provide information about function rather than anatomy aids diagnosis in the presence of a normal CT scan.

## CHAPTER CONTENTS

# 5.1 ANATOMY

## 5.1.1 Anatomical regions of the brain

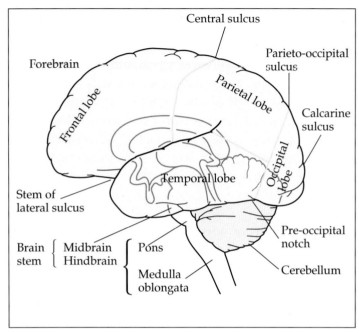

a  *Sagittal*

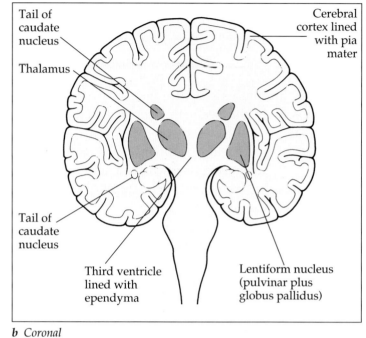

b  *Coronal*

**Fig. 5.1**

*(a) Diagram showing the general layout of the major components of the brain in the sagittal section. (b) Diagram of a coronal section through the cerebrum and brainstem, showing the general relationships of the deep masses of grey matter.*

# 5.1.2 Cerebral vasculature

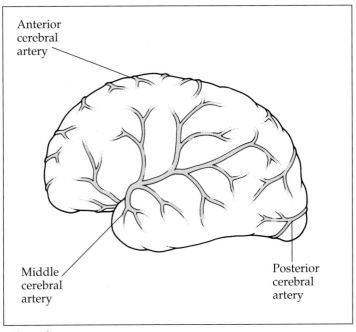

Anterior
cerebral
artery

Middle
cerebral
artery

Posterior
cerebral
artery

*a Lateral*

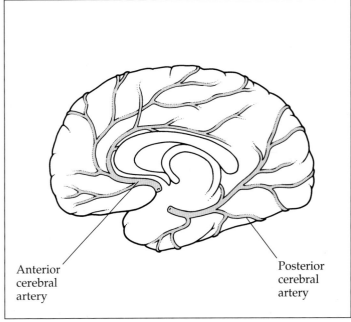

Anterior
cerebral
artery

Posterior
cerebral
artery

*b Medial*

**Fig. 5.2**

*Diagrams demonstrating the blood supply to the cerebral
hemispheres: (a) lateral view; (b) medial view.*

*The three arteries of the cerebral hemispheres, the anterior,
middle and posterior cerebral arteries, are connected via the Circle
of Willis.*

# 5.2  RADIOPHARMACEUTICALS

*Table 5.1  Radiopharmaceuticals for brain imaging*

| Radiotracer | Site localization | Pathological localization | Agent of choice in investigation of: |
|---|---|---|---|
| *Blood–brain barrier agents*<br>$^{99m}TcO_4$<br>$^{99m}Tc$ DTPA<br>$^{99m}Tc$ GHA | Localize in the intravascular space | Localize in regions where BBB breakdown occurs. Show abnormal blood pools | Primary and secondary brain tumours<br>Herpes encephalitis<br>Subdurals<br>Carotid stenosis<br>AVMS |
| *Cerebral perfusion agents*<br>$^{99m}Tc$ HMPAO<br>$^{123}I$ IMP<br>$^{99m}Tc$ ECD | Taken up by the brain | Decreased uptake seen in areas of hypoperfusion or hypofunction | Cerebral infarction and haemorrhage<br>TIAS<br>Epilepsy<br>Dementia<br>Head trauma |
| *CSF agents*<br>$^{111}In$ DTPA<br>$^{99m}Tc$ DTPA | Remain in CSF | Enter abnormally dilated ventricles communicating with CSF. Show abnormal CSF dynamics, leaks and shunts | Dilated ventricles<br>CSF leaks<br>Shunt patency |
| *Tumour agents*<br>$^{201}Tl$ | Extracellular fluid | Tumours | Tumour recurrence vs fibrosis/necrosis |

DTPA, diethylenetriamine pentaacetic acid;  GHA, glucoheptonate; HMPAO, hexamethylpropyleneamine oxime; IMP, iodoamphetamine; ECD, ethyl cysteinate dimer

# Localization of blood–brain barrier (BBB) agents

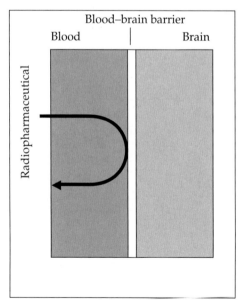

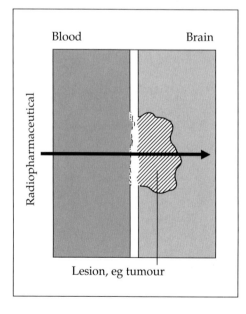

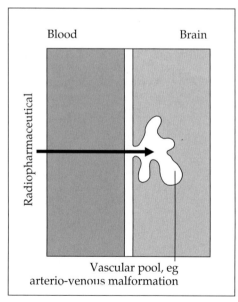

*Fig. 5.3*

*Normal mechanism*

*Fig. 5.4*

*Abnormal mechanism: breakdown of BBB/ presence of new ('leaky') capillaries.*

*Fig. 5.5*

*Abnormal mechanism: presence of vascular pool.*

## Normal distribution of uptake

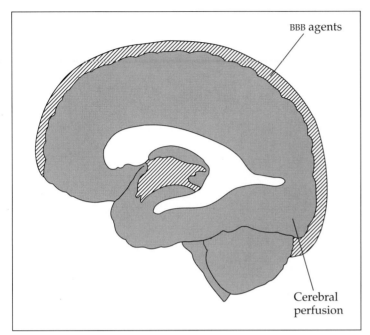

**Fig. 5.6**

*Diagram showing normal distribution of uptake.*

## Uptake of cerebral perfusion agents

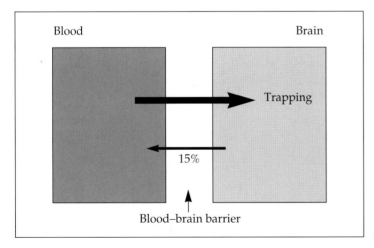

**Fig. 5.7**

*Passive uptake of lipophilic tracer with 70–80% first pass extraction. Active trapping in brain, with only a small amount of tracer returned to circulation ($^{99m}$Tc HMPAO). With $^{123}$I IMP, some redistribution of the radiotracer takes place, and so scanning must be completed within the first hour.*

# 5.3 NORMAL SCANS WITH VARIANTS AND ARTEFACTS

## 5.3.1 Normal BBB agent ($^{99m}$Tc DTPA) scan

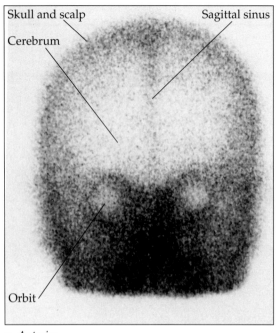

*a Anterior*

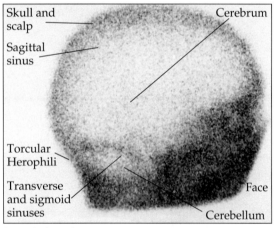

*b Right lateral*

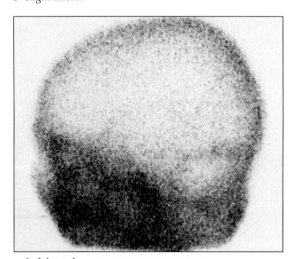

*c Left lateral*

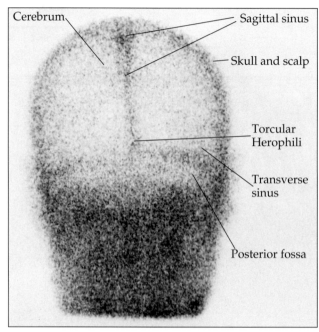

*d Posterior*

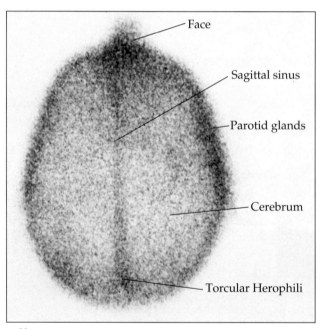

*e Vertex*

**Fig. 5.8**

*(a–e) The normal brain scan imaged 1–2 hours after an intravenous injection of $^{99m}$Tc DTPA.*

# 5.3.2 Normal $^{99m}$Tc DTPA: dynamic vascular study

The dynamic brain scan is obtained by accumulating images during the first passage of the injected bolus of radiopharmaceutical through the brain. Images may be displayed in a variety of ways (eg 1–2 per second or by adding the arterial and venous phases separately).

Time–activity (T/A) curves can be generated from regions of interest (ROIS). Individual vessels should be noted, and abnormal areas on the static brain scan assessed in conjunction with vascularity.

## Anterior view

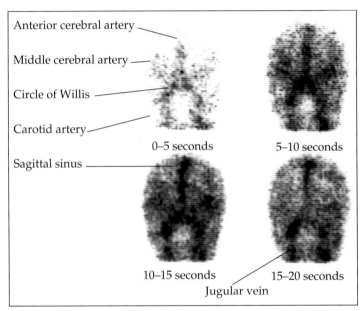

Anterior cerebral artery

Middle cerebral artery

Circle of Willis

Carotid artery

Sagittal sinus

0–5 seconds   5–10 seconds

10–15 seconds   15–20 seconds

Jugular vein

*a* Anterior

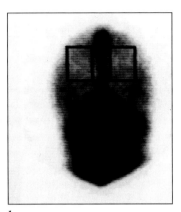

*b*

**Fig. 5.9**

**(a)** *Anterior images obtained during the first 30 seconds following a bolus intravenous injection of radionuclide.* **(b)** *ROIS over cerebral hemisphere.* **(c)** *T/A curves from ROIS.*

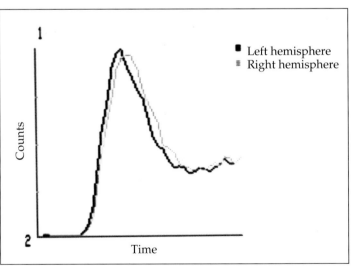

Counts

Time

■ Left hemisphere
▤ Right hemisphere

*c*

# NORMAL SCANS WITH VARIANTS AND ARTEFACTS

## Posterior view

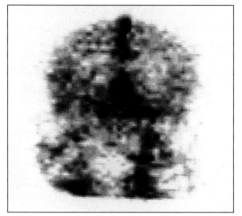

*a* Posterior

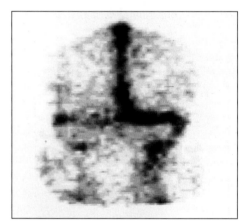

*c* Posterior

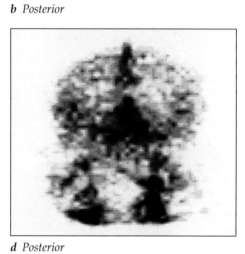

*b* Posterior

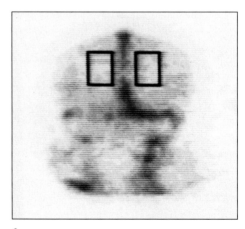

*d* Posterior

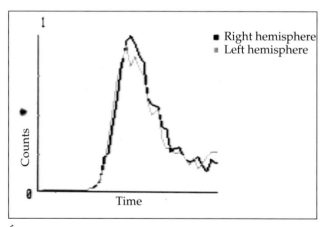

*e*

*f*

*Fig. 5.10*

*(a–d)* Posterior dynamic images. *(e)* ROI over hemispheres. *(f)* T/A curves from ROIs.

# NORMAL SCANS WITH VARIANTS AND ARTEFACTS

## Vertex view

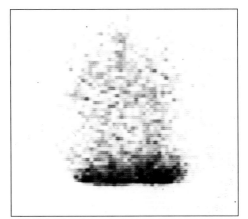

*a* Vertex

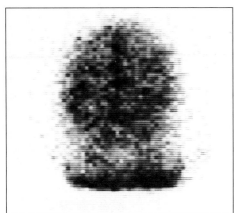

*b* Vertex

### Fig. 5.11

*(a–d)* Vertex view images, obtained during the first 30 seconds after injection. *(e)* ROIS over cerebral hemisphere. *(f)* T/A curves from ROIS.

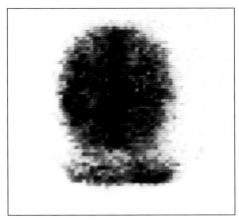

*c* Vertex

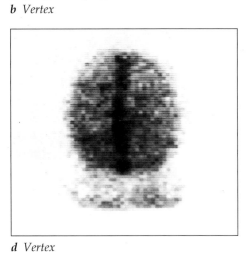

*d* Vertex

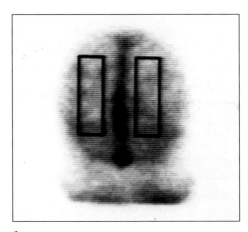

*e*

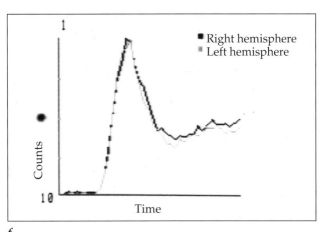

■ Right hemisphere
≡ Left hemisphere

Counts

Time

*f*

## 5.3.3   Normal regional cerebral perfusion study ($^{99m}$Tc HMPAO)

Following intravenous injection, $^{99m}$Tc HMPAO and $^{123}$I IMP are taken up into the brain tissue in proportion to the regional blood flow. The exact mechanisms remain somewhat unclear. Thus areas with a high blood flow, such as grey matter and basal ganglia, will show relatively avid uptake of tracer, whereas white matter will take up much less.

### *Transaxial slices*

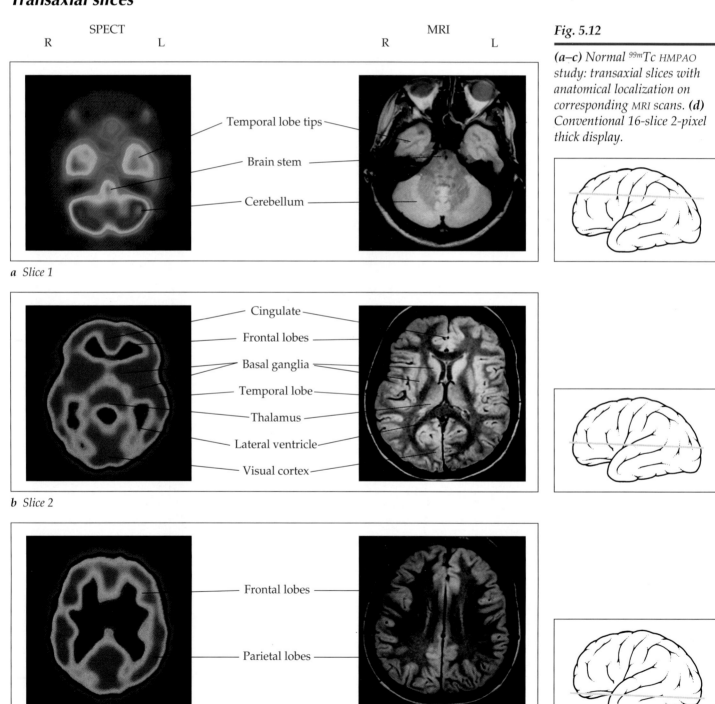

*Fig. 5.12*

(a–c) Normal $^{99m}$Tc HMPAO study: transaxial slices with anatomical localization on corresponding MRI scans. (d) Conventional 16-slice 2-pixel thick display.

a  Slice 1

b  Slice 2

c  Slice 3

# NORMAL SCANS WITH VARIANTS AND ARTEFACTS

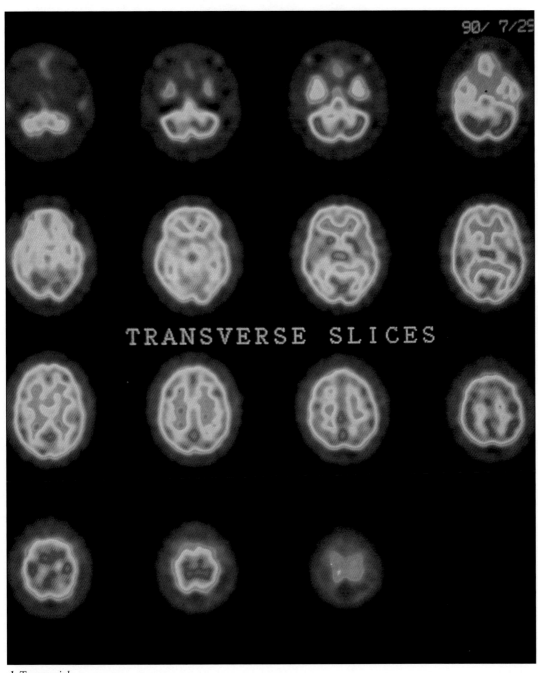

*d Transaxial*

## Coronal slices

SPECT                                    MRI
R              L                   R              L

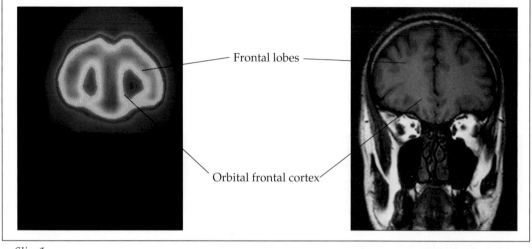

Frontal lobes

Orbital frontal cortex

*a* Slice 1

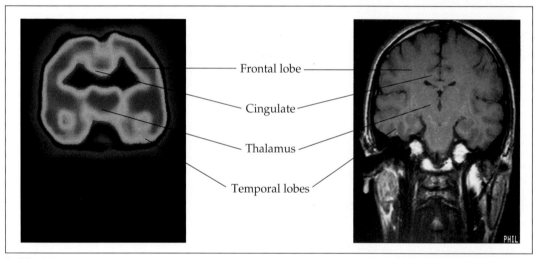

Frontal lobe

Cingulate

Thalamus

Temporal lobes

*b* Slice 2

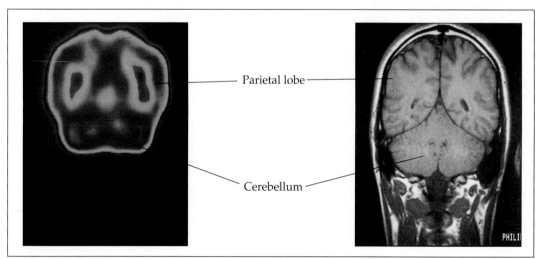

Parietal lobe

Cerebellum

*c* Slice 3

*Fig. 5.13*

**(a–d)** *Normal* [99m]*Tc* HMPAO *study: coronal slices with anatomical localization on corresponding* MRI *scans.* **(d)** *Conventional 16-slice, 2-pixel thick display.*

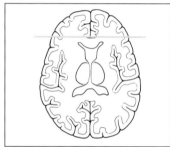

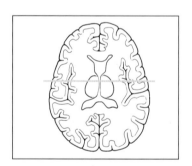

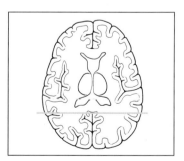

# NORMAL SCANS WITH VARIANTS AND ARTEFACTS

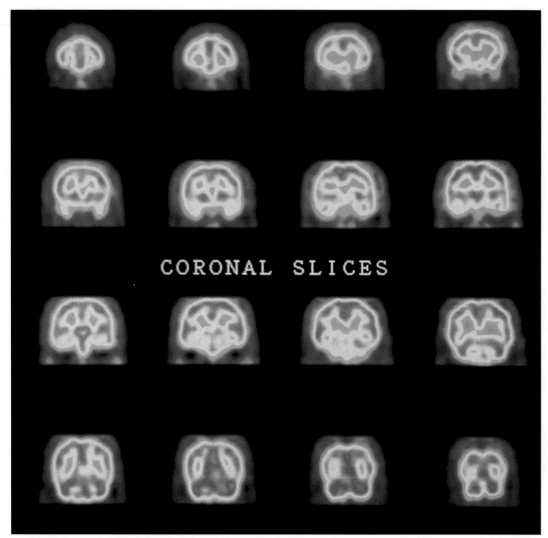

d Coronal

## *Sagittal slices*

SPECT                              MRI
R                    L        R                L

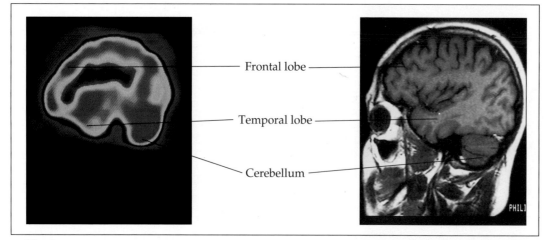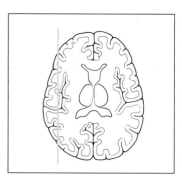

Frontal lobe

Temporal lobe

Cerebellum

*a*  *Slice 1*

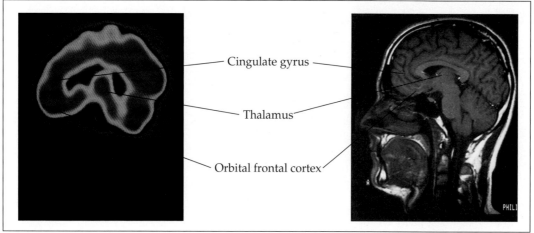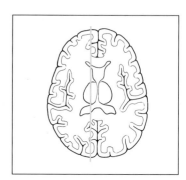

Cingulate gyrus

Thalamus

Orbital frontal cortex

*b*  *Slice 2*

### Fig. 5.14

*(a, b) Normal ⁹⁹ᵐTc HMPAO study: sagittal slices with anatomical localization on corresponding MRI scans. (c) Conventional 16-slice, 2-pixel thick display.*

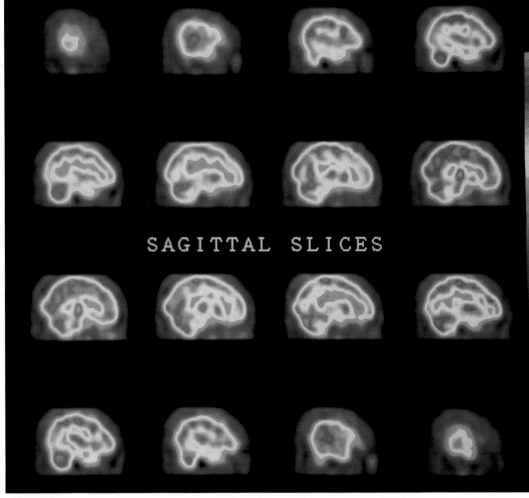

c  Sagittal

Fig. 5.14 (cont.)

## *Temporal lobe slices*

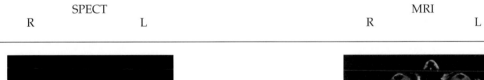

Fig. 5.15

Normal $^{99m}$Tc HMPAO study: temporal lobe slices.

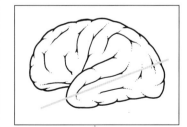

**NORMAL SCANS WITH VARIANTS AND ARTEFACTS**

## 5.3.4 Cerebral perfusion agents: normal planar images

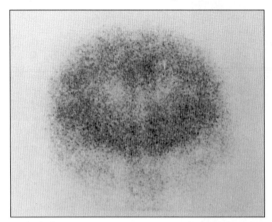

*a Anterior*

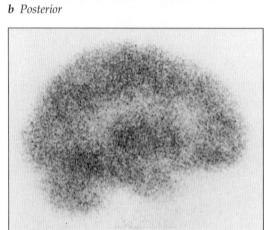

*b Posterior*

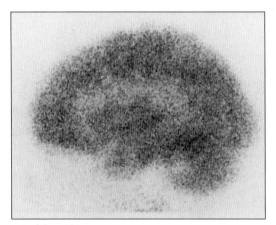

*c Left lateral*

*d Right lateral*

*Fig. 5.16*

*(a–d)* Normal planar $^{99m}Tc$ HMPAO *images.*

# 5.3.5 Variations and artefacts in SPECT imaging

Unfortunately, because of the complex nature of SPECT imaging, artefacts are easily introduced during the acquisition or processing, and may lead to misinterpretation of studies if not recognized. It is therefore important to be aware of these potential artefacts when interpreting brain SPECT studies.

## *Misinjection/delayed injection*

$^{99m}$Tc HMPAO is unstable and must be injected within 30 minutes of preparation. Injection after this time will result in a high proportion of the tracer existing in the hydrophilic form, which is not taken up by the brain but accumulates in soft tissues. This is easily recognized by the high activity in the parotid gland, and the low brain activity (Fig. 5.17). The same can occur if a dose is misinjected, and occasionally if blood is withdrawn into the syringe prior to injection.

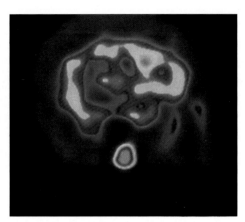

*Fig. 5.17*

*High activity in the parotid gland and low activity in the brain due to delay in injecting $^{99m}$Tc HMPAO, resulting in a significant fraction of the tracer being present in a hydrophilic form.*

Careful quality control is necessary, including paper chromatography of the $^{99m}$Tc HMPAO prior to injection. Injection should be performed immediately after preparation, preferably into a free flowing iv line. Blood should not be withdrawn into the syringe prior to injection.

## *Movement*

Movement of the patient's head during a study can produce significant artefacts, which may mimic focal defects (Fig. 5.18). Often these will prevent interpretation of the study, or may lead to false interpretation if the clinician is unaware of the problem.

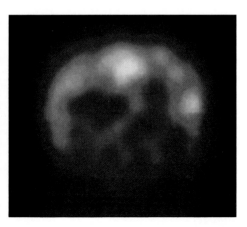

*Fig. 5.18*

*$^{99m}$Tc HMPAO SPECT scan obtained in a child with epilepsy.*

*Marked movement during the study has resulted in significant artefact.*

The patient's head should always be immobilized firmly with tape or velcro to the head-rest prior to the study. Small children or severely demented patients may require sedation, which should be given after the tracer injection, but before scanning. The patient should not be left unattended.

## Positioning

Mispositioning of the head, producing tilt, can make interpretation of SPECT studies very difficult, since asymmetry is used as a measure of abnormality. This can be particularly difficult when assessing for temporal lobe asymmetry, eg in patients with temporal lobe seizures.

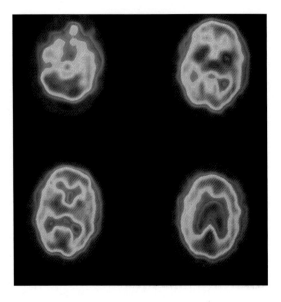

**Fig. 5.19**

*99mTc HMPAO SPECT scan in patient with temporal lobe epilepsy.*
*Severe head tilt in two directions makes interpretation of the right temporal lobe hypoperfusion uncertain.*

**Strenuous attempts should be made to ensure correct positioning. Some cameras contain laser light beams which help. Some also contain software which can perform a degree of tilt correction. The patient's position should be checked from the foot of the table.**

## Low count rate

Low count rates through injection of insufficient activity or partial infiltration are much more of a problem in SPECT than in planar studies. Very noisy studies are obtained, which may produce artefacts (Fig. 5.20).

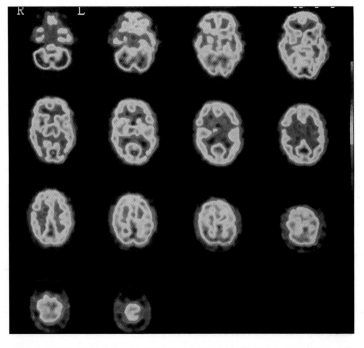

**Fig. 5.20**

*99mTc HMPAO SPECT scan which had only half the expected count rate. Note the noisiness of this study.*

**The usual count rate obtained on the camera should be recorded with brain SPECT studies at the beginning of acquisition. If the count rate in a study falls significantly below the expected, the scanning time per frame should be increased proportionally.**

## NORMAL SCANS WITH VARIANTS AND ARTEFACTS

## *Uniformity and centre of rotation*

In SPECT the field uniformity must be maintained within much closer limits (usually <2%) than can be tolerated with planar imaging. The centre of rotation of the camera must also be regularly checked; otherwise 'bulls eye' artefacts will be induced.

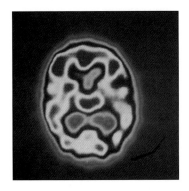

**Fig. 5.21**

$^{99m}Tc$ *HMPAO SPECT scan obtained in a normal volunteer with a non-uniform field.*

**Regular checking of high-count-rate phantoms (both planar and SPECT) is essential, as are regular centre of rotation corrections.**

## *Slice angle*

The angle at which the transaxial slices in brain SPECT studies are produced can have significant effects on the appearance of a study (Fig. 5.22). This is particularly important if patients are having repeated studies. Sometimes special slices such as those orientated along the long axis of the temporal lobes need to be generated in addition to transaxial, coronal and sagittal slices.

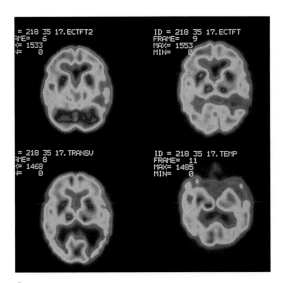

*a*

*b*

**Fig. 5.22**

*(a) Transaxial slices from the same study of a patient with Alzheimer's disease, showing the effect of slicing at the different angles shown in (b).*

**It is important to standardize the angle at which transaxial slices are produced. One way is to use a plane from a line connecting the inferior surfaces of the frontal and occipital lobes on a sagittal or lateral image (Fig. 5.22). External markers may also be placed on the patient's face to mark a line connecting the external canthus of the eye with the tragus of the ear.**

## Processing: attenuation correction and smoothing

Varying the processing of brain SPECT studies can radically affect the appearance of the scan. Increasing attenuation correction makes subcortical structures appear more intense (Fig. 5.23a). Decreased filtering ('smoothing') of images increases the resolution of structures at the expense of increased noise (Fig. 5.23b).

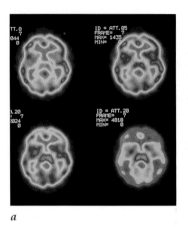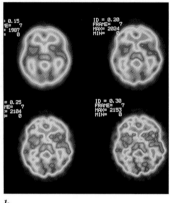

*a*                    *b*

**Fig. 5.23**

*(a)* Illustration of the effect of increasing calculated attenuation (from top left to bottom right). Note the prominence of basal ganglia in the lower right image. A consistent attenuation correction factor should thus be used. *(b)* Illustration of the effect of decreased filtering from top left to bottom right. Note the increased noise but improved resolution with the decreased filtering.

**The processing parameters used will depend on the camera and the type and injected dose of radiotracer. To obtain the optimum combination, trial and error is usually required initially, together with the advice of the camera manufacturer, but, once found, it should be adhered to wherever possible.**

## Display

The display of SPECT images, especially when using different colour schemes, can lead to both false positive and false negative interpretations. Some monochromatic and black-and-white colour schemes tend to underestimate abnormalities; conversely multicoloured schemes tend to overestimate abnormalities (see Fig. 5.24).

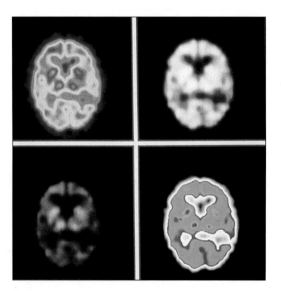

**Fig. 5.24**

*Display of SPECT images using different multicoloured schemes.*

**The user should adhere to a single colour scheme. In this way each user's level of 'normality' will gradually be set for this scheme. Where possible, images should be viewed on the monitor, since this reduces the problem of image saturation. Images should be viewed in all slices, with the display set to the maximum in the entire study, not on a frame-by-frame basis. If CT or MRI studies are available, they should be viewed concurrently. The colour scale should always be displayed and changes in colour (eg red to yellow) should be correlated with percentage changes in cerebral blood flow.**

## 5.3.6   Normal ¹¹¹In DTPA cisternogram

Following introduction of tracer into the CSF via lumbar puncture, it will appear in the basal cisterns after about 2 hours. Subsequent images at 6 and 24 hours will demonstrate rapid flow of CSF through the Sylvian fissure to the cortex, where it is absorbed in the parasagittal region.

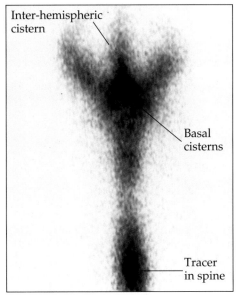

*a  Anterior, 3 hours*

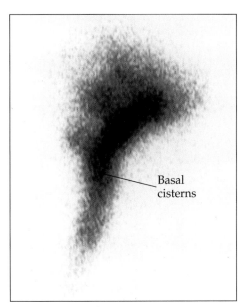

*b  Right lateral, 3 hours*

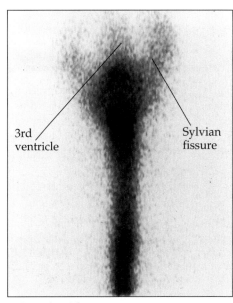

*c  Posterior, 3 hours*

**Fig. 5.25**

*(a–e) Normal ¹¹¹In DTPA cisternogram.*

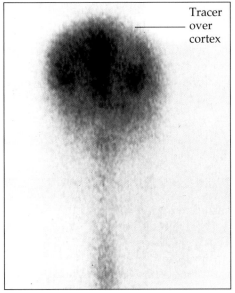

*d  Anterior, 24 hours*

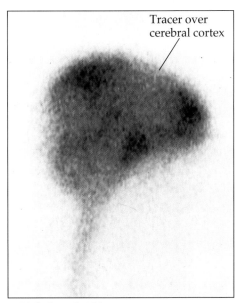

*e  Right lateral, 24 hours*

**In a normal study:**
• **No tracer should enter lateral ventricles**
• **Tracer should have flowed over the cerebral cortex by 24 hours.**

# 5.4 CLINICAL APPLICATIONS

Although the anatomical resolution of x-ray computed tomography (CT) and magnetic resonance (MR) brain imaging has far superseded that of radionuclide brain imaging, important roles remain for the latter when there is limited access to CT or MRI, when information about cerebral blood flow is required and when information about the dynamics of CSF flow is needed.

The more important indications for brain imaging with radionuclides are listed below, and examples of the various clinical problems are given on subsequent pages.

**5.4.1 Suspected cerebral infarction**
BBB agents
Features of cerebral infarction
Cerebral perfusion agents with SPECT
Appearance of middle cerebral artery (MCA) infarction
Appearance of posterior cerebral artery (PCA) infarction
Appearance of anterior cerebral artery (ACA) infarction
Appearance of basal ganglia infarction
Features that may help in the diagnosis of stroke
'Luxury' perfusion
Progress and resolution of scan appearances with time

**5.4.2 Intracerebral haemorrhage**
Cerebral perfusion agents

**5.4.3 Transient ischaemic attacks**
Cerebral perfusion agents

**5.4.4 Carotid artery stenoses**
BBB agents
Cerebral perfusion agents

**5.4.5 Subarachnoid haemorrhage**
Cerebral perfusion imaging

**5.4.6 Arterio-venous malformations**
BBB agents
Cerebral perfusion agents

**5.4.7 Brain death**
BBB agents
Cerebral perfusion agents

**5.4.8 Suspected cerebral infection**
Cerebral abscesses
Localized encephalitis
Generalized encephalitis
Ventriculitis

**5.4.9 Suspected chronic subdural haematoma**
Unilateral subdural haematoma
Bilateral subdural haematoma
Subdural haematoma
Extradural haematoma
Trauma

**5.4.10 CSF leaks**

**5.4.11 CSF shunts**

**5.4.12 Evaluation of dementia or personality change**
Alzheimer's disease
Early Alzheimer's disease
Asymmetric Alzheimer's disease
Progression of disease
Dementia with combined aetiologies
Multiple infarct dementia
Pick's disease
Communicating hydrocephalus (normal pressure hydrocephalus)
Advanced normal pressure hydrocephalus
Obstructive hydrocephalus
Jakob–Creutzfeld disease
Cerebral atrophy

**5.4.13 Investigation of seizures**
Interictal study
Frontal lobe seizures
Ictal study
Seizures caused by space-occupying lesions

**5.4.14 Suspected intracerebral space-occupying lesions**
Primary intracerebral tumour
Frontal lobe
Occipital lobe
Parietal lobe
Sphenoid ridge
Temporal lobe
Posterior fossa
Lateral ventricles
Improved localization and detection with SPECT
$^{201}$Tl SPECT imaging for localization of brain tumours

**5.4.15 Suspected cerebral metastases**
Features of cerebral metastases on the BBB brain scan
Brain metastases demonstrated by $^{99m}$Tc HMPAO SPECT imaging
Lymphoma
Features helping in the diagnosis of space-occupying lesions
Shape and position
Value of delayed views

**5.4.16 The donut sign**

**5.4.17 Skull and scalp lesions**
Bruising
Sebaceous cyst

# 5.4.1 Suspected cerebral infarction

A clinical diagnosis of stroke (cerebral infarct) or haemorrhage is usually adequate, and imaging investigations are not required. Occasionally, there may be some doubt about the diagnosis, in which case a brain scan is a valuable investigation.

When scanning with BBB agents, a stroke will appear as a region of decreased flow on the dynamic image, and will appear positive on delayed imaging owing to diffusion of the radiotracer across the leaky blood–brain barrier as well as accumulation of extracellular fluid in and around the infarct. With cerebral perfusion agents, decreased activity will be seen in accordance with the decreased perfusion to the region of the stroke. With both types of agents, the abnormalities follow vascular territories, and will indicate the vessels involved and assist in the differential diagnosis.

## *BBB agents*

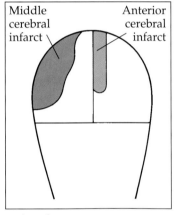

*a Anterior*

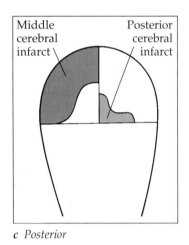

*b Lateral*

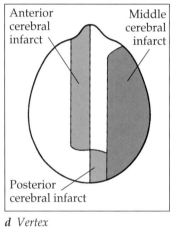

*c Posterior*

*d Vertex*

**Fig. 5.26**

*(a–d) Diagrammatic representation of localization of abnormalities seen in cerebral infarction.*

## *Features of cerebral infarction*

• The area of uptake will correspond to the anatomical territory of a blood vessel
• The uptake will increase with time from injection to imaging
• Usually, the dynamic blood flow study shows decreased blood flow, but increased blood flow may also occur (luxury perfusion)

• A static brain scan (but not the dynamic) may be negative immediately after the onset of a stroke. The positivity of the brain scan reaches a peak seven days after the onset.

## Cerebral perfusion agents with SPECT

*Transaxial slice*

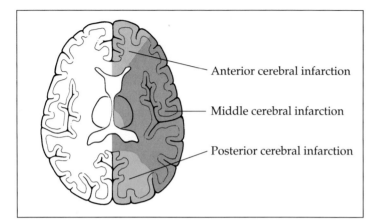

Anterior cerebral infarction

Middle cerebral infarction

Posterior cerebral infarction

**Fig. 5.27**

*Diagrammatic representation of regional abnormalities seen in cerebral infarction.*

*Coronal slice*

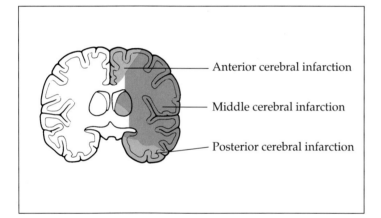

Anterior cerebral infarction

Middle cerebral infarction

Posterior cerebral infarction

*Sagittal slice*

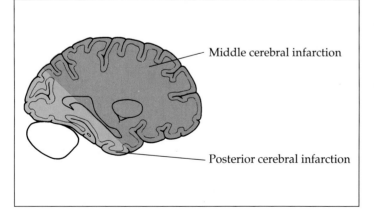

Middle cerebral infarction

Posterior cerebral infarction

- An infarct may not involve an entire vascular territory
- Vascular territories show some variation between individuals

## Appearance of middle cerebral artery (MCA) infarction

### BBB agents

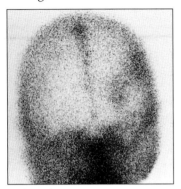 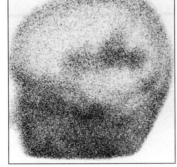 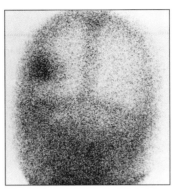 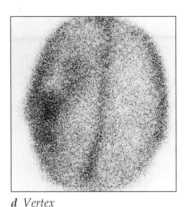

*a* Anterior      *b* Left lateral      *c* Posterior      *d* Vertex

**Fig. 5.28**

*(a–d)* $^{99m}$Tc DTPA *brain scan.*

*There is a massive area of abnormal tracer accumulation lying in the distribution of the left middle cerebral artery, with clear sparing of the anterior cerebral territory. The scan findings represent extensive infarction in the distribution of the left middle cerebral artery. A dynamic scan will often contribute to the diagnosis by showing an area of decreased blood flow.*

### Cerebral perfusion agents

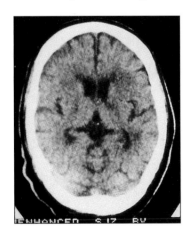

**Fig. 5.29**

*A 69-year-old man who presented with sudden onset of confusion and a right-sided weakness. CT showed only mildly decreased attenuation in the left hemisphere.*

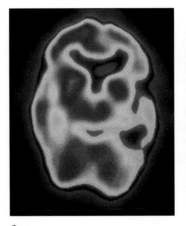 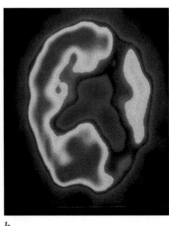

*a*      *b*

**Fig. 5.30**

 **Cerebral perfusion studies are abnormal immediately following the stroke, and often 24–48 hours before CT or MRI abnormalities appear**

*(a, b)* $^{99m}$Tc HMPAO SPECT *scan, showing extensive hypoperfusion involving the entire distribution of the left MCA, including the left basal ganglia. Two slices in the same patient:* *(a)* *through the temporal lobes;* *(b)* *through the parietal lobes.*

## Appearance of posterior cerebral artery (PCA) infarction

### BBB agents

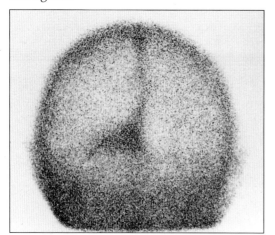

*a* Posterior

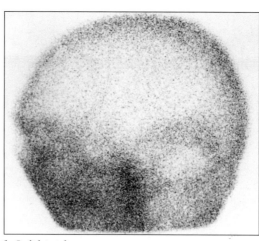

*b* Left lateral

**Fig. 5.31**

**(a, b)** *99mTc DTPA brain scan.*

The images show an area of increased tracer accumulation adjacent to, and to the left of, the torcular Herophili. The scan findings were due to a posterior cerebral infarct.

### Cerebral perfusion agents

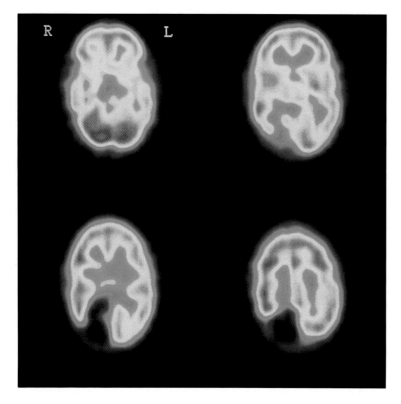

**Fig. 5.32**

*99mTc HMPAO SPECT scan from a child who suffered a right PCA infarct as a neonate.*

The patient has a left homonymous hemanopsia. Marked hypoperfusion is seen in the right occipital and medial temporal lobe, including the visual cortex.

## CLINICAL APPLICATIONS

## *Appearance of anterior cerebral artery (ACA) infarction*

### *BBB agents*

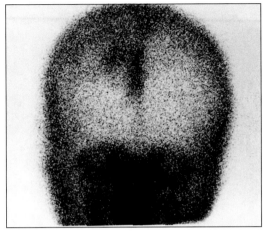

*a Anterior*

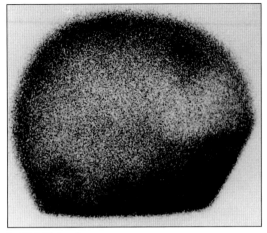

*b Right lateral*

**Fig. 5.33**

**(a, b)** $^{99m}$*Tc DTPA brain scan.*

*There is a focal area of increased tracer uptake seen in the right frontal region, arising from the midline and extending outwards. The scan findings are typical of an anterior cerebral infarct.*

## *Appearance of basal ganglia infarction*

### *Cerebral perfusion agents*

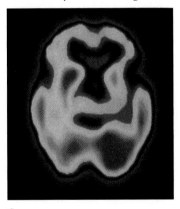

*a*

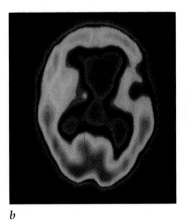

*b*

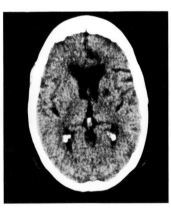

*c*

**Fig. 5.34**

**(a, b)** *Two transaxial slices from a* $^{99m}$*Tc HMPAO SPECT study of a 54-year-old woman.*

*Hypoperfusion is seen involving the left basal ganglia, both frontal lobes (more marked on the left), and the right cerebellum. The CT scan (c) shows only a left basal ganglia infarct.*

- The extent of abnormalities seen on brain SPECT imaging often exceeds those seen on CT/MRI.
- Hypoperfusion of the contralateral cerebellar hemisphere is often seen — so-called 'crossed cerebellar diaschisis'. This occurs most commonly in motor cortex infarcts, but can be seen in other conditions.

## Features that may help in the diagnosis of stroke

### Blood flow

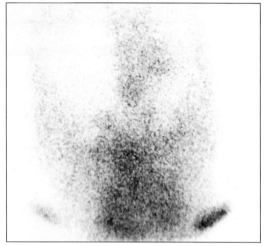

a  Anterior

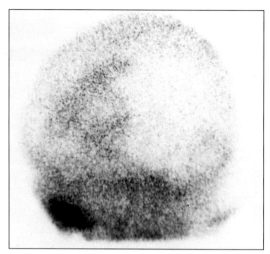

b  Left lateral

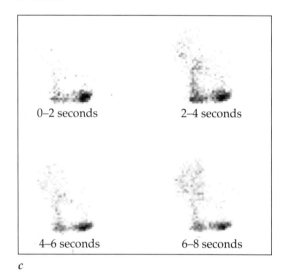

0–2 seconds  2–4 seconds

4–6 seconds  6–8 seconds

c

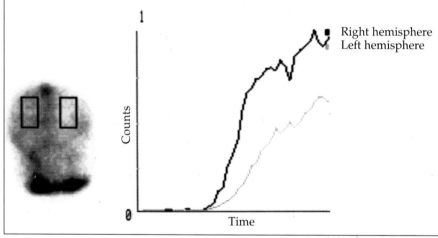

Right hemisphere
Left hemisphere

Counts

Time

d

### Fig. 5.35

*⁹⁹ᵐTc DTPA brain scan: (a) anterior view; (b) left lateral view; (c) dynamic study; (d) computer-generated curves.*

*On the delayed static images there is a large area of increased tracer uptake on the left in the frontal region, extending out from the midline in the territory of the anterior cerebral artery. The dynamic study shows decreased flow to much of the left cerebral hemisphere, but particularly in the distribution of the anterior cerebral artery. The computer-generated curves show a marked delay in peak activity on the left. The scan findings represent a large left-sided cerebral infarct in the distribution of the anterior cerebral artery. Nevertheless, the size of the lesion raises the possibility of some middle cerebral artery territory involvement.*

• When the static brain scan images are atypical, as in the case illustrated in Fig. 5.35, the presence of markedly decreased blood flow to that area will increase the probability of a cerebral infarct, because the main differential diagnosis, a glioma, will almost always have increased blood flow.
• When the static radionuclide brain scan is equivocally abnormal, with no specific features, the clear-cut loss of right middle cerebral perfusion makes an acute cerebral infarct almost certain.

## CLINICAL APPLICATIONS

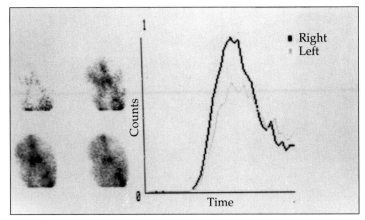

*a*

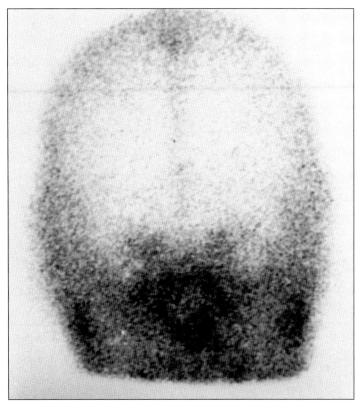

*b Anterior*

### *Fig. 5.36*

$^{99m}Tc$ DTPA *brain scan:* **(a)** *dynamic flow study with computer-generated curves;* **(b)** *anterior and* **(c)** *left lateral static views.*

*The static brain scan is normal. However, the flow study shows grossly diminished blood flow to the left cerebral hemisphere. The scan findings were due to a left-sided cerebrovascular accident, at a time when changes had not yet developed on the static brain scan.*

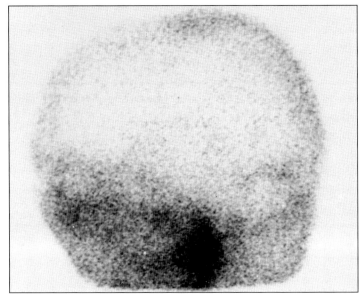

*c Left lateral*

Occasionally, the static brain scan may be completely normal, as in the case illustrated in Fig. 5.36. The vascular study showing loss of blood flow to the left side in a patient who has recently developed right-sided paresis will exclude a malignant space-occupying lesion as the cause with a high degree of certainty.

## 'Luxury' perfusion

### BBB imaging

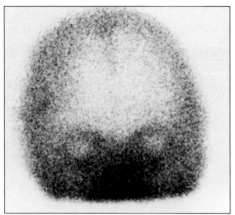 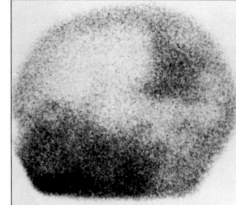 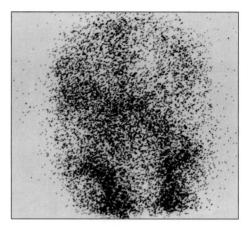

a  Anterior

b  Right lateral

c  Anterior, 10–12 seconds

**Fig. 5.37**

*(a, b) Static $^{99m}$Tc DTPA brain scan.
(c) Anterior dynamic flow study, 10–12 seconds.*

*On the static brain scan there is a focal area of increased tracer accumulation in the distribution of the posterior branches of the right middle cerebral artery. The dynamic study shows some increased perfusion to the right cerebral hemisphere. The scan findings were due to a cerebral infarct in the right hemisphere, with some 'luxury' perfusion.*

Most cerebral infarcts show decreased blood flow. However, the right-sided cerebral infarct seen in Fig. 5.37 shows increased blood flow, so-called 'luxury' perfusion. The clinician must be aware of this possibility so as to avoid reporting an infarct as a probable tumour. An important differential point in this case is the shape of the lesion on the lateral view and the fact that it lies discretely within the posterior branches of the middle cerebral artery territory.

### Cerebral perfusion imaging

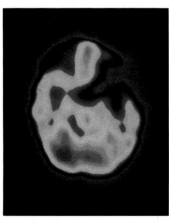 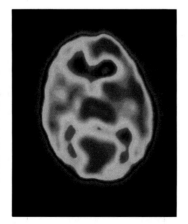

a

b

**Fig. 5.38**

*(a) Hypoperfusion is seen in the left temporal tip of a 53-year-old woman, 10 days post temporal lobe infarct. (b) Increased perfusion is seen in the cortex surrounding the infarct on a higher slice.*

Increased perfusion ('luxury' perfusion) can sometimes be seen in subacute infarcts. It is maximal at about 20 days, and is probably due to peri-infarct loss of vasomotor control and ingrowth of new capillaries.

# CLINICAL APPLICATIONS

## *Progress and resolution of scan appearances with time*

Frequently the cause of an equivocally abnormal scan becomes clear on a repeat study a few days or weeks later. This may particularly apply to cerebral infarcts scanned too early with BBB agents, which are maximally abnormal at 4–7 days, although the abnormalities may last several months or even years. Cerebral perfusion images of strokes are immediately abnormal, and may show partial resolution with time.

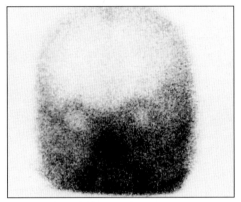

*a Anterior, 0 weeks*

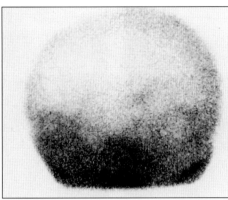
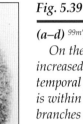

*b Left lateral, 0 weeks*

### Fig. 5.39

*(a–d)* ⁹⁹ᵐTc DTPA *brain scan.*

*On the original study there is a focus of increased tracer uptake lying in the left temporal parietal region. While the lesion is within the territory of the posterior branches of the middle cerebral artery, its precise nature is not clear. On the repeat study 3 weeks later there has been marked progression of disease, and the typical changes associated with a middle cerebral infarct are now apparent.*

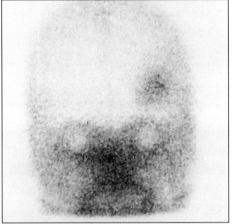

*c Anterior, 3 weeks*

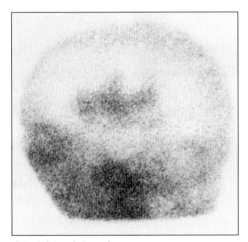

*d Left lateral, 3 weeks*

Not all BBB brainscans of cerebral infarcts resolve, and some may remain positive indefinitely. Therefore the presence of an infarct on the scan does not indicate a recent event.

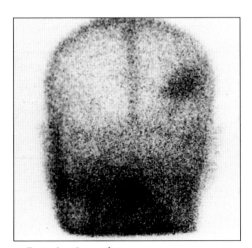

*a Posterior, 0 months*

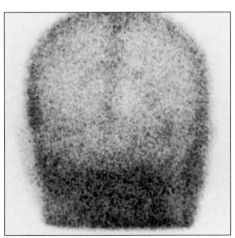

*b Posterior, 2 months*

### Fig. 5.40

*(a, b)* ⁹⁹ᵐTc DTPA *brain scan.*

*On the original study there is a well-delineated area of increased tracer uptake in the right parietal occipital region. This clearly lies within the distribution of the posterior branches of the middle cerebral artery. The repeat study 2 months later is normal. The scan findings represented resolution of a cerebral infarct.*

## 5.4.2   Intracerebral haemorrhage

### Cerebral perfusion agents

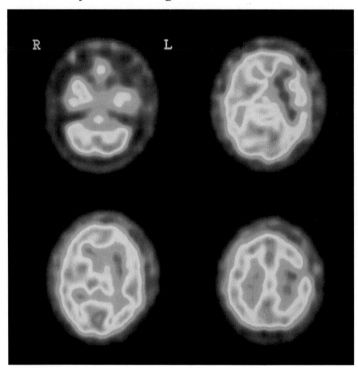

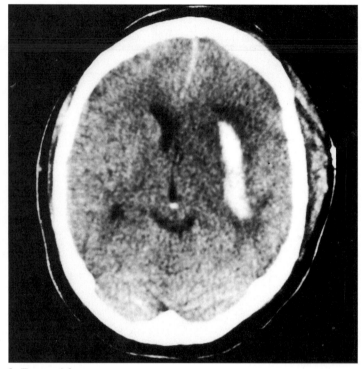

*a* Transaxial SPECT

*b* Transaxial CT

### Fig. 5.41

*(a)* ⁹⁹ᵐTc HMPAO SPECT scan of a 72-year-old man who had suffered a left intracranial haemorrhage. Dilatation of the left lateral ventricle is seen as well as absent perfusion to the left basal ganglia and mild hypoperfusion of the left cerebral cortex. The CT scan *(b)* shows intraventricular haemorrhage without cortical infarction.

• The distribution of cerebral haemorrhage may cross vascular territories.
• Marked white matter hypoperfusion, with retained cortical hypoperfusion, suggests haemorrhage or white matter infarction.

## 5.4.3   Transient ischaemic attacks

### *Cerebral perfusion agents*

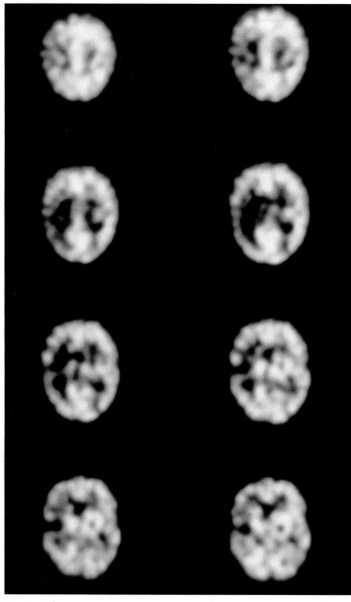

*Transaxial*

**Fig. 5.42**

*99mTc HMPAO scan in a patient with recurrent episodes of left-sided weakness. Scan shows diffuse hypoperfusion in the right hemisphere. (Courtesy of Dr M Devous, Texas, USA.)*

- BBB agent scans are usually normal in patients with TIAS unless there is a severe carotid stenosis.
- Scans with cerebral perfusion agents are only abnormal in 50–70% of cases in the absence of infarction.
- Positive scans are more likely to be obtained if the patient is scanned while symptomatic, or soon after recovery.
- Abnormalities should follow vascular territories.
- Some centres advocate the use of cerebral vasodilator agents such as $CO_2$ or acetazolamide to increase the sensitivity of HMPAO scans in TIAS/carotid stenoses.

## 5.4.4   Carotid artery stenoses

### BBB agents

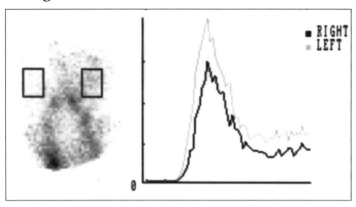

a

**Fig. 5.43**

---

*(a, b) First pass study, showing reduced blood flow to right hemisphere in a patient with right carotid artery stenosis.*

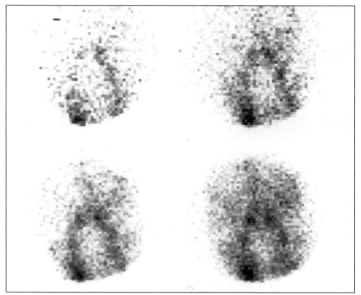

b

### Cerebral perfusion agents

Stenoses of the internal carotid artery may produce unilateral hypoperfusion if there is insufficient collateral flow via the Circle of Willis.

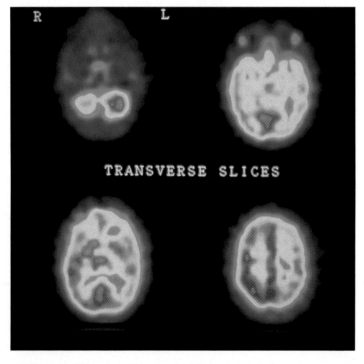

**Fig. 5.44**

---

*99mTc HMPAO SPECT scan from a 28-year-old woman with an asymptomatic iatrogenic 100% left internal carotid artery occlusion. Marked hypoperfusion is seen in the left hemisphere, mostly affecting left middle cerebral artery territory. Crossed cerebellar diaschisis is also seen. The CT was normal.*

# 5.4.5 Subarachnoid haemorrhage

## Cerebral perfusion imaging

The presence of blood in the CSF may produce vasospasm, which will decrease cerebral perfusion. This will usually follow vascular territories, unlike direct compressive effects from haematomas.

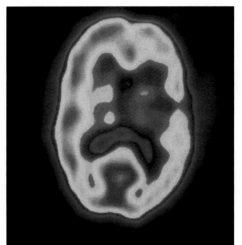

*a Transaxial HMPAO*

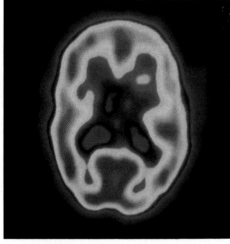

*b Transaxial HMPAO*

**Fig. 5.45**

(*a, b*) *Two* $^{99m}$*Tc HMPAO SPECT studies. Transaxial slices from a 29-year-old woman (*a*) 4 days and (*b*) 7 days after a subarachnoid haemorrhage. In (*a*) vasospasm of the left middle cerebral artery is producing diffusely decreased perfusion in the left hemisphere. The patient's vasospasm was successfully treated, as shown on the normal follow-up study (*b*). (*c, d*) Angiograms taken at the time of the SPECT studies show respectively the presence and resolution of the vasospasm. The CT scan (*e*) was normal.*

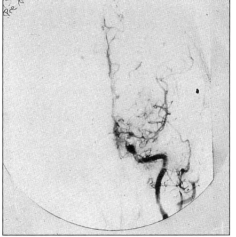

*c Angiogram*

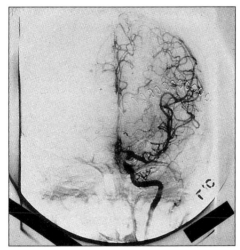

*d Angiogram*

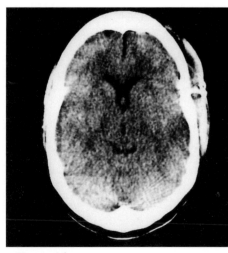

*e Transaxial CT*

## CLINICAL APPLICATIONS

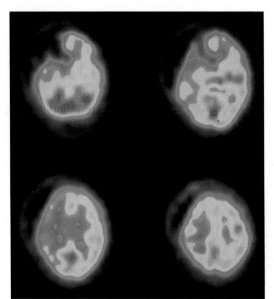

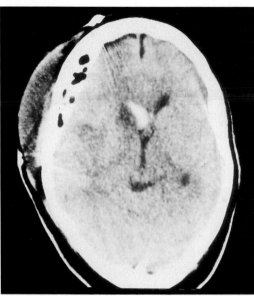

*a* Transaxial HMPAO

*b* Transaxial CT

### Fig. 5.46

*(a) Severe widespread vasospasm affecting both hemispheres in a patient with an intrapartum subarachnoid haemorrhage. Soft tissue swelling is seen due to attempted surgery. The CT (b) shows the presence of a right subdural collection and blood in the ventricle; the left hemisphere appears normal. The patient died from progressive vasospasm.*

- Brain perfusion studies may be used to detect vasospasm and to monitor therapy.
- Severe vasospasm is associated with a poor prognosis.
- BBB agent studies are normal in subarachnoid haemorrhage.

# 5.4.6 Arterio-venous malformations

### *BBB agents*

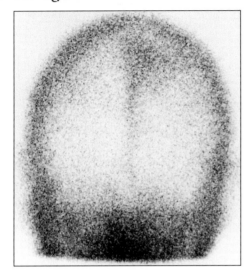 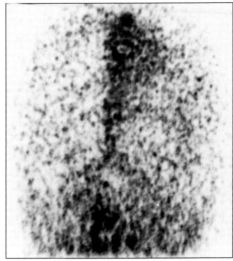

*a* Anterior                    *b*

Increased blood flow with a disproportionally massively increased blood volume is typical of an angiomatous malformation.

**Fig. 5.47**

*(a) Brain scan. (b) Dynamic image.*
*On the static brain scan views there is a single focal area of increased tracer uptake seen in the mid-parietal region, just to the left of the midline. The dynamic and blood pool images show that the lesion is extremely vascular. The scan findings were due to an angiomatous malformation.*

### *Cerebral perfusion agents*

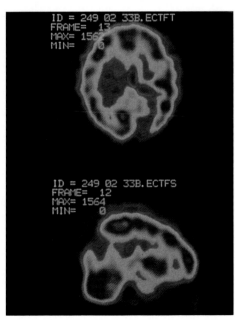

**Fig. 5.48**

*⁹⁹ᵐTc HMPAO SPECT scan (transaxial and sagittal views) of a 54-year-old man who presented with seizures and was found to have a homonymous quadrantopia.*
*The small area of markedly decreased perfusion seen in the left occipital lobe might have been caused by a small left PCA infarct, or even a tumour, but was found to be an AVM on CT scanning.*

AVMs do not accumulate ⁹⁹ᵐTc HMPAO, and so appear as space-occupying lesions.

## CLINICAL APPLICATIONS

# 5.4.7 Brain death

### BBB agents

These are conventionally used as an adjunct in cases of suspected brain death.

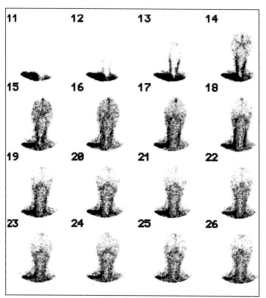

a Dynamic, normal

d Dynamic, brain death

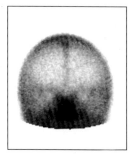

b Anterior, normal    c Posterior, normal    e Anterior, brain death    f Posterior, brain death

**Fig. 5.49**

*Brain scans: (a) normal dynamic and (b, c) normal static studies; (d–f) brain death studies. This 67-year-old male on anticoagulants had a spontaneous intracerebral haemorrhage. The brain scan shows only perfusion of the scalp veins.*

**Criteria for brain death:**
- No intracerebral arterial, capillary or venous flow on dynamic study
- No visualization of sagittal sinus on immediate post-injection images.

## CLINICAL APPLICATIONS

# *Cerebral perfusion agents*

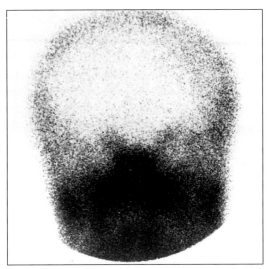

*a Anterior* HMPAO

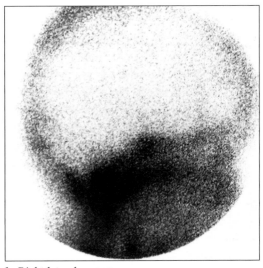

*b Right lateral* HMPAO

### Fig. 5.50

*(a, b) Planar* $^{99m}Tc$ HMPAO *scans in a patient who is brain dead following an accident, showing total absence of cerebral uptake. The increased uptake in the left parietal region is due to a scalp contusion. (Courtesy of Dr JE Powe, Canada and RH Reid, Canada.)*

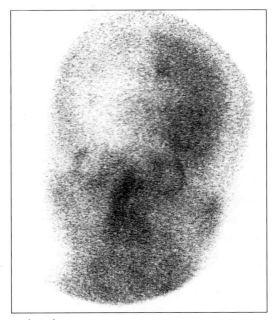

*a Anterior* HMPAO

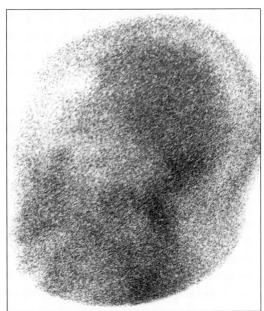

*b Lateral* HMPAO

### Fig. 5.51

*(a, b) Planar* $^{99m}Tc$ HMPAO *scans in a patient after a severe head injury who was suspected of brain death. Significant uptake is still seen in the left hemisphere — a negative study. (Courtesy of Dr JE Powe, Canada and RH Reid, Canada.)*

$^{99m}Tc$ HMPAO **is preferred to a** BBB **agent to assess brain death.**

# 5.4.8  Suspected cerebral infection

Intracerebral infection is usually suspected when an underlying or predisposing condition such as septicaemia or cyanotic heart disease is present.

## *Cerebral abscesses*

### *Features of cerebral abscesses*

- They are frequently multiple
- They frequently demonstrate the donut sign because of central necrosis
- A blood flow study is usually normal, but may be decreased. Increased blood flow is extremely rare.

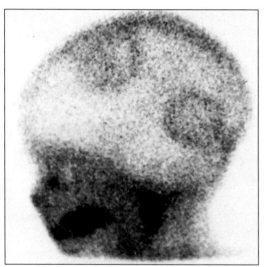

*a Left lateral*

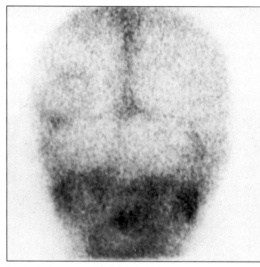

*b Posterior*

*Fig. 5.52*

*(a, b) ⁹⁹ᵐTc DTPA brain scan.*
*There are two large spherical lesions present in the left cerebral hemisphere. The first lies in the frontoparietal region, the second in the parietal occipital region. Both lesions have a central, relatively photon-deficient area, ie they demonstrate the donut sign. The scan findings were due to multiple intracerebral abscesses.*

## Localized encephalitis

Focal viral encephalitis is frequently negative on a CT scan, and is one of the few focal pathologies that is more often positive on a radionuclide brain scan.

*Features of focal encephalitis*

- Tracer uptake is rarely intense
- Uptake is diffuse and poorly demarcated
- Blood flow studies are usually normal.

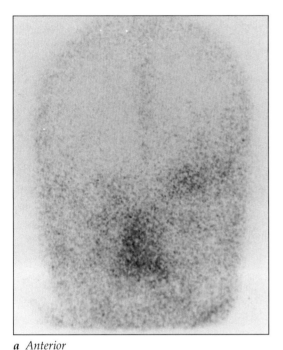

*a Anterior*  *b Left lateral*

**Fig. 5.53**

*(a, b)* $^{99m}$Tc DTPA *brain scan. There is increased tracer accumulation over the periphery of the left temporal lobe. The scan findings are in keeping with inflammation of the left temporal lobe, and were due to herpes encephalitis.*

## Generalized encephalitis

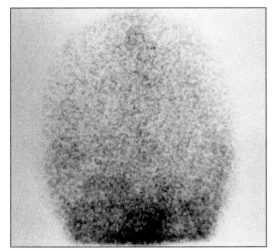
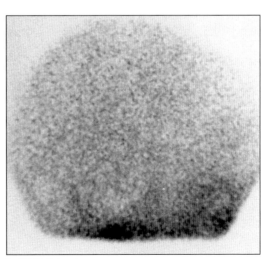

*a Anterior*  *b Right lateral*

**Fig. 5.54**

*(a, b)* $^{99m}$Tc DTPA *brain scan. There is diffusely increased tracer uptake throughout both cerebral hemispheres. This patient had viral encephalitis.*

## *Ventriculitis*

Ventriculitis may be associated with any extensive infection, but tuberculosis is most common.

### *Features of ventriculitis*

• Distribution of tracer uptake is usually bilateral and follows the shape and position of the ventricles
• The blood flow study is usually normal.

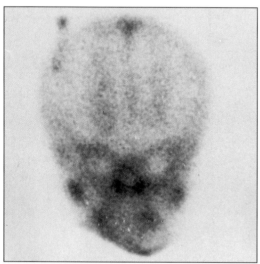

*a  Anterior*

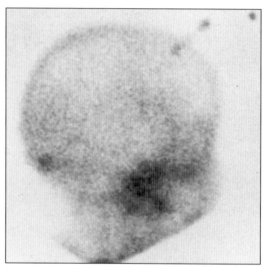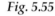

*b  Right lateral*

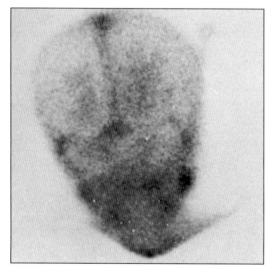

*c  Posterior*

*Fig. 5.55*

*(a–c)* $^{99m}$*Tc* DTPA *brain scan.*
*There is increased tracer uptake in the region of both ventricles, best seen on the anterior and posterior views. This child has* TB *meningitis with ventriculitis.*

# 5.4.9 Suspected chronic subdural haematoma

Subdural haematomas usually follow cerebral trauma. However, in children and old people a history of trauma is frequently absent. Slowly progressive focal signs and intermittent decreased consciousness are indications for a brain scan. The first investigation is a CT scan, but, if this is not immediately available, the radionuclide brain scan with dynamic flow is 90% sensitive and may be used as an alternative. A dynamic study should always be obtained, since this increases the sensitivity of detection.

## Unilateral subdural haematoma

*BBB agents*

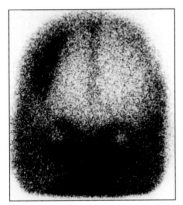 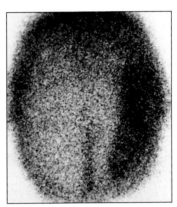 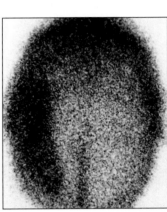

*a Anterior*     *b Right lateral*     *c Posterior*     *d Vertex*

**Fig. 5.56**

*(a–d)* $^{99m}$*Tc DTPA brain scan.*
  *There is a large area of increased tracer accumulation lying peripherally over the right hemisphere. The cerebral blood flow study shows this area to be of reduced vascularity. The scan shows the classic appearances of a huge, right-sided chronic subdural haematoma.*

## Features of a subdural haematoma

• Typically, a crescent-shaped area of increased tracer uptake is seen over the cerebral hemispheres, best visualized on the anterior and posterior views. Especially in small subdural haematomas, the lateral view may be virtually normal. This occurs because of a relatively thin layer of blood surrounding the cerebral hemisphere, whereas on anterior and posterior views the scan image is made through tissue 'thickness'.

• The scan shows progressive increased tracer uptake with time after injection.
• The dynamic study may show typical appearances of distortion of the middle cerebral vessel and compression of the cerebral cortex.
• A subdural haematoma may occasionally be isodense and appear normal on a CT scan.

**CLINICAL APPLICATIONS**

## Bilateral subdural haematoma

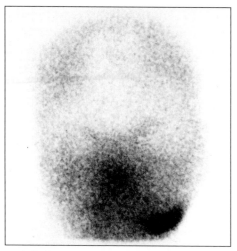

*a Anterior*

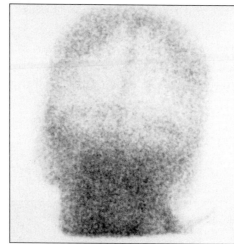

*b Posterior*

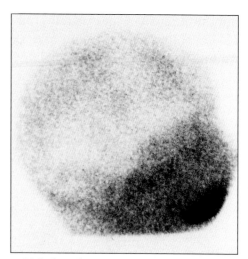

*c Right lateral*

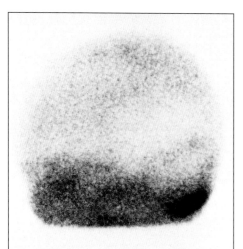

*d Left lateral*

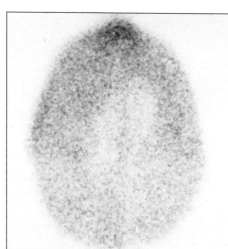

*e Vertex*

*Fig. 5.57*

*(a–e)* $^{99m}Tc$ DTPA *brain scan.*
*There are areas of diffusely increased tracer accumulation lying peripherally over both cerebral hemispheres. Bilateral 'crescent' signs are present, and the scan findings were due to bilateral subdural haematoma.*

Small bilateral chronic subdural haematomas may easily be missed because of their symmetrical appearances. Points to note are:

• The blood flow study showing compression of the cerebral cortex
• On delayed images, the loss of frontal lucency on the lateral view, since the region at the frontal lobe should normally be more photon-deficient than the parietal and temporal lobes.

## Subdural haematoma

### Cerebral perfusion agents

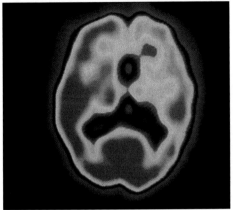

*a  Transaxial HMPAO*

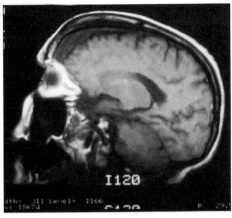

*b  Sagittal MRI*

**Fig. 5.58**

*(a) Transaxial slice from ⁹⁹ᵐTc HMPAO SPECT scan of a 78-year-old woman with rapid mental deterioration. Focal hypoperfusion is seen in the left frontal lobe. The sagittal MRI (b) confirms the presence of a significant subdural haematoma.*

- **Focal unilateral or bilateral hypoperfusion in the frontal or parietal regions in a non-vascular distribution is suspicious of subdural/extradural haematomas.**
- **The presence of hypoperfusion suggests that a known haematoma is of sufficient size to compromise cerebral perfusion.**

## Extradural haematoma

### BBB agents

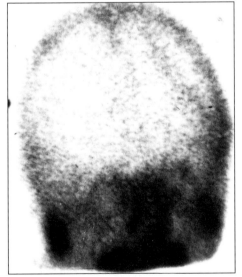

*a  Anterior*

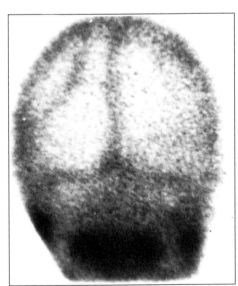

*b  Posterior*

**Fig. 5.59**

*(a, b) ⁹⁹ᵐTc DTPA brain scan.*

*This study shows the appearances of an extradural haematoma, which are the same as those of an acute massive subdural haematoma. The rim of increased activity representing superficial blood vessels is characteristic. A CT scan is indicated if an extradural is suspected.*

## Trauma

### Brain contusion: BBB agents

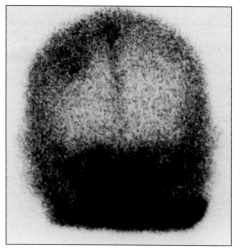

*a Anterior*

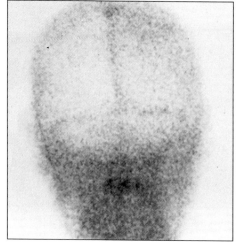

*b Posterior*

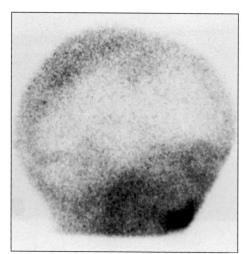

*c Right lateral*

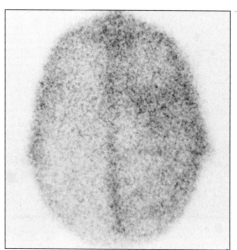

*d Vertex*

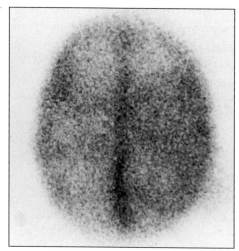

*e Vertex*

**Fig. 5.60**

(*a–d*) ⁹⁹ᵐTc DTPA brain scan. (*e*) Blood pool image.

There is some diffusely increased tracer uptake present in the right parietal area, lying peripherally. The blood pool image shows relatively increased tracer uptake at that site. This patient, who was in her sixties, had sustained trauma to her head and presented with drowsiness and persistent headaches. A subdural haematoma was suspected, but the scan findings, while abnormal, were not typical of this, in the light of the blood pool study. It was considered that this patient had sustained brain contusion. The repeat brain scan 3 months later was completely normal.

*Brain contusion: cerebral perfusion agents*

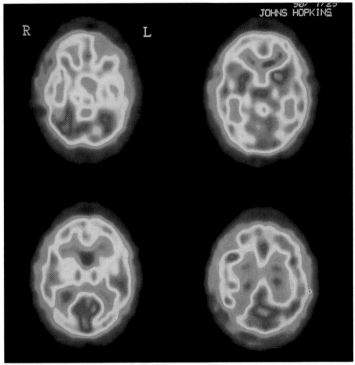

*a  Transaxial* HMPAO

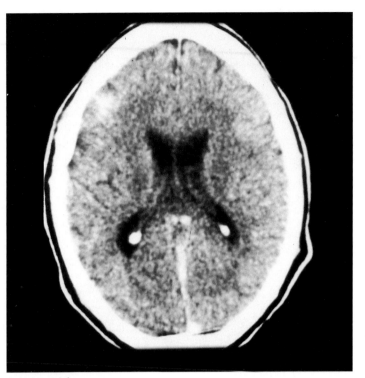

*b  Transaxial* MRI

**Fig. 5.61**

*(a) Brain* SPECT *from a 40-year-old man 6 months after a moderately severe head injury, who was suffering from headaches and memory problems. Focal defects are seen in the left frontal, right frontal and right parietal regions. The* CT *(b) only revealed the right frontal abnormality.*

- • **Brain perfusion studies are very sensitive in localizing cerebral contusions in acute and chronic head injuries.**
- • **Abnormalities are usually focal and asymmetrical.**
- • **Abnormalities are often more extensive and numerous than the** CT **abnormalities.**

## 5.4.10 CSF leaks

Radionuclide cisternography can be used to confirm and localize suspected CSF leaks.

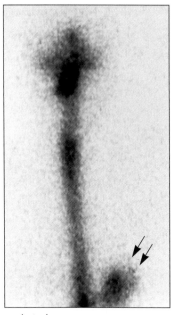

*a* Anterior

*b* Right lateral

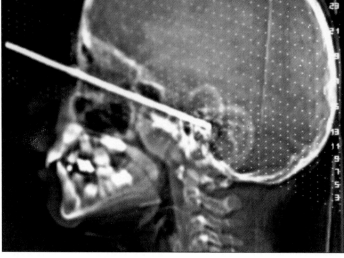

*c*

**Fig. 5.62**

*(a, b) Cisternogram obtained at 6 hours in a child with rhinorrhoea following a penetrating injury to the skull base (CT scan (c)). Abnormal CSF collections are seen in the nasopharynx (arrow) and in the stomach (double arrows) due to swallowed tracer. (Reproduced with permission from* Eur J Nucl Med *(1990)* 17: 365–8.)

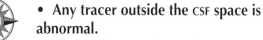

- Any tracer outside the CSF space is abnormal.
- Pledgets inserted into the nasopharynx which are removed at 6 hours and counted along with a sample of blood increase the sensitivity for small leaks. Pledget/serum ratios should be less than 1.3:1.
- Tilting the head forward or performing a valsalva manoeuvre may increase sensitivity.
- Spinal dural leaks can also be localized.
- An image should be obtained of the spinal injection site, since infiltrated tracer will affect results.

# 5.4.11 CSF shunts

By injecting ¹¹¹In DTPA (using sterile technique) into the reservoir of a ventriculo-peritoneal, ventriculo-atrial or lumbo-peritoneal shunt, the patency of the shunt can be assessed.

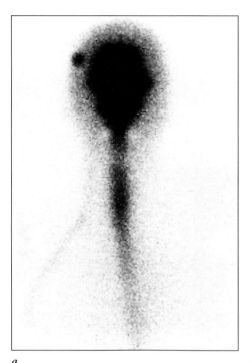

*a*

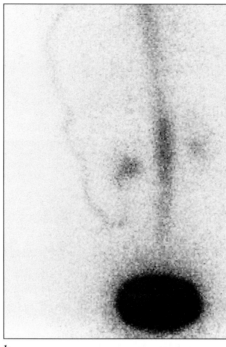

*b*

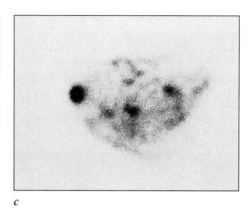

*c*

**Fig. 5.63**

*(a) Head and (b) abdominal views of a patent ventriculo-peritoneal shunt at 45 minutes, showing passage of the radiotracer down the tubing. Four-hour abdominal images (c) reveal significant accumulation of tracer in the peritoneal cavity.*

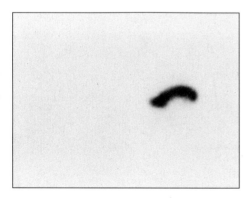

**Fig. 5.64**

*Anterior head image of blocked shunt at 4 hours. Tracer is seen to remain in the reservoir, with no distal or proximal passage.*

- There should be rapid passage of the tracer distally with appearance in the peritoneum or circulation (eg kidneys). The speed will depend on the CSF pressure and flow rate, but should be seen within 1–2 hours.
- Proximal flow of tracer may or may not be seen, depending on the reservoir valve type.
- It is important to check for misinjection in the scalp, since this can produce systemic uptake.
- Lumbar-peritoneal shunts can be checked by lumbar subarachnoid injection and following tracer passage into the peritoneum.

**CLINICAL APPLICATIONS**

## 5.4.12   Evaluation of dementia or personality change

Brain perfusion agents are the tracers of choice for assessing patients with dementia. BBB scans are usually normal in dementia unless space-occupying lesions are present. If hydrocephalus is present, cisternography should be performed.

### Alzheimer's disease

Alzheimer's disease is a progressive degenerative disease of the brain. Sensitive and specific abnormalities are seen on brain perfusion studies, even early in the disease, often in the absence of CT or MRI atrophy.

**Fig. 5.65**

*(a) Transaxial and (b) sagittal slices of a ⁹⁹ᵐTc HMPAO SPECT study in a 72-year-old man with severe memory loss. Marked bilateral temporo-parietal hypoperfusion is seen. The MRI scan (c) shows mild atrophy.*

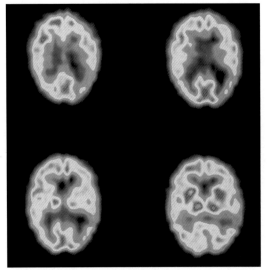

*a  Transaxial HMPAO*

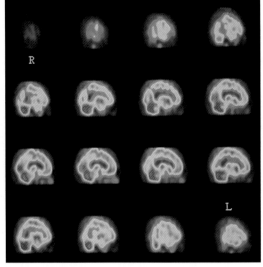

*b  Sagittal HMPAO*

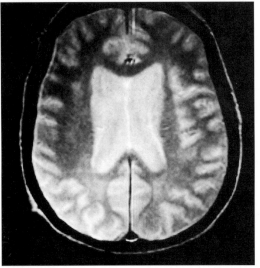

*c  Transaxial MRI*

• Typically, bilateral temporal and parietal hypoperfusion is seen in Alzheimer's disease.
• Perfusion is usually retained in the frontal lobes in early disease, as well as in the basal ganglia, visual and sensorimotor cortex and cerebellum.

## Early Alzheimer's disease

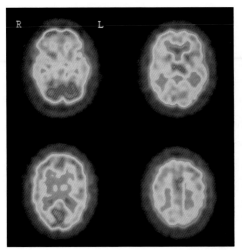

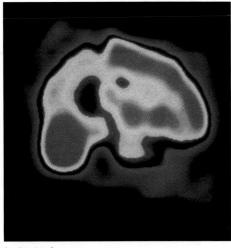

*a Transaxial HMPAO*

*b Sagittal HMPAO*

**Fig. 5.66**

*Transaxial (a) and (b) sagittal slices of brain SPECT from a 54-year-old man with a 1-year history of memory loss. Mild hypoperfusion is seen in the temporo-parietal regions bilaterally. MRI was normal.*

## Asymmetric Alzheimer's disease

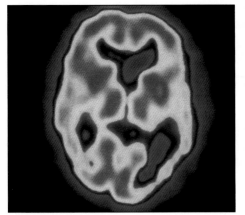

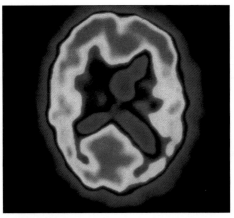

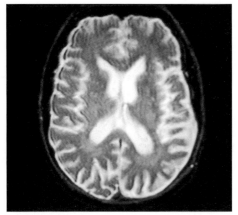

*a Transaxial HMPAO*

*b Transaxial HMPAO*

*c Transaxial MRI*

**Fig. 5.67**

*(a, b) Transaxial slices from a ⁹⁹ᵐTc HMPAO SPECT scan from an 82-year-old man with dementia. The temporal and parietal hypoperfusion is significantly worse on the left. The MRI scan (c) shows only left-sided atrophy.*

• The abnormalities in early disease are often subtle, and are best seen on the sagittal slices.
• Asymmetric disease is common, but a purely unilateral abnormality should raise the possibility of stroke or even subdural haematoma.

## Progression of disease

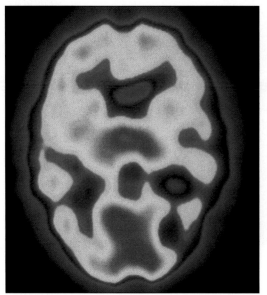

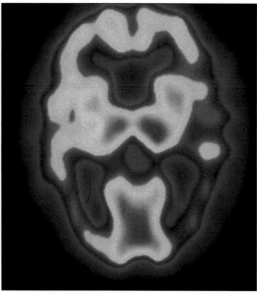

*a* Transaxial HMPAO

*b* Transaxial HMPAO

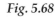

**Fig. 5.68**

*Scan (a) was obtained in a 55-year-old woman with a 3-year history of dysphasia and memory loss. Abnormalities typical of Alzheimer's disease are seen, with bilateral temporo-parietal hypoperfusion. Scan (b) was taken 1 year later. The hypoperfused areas can be seen to have worsened, with progression to involve the frontal lobes.*

The frontal lobes may be involved in severe disease. Eventually, a pattern of marked pan-cortical hypoperfusion may be seen in very advanced cases.

## Dementia with combined aetiologies

### Alzheimer's disease and stroke

Stroke, being very common in the elderly, may co-exist with Alzheimer's disease. Usually this is obvious on the scan; however, confusion can arise particularly in parietal strokes. Sagittal slices of the non-stroke hemisphere may be helpful.

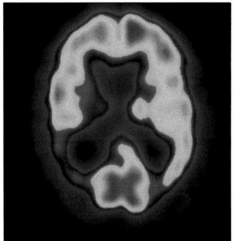

*a  Transaxial* HMPAO

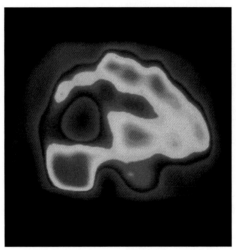

*b  Sagittal* HMPAO

**Fig. 5.69**

*An 82-year-old man with a known right parietal stroke, who presented with gradual further memory loss. (a) Transaxial slice from a $^{99m}$Tc HMPAO SPECT scan showing R>>L parietal hypoperfusion. (b) Left sagittal slice confirms that the left parietal lobe is also significantly abnormal.*

### Parkinson's disease and dementia

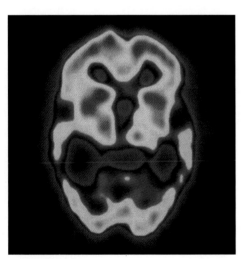

*Transaxial* HMPAO

**Fig. 5.70**

*A 77-year-old woman with Parkinson's disease and dementia. This study is indistinguishable from those obtained in patients with Alzheimer's disease. Note the normal basal ganglia perfusion.*

• Similar patterns to Alzheimer's disease can be seen in bilateral parietal subdurals or strokes. CT scanning may be required to exclude these.

• Parkinson's disease with dementia appears similar to Alzheimer's disease on brain perfusion imaging. The basal ganglia are typically normally perfused.

## *Multiple infarct dementia*

Multiple infarct dementia (MID) accounts for approximately 15% of cases of dementia and is caused by progressive neuronal loss through repeated small strokes.

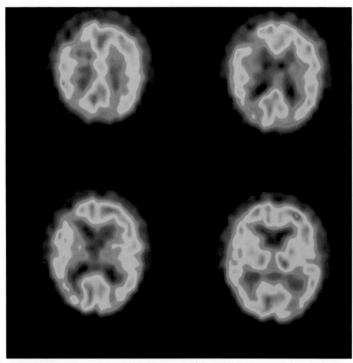

*Transaxial HMPAO*

### Fig. 5.71

*99mTc HMPAO SPECT scan from a 64-year-old man with known coronary artery disease and memory loss.*

*Focal perfusion defects are seen in the right frontal, right parietal and left parietal lobes.*

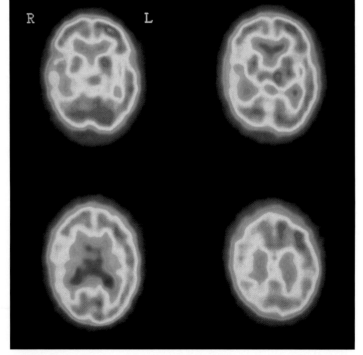

*Transaxial HMPAO*

### Fig. 5.72

*99mTc HMPAO SPECT scan from a 68-year-old woman with dementia.*

*A single focal lesion is seen in the right temporal lobe. No other cause for her dementia was found.*

**CLINICAL APPLICATIONS**

## Extensive multiple infarcts

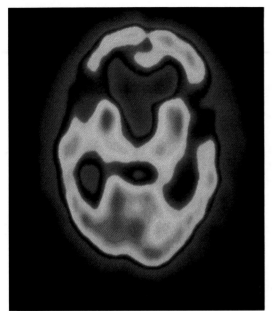

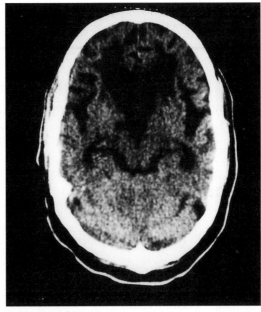

*a* Transaxial HMPAO

*b* Transaxial CT

**Fig. 5.73**

*An 80-year-old man with severe dementia and frontal lobe signs, known long-term hypertension and coronary artery disease.*

*The SPECT scan (a) shows severe but patchy cortical and subcortical hypoperfusion. The CT scan (b) shows diffuse white matter infarction and atrophy. This is an example of Binzwanger's disease — extensive white matter infarction.*

- **The lesions of MID are focal, usually in both hemispheres and asymmetrical.**
- **Lesions should remain within vascular territories if there is cortical involvement.**
- **The number of focal perfusion defects will vary considerably from apparently single lesions to widespread abnormalities (eg Binzwanger's disease).**

## Pick's disease

Pick's disease is a frontal lobe dementing syndrome. Abnormalities may be seen on cerebral perfusion studies before frontal atrophy is recognized on CT.

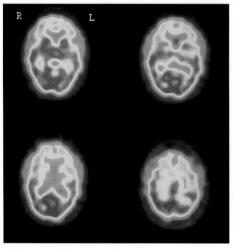

*a* Transaxial HMPAO

*b* Sagittal HMPAO

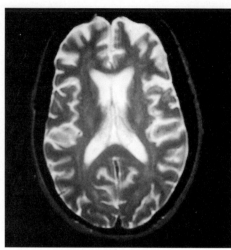

*c* Transaxial MRI

**Fig. 5.74**

*(a) Transaxial slices and (b) sagittal slice from a $^{99m}$Tc HMPAO SPECT scan of a 68-year-old woman with dementia, speech problems and frontal lobe signs. Marked hypoperfusion is seen involving the entire frontal lobes. The MRI scan (c) shows mild diffuse atrophy.*

## A case of personality change

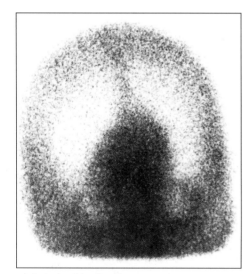

*a* Anterior, blood pool

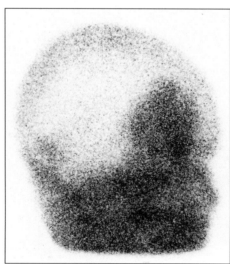

*b* Right lateral, delayed

**Fig. 5.75**

*Hypervascular primary tumour. $^{99m}$Tc DTPA brain scan: (a) blood pool image; (b) right lateral view.*

*Static brain scan images show massive abnormal radionuclide accumulation in the mid-line involving both frontal lobes. The perfusion studies show this lesion to have a very high blood flow and blood pool. The scan findings were due to a primary intracerebral tumour.*

 **Personality change may be the only feature of a frontal lobe tumour, and there may not be any obvious focal neurological signs.**

**CLINICAL APPLICATIONS**

## Communicating hydrocephalus (normal pressure hydrocephalus)

Communicating hydrocephalus is suggested when progressive dementia and gait disturbances are seen, particularly when this follows cerebral trauma or meningeal irritation (meningitis, arachnoiditis or subarachnoid haemorrhage). A CT scan should always be performed before the radionuclide cisternogram. An increase in size of the ventricles out of proportion to a degree of cerebral atrophy on CT is a further indication of possible communicating hydrocephalus.

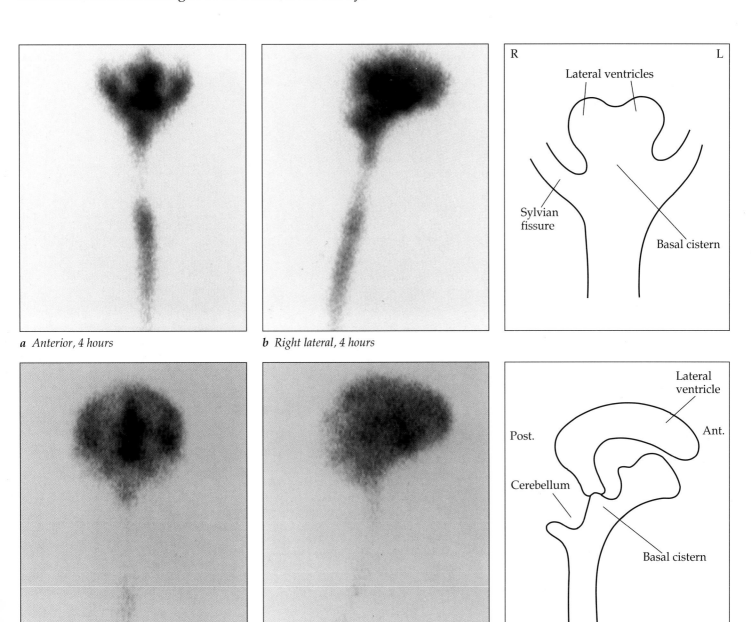

*a Anterior, 4 hours*

*b Right lateral, 4 hours*

*c Anterior, 24 hours*

*d Right lateral, 24 hours*

**Fig. 5.76**

*(a–d)* [111]*In cisternograms in a 72-year-old woman with dementia and ataxia. Radiotracer is seen in the lateral ventricles at 4 hours, still remaining at 24 hours. An incidental cervical spinal stenosis is noted. In this patient with relatively mild disease, activity is seen over the cerebral hemispheres at 24 hours.*

## Advanced normal pressure hydrocephalus

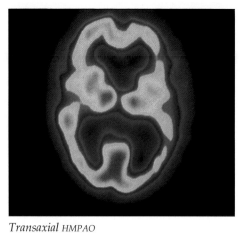

*Transaxial HMPAO*

**Fig. 5.77**

*$^{99m}$Tc HMPAO SPECT scan from a 69-year-old woman with dementia.*
*Diffuse cortical hypoperfusion is seen, with dilated ventricles (note separation of thalami).*

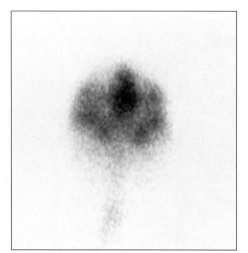

***a*** *Anterior, 24 hours, $^{111}$In DTPA*

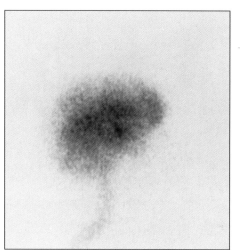

***b*** *Right lateral, 24 hours, $^{111}$In DTPA*

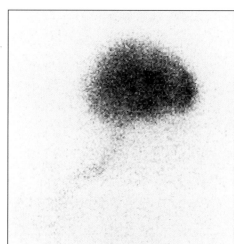

***c*** *Anterior, 48 hours, $^{111}$In DTPA*

**Fig. 5.78**

*$^{111}$In cisternogram in the same patient as in Fig. 5.77.*
*The 24-hour images (**a, b**) show entry of the radiotracer into the lateral ventricles, with delayed ascent over the cerebral hemispheres until 48 hours (**c**).*

- Tracer in the ventricles is always abnormal.
- In communicating hydrocephalus tracer is seen in the lateral ventricles at 4 hours, remaining at 24 hours.
- Delayed imaging at 48 hours is occasionally required.
- In severe disease there may be delayed ascent of the tracer over the hemispheres.
- In cerebral atrophy radiotracer may pass into the lateral ventricles, but it rapidly empties.

## Obstructive hydrocephalus

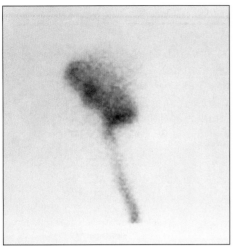 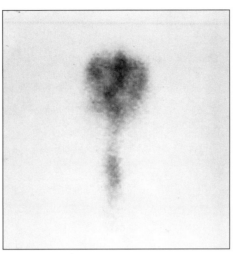 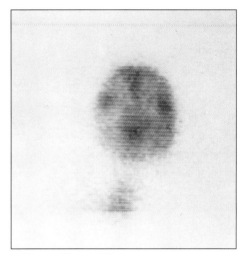

*a  Lateral, 6 hours, ¹¹¹In DTPA*     *b  Anterior, 6 hours, ¹¹¹In DTPA*     *c  Vertex, 6 hours, ¹¹¹In DTPA*

### Fig. 5.79

**(a–c)** ¹¹¹In DTPA *cisternogram.*

This patient presented with dementia, and was found to have dilated ventricles. On the cisternogram it is seen that there is no entry of tracer into the dilated ventricles, which indicates that obstructive hydrocephalus must be present. The cause of obstruction was a third ventricle tumour.

## Jakob–Creutzfeld disease

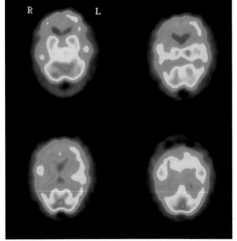 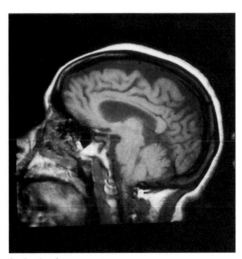

*a  Transaxial HMPAO*     *b  Sagittal MRI*

### Fig. 5.80

**(a)** ⁹⁹ᵐTc HMPAO SPECT *scan from a 69-year-old woman with rapid onset dementia and myoclonus. The scan shows marked diffuse cortical hypoperfusion, with sparing of the basal ganglia, sensorimotor and visual cortex. The* MRI **(b)** *shows moderate cortical atrophy.*

## CLINICAL APPLICATIONS

## *Cerebral atrophy*

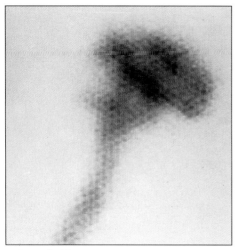 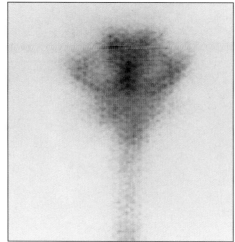

*a  Lateral, 6 hours*          *b  Anterior, 6 hours*

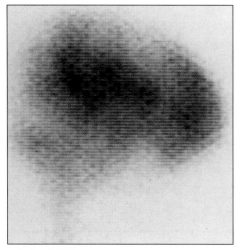 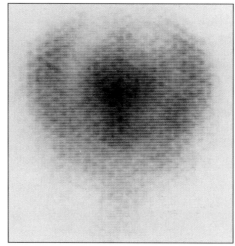

*c  Lateral, 24 hours*        *d  Anterior, 24 hours*

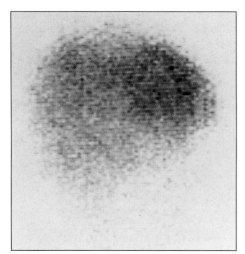 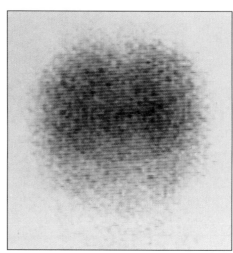

*e  Lateral, 48 hours*        *f  Anterior, 48 hours*

### Fig. 5.81

*(a–f)* $^{111}$In DTPA *cisternogram.*
  *This patient presented with dementia and an uncoordinated gait. A CT scan showed ventricular atrophy, and communicating hydrocephalus was suspected. Note, however, how the tracer refluxes into the ventricles, but rapidly empties.*

**CLINICAL APPLICATIONS**

# 5.4.13   Investigation of seizures

Epilepsy may sometimes be associated with a focal space-occupying lesion, which may be localized by BBB imaging. Often, CT or MRI is normal, and in these cases a seizure focus may be localized by a cerebral perfusion scan. This is helpful in planning surgery.

## *Interictal study*

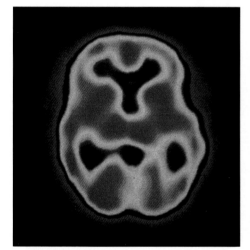

*a  Transaxial* HMPAO

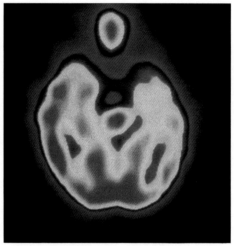

*b  Transaxial* HMPAO

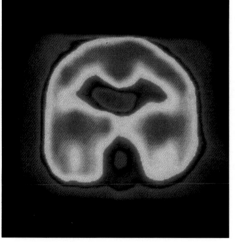

*c  Coronal* HMPAO

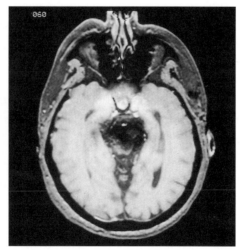

*d  Transaxial* MRI

### Fig. 5.82

$^{99m}Tc$ HMPAO *study of a 45-year-old woman with a 5-year history of temporal lobe seizures. The transaxial slice* (**a**)*, the temporal lobe slice* (**b**) *and the coronal slice* (**c**) *all show hypoperfusion of the left temporal lobe. Depth electrodes confirmed this as the site of seizures. The* MRI (**d**) *shows bilateral medial temporal lobe sclerosis.*

## CLINICAL APPLICATIONS

### Frontal lobe seizures

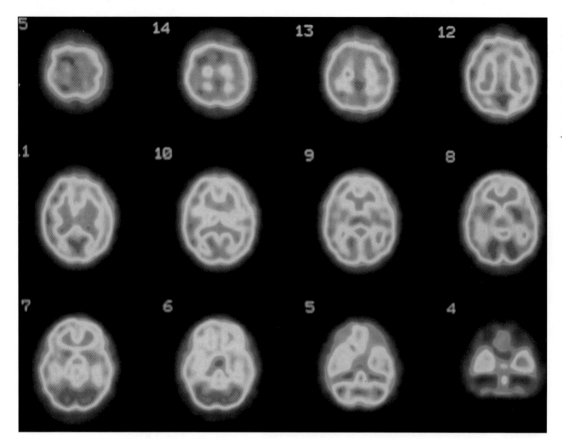

**Fig. 5.83**

*$^{99m}Tc$ HMPAO SPECT study of a 21-year-old woman with atypical seizures. CT was normal. A focus of hypoperfusion is seen in the left frontal lobe, corresponding to the seizure focus.*

- Interictal scans show hypoperfusion at the site of the seizure focus in 60–75% of patients with focal seizures.
- The commonest site is the temporal lobe.
- The abnormality often involves an extensive area.
- Slices orientated along the axis of the temporal lobe are helpful, as are coronal slices.

## CLINICAL APPLICATIONS

### *Ictal study*

If an interictal study is non-localizing, a patient may be injected during a seizure (ictal study). This may occur incidently, and if so must be noted, otherwise misinterpretation of the study may occur.

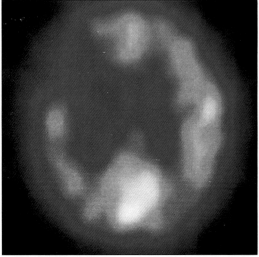

*a Transaxial* HMPAO

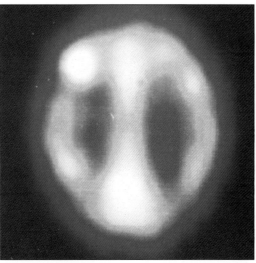

*b Transaxial* HMPAO

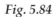

**Fig. 5.84**

*Interictal (a) and ictal (b) $^{99m}Tc$ HMPAO SPECT scans from a 6-year-old boy with epilepsia partialis continua. Study (a) shows hypoperfusion in the right frontal lobe, while study (b) shows hyperperfusion in the same region.*

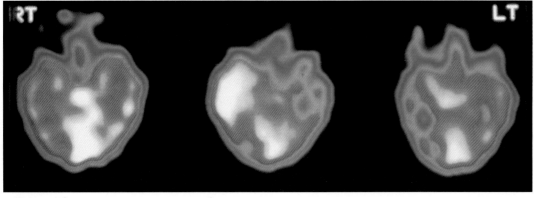

*a Transaxial*     *b*     *c*

**Fig. 5.85**

*Interictal (a), ictal (b) and immediately post-ictal (tracer injected within 1 minute post-seizure) (c) scans from a patient with seizures arising in the right temporal lobe. Note the improved localization in the ictal and post-ictal studies.*

- Hyperperfusion is seen at the site of the seizure focus in an ictal study.
- An extensive area of brain may be involved, especially if the seizure becomes generalized, and caution must be used in interpretation.
- Occasionally bilateral abnormalities are seen to be secondary activation of other areas. The interictal study may be helpful in this case.
- Early post-ictal (within 1–5 minutes) studies may localize more accurately.
- EEG monitoring at the time of injection is required for accurate interpretation of ictal studies.

## Seizures caused by space-occupying lesions

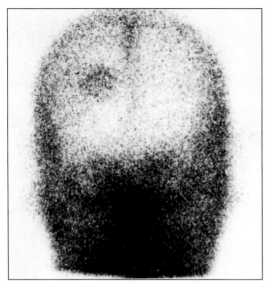

*a* Anterior

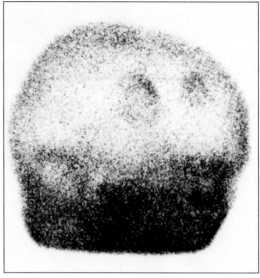

*b* Right lateral

### Fig. 5.86

*(a–c)* $^{99m}$Tc DTPA *brain scan.*

This patient with known carcinoma of the lung developed focal seizures involving the left arm. The brain scan shows multiple lesions in the parietal and frontal lobes on the right, caused by metastatic deposits.

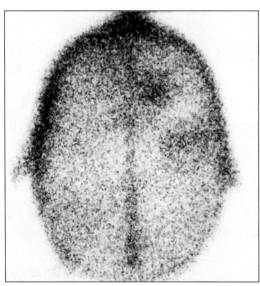

*c* Vertex

# 5.4.14   Suspected intracerebral space-occupying lesions

Space-occupying lesions are most commonly due to tumours, although abscesses, arterio-venous malformations and subdural haematomas may present similarly. Tumours may either be primary or secondary from metastatic disease. Occasionally, they may be the presenting symptom from an unknown primary elsewhere. Lung, breast and colon are the commonest tumours metastasizing to the brain. Single metastatic lesions cannot be differentiated from primary tumours on radionuclide scans, although the presence of multiple lesions is almost always due to metastases. BBB agent scans may be helpful as a primary investigation in the patient with a suspected intracerebral space-occupying lesion.

## *Primary intracerebral tumour*

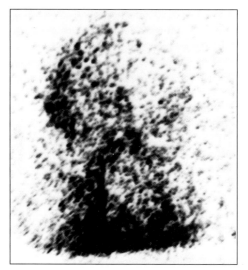

*a Anterior, dynamic*

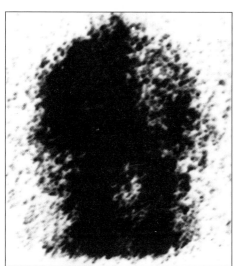

*b Anterior, dynamic*

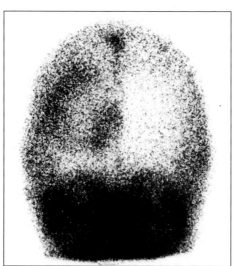

*c Anterior, delayed*

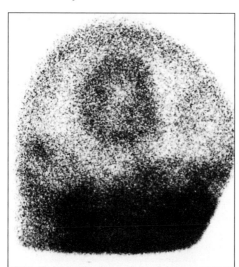

*d Right lateral, delayed*

**Fig. 5.87**

*99mTc DTPA brain scan: (a, b) anterior dynamic flow study; (c) anterior and (d) right lateral delayed views.*

*This patient with a large glioma presented with progressive left-sided weakness. The dynamic flow study shows increased blood flow associated with a space-occupying lesion.*

• Although the CT scan has a higher sensitivity than the radionuclide study for detection of cerebral space-occupying lesions, the sensitivity of the radionuclide study is nevertheless still high, at greater than 90%. The radionuclide study is usually not as good at defining the pathological entity as CT.

• A very large solitary space-occupying lesion in the brain is much more likely to be a primary tumour than a secondary deposit. The latter lesion is more frequently small and multiple.

## Frontal lobe

Presentation of a frontal lobe tumour is usually that of progressive dementia, which often manifests itself initially as a personality disorder. A contralateral grasp reflex may be present.

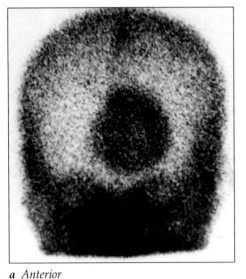

*a* Anterior    *b* Vertex

**Fig. 5.88**

*(a, b) ⁹⁹ᵐTc DTPA brain scan.*

*There is a massive focal area of increased tracer accumulation in the frontal region, predominantly in the left, but extending across the midline to the right. This lesion was found to be a meningioma, but it should be noted that it is extremely unusual for a benign lesion to cross the midline, and when this is seen it is usually strong evidence in favour of malignancy.*

## Occipital lobe

Occipital lobe tumours may present with visual hallucinations, and there is usually an associated contralateral homonymous hemianopia.

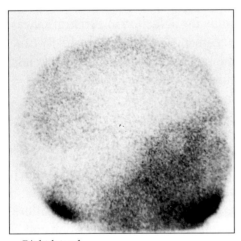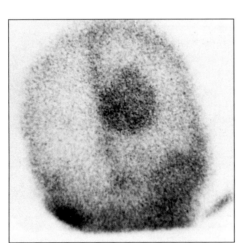

*a* Right lateral    *b* Posterior

**Fig. 5.89**

*(a, b) ⁹⁹ᵐTc DTPA brain scan.*

*There is a large, well-circumscribed area of increased tracer uptake in the right occipital region. The scan findings were due to a metastasis.*

 **Benign lesions very rarely cross the midline.**

**CLINICAL APPLICATIONS**

## *Parietal lobe*

Parietal lobe lesions usually present with contralateral limb weakness, and focal motor fits are relatively common.

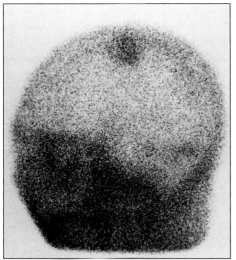 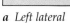 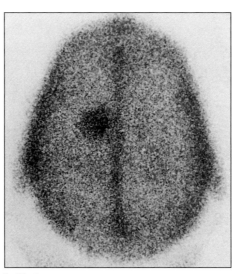

*a  Left lateral*

*b  Vertex*

**Fig. 5.90**

*(a, b)* $^{99m}$*Tc* DTPA *brain scan.*
   *There is a focus of increased tracer accumulation lying somewhat superficially in the left parietal cortex in the parasagittal region. This patient presented with focal left-sided motor fits caused by cerebral metastasis from a bronchogenic neoplasm.*

## *Sphenoid ridge*

A sphenoid ridge meningioma may protrude into the orbit, with unilateral proptosis and optic atrophy. Ptosis and diplopia may also occur.

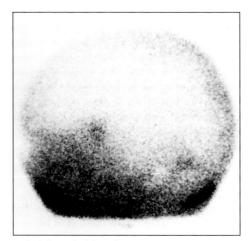 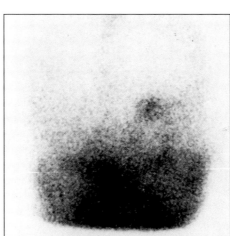

*a  Left lateral, delayed*

*b  Anterior, blood pool*

**Fig. 5.91**

$^{99m}$*Tc* DTPA *brain scan: (a) delayed left lateral image; (b) blood pool image.*
   *There is a discrete focal area of increased tracer uptake in the region of the left sphenoid ridge. On the blood pool image it is seen that the lesion has high vascularity. The scan findings were due to a sphenoid ridge meningioma.*

## Temporal lobe

Temporal lobe lesions usually present with temporal lobe epilepsy. Focal epilepsy affecting the contralateral hand and sometimes weakness of the hand and arm are also seen. If the lesion extends posteriorly, an upper quadrantic field defect or sensory aphasia may also be present.

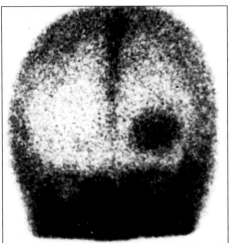
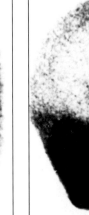

*a Anterior*

*b Left lateral*

**Fig. 5.92**

*(a, b) $^{99m}$Tc DTPA brain scan.*
*There is a left temporal lobe lesion caused by a metastasis from carcinoma of the breast.*

## Posterior fossa

### Cerebellum

The typical presentation of a lesion in the cerebellum is cerebellar ataxis in the limbs on the side of the tumour, with nystagmus on lateral gaze to the contralateral side.

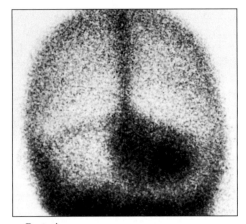

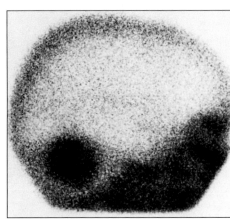

*a Posterior*

*b Right lateral*

**Fig. 5.93**

*(a, b) $^{99m}$Tc DTPA brain scan.*
*There is a massive focal area of increased tracer accumulation in the right posterior fossa, reaching and extending slightly across the midline. The scan findings were due to a cerebellar astrocytoma.*

 **The brain scan will be normal in a patient with cerebellar signs due to a paraneoplastic syndrome.**

## Vermis

A typical presentation of a midline vermis lesion is gait disturbance and truncal ataxia, usually without any nystagmus and often no ataxia in the limbs. Frequently there is associated vomiting and papilloedema caused by obstructive hydrocephalus.

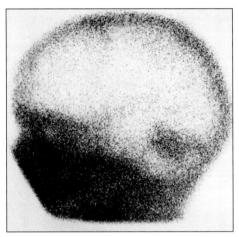

*a* Left lateral

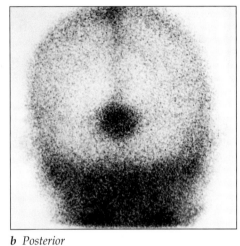

*b* Posterior

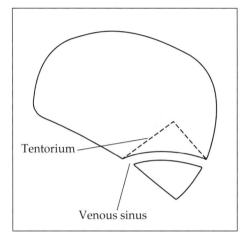

*Fig. 5.94*

(*a, b*) ⁹⁹ᵐTc DTPA brain scan.
There is a round focal area of increased tracer accumulation seen centrally in the posterior fossa. The scan findings were due to a benign astrocytoma involving the vermis.

The posterior fossa is bounded superiorly by the tentorium, not by the venous sinuses. Therefore, as in the case illustrated in Fig. 5.94, the vermis lesion may appear to be above the posterior fossa.

## Cerebellopontine angle

A cerebellopontine angle tumour usually presents with unilateral nerve deafness and vertigo. Unilateral facial sensory loss with an absent corneal reflex is often seen.

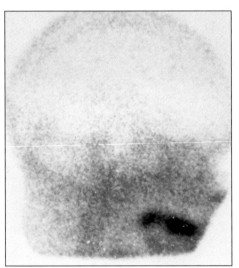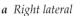

*a* Right lateral

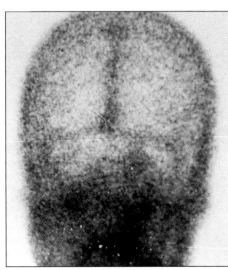

*b* Posterior

*Fig. 5.95*

(*a, b*) ⁹⁹ᵐTc DTPA brain scan.
There is a single focal area of increased tracer accumulation in the right cerebellopontine angle. No other abnormality is seen. The scan findings are typical of acoustic neuroma, which was subsequently confirmed.

## Lateral ventricles

A glioma may arise from the corpus callosum and grow to involve the ventricles. The scan appearances may be those of a 'butterfly' glioma. Presentation is often non-specific, but progressive apathy, drowsiness, occasional memory disorders and general convulsions followed by bilateral parietal lobe signs may be seen.

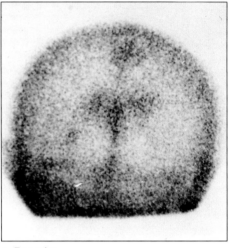

*a Posterior*

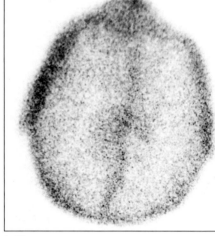

*b Vertex*

### Fig. 5.96

**(a, b)** ⁹⁹ᵐTc DTPA *brain scan.*
*There is abnormal radionuclide accumulation extending from the midline bilaterally in the region of both ventricles. The scan findings are due to a butterfly glioma.*

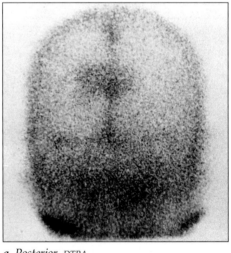

*a Posterior, DTPA*

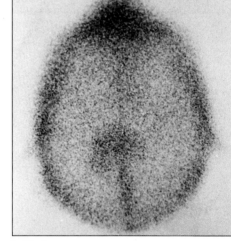

*b Vertex, DTPA*

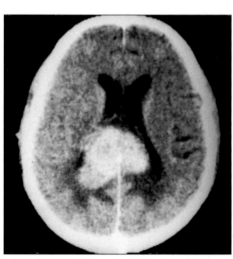

*c Transaxial CT*

### Fig. 5.97

**(a–c)** ⁹⁹ᵐTc DTPA *brain scan.* **(d)** CT *scan.*
*The brain scan shows a large focal area of increased tracer uptake in the region of the corpus callosum, crossing the midline. The scan appearances are those of a large space-occupying lesion (butterfly tumour). This is confirmed on the CT scan. This elderly man had a bronchogenic neoplasm, and the scan appearances were due to a metastasis.*

## CLINICAL APPLICATIONS

### *Improved localization and detection with SPECT*

SPECT may be performed using BBB agents as well as cerebral perfusion agents. This may significantly improve the rate of detection and the localization of small lesions.

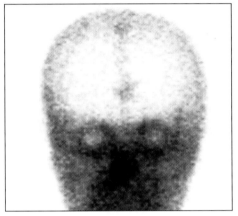

*a  Anterior*

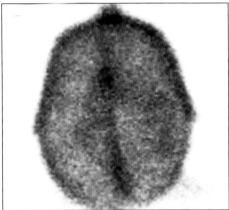

*b  Right lateral*

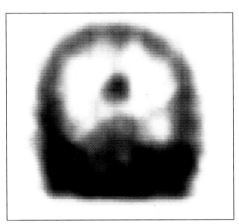

*c  Posterior*

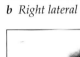

*d  Vertex*

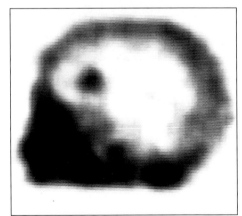

*e  Coronal*

*f  Sagittal*

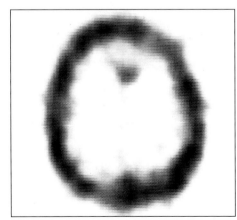

*g  Transaxial*

**Fig. 5.98**

*(a–d)Planar $^{99m}$Tc DTPA brain scan. (e–g) $^{99m}$Tc DTPA SPECT scan.*

*On the brain scan study a midline metastasis is faintly visualized. However, the SPECT reconstructed slices allow the lesion to be seen more clearly and demonstrate how this technique may assist in the localization of lesions.*

## $^{201}Tl$ SPECT *imaging for localization of brain tumours*

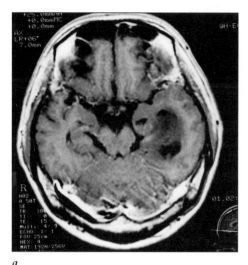 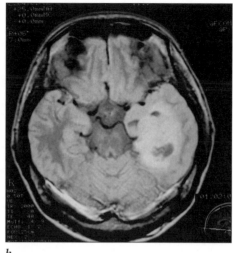 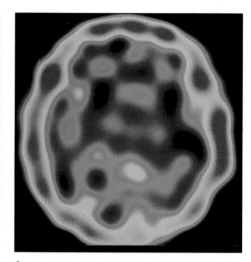

*a*                 *b*                 *c*

### Fig. 5.99

*A 45-year-old male with astrocytoma grade II in the left temporal lobe. The astrocytoma is identified as a low-intensity area on T1-weighted MRI (a) and a high-intensity area on proton density MRI (b). There is relatively low accumulation in the tumour on the $^{201}Tl$ SPECT early image (c). (Courtesy of Dr T Ueda, Miyazaki, Japan.)*

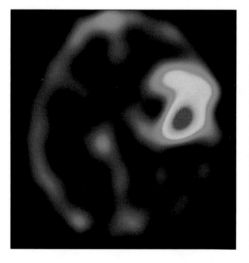 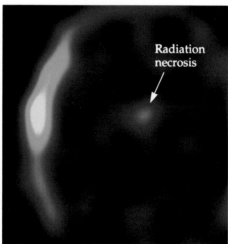

Radiation
necrosis

• $^{201}Tl$ is a non-specific tumour imaging agent.
• $^{201}Tl$ may be useful in distinguishing a malignant lesion from an infection or necrosis.
• Low-grade tumours may exhibit low $^{201}Tl$ uptake.

### Fig. 5.100

*A 55-year-old female with a glioblastoma multiforme in the left temporal lobe. There is high accumulation in the tumour on the $^{201}Tl$ SPECT image. (Courtesy of Dr T Ueda, Miyazaki, Japan.)*

### Fig. 5.101

*A 33-year-old male with a radiation-induced necrosis in the hypothalamic region. There is a small amount of accumulation in the lesion on the $^{201}Tl$ SPECT image (arrow). (Courtesy of Dr T Ueda, Miyazaki, Japan.)*

# 5.4.15   Suspected cerebral metastases

### Features of cerebral metastases on the BBB brain scan

• When multiple lesions are present, the most likely diagnosis is cerebral metastases
• Multiple lesions may be inferred when the site of the brain scan lesion does not correspond to the anatomical origin of the symptom or sign, and hence the probability of metastases is increased

• Uptake of tracer is usually only moderate and not intense
• Uptake of tracer will increase with increasing time interval between injection and imaging
• The blood flow study is usually normal

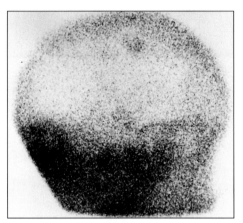
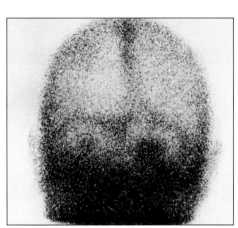

*a  Left lateral*          *b  Posterior*

**Fig. 5.102**

*(a, b) ⁹⁹ᵐTc DTPA brain scan of a patient with bilateral cerebellar tumours and a left parietal tumour. The primary originated from a breast carcinoma.*

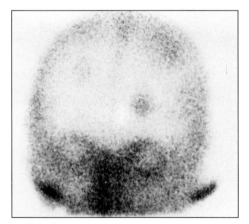
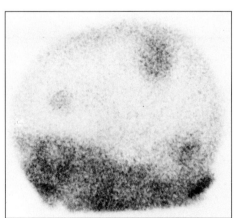

*a  Anterior*          *b  Left lateral*

**Fig. 5.103**

*(a, b) ⁹⁹ᵐTc DTPA brain scan.*
*There are multiple focal lesions throughout both cerebral hemispheres, and the scan appearances are typical of multiple intracranial metastases.*

In any patient with a known neoplasm that may metastasize, almost any neurological sign or symptom justifies a brain scan, since the presentation of a cerebral metastasis is extremely variable.

# Brain metastases demonstrated by $^{99m}Tc$ HMPAO SPECT imaging

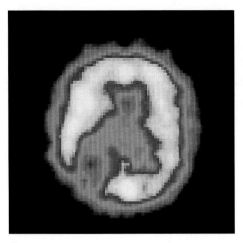
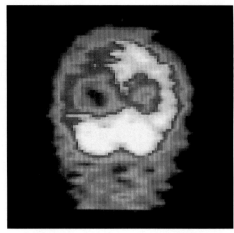
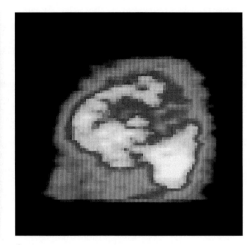

a                     b                     c

**Fig. 5.104**

*(a–c) Cerebral blood flow study ($^{99m}Tc$ HMPAO SPECT) in a patient with primary breast carcinoma who presented with visual disturbance.*

*Transaxial (a), coronal (b) and sagittal (c) sections through the left occipital lobe show the loss of normal blood flow to the occipital cortex caused by a small deep metastasis.*

Cerebral tumours usually appear as non-specific focal perfusion defects on brain perfusion imaging. Occasionally the tumours may have uptake equal to or in excess of the surrounding cortex. If the defects cross vascular territories, metastases rather than multiple infarctions should be suspected.

# Lymphoma

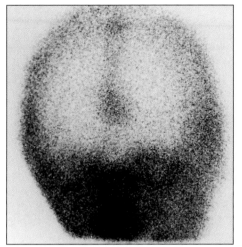

*a  Anterior, 0 weeks*

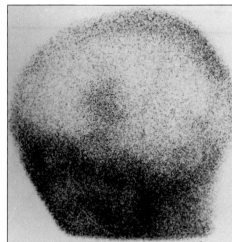

*b  Left lateral, 0 weeks*

### Fig. 5.105

*(a–f)* $^{99m}$Tc DTPA *brain scan.*

*This patient with known lymphoma presented with drowsiness and slight neck rigidity. The original study shows an abnormal focal area of tracer accumulation in the region of the thalamus. The scan findings were due to a lymphoma deposit in the thalamus. The patient received radiotherapy, and the repeat study 2 weeks following therapy showed some improvement. A further scan 2 months later was normal.*

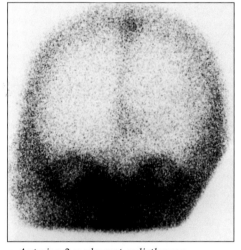

*c  Anterior, 2 weeks post-radiotherapy*

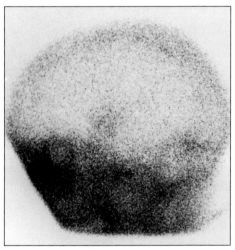

*d  Left lateral, 2 weeks post-radiotherapy*

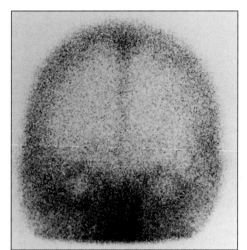

*e  Anterior, 2 months*

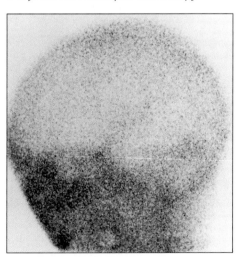

*f  Left lateral, 2 months*

## Features helping in the diagnosis of space-occupying lesions

### Blood flow

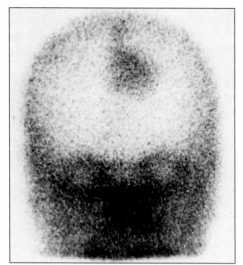

*a  Anterior, delayed*

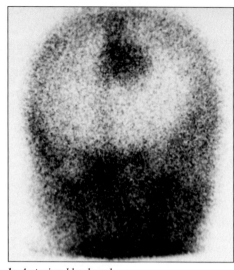

*b  Anterior, blood pool*

**Fig. 5.106**

(*a*) ⁹⁹ᵐTc DTPA *delayed brain scan.* (*b*)
*Blood pool image.*
   *There is a large spherical area of
increased tracer uptake lying to the left of
the midline in the frontal lobe. There is
marked increased blood pool associated
with this lesion. The scan findings are
typical of meningioma.*

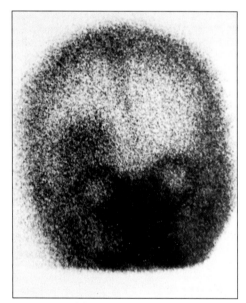

*a  Anterior, delayed*

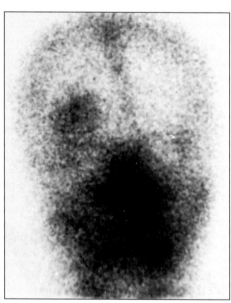

*b  Anterior, blood pool*

**Fig. 5.107**

(*a*) ⁹⁹ᵐTc DTPA *delayed brain scan.* (*b*)
*Blood pool image.*
   *There is a solitary, well-circumscribed
large lesion in the right frontal temporal
region. It is seen that the lesion has
markedly increased blood volume. The scan
findings are those of a highly vascular
cerebral neoplasm.*

• As demonstrated in the cases in Figs 5.106 and 5.107, the meningioma arises from the meninges, whereas the glioma arises from brain tissue expanding concentrically from this. Both tumours, however, have equally increased blood flow, although frequently the meningioma has a blood flow which is greater than that of an average glioma.

• Differentiation between a meningioma and an intracerebral infarct can be difficult. Differential points to note are that in at least one view (the lateral) the meningioma is apparently spherical, whereas the cerebral infarct keeps to the distribution of the middle cerebral artery territory. Further, on the posterior view, the meningioma appears to be extending towards the midline. Blood flow studies are also of value, as these show increased blood flow to a meningioma and decreased blood flow to an infarct.

**CLINICAL APPLICATIONS**

## Tumour causing hypovascularity

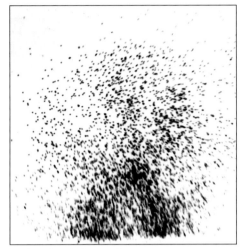

*a Anterior, 0–3 seconds*

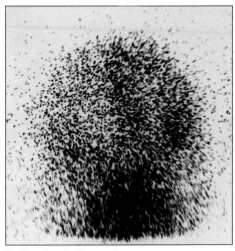

*b Anterior, 3–6 seconds*

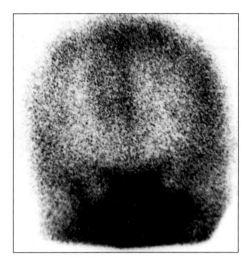

*c Anterior, blood pool*

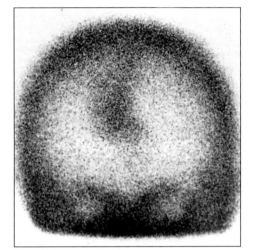

*d Anterior, delayed*

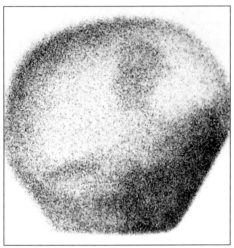

*e Right lateral, delayed*

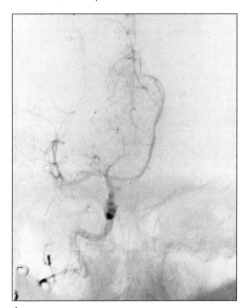

*f*

**Fig. 5.108**

*Glioma with hypovascularity, caused by a shift of the anterior cerebral artery away from the lesion. ⁹⁹ᵐTc DTPA dynamic flow study: (a) 0–3 seconds; (b) 3–6 seconds; (c) blood pool image. Static brain scan: (d) anterior and (e) right lateral views. (f) Arteriogram.*

*There is a focal area of increased tracer accumulation in the right frontoparietal region. On the dynamic study there is reduced perfusion to the right cerebral hemisphere. The scan findings are suggestive of a right anterior cerebral artery infarct, but on this occasion were due to a glioma, which was causing shift of the anterior cerebral artery away from the lesion, as is seen on the arteriogram.*

Unfortunately, not all gliomas have an increased blood supply. Figure. 5.108 shows an example of a hypovascular glioma, simulating an anterior cerebral infarct. This is a rare finding, but an important potential pitfall. A useful point of differentiation is the fact that the lesion on the anterior view crosses the midline to the left side.

## Shape and position

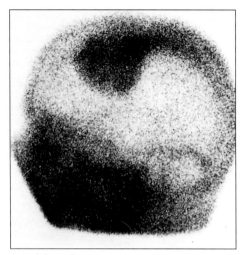

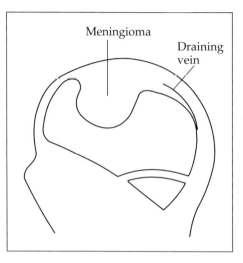

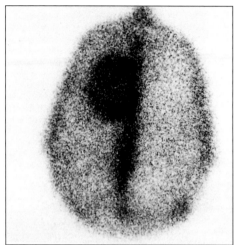

*a* Left lateral

*b* Vertex

**Fig. 5.109**

*(a, b)* ⁹⁹ᵐTc DTPA *brain scan.*

   *The brain scan shows a massive accumulation of tracer in the left frontal lobe adjacent to the midline, with a large draining vein seen on all three views. The scan findings are typical of a meningioma.*

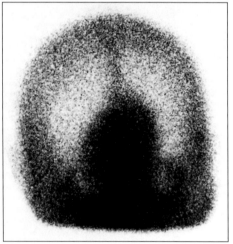

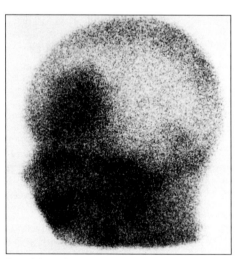

*a* Anterior

*b* Left lateral

**Fig. 5.110**

*(a, b)* ⁹⁹ᵐTc DTPA *brain scan.*

   *There is a massive focus of increased tracer uptake seen extending across the midline. The scan findings were due to a malignant glioma.*

The two cases in Figs 5.109 and 5.110 illustrate some of the differences between a meningioma and a malignant glioma. Meningioma does not cross the midline, and arises from a site in the meninges, and there is a massive drainage vein associated with it. Glioma, on the other hand, can be clearly seen invasively crossing the midline, which would be rare for a meningioma.

## CLINICAL APPLICATIONS

## Value of delayed views

Delayed views following a routine BBB agent brain scan may help to differentiate between the presence and absence of a lesion, and, to some extent, between different lesions. The extent to which any single lesion becomes more or less prominent with time following injection depends largely on whether a positive brain scan is mainly dependent on blood volume or a breakdown of the blood–brain barrier. As tracer leaves the blood into the larger volume of the extracellular fluid, lesions that are dependent on visualization because of blood volume will become relatively less prominent, while lesions produced by blood–brain barrier breakdown will become more prominent.

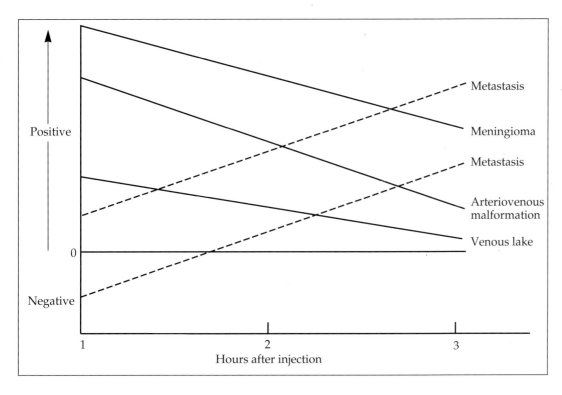

### Fig. 5.111

*Diagrammatic representation of the value of delayed views following a routine BBB agent brain scan.*

**Table 5.2   *Differentiation of lesions based on changes in tracer uptake with time after injection***

| Decrease with time after injection | Increase with time after injection |
|---|---|
| Vascular tumours | Most metastases |
| Arterio–venous malformation | Gliomas |
| Angiomatous malformation | Subdural haematoma |
| Skull and scalp lesions | Cerebrovascular accident |
| | Abscess |

## CLINICAL APPLICATIONS

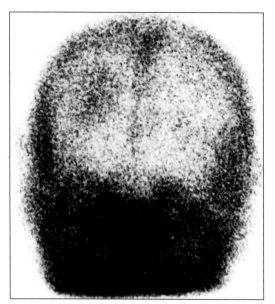

*a  Anterior, 1 hour post-injection*

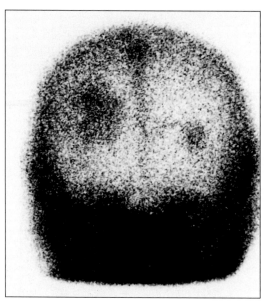

*b  Anterior, 3 hours post-injection*

### Fig. 5.112

*(a) Initial brain scan.*
*(b) Delayed image.*
    On the original study there is a clear-cut focal lesion present in the right temporal parietal region. On the delayed image the right-sided lesion has become more obvious, but it is now apparent that there are multiple intracranial lesions, increasing the probability of metastatic disease.

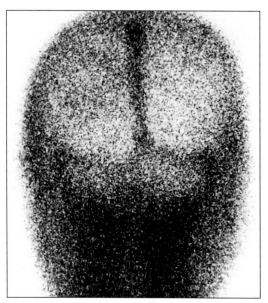

*a  Posterior, 1 hour post-injection*

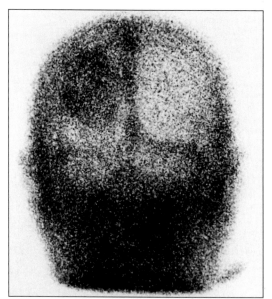

*b  Posterior, 3 hours post-injection*

### Fig. 5.113

*(a) Initial brain scan.*
*(b) Delayed image.*
    The initial scan shows only a faint, diffuse uptake in the left occipital parietal area, which is non-specific. The delayed image shows a massive area of increased tracer uptake which does not respect the vascular boundaries and therefore is unlikely to be a cerebral infarct. The scan findings were due to a glioma.

**Many lesions will become progressively more prominent as a result of relatively greater tracer avidity; however, because the half-life of $^{99m}$Tc is only 6 hours, there is a limit to the benefit which will be obtained from more prolonged waiting.**

## 5.4.16　The donut sign

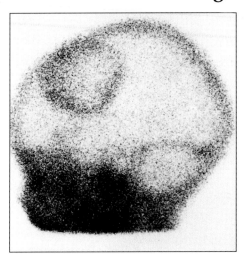

*Left lateral*

**Fig. 5.114**

*Donut sign caused by a cerebral abscess.*

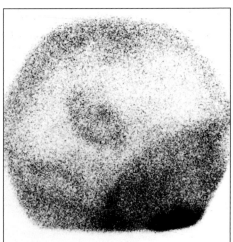

*Right lateral*

**Fig. 5.115**

*Donut sign caused by a lymphoma.*

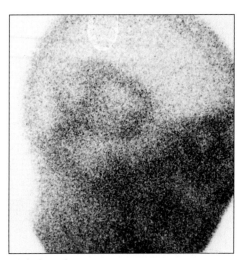

*Right lateral*

**Fig. 5.116**

*Donut sign caused by middle cerebral artery infarct.*

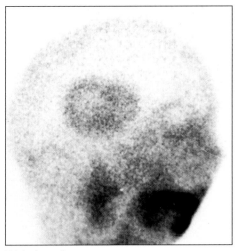

*Right lateral*

**Fig. 5.117**

*Donut sign caused by a glioma.*

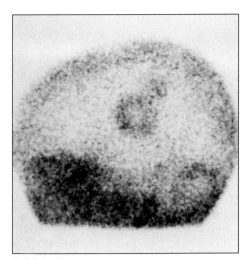

*Left lateral*

**Fig. 5.118**

*Donut sign caused by a cerebral metastasis.*

It has often been said that the appearance of a donut sign indicates a cerebral abscess. While cerebral abscesses may indeed show this sign, the finding is non-specific, as illustrated by the cases in Figs 5.114–5.118. Because of the prevalence of disease, the donut sign will more often be found in association with tumour.

## 5.4.17   Skull and scalp lesions

Scalp and cranial lesions provide some of the most difficult complicating factors in the interpretation of a radionuclide brain scan. Points to be aware of in differentiating them from an intracranial lesion are:

• They tend to decrease with time because they usually represent an increased blood pool

• They are often rather diffuse
• It is often difficult to locate them clearly in three dimensions
• In at least one view they often appear to distort the outer curvature of the skull.

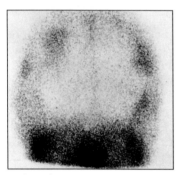

*a Anterior*

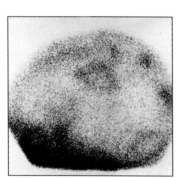

*b Left lateral*

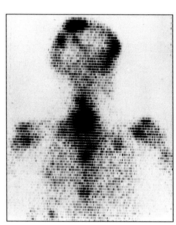

*c Bone scan*

**Fig. 5.119**

**(a, b)** ⁹⁹ᵐTc DTPA *brain scan.* **(c)** *Bone scan image.*

*This patient with carcinoma of the breast developed headaches and some focal neurological signs. While the brain scan shows multiple deposits, some of these are due to skull lesions, as shown on the bone scan, and it is not possible to discern which lesions, if any, represent intracerebral disease. This clinical situation demands a* CT *scan rather than a radionuclide brain scan.*

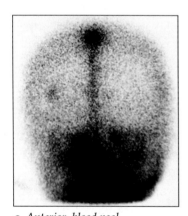

*a Anterior, blood pool*

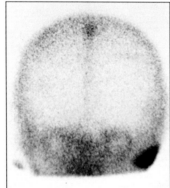

*b Anterior, delayed*

**Fig. 5.120**

⁹⁹ᵐTc DTPA *brain scan:* **(a)** *anterior blood pool image;* **(b)** *anterior delayed view.*

*There is a single focal area of increased tracer uptake seen only on the blood pool image in the right frontal region. The delayed image is normal. The lesion corresponded to a palpable nodule in bone which, on x-ray, was shown to be lytic. In this case there was no evidence of intracerebral metastases, and the blood pool accumulation on the brain scan was due to a skull metastasis.*

• Bony involvement of the skull is a well-recognized cause of a false-positive brain scan for subdural collection, and is most often seen in association with either metastases or Paget's disease. A radionuclide bone scan will often clarify the situation.
• Most non-cerebral, ie skull and scalp, lesions are prominent because of the vascular space within them. Therefore most of these lesions will show decreased tracer uptake with increasing time between injection and imaging, as in the example in Fig. 5.120.

**CLINICAL APPLICATIONS**

## *Bruising*

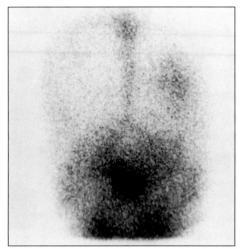
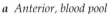
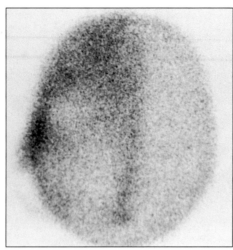

*a  Anterior, blood pool*

*b  Vertex, delayed*

**Fig. 5.121**

*⁹⁹ᵐTc DTPA brain scan: **(a)** anterior blood pool image; **(b)** vertex view.*

*There is an area of increased tracer uptake lying superficially in the left frontal region. There is increased vascularity to this area. The scan findings were due to skull bruising, and there was no evidence of intracranial pathology.*

## *Sebaceous cyst*

Any superficial scalp lesion may cause an abnormal brain scan. This example of a sebaceous cyst is a typical example.

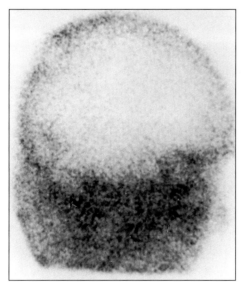
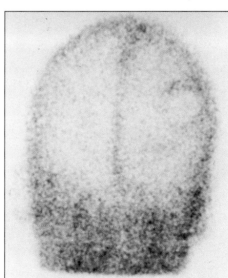

*a  Right lateral, delayed*

*b  Posteror, delayed*

**Fig. 5.122**

*(a, b) ⁹⁹ᵐTc DTPA brain scan.*

*There is an apparent photon-deficient area in the right side of the skull posteriorly, involving the outer table of the skull, but with no defect lying within. The scan findings were due to a large sebaceous cyst.*

• The importance of clinical examination once the study has been performed is illustrated by the two cases in Figs 5.121 and 5.122. Both lesions could be easily localized by manual palpation.

• Skull and scalp lesions may often provide a clue as to their origin by distorting the smooth outer margin of the skull on one of the brain scan views. Intracerebral lesions never do this.

# CHAPTER 6

# CARDIAC

Imaging the heart using radionuclide techniques provides unique non-invasive functional information which is complementary to the more invasive and essentially structural information obtained from the radiological investigations of coronary angiography and ventriculography. There are a variety of nuclear medicine techniques available, each of which may provide different functional information. These include: first pass studies for assessing the sequences of chamber filling and for the measurement of intracardiac shunting, as well as for the measurement of ventricular function; myocardial perfusion with thallium-201 ($^{201}$Tl) and technetium-99m ($^{99m}$Tc) radiopharmaceuticals for the assessment of regional perfusion abnormalities caused by coronary artery disease; 'hot spot' imaging with $^{99m}$Tc pyrophosphate and radiolabelled myoscint antibodies for demonstrating recent myocardial infarction; gated equilibrium blood pool imaging, which is the only technique allowing the assessment of regional and total ventricular function following repeated physiological interventions; and, finally, $^{99m}$Tc-labelled microspheres, which may be used to measure the size of right to left shunts and regional pulmonary blood flow. Because of this wide choice and because the techniques are often difficult to perform well, it is even more important in nuclear cardiology than in other branches of nuclear medicine to make a critical assessment of the clinical problem before deciding which method to use and the way in which it should be performed. Close collaboration between nuclear medicine practitioners and cardiologists is essential for the most effective use of radionuclide techniques, and will ultimately determine their value in patient management.

In this chapter the normal appearances of the commonly performed investigations are illustrated, together with main points to note when interpreting studies. Several important clinical problems which may be resolved by radionuclide techniques are highlighted to demonstrate how the use of appropriate techniques can be applied to individual cases.

## CHAPTER CONTENTS

# 6.1 ANATOMY/PHYSIOLOGY

## 6.1.1 Normal gated blood pool radionuclide angiogram

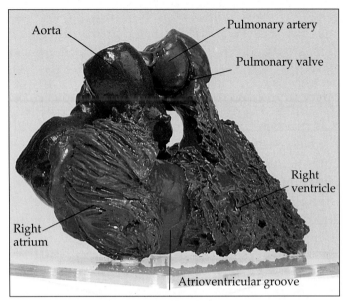

*a* RAO

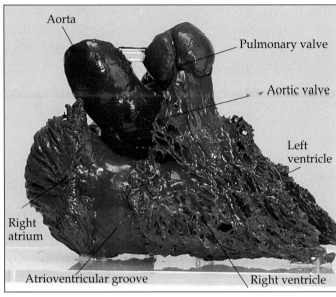

*b* Anterior

### Fig. 6.1

*(a–e) Wax casts of the cardiac chambers (right side in blue, left side in red) are shown in various views to facilitate the functional assessment of the gated blood pool study. (Courtesy of Dr Michael Hutchinson, London, UK.)*

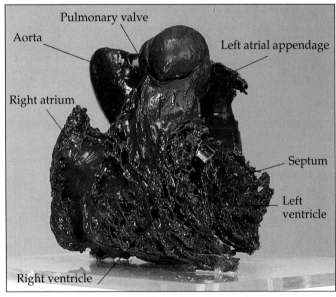

*c* LAO

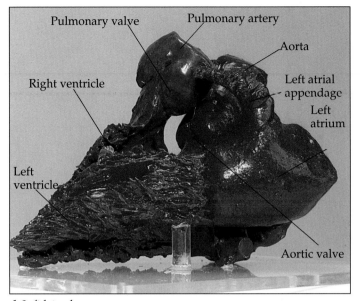

*d* Left lateral

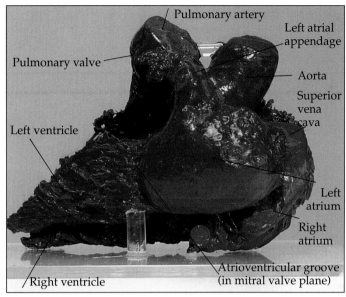

*e* LPO

## 6.1.2   Normal coronary artery anatomy

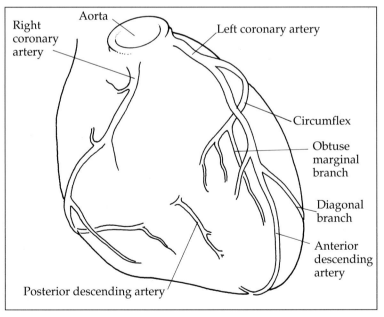

*Fig. 6.2*

*Normal coronary artery anatomy.*

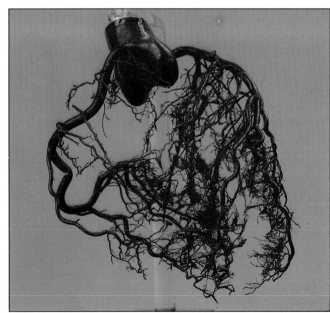

*Fig. 6.3*

*Cast of the normal coronary tree.*

## Coronary artery territories on planar views

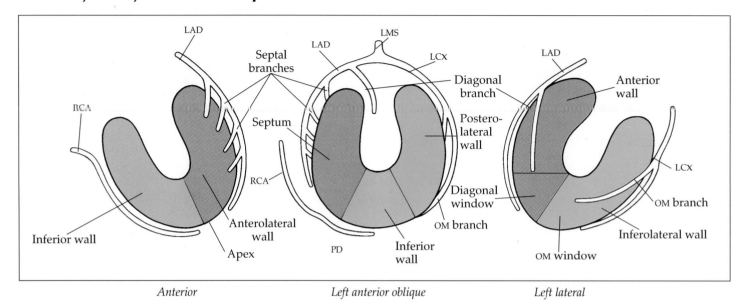

Anterior                Left anterior oblique                Left lateral

**Fig. 6.4**

Normal coronary artery territories in left ventricle corresponding to ²⁰¹Tl myocardial planar views.
LAD, left anterior descending artery; RCA, right coronary artery; LMS, left main stem; LCX, left
circumflex artery; PD, posterior descending artery; OM obtuse marginal artery.

## Coronary artery territories on SPECT views

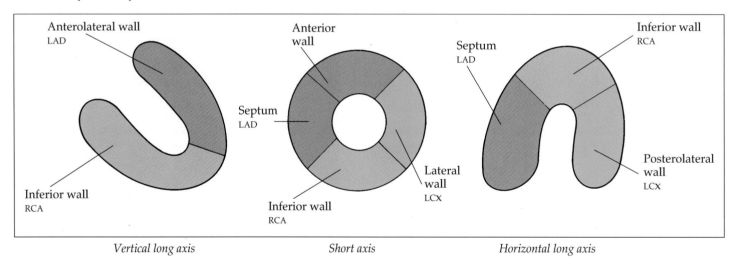

Vertical long axis                Short axis                Horizontal long axis

**Fig. 6.5**

Normal coronary artery territories in the left ventricle corresponding to ²⁰¹Tl myocardial SPECT views.
LAD, left anterior descending artery; RCA, right coronary artery; LCX, left circumflex artery.

# 6.2  RADIOPHARMACEUTICALS

*Table 6.1  Method and radiopharmaceuticals*

| Cardiac function | Method | Radiopharmaceutical |
|---|---|---|
| Myocardial perfusion | Exercise or dipyridamole stress perfusion scan | $^{201}$Tl chloride<br>$^{99m}$Tc isonitriles |
| Ventricular function | First pass or gated blood pool radionuclide angiogram | $^{99m}$Tc-labelled red blood cells (RBC) |
| Intracardiac shunt measurement | First pass angiogram (L → R shunt)<br>Microsphere trapping (R → L shunt) | $^{99m}$TcO$_4^-$ or $^{99m}$Tc RBC<br>$^{99m}$Tc microspheres |
| Cardiac chamber filling sequence | First pass angiogram | $^{99m}$TcO$_4^-$, $^{99m}$Tc DTPA or $^{99m}$Tc RBC |
| Visualization of recently infarcted muscle | Tracer uptake ('hot spot' imaging) | $^{99m}$Tc pyrophosphate<br>$^{111}$In-antimyosin antibody |

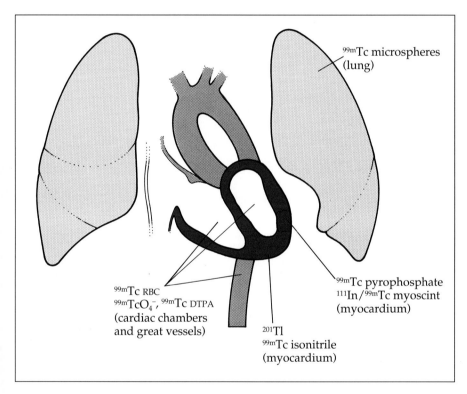

$^{99m}$Tc microspheres (lung)

$^{99m}$Tc RBC
$^{99m}$TcO$_4^-$, $^{99m}$Tc DTPA
(cardiac chambers and great vessels)

$^{99m}$Tc pyrophosphate
$^{111}$In/$^{99m}$Tc myoscint (myocardium)

$^{201}$Tl
$^{99m}$Tc isonitrile (myocardium)

*Fig. 6.6*

*Radiopharmaceuticals for cardiac imaging.*

# 6.3 NORMAL SCANS WITH VARIANTS

## 6.3.1 First pass studies

The success of a first pass study depends on the rapid injection of a single bolus of a radionuclide. Immediate imaging provides information on the sequence with which the cardiac chambers are filled, and the presence of intracardiac shunts. Quantitation of the pulmonary time–activity (T/A) curve will allow measurement of the size of the shunt. $^{99m}$Tc red blood cells is the radio-pharmaceutical of choice, since this permits subsequent assessment of ventricular function using the gated blood pool technique.

### Normal first pass study

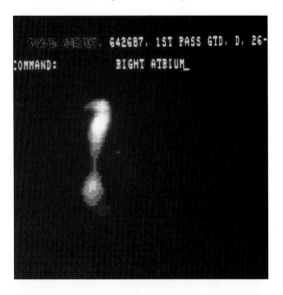

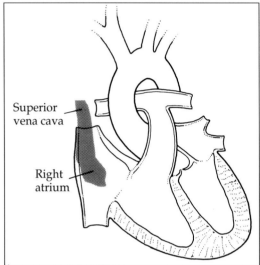

Superior vena cava

Right atrium

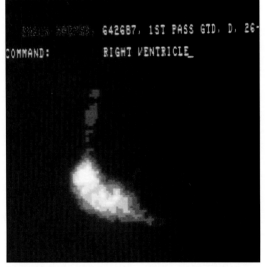

Right atrium

Right ventricle

b

**Fig. 6.7**

*(a–e) Serial images from a two frame per second first pass cardiac study using $^{99m}$Tc-labelled red blood cells, formatted to demonstrate the serial passage of the bolus through the cardiac chambers.*

# NORMAL SCANS WITH VARIANTS

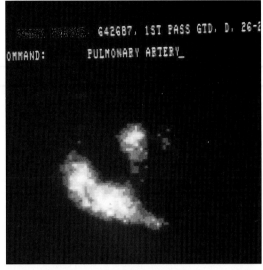

*c*

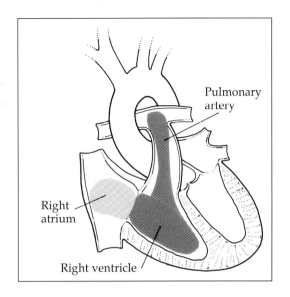

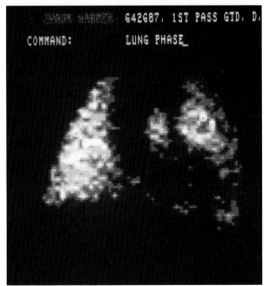

*d*

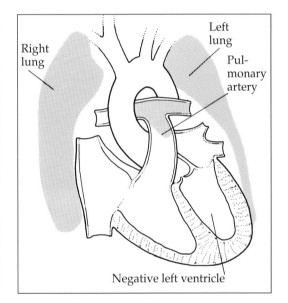

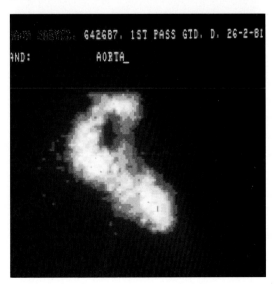

*e*

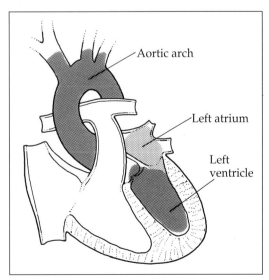

## Normal first pass study T/A curve

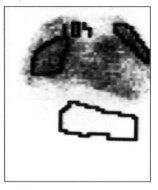

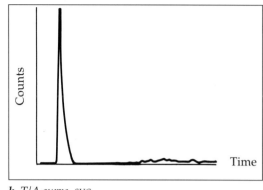

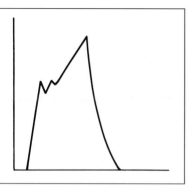

*a* ROIS  *b* T/A curve, SVC  *c* T/A curve, SVC

*Fig. 6.8*

*T/A curve from the superior vena cava (SVC) is essential for quality control, to assess the adequacy of a bolus, particularly when quantitation of a shunt is undertaken. (**a**) ROIS (SVC, right and left lungs, aorta). (**b**) Good SVC bolus. (**c**) Poor SVC bolus.*

## Lung and aortic T/A curves

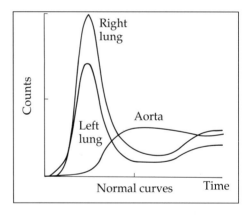

*Fig. 6.9*

*The lung curve should be symmetrical in the absence of shunting. The activity in the aorta should not appear before most of the tracer has left the lungs. Early appearance in the aorta indicates right to left shunting.*

**A poor bolus will usually invalidate quantitation of shunt size and make qualitative assessment difficult.**

## Points in assessing a first pass study

- Is the bolus compact? Assess either visually or by the T/A curve from the superior vena cava.
- Does the tracer then enter the right atrium and right ventricle with no dilution?
- As the tracer enters the lungs, is there a clearly negative (empty) left ventricle?
- Before the tracer enters the left ventricle, is there any tracer below the diaphragm which would suggest a right to left shunt?
- As the tracer enters the left ventricle, does activity

'clear' from the lung fields? Lack of clearance suggests recirculation, ie, left to right shunting.
- Is the pulmonary perfusion uniform? Are there any large areas of pulmonary hypoperfusion or asymmetry between the two lungs?
- Is the aortic arch clearly visualized? Poor visualization suggests high background activity caused by left to right shunting.
- Are the sizes of the ventricles approximately normal?

## NORMAL SCANS WITH VARIANTS

### Normal gated first pass studies for the assessment of right and left ventricular function

*Right ventricle*

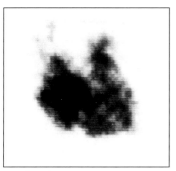

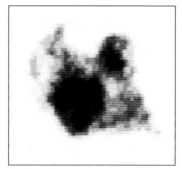

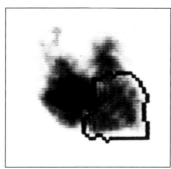

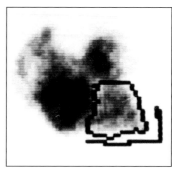

*a Diastole*  *b Systole*  *c Diastolic ROI*  *d Systolic ROI with background*

**Fig. 6.10**

*Gating the first pass study allows assessment of the right ventricular outline without it being obscured by the left side of the heart. Changes in right ventricular counts can be used to measure the right ventricular ejection fraction (RVEF). (a) Diastole. (b) Systole. (c) Right ventricular region of interest (ROI). (d) Background ROI. (e)T/A curve from right ventricular ROI.*

Counts

5 seconds

*e T/A curve*

*Formula for measuring RVEF*

$$\text{Ejection fraction (\%)} = \frac{\text{Counts at end-diastole} - \text{counts at end-systole}}{\text{Counts at end-diastole} - \text{background}} \times 100$$

Normal values RVEF: mean 55% range 45–65%

*Left ventricle*

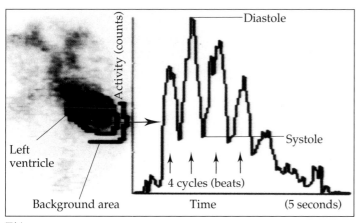

*T/A curve*

**Fig. 6.11**

*T/A curve from the left ventricle, showing the beat to beat variation of counts in the left ventricle which is used to calculate the ejection fraction (LVEF).*

*Formula for measuring LVEF*

$$\text{Ejection fraction (\%)} = \frac{\text{Diastole counts (mean of 3 beats)} - \text{systolic counts}}{\text{Diastolic counts} - \text{background}} \times 100$$

Normal values LVEF: mean 65%, range 55–75%.

## NORMAL SCANS WITH VARIANTS

## *Delayed pulmonary transit simulating a shunt*

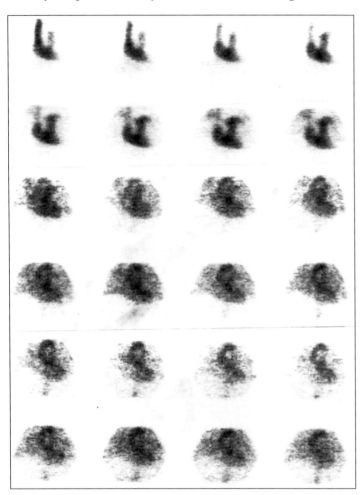

*a*

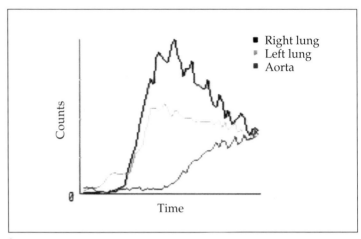

*b*

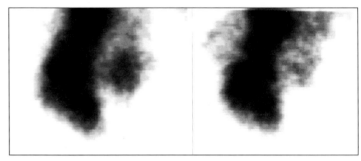

*c*

**Fig. 6.12**

*(a) Sequence of first pass images (two frames per second), showing a dilated right ventricle and pulmonary artery and slow pulmonary clearance of tracer. (b) T/A curve from lungs and aorta, showing the asymmetric lung curve usually associated with left to right intracardiac shunting. (c)* LAO *gated blood pool study, showing large dilated right ventricle and small volume left ventricle usually associated with a large* ASD.

*This man presented with right ventricular failure and was suspected of having a shunt. There are many features to suggest an* ASD, *but these were caused by pulmonary hypertension with right ventricular overload.*

**Any cause of slow pulmonary transit of blood may cause a false positive diagnosis of left to right shunt.**

# 6.3.2 Gated blood pool studies

There is a constant relationship between the electrical and mechanical phases of the heart.

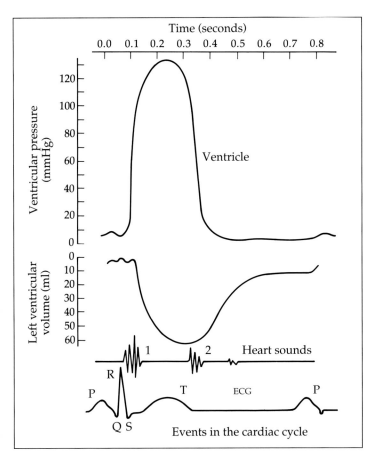

*Fig. 6.13*

*Events in the cardiac cycle.*

Linking the ECG with the gamma camera and computer system permits images to be obtained of the heart cavities from 2 (systole and diastole) to multiple (typically 16–32) moments in time throughout the cardiac cycle. This is achieved by storing data from each part of the cycle into a different memory of the data system until enough can be summed to produce a statistically satisfactory image (typically 5–10 minutes).

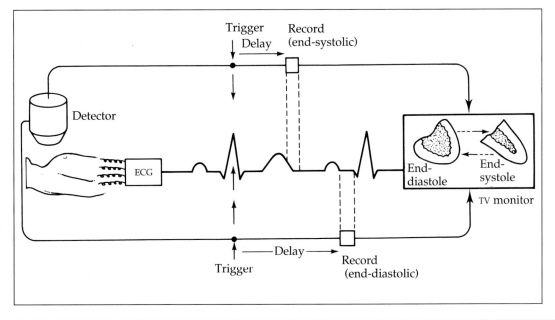

*Fig. 6.14*

*ECG: simple two-gate system for systole and diastole.*

# NORMAL SCANS WITH VARIANTS

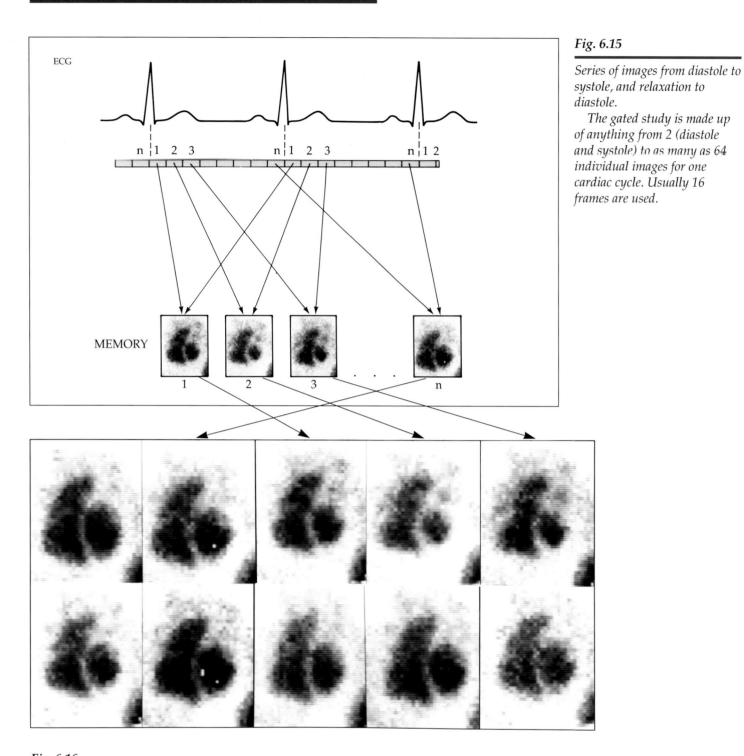

ECG

MEMORY

1    2    3    n

**Fig. 6.15**

Series of images from diastole to systole, and relaxation to diastole.

The gated study is made up of anything from 2 (diastole and systole) to as many as 64 individual images for one cardiac cycle. Usually 16 frames are used.

**Fig. 6.16**

LAO view, showing the changes from diastole to systole, and then relaxation.

## NORMAL SCANS WITH VARIANTS

### *Normal gated blood pool study*

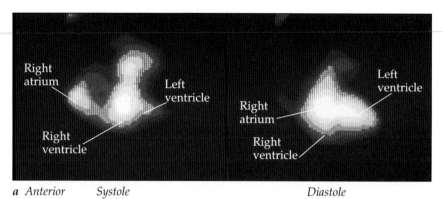

Right atrium

Left ventricle

Right ventricle

*a* Anterior    Systole

Left ventricle

Right atrium

Right ventricle

Diastole

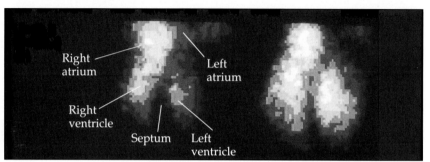

Right atrium

Left atrium

Right ventricle

Septum    Left ventricle

*b* LAO    Systole    Diastole

*Fig. 6.17*

*(a, b) Normal gated blood pool study.*

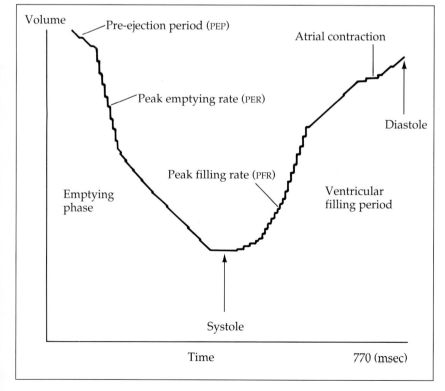

Volume

Pre-ejection period (PEP)

Atrial contraction

Peak emptying rate (PER)

Diastole

Peak filling rate (PFR)

Emptying phase

Ventricular filling period

Systole

Time    770 (msec)

*Fig. 6.18*

*T/A curve from the left ventricle, showing the activity changes in the left ventricle during a cardiac cycle. This T/A curve contains data from approximately 300 cardiac cycles.*

## *Points to note in evaluating a gated study*

- What is the relative volume of the cardiac chambers?
- Do the ventricles contract normally? Assess the end-diastolic and end-systolic volumes of the left and right ventricle. Assess the long axis shortening of the left ventricle on the anterior view. Are there any regional wall motion abnormalities (hypokinesis, akinesis, paradoxical movement)?

- Are the atria contracting? This is the best way to assess the quality of the gating.
- Do the ventricles contract simultaneously, ie, could there be a conduction defect?
- What changes occur during the stress studies?

## *Calculation of ejection fraction*

The left ventricular ejection fraction (LVEF) is calculated by defining the left ventricular region of interest (ROI) and a background region. These ROIs are defined anatomically using standard computer processing software. Threshold and second derivative methods are generally used. From the derived, background-corrected time–activity curve, the ejection fraction may be calculated. Again, this value is automatically calculated using standard nuclear medicine software.

It is essential that adequate counts/frame are obtained to accurately define the left ventricular region.

The following parameters may also be calculated if adequate frames/cycle are acquired:

- LV peak emptying rate
- LV peak filling rate
- Time to end-systole
- Time from end-systole to diagnosis

$$\text{Left ventricular ejection fraction (LVEF)} = \frac{\text{Counts in LV at end-diastole} - \text{counts in LV at end-systole}}{\text{Counts in LV at end-diastole} - \text{background counts}}$$

*Table 6.2   Errors in ejection fraction measurement*

| | |
|---|---|
| *Overestimation* | Too much background subtraction (eg background ROI over spleen, aorta)<br>End-diastolic ROI too large |
| *Underestimation* | Including the left atrium in left ventricle ROI in systole, especially when the left atrium is enlarged<br>Poor separation of right and left ventricles<br>Fixed (non-variable) background ROI<br>Too little background subtraction (eg LVH, pleural or pericardial effusion)<br>Variable gating<br>Presence of anterior aneurysm |

LVH, left ventricular hypertrophy.

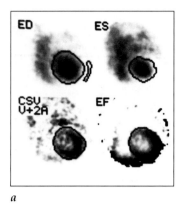

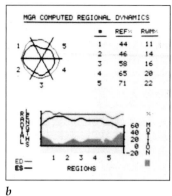

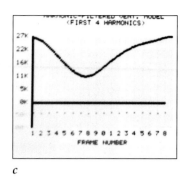

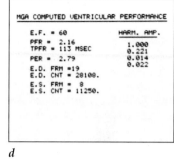

*a*             *b*            *c*           *d*

**Fig. 6.19**

*Automatic ejection fraction determination.*

*(a) The end-diastolic, end-systolic and background ROIs are demonstrated. The end-diastolic region is also displayed on the stroke volume and regional ejection fraction parametric images. (b) Computed regional dynamics. (c) The resultant background-corrected left ventricular T/A curve. (d) Computed ventricular performance.*

## Functional images

To obtain functional (phase and amplitude) images from a gated blood pool study, T/A curves are generated for each individual pixel. Using Fourier analysis, whereby a sine wave is fitted to each point, regional contraction patterns can be shown in colour or shades of grey to represent either *amplitude*—a measure of the size of the difference between the maximum and the minimum counts at each pixel, irrespective of the time when the difference occurs—or *phase*—the time when maximum change occurs.

In general, a large amplitude will indicate a well-contracting ventricle, but will also be seen in a region of gross paradox; however, the latter would be identified on the phase study, since the timing of contraction would be quite different. It is apparent that phase and amplitude images should be interpreted together to obtain optimal information.

### Amplitude image

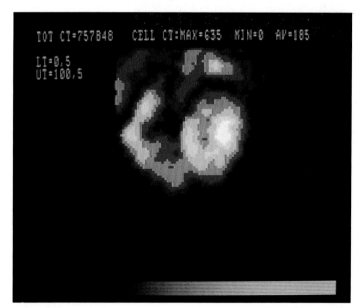

**Fig. 6.20**

*Amplitude image, showing that the major contraction occurs in the left ventricle, which is represented by a uniform U-shaped appearance.*

## Phase image

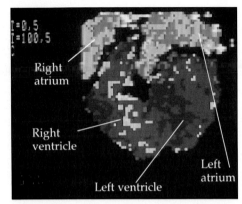

*a*

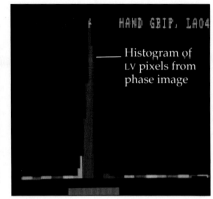

*b*

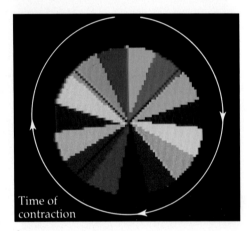

*c*

### Fig. 6.21

*(a–c) Phase image.*
  *Note that the two ventricles contract simultaneously, and 180° out of phase with the atria. Quantitatively, the left ventricle phase can be represented by a histogram (b), which, if there is almost simultaneous contraction throughout the ventricle, will be a narrow band, but will become broader with increasing regional dyskinesia or the appearance of an aneurysm.*

# NORMAL SCANS WITH VARIANTS

## Gated blood pool study with stress

The evaluation of cardiac function under conditions causing increased myocardial workload provides information about myocardial reserve and the ability of coronary blood flow to increase from the resting state. This provides the most sensitive means of identifying myocardial ischaemia.

### Cardiac stress protocols

#### Dynamic exercise
- Supine or erect bicycle ergometer
- Increase workload by 25 watts every 2 minutes
- Attain maximum workload possible
- Achieve greater than 85% of predicted heart rate
- Image throughout at each interval

#### Isometric hand grip
- Supine hand grip exercise
- Apply hand grip
- Check maximum pressure achievable
- Maintain pressure at approximately 50% of maximum for 4 minutes

Note that blood pressure and pulse rate are monitored at 1-minute intervals during stress. If two stress methods, eg cold pressor and isometric hand grip, are used, allow the haemodynamic response to return to baseline between studies.

#### Cold pressor
- Hand and wrist immersed in bucket of iced water
- Wait approximately 30 seconds to 1 minute
- Collect data for 4 minutes

## NORMAL SCANS WITH VARIANTS

*Table 6.3   Choice of stress*

| Stress | Effect | Advantages | Disadvantages | Values for LVEF response | | |
| --- | --- | --- | --- | --- | --- | --- |
| | | | | Resting value | Normal | Abnormal |
| Dynamic supine or erect bicycle exercise | ↑ BP and PR ↑ EF | Physiological | Technically difficult because of patient movement Sensitivity drops rapidly below maximum effort Requires cooperation and agility | 55–75% | <5% rise or fall | >5% Fall in EF |
| Isometric stress | ↑ BP Slight ↑ EF | Simple, no patient movement | May not be sustained for long enough to collect data | 55–75% | Rise or <5% fall | >5% fall in EF |
| Cold pressor test | ↑ BP Slight ↑ EF | Does not require cooperation | May be painful Variable haemodynamic response | | | |

BP, blood pressure; PR, pulse rate; EF, ejection fraction.

- For dynamic exercise to be effective, maximum work must be achieved.
- During cold pressor and isometric hand grip stress, the haemodynamic response decays over 4 minutes, and therefore collection of data must be completed rapidly.
- If there is no rise in blood pressure with cold pressor or isometric hand grip stress, and the test result is negative, then this result should be considered unreliable.

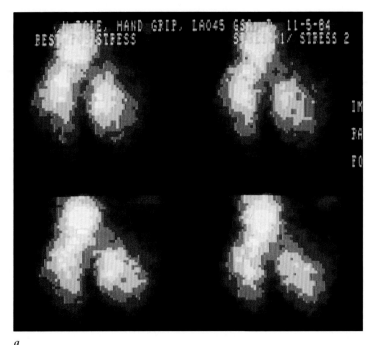

*a*

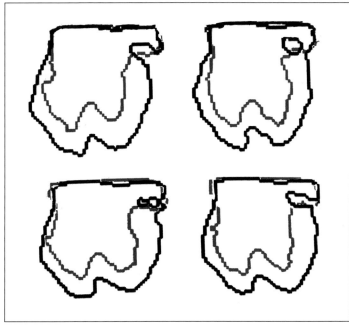

*b*

## Fig. 6.22

LAO *views during normal stress study.* **(a)** *Diastolic images.* **(b)** *Diastolic and systolic ventricular outlines. The key to the images is shown below* **(b)**.

| Rest | Cold pressor |
|---|---|
| Post-stress rest | Hand grip |

## Quantitation of stress data

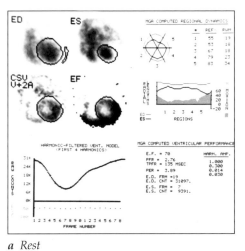

*a Rest*

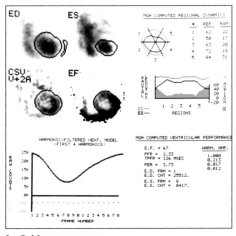

*b Cold pressor stress*

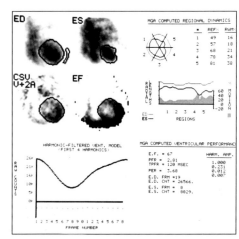

*c Isometric hand grip stress*

## Fig. 6.23

**(a)** *Rest quantitation.* **(b)** *Cold pressor stress quantitation.* **(c)** *Isometric hand grip quantitation.*

The LVEF *is normal at rest (70%)* **(a)**. *With cold pressor* **(b)** *and isometric hand grip stress* **(c)**, *there is a non-significant fall in ejection fraction to 67%.*

# NORMAL SCANS WITH VARIANTS

## Points to note during the stress study

- Whether there is any significant ventricular dilatation
- Whether the ejection fraction drops
- Whether there are any focal areas of myocardium which become hypokinetic, akinetic or even paradoxical.

It is also important to ensure that the haemodynamic response to the stress is adequate.

Gated cardiac studies, particularly, with stress, are difficult to perform and interpret. Table 6.4 shows some of the factors to be taken into account in the interpretation.

*Table 6.4 Factors influencing results in ventricular function studies*

| Patient | Technical |
| --- | --- |
| Cardiac disease (response is non-specific) | Labelling efficiency |
| Choice of stress | Patient positioning |
| Haemodynamic response to stress (BP and PR) | Patient movement |
| Drug treatment (eg beta-blockers) | Choice of ROI |
| Ageing (decreases the ejection fraction response) | Data collection time |
| Regular heart rate | Number of views |
| | Frame rate |

*Table 6.5 Advantages and disadvantages of first pass versus gated blood pool techniques*

| | First pass | Gated |
| --- | --- | --- |
| *Advantages* | Direct assessment of each cardiac chamber without activity from overlying chambers<br>Rapid (less than 30 seconds)<br>Beat to beat analysis<br>Patient movement is not a problem<br>Better for assessment of right ventricle function<br>Can assess and evaluate the size of shunts | Multiple studies possible<br>Multiple views possible<br>Intervention studies possible |
| *Disadvantages* | Single study only<br>One view only<br>Bolus quality is critical | Lower target to background ratio<br>Long acquisition (2–10 minutes)<br>Patient movement is a problem with exercise studies<br>Unreliable with significant R:R variations |

# 6.3.3 Myocardial perfusion imaging studies

## Concept of stress myocardial imaging

Myocardial blood flow distal to coronary artery stenosis is normal at rest unless occlusion is greater than 90% of luminal diameter, or a myocardial infarct is present. However, following the maximal stress, the normal increase in myocardial blood flow becomes impaired distal to stenosis of approximately 45–50%, or greater.

Myocardial perfusion studies are performed by injecting $^{201}$Tl or $^{99m}$Tc isonitrile intravenously after increased coronary flow has been induced by maximal exercise. Images are obtained within 10 minutes of injection using planar or tomographic imaging. With $^{201}$Tl, redistribution images are obtained 3–4 hours later to allow comparison of regional blood flow at rest and exercise. With $^{99m}$Tc isonitrile, a separate study at rest must be performed, or a further injection of $^{99m}$Tc isonitrile should be given to obtain the rest images.

## $^{201}$Tl perfusion imaging

### Mechanism of myocardial uptake of $^{201}$Tl

- Myocardial blood flow
- Integrity of ATP-ase dependent sodium–potassium pump.

Thus, while thallium images generally reflect myocardial perfusion, they also reflect myocardial cell function.

### Limitations of $^{201}$Tl

- Low photon energy — diminished resolution
  — tissue absorption
  — patient scatter

Low fractional myocardial uptake

Long half-life (73.5 hours) — high radiation dose

### Drug effects on $^{201}$Tl uptake

- Digoxin and beta-blockers reduce myocardial extraction of tracer, but this does not generally seem to affect image quality
- Dipyridamole causes coronary vasodilatation and increases myocardial uptake or tracer. This is used clinically (see page 418).

### Uptake of $^{201}$Tl

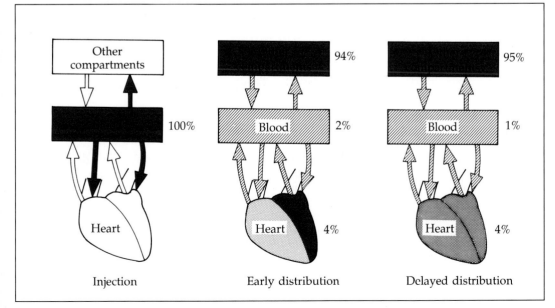

| Injection | Early distribution | Delayed distribution |

*Fig. 6.24*

$^{201}$Tl uptake: relative intensity of shading = concentration of $^{201}$Tl.

Percentage uptake
in heart                 4%
Extraction efficiency 80%
Peak uptake
after injection          10 min
Myocardial
clearance rate           7–8 hours

$^{201}$Tl is not an ideal isotope for imaging. Although it does have gamma-rays (137 and 167 keV), imaging is performed using the 80 keV x-rays, which are seven times as abundant as the gamma-rays.

*Exercise test*

*Contraindications to performing a $^{201}$Tl exercise test*
- Unstable angina or rest pain
- Cardiac failure
- Severe valve disease
- Uncontrolled hypertension
- Ventricular arrhythmias at rest
- Heart block (2nd or 3rd degree).

If a patient is unable to exercise, the stress thallium study can be performed using dipyridamole, which is a coronary vasodilator.

*Points to note during an exercise test*
- Appearance of ST segments—horizontal or down-sloping shift of 1 mm or more persisting for 3 minutes into the recovery period, constitutes a positive exercise test
- Reason for discontinuing the test
- Presence of chest pain
- Duration and total work achieved
- Haemodynamic response (blood pressure and pulse rate).

*End points to discontinue an exercise test*
- Severe angina
- Fatigue
- Severe dyspnoea
- ≥5 mm ST depression
- Frequent multifocal or paired ventricular ectopic beats (≥10 per minute)
- Three or more consecutive ventricular ectopic beats
- Blood pressure falls below resting level
- Dizziness or syncope.

- **An exercise test for a $^{201}$Tl scan differs from a diagnostic exercise test; the end point is not evidence of ischaemia, but when the greatest amount of work has been achieved within the limits of safety.**
- **Submaximal stress will result in a false negative result in some patients with coronary artery disease.**

*Dipyridamole test*

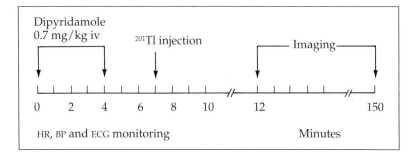

**Fig. 6.25**

*Dipyridamole protocol.*

- **Patients may not be able to achieve adequate exercise levels or pulse rates because of:**
(a) **Leg claudication**
(b) **Physical inability, eg only one leg**
(c) **Unwillingness to make the physical effort necessary**
(d) **Unfamiliarity with a bicycle if a bicycle ergometer is used.**
- **In these circumstances using dipyridamole stress instead of exercise will give better results.**
- **Dopamine and adenosine may also be used as pharmacological stress agents.**

## NORMAL SCANS WITH VARIANTS

*Normal thallium myocardial perfusion scan with planar imaging*

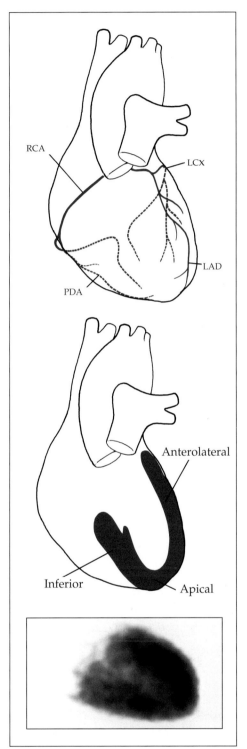

*a Anterior*

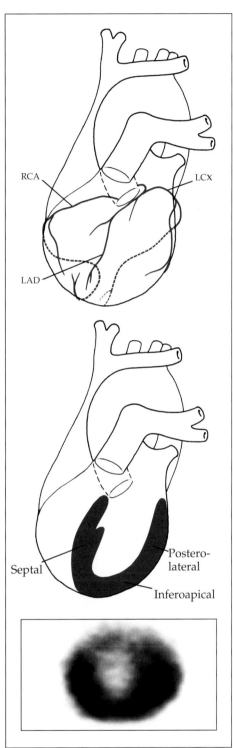

*b LAO (45°–50°)*

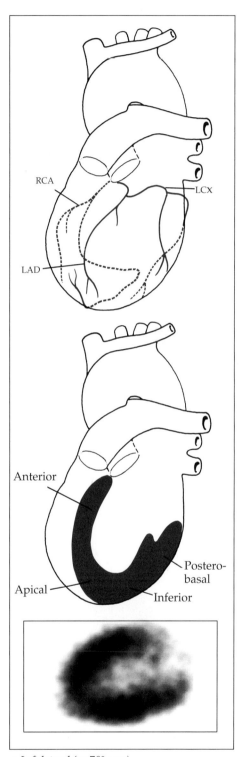

*c Left lateral (or 70° LAO)*

**Fig. 6.26**

*(a–c) Normal ²⁰¹Tl myocardial perfusion scan with planar imaging: RCA, right coronary artery; PDA, posterior descending artery; LCX, left circumflex artery; LAD, left anterior descending artery.*

*Points to note when evaluating a ²⁰¹Tl perfusion study*

- Is the cavity size of the left ventricle normal?
- Is the distribution of ²⁰¹Tl in the left ventricular myocardium normal?

- Is there abnormal uptake in the right ventricular myocardium?
- Is there significant change in regional distribution of tracer between exercise and rest views?

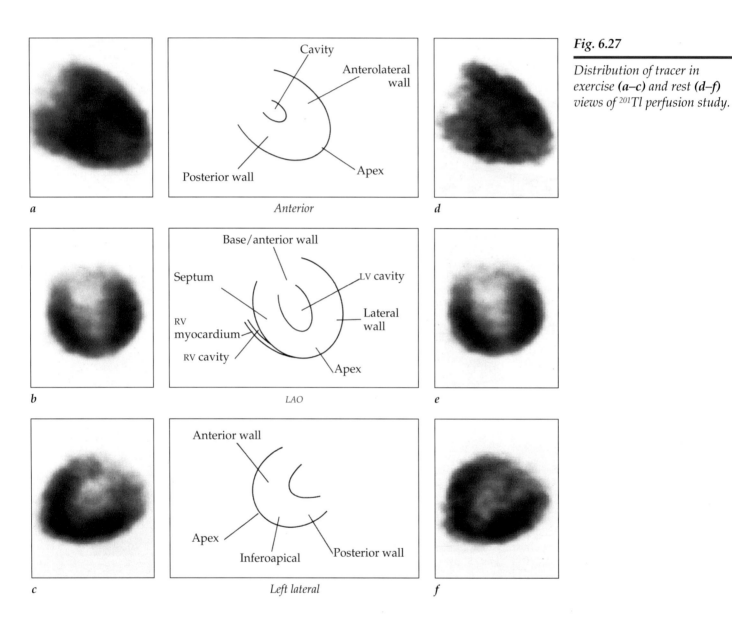

**Fig. 6.27**

*Distribution of tracer in exercise (a–c) and rest (d–f) views of ²⁰¹Tl perfusion study.*

## NORMAL SCANS WITH VARIANTS

*Variation in LAO view appearance*

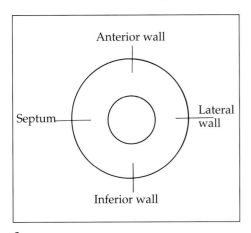

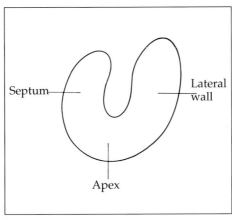

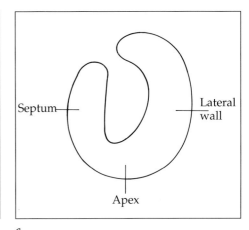

*a*

*b*

*c*

**Fig. 6.28**

*(a) True 'short axis' view looking 'through' the apex. (b, c) Less caudal tilt of camera, so a 'defect' is seen where the anterior wall would be.*

**The right ventricle will be easily seen on the ²⁰¹Tl study when there is:**

- **Right ventricular hypertrophy**
- **Pulmonary arterial hypertension**
- **Global decrease in left ventricular uptake.**

### ²⁰¹Tl washout

Data may be improved by semi-quantitative assessment of relative uptake of ²⁰¹Tl at rest and exercise, and by measuring the percentage washout of tracer. The initial uptake of tracer in the myocardium is proportional to the coronary blood flow induced by maximal exercise. When exercising is discontinued, coronary blood flow reverts to the resting level, and during the next 3–4 hours a new equilibrium is reached, with a lower level of tracer concentration in all areas, but with the same relative concentrations. Thus the stress and redistribution images of a normal person look identical, but at a low overall level of activity. This can be expressed graphically by count profiles, constructed in the same way as the count contours.

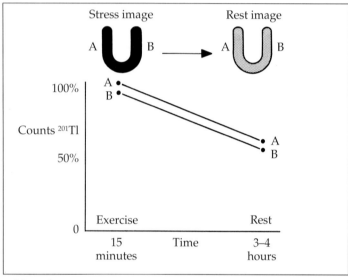

*a Normal*

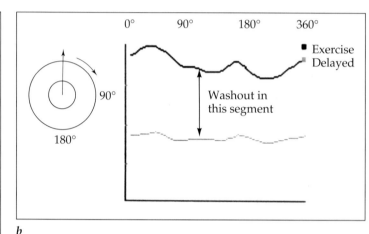

*b*

**Fig. 6.29**

*(a, b) Diagrammatic illustration of ²⁰¹Tl washout during the post-injection period.*

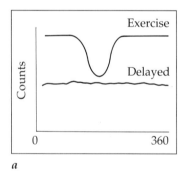

*a*

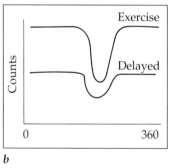

*b*

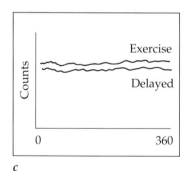

*c*

**Fig. 6.30**

*Diagrammatic illustration of three common washout profile abnormalities: **(a)** ischaemia; **(b)** infarct; **(c)** poor exercise or global reduction of ²⁰¹Tl uptake (which may occur with triple vessel disease).*

### Causes of slow myocardial ²⁰¹Tl washout

- Myocardial ischaemia
- Low exercise heart rate (less than 75% of the predicted maximum)
- Subcutaneous infiltration of thallium
- Failure to collect rest/stress images for the same time, or failure to correct for the time.

## Normal $^{201}$Tl myocardial scan with tomographic imaging

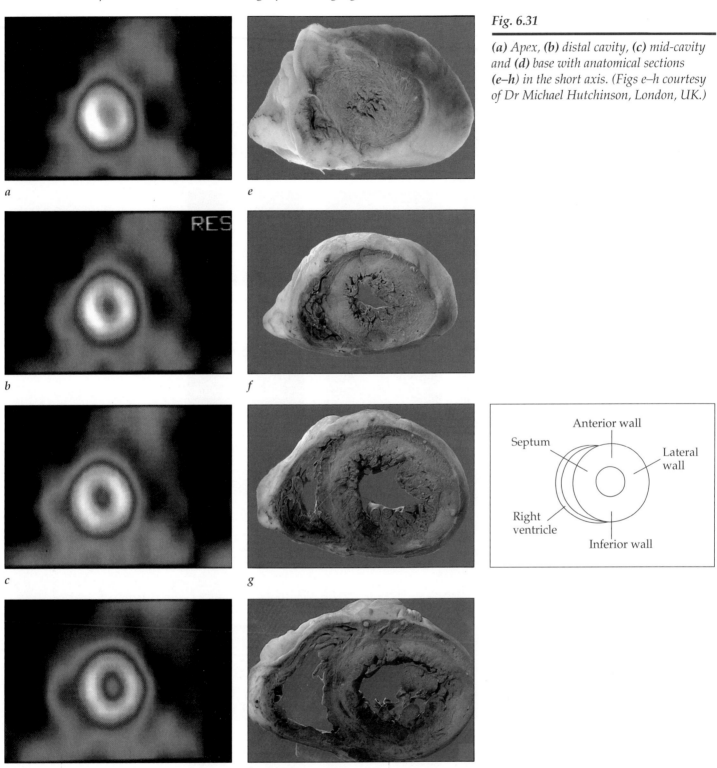

**Fig. 6.31**

*(a)* Apex, *(b)* distal cavity, *(c)* mid-cavity and *(d)* base with anatomical sections *(e–h)* in the short axis. (Figs e–h courtesy of Dr Michael Hutchinson, London, UK.)

## NORMAL SCANS WITH VARIANTS

Visual comparison of the exercise and rest slices should be made after ensuring that they are comparable in anatomical position.

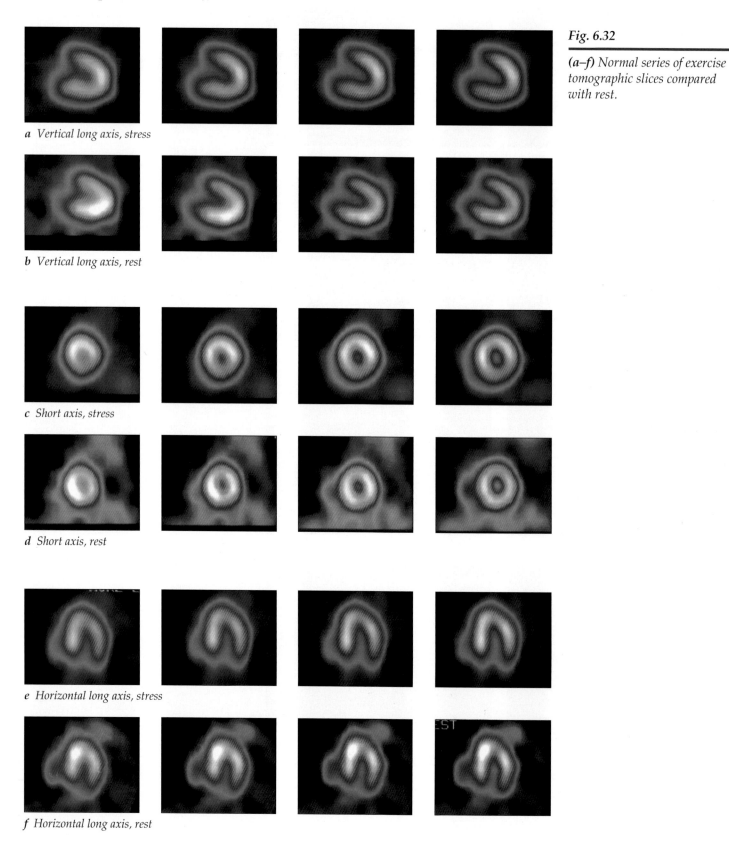

a  Vertical long axis, stress

b  Vertical long axis, rest

c  Short axis, stress

d  Short axis, rest

e  Horizontal long axis, stress

f  Horizontal long axis, rest

**Fig. 6.32**

*(a–f) Normal series of exercise tomographic slices compared with rest.*

## NORMAL SCANS WITH VARIANTS

### Causes of a false negative $^{201}$Tl study

- Patient not exercised adequately
- If imaging is continued for more than 30 minutes after injection of tracer, there may be some reversal of a defect
- Adequate collateral blood supply (study is false negative for coronary stenosis but accurate for myocardial blood flow)
- Rarely, with triple vessel disease, when there is global reduction of tracer uptake throughout the myocardium equally in each vessel distribution. Images may appear normal, although there is an absolute reduction of tracer uptake which may be detected by quantitative techniques.

### Causes of a false positive $^{201}$Tl study

- Accepting coronary arteriography findings as the 'gold standard', the interpretation of which is usually a subjective evaluation
- Soft tissue attenuation, especially breast tissue
- Normal apical thinning interpreted as a defect
- Decreased uptake in upper septum caused by aortic valve and membranous septum
- Myocardial disease.

- **Adequate exercise and pulse rate response are necessary to increase the myocardial blood flow to normal myocardium sufficiently to bring out the contrast between normal and abnormal myocardium, where the blood flow cannot increase because of the stenosed supplying vessel.**
- **Decreased tracer uptake at rest is almost always due to an infarct, because, even with severe ischaemic lesions, the coronary blood flow is rarely significantly decreased at rest.**
- **A 'reversible' defect has a high specificity for myocardial ischaemia induced by occlusive coronary disease. However, $^{201}$Tl uptake in the myocardium is partially cell-dependent and may, on occasion, be seen in other disorders such as myocarditis.**
- **Redistribution image at 3 hours after stress study is comparable, but not exactly the same as, a rest image. Decreased uptake on the redistribution image does not always signify an infarct, ie the fixed lesion may be over-reported.**

## NORMAL SCANS WITH VARIANTS

### Redistribution, rest imaging or reinjection?

A redistribution image is generally acquired four hours following the $^{201}$Tl injection at peak stress. Redistribution imaging usually shows some impairment in relative tracer uptake in patients with myocardial ischaemia, but redistribution is usually incomplete, ie the fixed component of a defect is overestimated, particularly in patients with a tight coronary artery stenosis. In practice, redistribution imaging at 3–4 hours is widely performed and is adequate to diagnose the presence of ischaemia. However, a separate rest study performed at 24 hours is required if it is necessary to quantitate accurately the degree of a fixed defect. There is evidence that a second injection of $^{201}$Tl before the study at 3–4 hours increases the sensitivity of the technique.

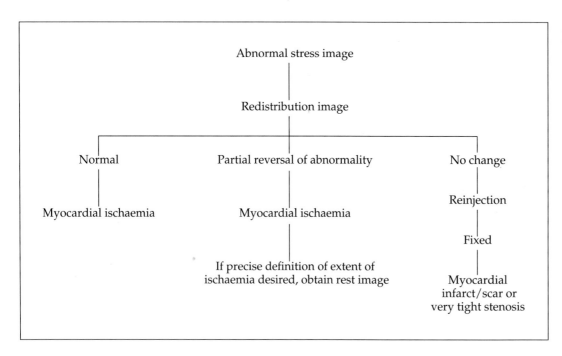

**Fig. 6.33**

*Use of stress, redistribution, and rest $^{201}$Tl imaging in the evaluation of coronary artery disease.*

**30–50% of apparently 'fixed' defects will reverse following reinjection of $^{201}$Tl on delayed imaging.**

## NORMAL SCANS WITH VARIANTS

### $^{99m}$Tc isonitrile studies

Unlike $^{201}$Tl, the isonitrile $^{99m}$Tc sestamibi is extracted by viable myocardial cells and is bound to cytosolic protein. There is minimal washout observed from normal segments. An image performed several hours after injection will be virtually unchanged from that immediately after injection.

*Table 6.6   Comparison of $^{99m}$Tc isonitrile with $^{201}$Tl*

| Advantages | Disadvantages |
|---|---|
| Better imaging characteristics of $^{99m}$Tc isonitrile compared with $^{201}$Tl. | Complex two stage preparation process. |
| Decay characteristics of $^{99m}$Tc isonitrile mean that higher administered doses of radiation can be used without increasing whole body radiation dose to the patient. | Cost. |
| Minimal washout simplifies imaging protocol, since there is no urgency to commence acquisition after injection. The stress part of the protocol can therefore be performed away from the department. | Minimal myocardial washout means that a second injection of radiopharmaceutical must be used to obtain the rest image. Rest and stress studies are ideally performed on separate days although low dose/high dose protocol for the same day studies are being used. |
| Minimal washout enables gated tomography to be performed so that both myocardial perfusion and regional wall motion can be studied simultaneously. | Gall bladder activity may interfere with image quality. |
| A first pass study can be performed at the time of injection of this radiopharmaceutical. | Possible lower sensitivity on planar imaging due to shine through from normal myocardium. |

# NORMAL SCANS WITH VARIANTS

## Normal isonitrile study

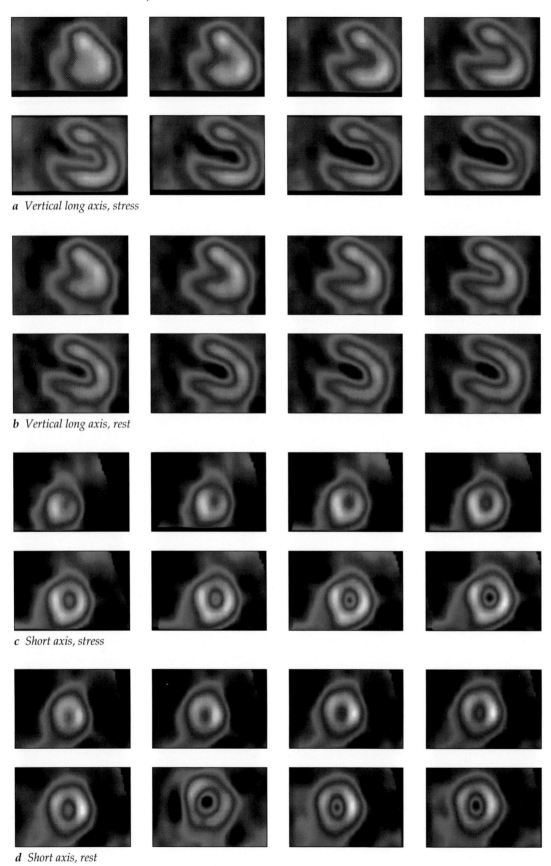

a Vertical long axis, stress

b Vertical long axis, rest

c Short axis, stress

d Short axis, rest

**Fig. 6.34**

*(a–f)* Normal isonitrile study in a 64-year-old man.

# NORMAL SCANS WITH VARIANTS

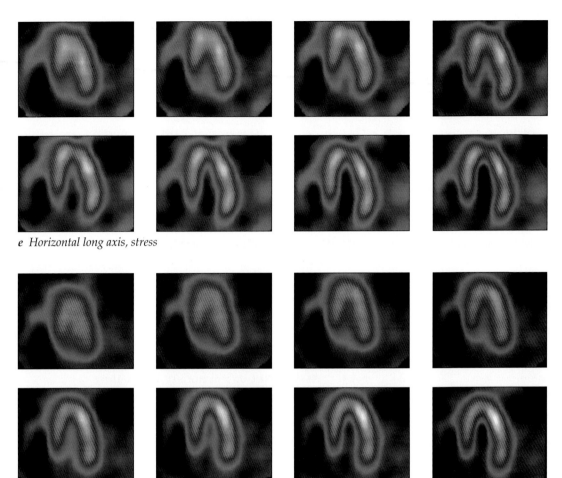

*e Horizontal long axis, stress*

*f Horizontal long axis, rest*

# 6.4 CLINICAL APPLICATIONS

In the investigation of cardiac problems it is perhaps more important than in any other area of nuclear medicine to know the patient's history in detail, the clinical questions to be answered and the management implications of the answers, in order to undertake such studies optimally. Each study must be individually tailored for the patient to answer the particular clinical problem. Ideally, these tests are performed in close consultation with the clinical cardiologist, both in deciding the study to be undertaken and in discussing the significance of the result.

The clinical applications of cardiac imaging are listed below, and examples of the various clinical problems are given on subsequent pages.

6.4.1 **Ischaemic heart disease**
Investigation of chest pain
Diagnosis of myocardial ischaemia
Investigation of myocardial ischaemia
Diagnosis of acute myocardial infarction
Diagnosis of non-acute myocardial infarction
Diagnosis and assessment of ventricular aneurysm
Follow-up after intervention
6.4.2 **Assessment of cardiac function**
Gated blood pool studies
6.4.3 **Congenital heart disorders**
Classification of principal congenital heart disorders
Clinical uses of functional radionuclide investigation in congenital heart disorders
First pass studies
Diagnosis of intracardiac left to right shunting: VSD

Intracardiac left to right shunt: gated cardiac study
Presentation with incidental murmur
Transposition of the great vessels
Tricuspid atresia with right to left shunt
Patent ductus arteriosus (PDA)
Measurement of intracardiac shunt size postoperatively
6.4.4 **Assessment of pulmonary blood flow**
Measurement of right to left shunt
Assessment of regional lung blood flow
6.4.5 **Identification of thrombus**
$^{111}$In-labelled platelets
$^{99m}$Tc fibrin monoclonal antibody
6.4.6 **Identification of cardiac tumour**
6.4.7 **Cardiac transplantation**

## CLINICAL APPLICATIONS

# 6.4.1 Ischaemic heart disease

## *Investigation of chest pain*

It is important to obtain a careful history before subjecting a patient with chest pain to radionuclide investigation. Often, the history combined with an exercise ECG will avoid the necessity of the more complicated and expensive use of nuclear cardiology investigations.

### *Common causes of chest pain*

- Angina (coronary artery disease)
- Musculoskeletal
- Pleuritic
- Neurological (eg intercostal nerve lesions)
- Oesophageal spasms
- Oesophageal reflux.

### *Risk factors for coronary artery disease*

- Family history of coronary artery disease
- Cigarette smoking
- Hypertension
- Obesity
- Lack of physical exercise.

The risk factors for ischaemic heart disease and the nature of the chest pain will determine the likelihood of coronary artery disease being present in an individual prior to undertaking any investigation. If the probability is high (above 90%) then radionuclide investigations will not contribute to establishing a diagnosis, and such tests are of most value when the pre-test probability lies between 30% and 70%.

*Gated cardiac study for the investigation of chest pain*

*Rest*

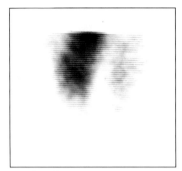

*a Diastolic*

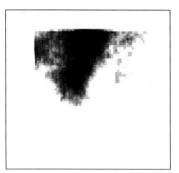

*b Systolic*

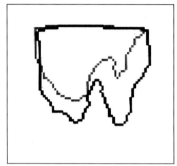

*c Outline*

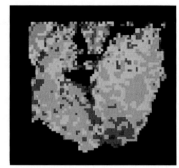

*d Phase image*

*Handgrip stress*

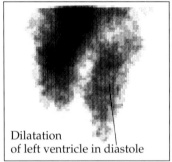

Dilatation
of left ventricle in diastole

*e Diastolic*

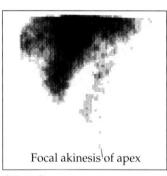

Focal akinesis of apex

*f Systolic*

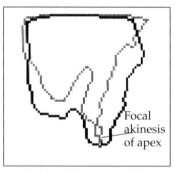

Focal
akinesis
of apex

*g Outline*

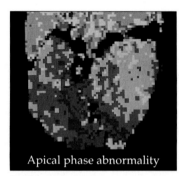

Apical phase abnormality

*h Phase image*

**Fig. 6.35**

*Gated cardiac study: (a, e) diastolic images; (b, f) systolic images; (c, g) outlines; (d, h) phase images.*
*This patient was referred for suspected myocardial ischaemia. He had a long history of chest pain typical of oesophageal reflux, which had been demonstrated on a barium meal. Treatment, however, had been unsuccessful. The possibility of ischaemic heart disease was therefore considered. The gated study shows normal function at rest, with an ejection fraction of 56% and no wall motion abnormalities. However, with isometric hand grip there is severe akinesis of the lower septum and apex, and the ejection fraction fell to 33%. This is a classic appearance of function disturbance secondary to coronary artery stenosis, brought on by afterload stress. Note the phase study, which shows the changes between rest and exercise, highlighting the abnormal akinetic area which appears during stress.*

**It is essential to be sure that maximum exercise is achieved if dynamic exercise is used, or that there is an adequate haemodynamic response to isometric hand grip or cold pressor, to avoid false negative studies.**

*Myocardial scan for the investigation of chest pain*

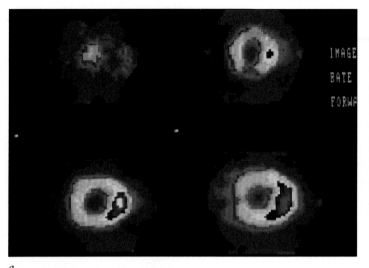

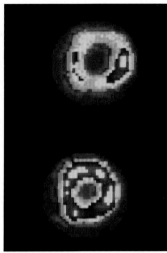

*a*

*b*

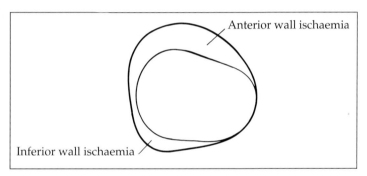

Anterior wall ischaemia

Inferior wall ischaemia

*c*

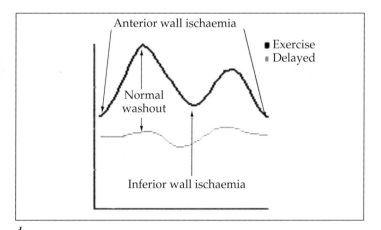

Anterior wall ischaemia

Normal washout

Inferior wall ischaemia

■ Exercise
▪ Delayed

*d*

*Fig. 6.36*

[201]Tl *myocardial scan:* (a) *tomographic exercise images;* (b) *exercise (top) and rest (bottom) compared;* (c) *relative uptake outlines;* (d) *washout curves. The key to the tomographic images in* (a) *is as follows.*

| Apex | Mid-cavity |
|------|------------|
| Mid-cavity | Base |

*This patient presented with chest pain, and was referred for investigation of possible coronary artery disease. He exercised well and had no chest pain during the exercise, and the* ECG *exercise test result was negative. The tomographic* [201]Tl *images demonstrate decreased tracer uptake in an extensive area involving the anterior, septal and part of the inferior walls. These findings confirmed ischaemic heart disease. The patient subsequently underwent coronary angiography, which demonstrated double vessel disease involving the left anterior descending and right coronary arteries, which was treated by bypass grafting.*

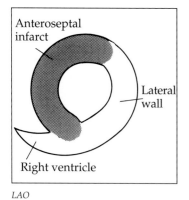

LAO

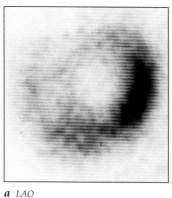

*a* LAO

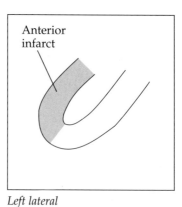

Left lateral

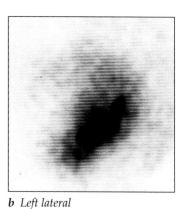

*b* Left lateral

**Fig. 6.37**

**(a, b)** $^{201}$Tl myocardial scan.

This patient was a 64-year-old man who was admitted to hospital with acute chest pain. A rest-injected $^{201}$Tl scan shows extensive loss of $^{201}$Tl uptake into the septum and anterior wall. This confirmed the diagnosis of massive acute myocardial infarction.

Absent $^{201}$Tl uptake on a rest image may be due to either recent or old infarction which cannot be differentiated.

*Pyrophosphate scan in the investigation of chest pain*

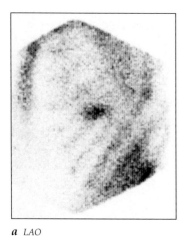

*a* LAO

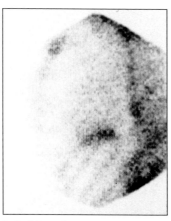

*b* Left lateral

**Fig. 6.38**

**(a, b)** Imaging with $^{99m}$Tc pyrophosphate to demonstrate recent myocardial infarction.

This patient was a 47-year-old man who was admitted to hospital with chest pain. The ECG showed left bundle branch block and the enzymes were equivocal. A $^{99m}$Tc pyrophosphate study was requested, which shows definite uptake of pyrophosphate due to a small recent posterior infarct. (See also page 458.) (Courtesy of Dr J Bingham, London, UK.)

The clinical indications for $^{99m}$Tc pyrophosphate imaging are few, but in certain clinical circumstances where the ECG is equivocal, pyrophosphate imaging may prove useful.

## CLINICAL APPLICATIONS

*Investigation of chest pain following previous myocardial infarction*

Following a myocardial infarction, many patients develop chest pain, and this may occur for a variety of reasons other than myocardial ischaemia, the most common being psychological, ie cardiac neurosis. In such circumstances, $^{201}$Tl scanning is a useful aid to diagnosis.

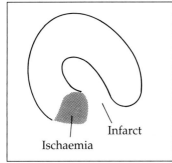

*Anterior*

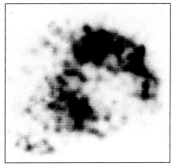

*a Anterior, stress*

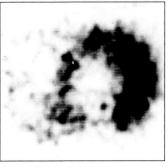

*b Anterior, rest*

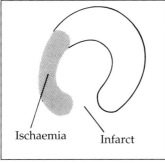

*LAO 45°*

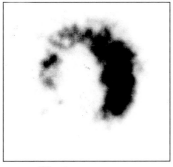

*c LAO 45°, stress*

*d LAO 45°, rest*

### Fig. 6.39

*(a–d)* $^{201}$Tl *myocardial scan.*
*This patient was known to have had a previous inferoseptal myocardial infarct and had made a good recovery. However, he subsequently developed atypical chest pain which was unrelated to exercise. The exercise* ECG *was not helpful because of the presence of bundle branch block. The* $^{201}$Tl *scan performed on stress (a, c) shows reduced uptake in the septum and inferior wall. On delayed imaging (b, d) there is reperfusion in the septum confirming ischaemia, but there is also a persistent defect seen in the inferior wall caused by an infarct at this site. This study therefore confirms that, in addition to the previous myocardial infarct, there was reversible myocardial ischaemia in the left anterior descending artery territory. This was subsequently treated by angioplasty.*

**Exercise ECG studies are usually non-diagnostic when there is a significant conduction defect present.**

*Use of dipyridamole in the investigation of chest pain*

Dipyridamole increases coronary blood flow, and can be substituted for dynamic exercise if a patient is unlikely to be able to achieve sufficient exercise.

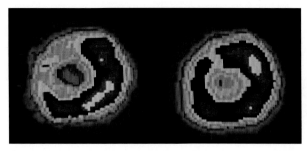

a

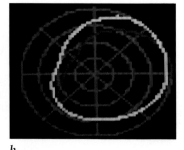

b

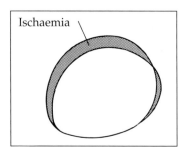

Ischaemia

Ischaemia

—— Exercise
—— Delayed

c

### Fig. 6.40

$^{201}Tl$ *myocardial study:* **(a)** *mid-cavity tomographic slice (exercise and rest);* **(b)** *relative uptake outlines;* **(c)** *washout curves.*

*This patient was a 60-year-old man with intermittent claudication who developed atypical chest pain at rest. As the claudication would restrict the amount of exercise achieved, and therefore the accuracy of the $^{201}Tl$ scan, a dipyridamole stress study was substituted. The immediate image shows decreased $^{201}Tl$ uptake in the anterior wall and septum. Scan findings revert to normal on the delayed view. Subsequent investigations confirmed a 70% stenosis of the left anterior descending artery.*

**A combination of dipyridamole and limited stress such as isometric hand grip or walking on the spot will increase the sensitivity of the study.**

## CLINICAL APPLICATIONS

### *Chest pain following coronary artery bypass grafting*

Chest pain is a frequent occurrence following coronary artery bypass grafting, and myocardial ischaemia is one, but not the only, possible explanation.

#### *Causes of chest pain after coronary artery bypass grafting*
- Angina caused by progression of native disease
- Functionally inadequate graft:
    graft stenosis
    poor distal run-off
- Deterioration of ventricular function
- Postoperative sternal pain
- Graft occlusion.

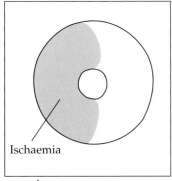

Ischaemia

*LAO 45°*

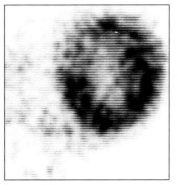

*a LAO 45°, stress*

*b LAO 45°, rest*

**Fig. 6.41**

***(a, b)*** ²⁰¹Tl *myocardial scan.*

*This patient had previously developed angina caused by a circumflex vessel lesion and a left anterior descending artery lesion. Postoperatively there was a complete remission of symptoms. However, after 18 months he returned with recurrence of the chest pain. The* ²⁰¹Tl *scan shows that the lateral wall remains well perfused, indicating patency of the circumflex graft. However, there is ischaemia in the distribution of the left anterior descending artery and the right coronary artery. Subsequent investigation showed that there was progression of native disease in the right coronary artery, and the left anterior descending artery bypass graft had become occluded.*

## Diagnosis of myocardial ischaemia

### $^{201}Tl$ myocardial imaging to diagnose myocardial ischaemia

The stress $^{201}$Tl image approximates closely to the regional myocardial blood flow at the time of injection. The contrast between normal and abnormal myocardium occurs because the coronary blood flow increases five to ten times during exercise, but the blood flow to the myocardium supplied by a stenotic vessel hardly increases at all. With time after injection, the distribution of $^{201}$Tl reaches a new equilibrium, approximating to the distribution of blood flow at rest, which may be the same in ischaemic and normal muscle. This occurs by a process of $^{201}$Tl washout from normal myocardium and, to a lesser extent, wash-in to ischaemic myocardium occurring simultaneously. Thus contrast between normal and abnormal myocardium decreases with time.

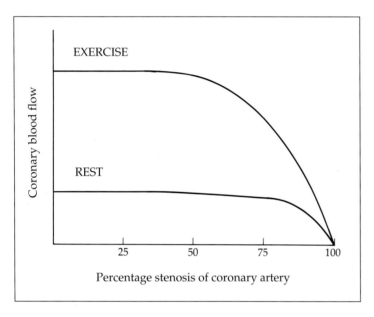

**Fig. 6.42**

*The effect of coronary stenosis on blood flow at rest and exercise.*

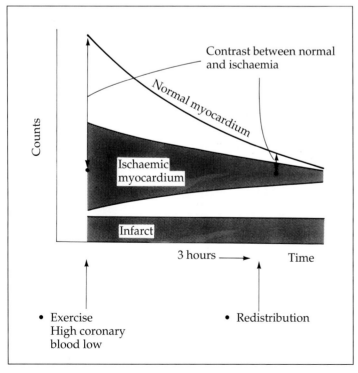

**Fig. 6.43**

*Diagrammatic representation of $^{201}$Tl uptake in myocardial ischaemia.*

438

Abnormalities of myocardial perfusion should always be attributed to the anatomical part of the heart, not to a specific vessel when the coronary anatomy is not known, because:

• There is great variability in territory of supply of individual vessels, especially in the dominance of the right coronary artery

• Variability in collateral vessel development may obscure the effect of even complete occlusion of a vessel.

The following cases illustrate examples of a variety of ischaemic and infarcted myocardial segments. The abnormality of the vessel can be inferred, but not definitely stated.

*Anteroseptal ischaemia: planar imaging*

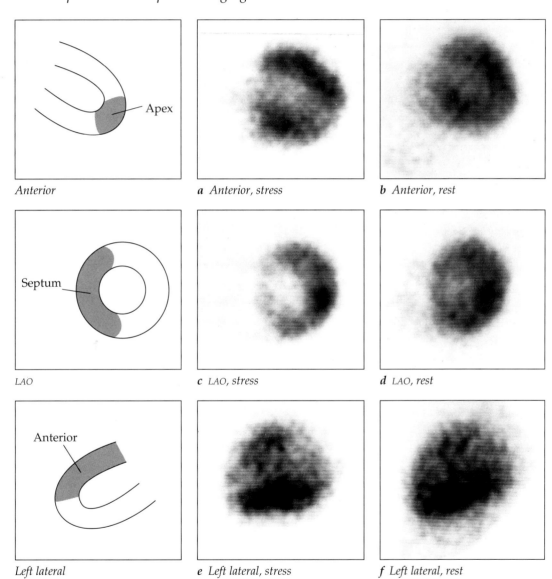

Anterior

*a Anterior, stress*

*b Anterior, rest*

LAO

*c LAO, stress*

*d LAO, rest*

Left lateral

*e Left lateral, stress*

*f Left lateral, rest*

**Fig. 6.44**

*(a–f)* $^{201}Tl$ *myocardial perfusion scan, showing anteroseptal disease.*

*There is reversible ischaemia of the septum and anterior wall in the areas shown. This scan appearance is typical of the distribution of septal branches of the left anterior descending artery and probably not of the right coronary artery, because the inferior wall on the anterior view is relatively normal.*

*Anteroseptal ischaemia: tomographic imaging*

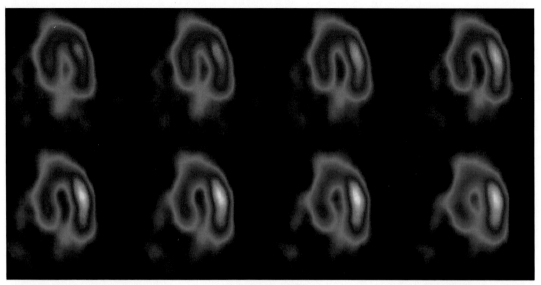

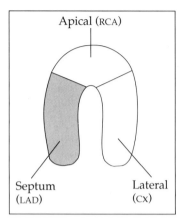

*a Horizontal long axis, stress*

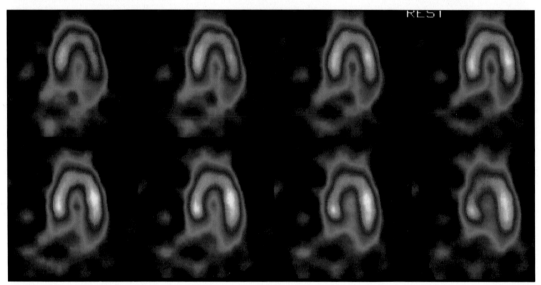

*b Horizontal long axis, rest*

**Fig. 6.45**

*(a, b) Horizontal long axis views. (c, d) Short axis views, at stress and rest.*

*There is reversible ischaemia identified in the anterior wall and septum consistent with LAD disease. There is also a non-reversible defect noted in the inferior wall on the short axis views.*

## CLINICAL APPLICATIONS

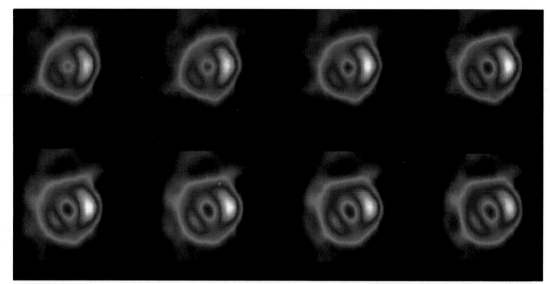

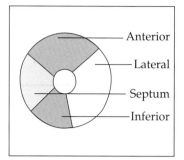

*c* Short axis, stress

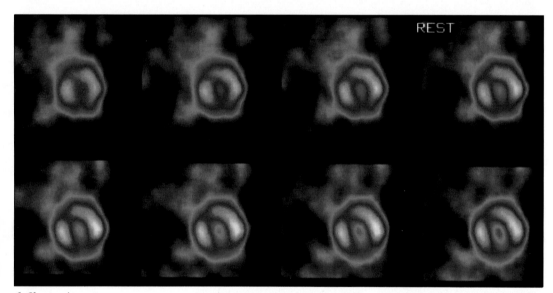

*d* Short axis, rest

### *LAD disease causing anteroseptal and lateral ischaemia*

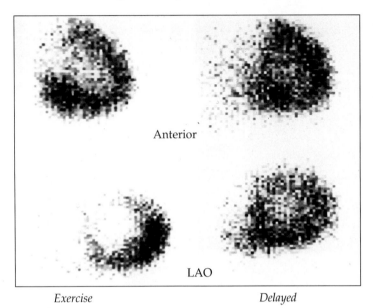

Anterior

LAO

*Exercise*                    *Delayed*

**Fig. 6.46**

*Typical appearance of a lesion of the left anterior descending artery on a $^{201}$Tl myocardial scan with planar imaging.*

*Note that the abnormality is seen on the anterolateral wall in the anterior view, and in the anterior and septal walls on the oblique view. When the exercise and delayed views are directly compared, it can be seen that the delayed view has returned to an entirely normal scan appearance.*

### *Anterolateral ischaemia*

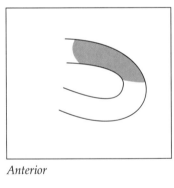

Anterior

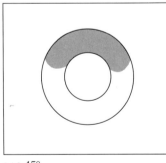

LAO 45°

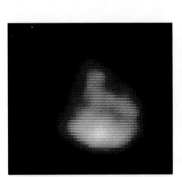

*a* Anterior, stress

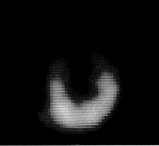

*c* LAO 45°, stress

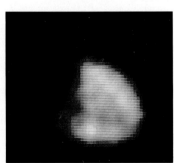

*b* Anterior, rest

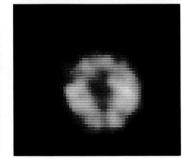

*d* LAO 45°, rest

**Fig. 6.47**

*(a–d) $^{201}$Tl myocardial scans.*

*This planar study shows the appearances of anterior reversible ischaemia. There is decreased $^{201}$Tl uptake seen on the anterior and LAO 45° views. This normalizes on the delayed redistribution images. In this case it was due to stenosis of the diagonal branch of the left anterior descending vessel after the septal branches to the septum.*

## CLINICAL APPLICATIONS

*Septal ischaemia*

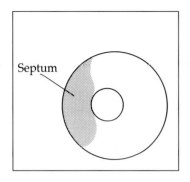

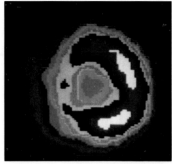

*a Stress*

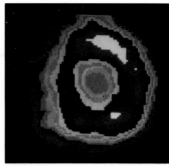

*b Rest*

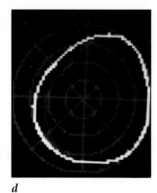

*c*

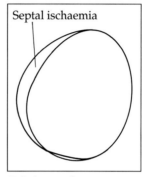

*d*                    *Relative uptake curves*

**Fig. 6.48**

²⁰¹*Tl myocardial scan: (**a, b**) mid-cavity tomographic slices showing reversible ischaemia; (**c**) washout curves; (**d**) relative uptake outlines.*

*The tomographic slice through the mid-cavity of the left ventricle shows grossly diminished* ²⁰¹*Tl uptake in the septum, in the exercise study (**a**). The delayed study (**b**) still shows the decreased uptake, but the relative difference between the septum and the rest of the myocardium is much less.*

## Septal and apical ischaemia

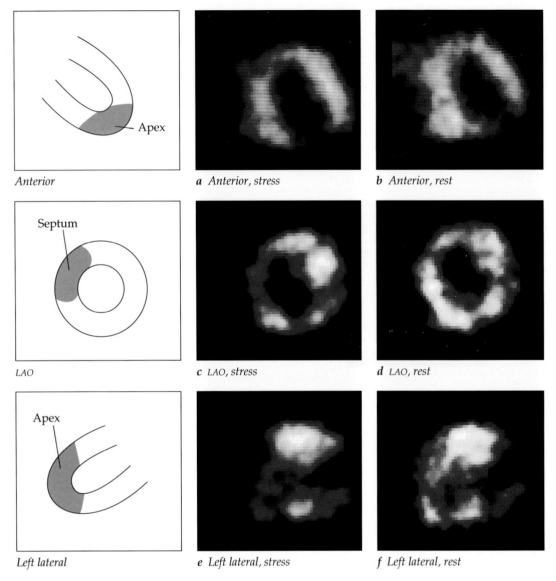

Anterior

*a* Anterior, stress

*b* Anterior, rest

LAO

*c* LAO, stress

*d* LAO, rest

Left lateral

*e* Left lateral, stress

*f* Left lateral, rest

**Fig. 6.49**

**(a–f)** Planar [201]Tl myocardial scan, showing septal and apical ischaemia.

The reversible ischaemia of the septum is best shown in the LAO view. The left lateral view shows the apical ischaemia, which is seen with lesions of the diagonal branches of the left anterior descending artery, and sometimes called the 'diagonal window'.

*Inferior ischaemia: planar study*

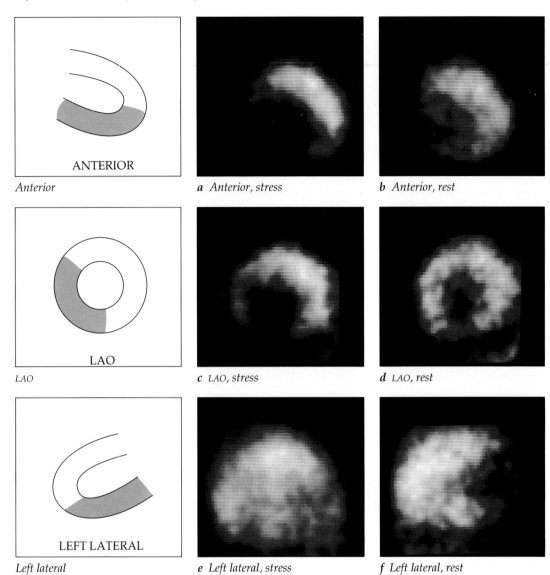

Anterior

*a Anterior, stress*

*b Anterior, rest*

LAO

*c LAO, stress*

*d LAO, rest*

Left lateral

*e Left lateral, stress*

*f Left lateral, rest*

*Fig. 6.50*

*(a–f) [201]Tl myocardial scan with planar imaging.*

*These planar views show the appearances of reversible ischaemia resulting from a right coronary artery stenosis. There is decreased [201]Tl uptake inferiorly on all views which reverses on the delayed rest study.*

*Inferior ischaemia: tomographic study*

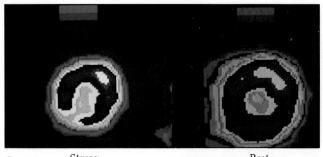

*a*          Stress                    Rest

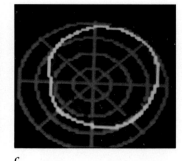

*c*

**Fig. 6.51**

[201]Tl *myocardial scan:*
*(a) tomographic slices; (b) washout curves; (c) relative uptake outlines.*

*The tomographic slices of the left ventricle show decreased* [201]Tl *uptake in the inferior septum and inferior wall, which is the territory supplied by the right coronary artery. Comparison of the exercise and delayed views shows that this area has returned to normal.*

*b*

## Inferoseptal ischaemia

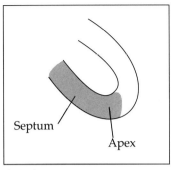

*Anterior*

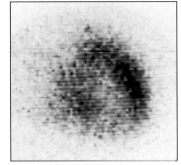

*a Anterior, stress*

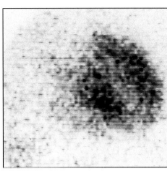

*b Anterior, rest*

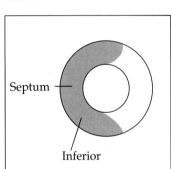

*LAO 45°*

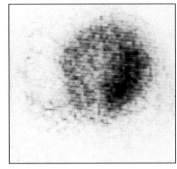

*c LAO, stress*

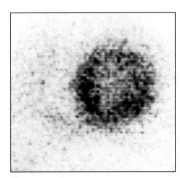

*d LAO, rest*

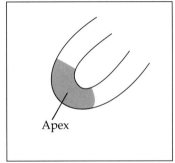

*Left lateral*

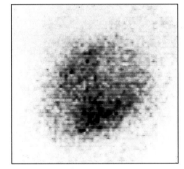

*e Left lateral, stress*

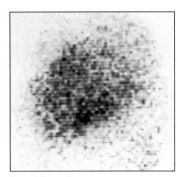

*f Left lateral, rest*

### Fig. 6.52

*(a–f)* 201Tl *myocardial scan, showing reversible ischaemia throughout the septum and extending inferiorly.*

*This scan appearance may be seen with ischaemia of the septal branches of the left anterior descending artery, if the vessel is dominant, or in double vessel disease (left anterior descending artery and right coronary artery disease).*

## CLINICAL APPLICATIONS

### Inferolateral ischaemia

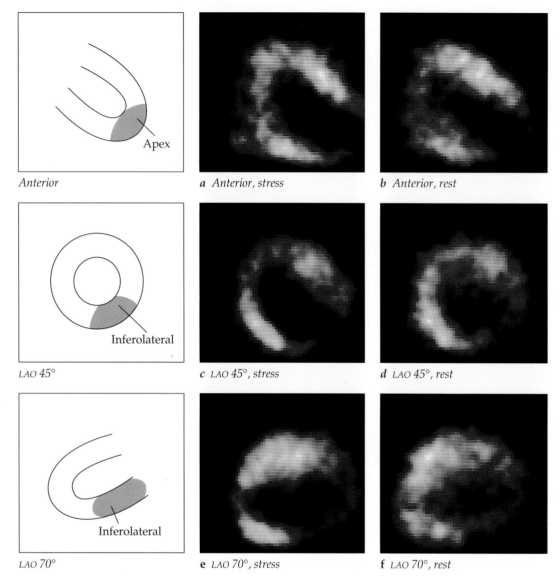

Anterior

a  Anterior, stress

b  Anterior, rest

LAO 45°

c  LAO 45°, stress

d  LAO 45°, rest

LAO 70°

e  LAO 70°, stress

f  LAO 70°, rest

*Fig. 6.53*

*(a–f) Planar $^{201}$Tl myocardial scan, showing evidence of reversible ischaemia inferolaterally, extending from the base to the apex.*

*This scan appearance is most often seen with a lesion in the territory of the circumflex vessel. Note that it does not revert completely to normal at rest, which indicates either a severe stenosis or associated infarction.*

*Double vessel disease*

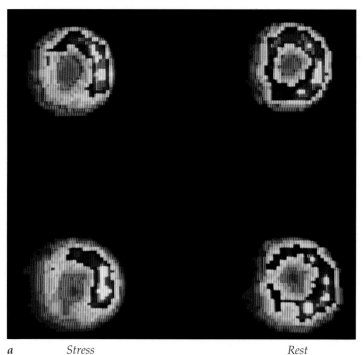

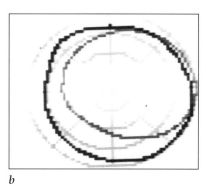

b

a  Stress       Rest

**Fig. 6.54**

$^{201}$Tl myocardial scan: (**a**) tomographic slices; (**b**) isocount contours.
 The tomographic slices through the mid-cavity of the left ventricle show decreased $^{201}$Tl uptake in the septum, and this extends round to the inferior wall. At rest there is significant reperfusion seen in the septum and inferior wall. The isocount contours confirm this extensive reversible change. In this case the scan appearance was due to a lesion of the left anterior descending artery and a lesion of the right coronary artery. However, a single lesion of the right coronary artery, if it is a very dominant vessel, can cause this appearance alone, and similarly, if the right coronary vessel is redundant, these appearances may be caused by disease of the left anterior descending artery.

## CLINICAL APPLICATIONS

*Triple vessel disease*

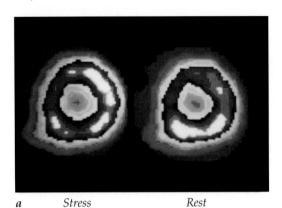 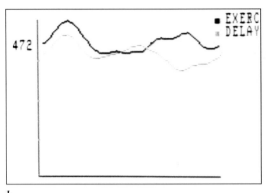

| | |
|---|---|
| *a* Stress Rest | *b* |

**Fig. 6.55**

²⁰¹Tl *myocardial scan:* (**a**) *tomographic slices;* (**b**) *washout curves.*

*The images of this patient who achieved a good workload are relatively normal, with no apparent ischaemia. However, the washout curves reveal almost no difference between exercise and rest. This indicates probable balanced disease. The patient was shown to have triple vessel disease including a 95% stenosis of the circumflex vessel.*

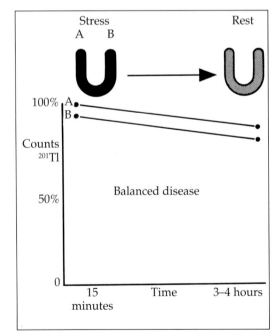

**Fig. 6.56**

*Diagrammatic representation of the scan appearance in balanced disease.*

• If exercise is inadequate, the scan appearance shown in Fig. 6.56 may be seen. If the disease is balanced, ie is approximately equal in all three vessel territories, and only the images are studied, abnormalities may be missed.
• If washout curves are used, errors in this group of patients will be diminished.

## CLINICAL APPLICATIONS

*Appearance of ischaemia using a $^{99m}$Tc-labelled isonitrile derivative as the radiopharmaceutical*

Because of the disadvantages of $^{201}$Tl, $^{99m}$Tc-labelled radiopharmaceuticals are being introduced which are showing promise as a replacement for $^{201}$Tl. They have the additional advantage that high-quality SPECT images can be obtained. The following case illustrates a right coronary artery lesion in three oblique SPECT views.

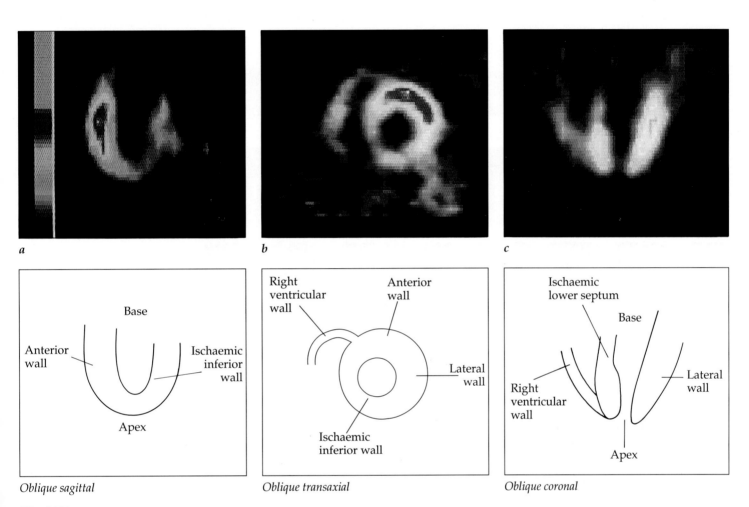

*a*                     *b*                     *c*

Base

Anterior wall — Ischaemic inferior wall

Apex

*Oblique sagittal*

Right ventricular wall         Anterior wall

Lateral wall

Ischaemic inferior wall

*Oblique transaxial*

Ischaemic lower septum

Base

Right ventricular wall

Lateral wall

Apex

*Oblique coronal*

**Fig. 6.57**

**(a–c)** *Oblique SPECT views, showing a right coronary artery lesion. These views were obtained by injecting 400 MBq of $^{99m}$Tc isonitrile at peak exercise and imaging after 1 hour.*

*Anteroseptal and inferoapical ischaemia:* $^{99m}$Tc *isonitrile study*

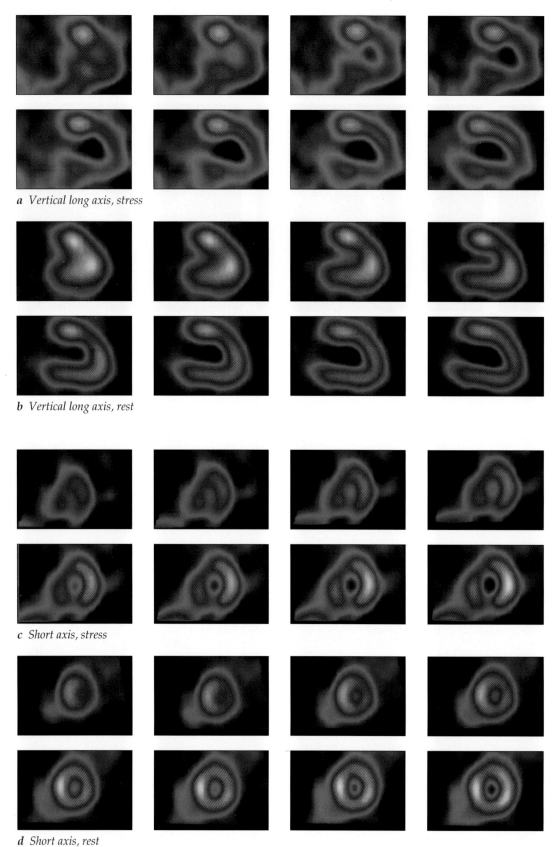

*a* Vertical long axis, stress

*b* Vertical long axis, rest

*c* Short axis, stress

*d* Short axis, rest

### Fig. 6.58

*A 45-year-old man with atypical chest pain.*

*The stress/rest isonitrile study (**a–f**) identifies reversible changes in the anteroseptal (LAD) and inferoapical (RCA) walls confirming two-vessel ischaemic heart disease.*

# CLINICAL APPLICATIONS

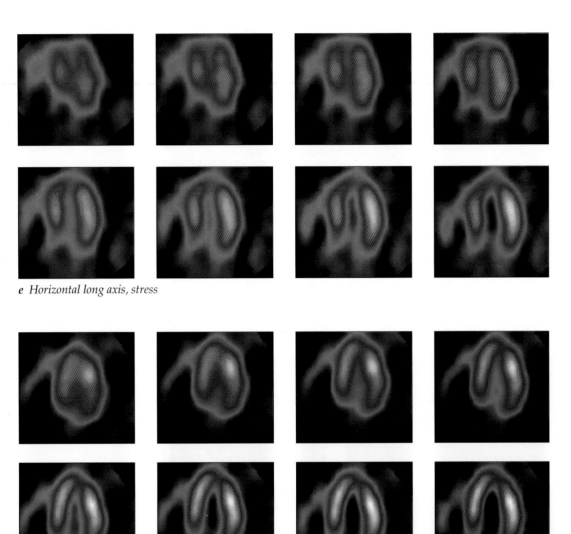

*e  Horizontal long axis, stress*

*f  Horizontal long axis, rest*

## Investigation of myocardial ischaemia

There are frequently times when the diagnosis of myocardial ischaemia is equivocal. The use of functional radionuclide methods can be the only direct way to establish the presence or significance of ischaemic lesions.

Radionuclide investigations can determine the following:

• Functional significance of an angiographically discovered coronary lesion

• Diagnostic significance of a positive exercise ECG test result
• Selection of patients with chest pain for further investigation
• Presence of ischaemia after myocardial infarction — to indicate whether surgical or angioplastic treatment might be indicated
• Presence of residual ischaemia after coronary artery bypass grafting or angioplasty.

### Functional significance of an angiographic lesion: $^{201}$Tl

The coronary angiogram may be difficult to interpret, and the exact size of a stenosis and its functional significance may not always be apparent. The $^{201}$Tl scan is useful because it provides information about the blood flow to the myocardium subtended by the involved coronary vessel.

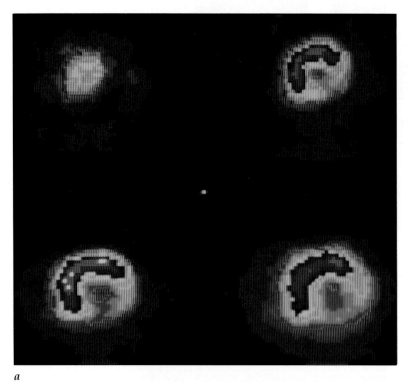

a

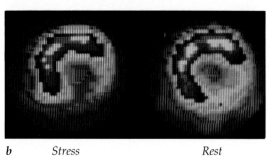

b    Stress                Rest

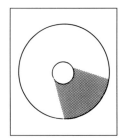

c

### Fig. 6.59

$^{201}$Tl myocardial scan: **(a)** four exercise tomographic slices; **(b)** exercise and rest compared; **(c)** relative uptake outlines. The key to the tomographic images in **(a)** is as follows:

| Apex | Mid-cavity |
|------|------------|
| Mid-cavity | Basal |

This patient underwent coronary angiography for the investigation of chest pain. A 50% lesion in the left circumflex vessel was identified, and the patient was referred for a $^{201}$Tl scan to determine whether this was functionally significant. The scan shows decreased $^{201}$Tl uptake in the inferolateral wall, which becomes somewhat more normal on the delayed view. This study therefore confirms that the angiographic lesion was haemodynamically significant and therefore likely to be the cause of the patient's symptoms.

## CLINICAL APPLICATIONS

### $^{201}$Tl study after myocardial infarction

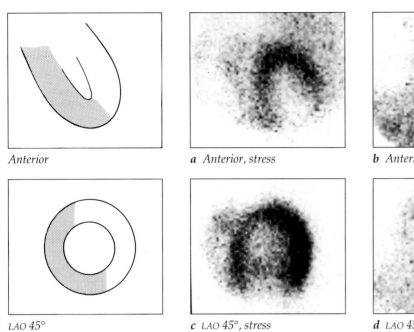

Anterior

**a** Anterior, stress

**b** Anterior, rest

LAO 45°

**c** LAO 45°, stress

**d** LAO 45°, rest

Left lateral

**e** Left lateral, stress

**f** Left lateral, rest

**Fig. 6.60**

**(a–f)** *Planar* $^{201}$*Tl myocardial study after myocardial infarction.*

*This patient was a 45-year-old man who had persistent pain after a myocardial infarction. Coronary angiography showed an occluded posterior descending vessel and stenoses of the right coronary and left anterior descending arteries, the significance of which were doubtful. A* $^{201}$*Tl scan was performed to assess these lesions. The study shows that there is reversible ischaemia of both vessels, and the patient was referred for bypass grafting.*

## Diagnostic significance of a positive exercise test result

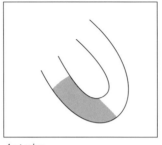

Anterior

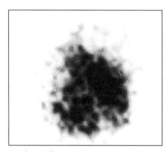

*a* Anterior, stress

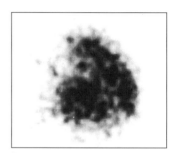

*b* Anterior, rest

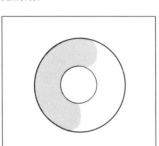

LAO 45°

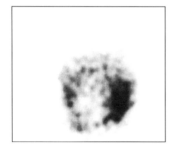

*c* LAO 45°, stress

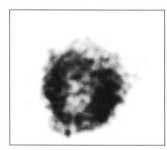

*d* LAO 45°, rest

**Fig. 6.61**

*(a–d)* Planar 201Tl myocardial scan.

This patient was an airline pilot attending a routine medical which included an exercise ECG test. This showed borderline results, with 1 mm of ST depression at maximal exercise. He was subsequently referred for a 201Tl scan to assess the significance of these findings. The planar 201Tl stress images show decreased tracer uptake inferiorly and in the septum, with redistribution of tracer, and there is a reversal to a normal pattern on the rest images. This study clearly shows reversible myocardial ischaemia in the left anterior descending artery and possibly also in the right coronary artery territory. The patient was subsequently referred for angiography and angioplasty.

## Preoperative assessment

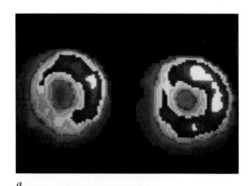

*a*

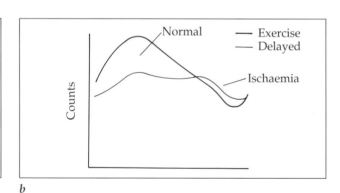

Stress

Ischaemia

*b*

— Exercise
— Delayed

Normal

Ischaemia

Counts

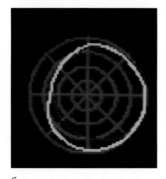

*c*

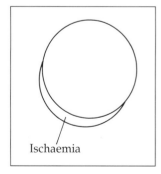

Ischaemia

**Fig. 6.62**

201Tl myocardial scan: *(a)* mid-cavity tomographic slices; *(b)* washout curves; *(c)* relative uptake outlines.

This patient has a previous history of atypical chest pain, but this had diminished when he became less mobile as the result of a back injury. He was referred for a lumbar vertebral fusion, but before this was performed a 201Tl scan was requested. As exercise could not be performed, a dipyridamole/201Tl study was undertaken which demonstrates inferoseptal ischaemia. After the back surgery, angina recurred, and he was successfully treated by angioplasty.

## CLINICAL APPLICATIONS

*Functional significance of an angiographic lesion: gated cardiac study*

An angiographic lesion is functionally significant if it results in relative ischaemia during exercise, and if it causes changes in ventricular contractility. The following case illustrates changes in contractility associated with a coronary stenosis.

*Rest*

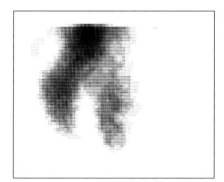

*a Diastolic*

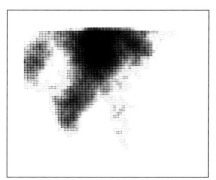

*b Systolic*

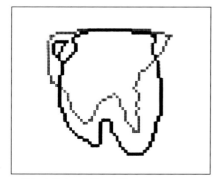

*c Diastolic/systolic outline*

*Stress*

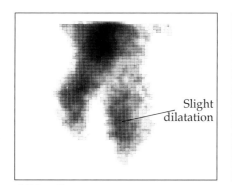

Slight dilatation

*d Diastolic*

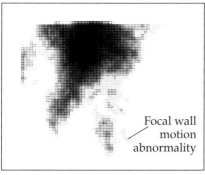

Focal wall motion abnormality

*e Systolic*

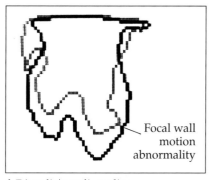

Focal wall motion abnormality

*f Diastolic/systolic outline*

**Fig. 6.63**

*Gated cardiac study: **(a, d)** diastolic images; **(b, e)** systolic images; **(c, f)** diastolic/systolic outlines.*

*This patient underwent a coronary arteriogram following a positive result from an exercise test performed as a routine investigation. A small lesion in the circumflex territory was noted but not thought to be clinically significant. A gated study shows normal ventricular function at rest, with a normal ejection fraction. However, with cold pressor stimulation, there is slight ventricular dilatation. In addition, the appearance of a dramatically positive wall motion abnormality in the lateral wall is seen, confirming the significance of the lesion.*

## CLINICAL APPLICATIONS

### *Diagnosis of acute myocardial infarction*

*Infarct imaging with $^{99m}$Tc pyrophosphate*

Pyrophosphate accumulates in recent myocardial infarction and has a role as an adjunct to conventional diagnostic methods (ECG and cardiac enzymes) in certain circumstances (see page 461). The scan is not positive immediately after an infarct, but becomes progressively so with time.

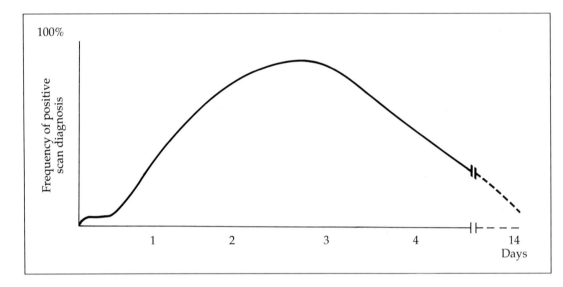

*Fig. 6.64*

$^{99m}$Tc pyrophosphate infarct imaging.

*Cardiac causes of $^{99m}$Tc pyrophosphate uptake*
- Myocardial infarction
- Left ventricular aneurysm
- Unstable angina
- Myocardial contusion
- Cardiomyopathy
- Valvular calcification

*Non-cardiac causes of $^{99m}$Tc pyrophosphate uptake*
- Rib fracture
- Muscle trauma, eg cardioversion
- Skin lesions
- Calcified costal cartilage
- High, persistent blood pool
- Breast disease, eg tumour

**Sensitivity of pyrophosphate imaging is maximum between 1 and 3 days.**

## CLINICAL APPLICATIONS

*Sites of pyrophosphate uptake and infarct localization*

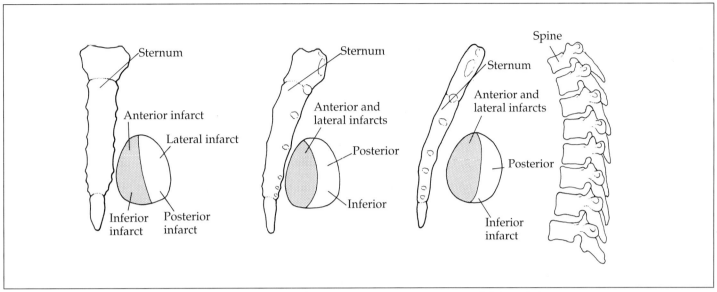

Anterior view                *LAO view*                *Left lateral view*

*Fig. 6.65*

*Localization of different infarcts by site of pyrophosphate uptake.*

*Classification of abnormal scans*
- Uptake pattern: focal or diffuse
- Intensity:   0   negative
                1+  equivocal uptake
                2+  definite uptake less than sternum
                3+  definite uptake equal to sternum
                4+  definite uptake greater than sternum
- Site: anterior, inferior, lateral, true posterior.

*Pyrophosphate imaging in myocardial infarction*

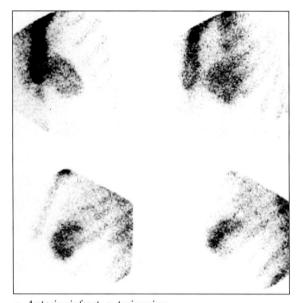

*a  Anterior infarct, anterior view*

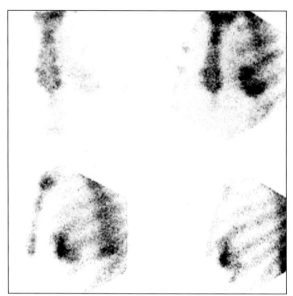

*b  Septal infarct, LAO 45° view*

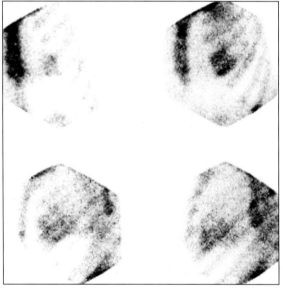

*c  Posterior infarct, LAO 70° view*

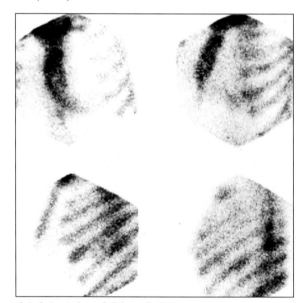

*d  Inferior infarct, left lateral view*

**Fig. 6.66**

*(a–d) Appearance of infarcts on different views using* $^{99m}$*Tc pyrophosphate. (Courtesy of Dr J Bingham, London, UK.)*

## 'Donut' appearance

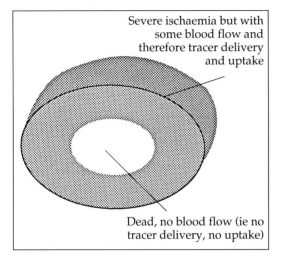

Severe ischaemia but with some blood flow and therefore tracer delivery and uptake

Dead, no blood flow (ie no tracer delivery, no uptake)

**Fig. 6.67**

*Cause of 'donut' appearance.*

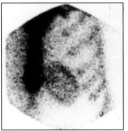 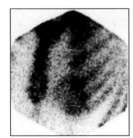

*a* Anterior     *b* LAO 45°

**Fig. 6.68**

*(a, b)* 'Donut' appearance on $^{99m}$Tc pyrophosphate scan. (Courtesy of Dr J Bingham, London, UK.)

 **A 'donut' appearance always indicates a large transmural infarct.**

## Possible uses of $^{99m}$Tc pyrophosphate scans

Myocardial scanning with $^{99m}$Tc pyrophosphate may be used in the following circumstances:

- Suspected recent infarction 1–7 days old
- Postoperative myocardial infarction
- Myocardial damage from trauma
- Localization of infarction (especially with bundle branch block)
- Unstable angina.

## CLINICAL APPLICATIONS

### *⁹⁹ᵐTc pyrophosphate study with tomography*

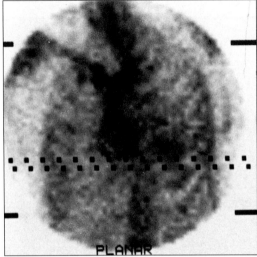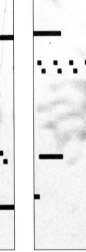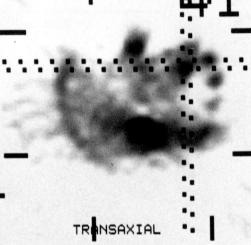

*a Planar*

*b Transaxial* SPECT

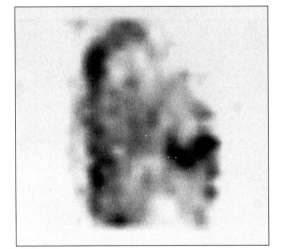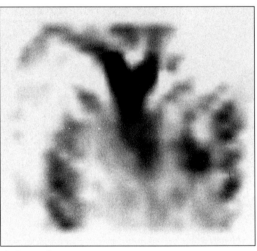

*c Sagittal* SPECT

*d Coronal* SPECT

**Fig. 6.69**

**(a–d)** *Pyrophosphate* SPECT *study in a 39-year-old man who presented with severe continuous chest pain.*

*The patient had no past history of angina and no possible risk factors for ischaemic heart disease. The* ECG *changes were equivocal but the pyrophsophate* SPECT *study confirms uptake in the inferoapical region of the left ventricle.* ECG *changes subsequently became frankly positive for a myocardial infarct.*

## CLINICAL APPLICATIONS

### Diagnosis of non-acute myocardial infarction

[201]Tl and [99m]Tc isonitrile may be used to diagnose chronic myocardial infarction. On delayed or test imaging there is no tracer seen in the region of absent uptake identified on the stress study. A reinjection technique may be required with [201]Tl studies to differentiate an infarction from a tight coronary artery stenosis.

## Anteroseptal myocardial infarction

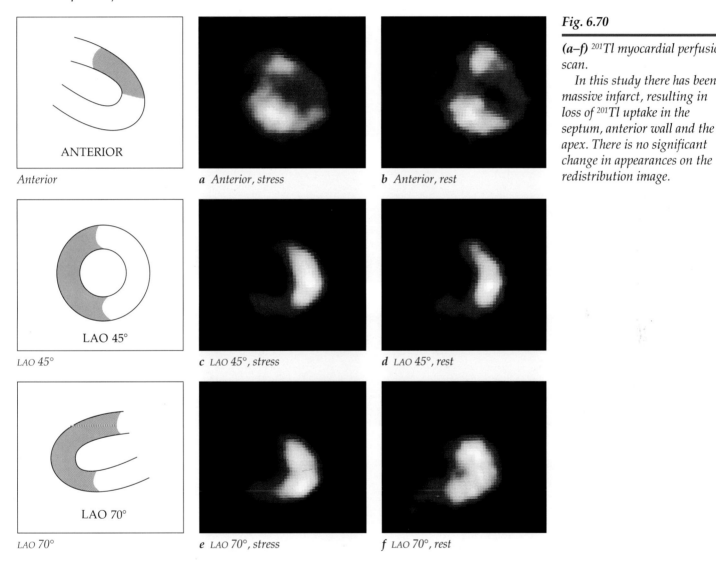

Anterior

ANTERIOR

*a Anterior, stress*

*b Anterior, rest*

*LAO 45°*

LAO 45°

*c LAO 45°, stress*

*d LAO 45°, rest*

*LAO 70°*

LAO 70°

*e LAO 70°, stress*

*f LAO 70°, rest*

### Fig. 6.70

*(a–f)* [201]Tl *myocardial perfusion scan.*

*In this study there has been a massive infarct, resulting in loss of* [201]Tl *uptake in the septum, anterior wall and the apex. There is no significant change in appearances on the redistribution image.*

## $^{201}$Tl tomography in septal and apical infarction

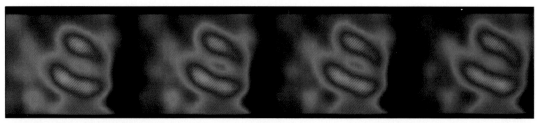

*a  Vertical long axis, stress*

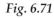
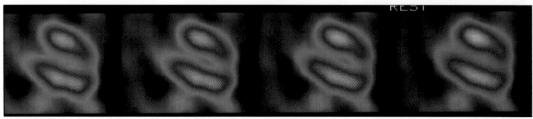

*b  Vertical long axis, rest*

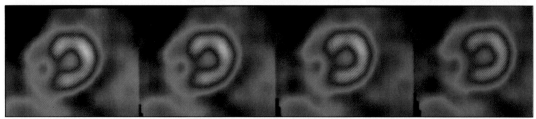

*c  Short axis, stress*

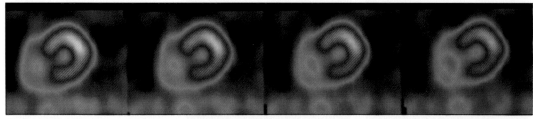

*d  Short axis, rest*

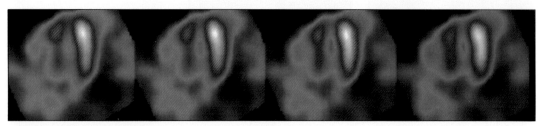

*e  Horizontal long axis, stress*

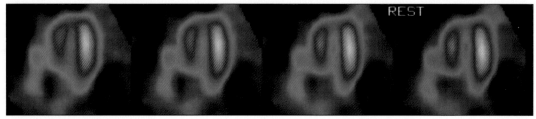

*f  Horizontal long axis, rest*

**Fig. 6.71**

**(a–f)** $^{201}$Tl myocardial scan performed with dipyridamole stress.

The tomographic slices show fixed abnormalities in the septum and apex. A coronary arteriogram performed 1 year before showed 100% stenosis of the LAD and 55% stenosis of the RCA. The study confirms the infarct in the septum and diagnoses that an infarct has also occurred in the RCA territory.

## CLINICAL APPLICATIONS

*Lateral infarction*

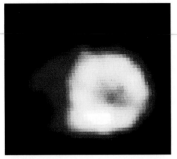

*a  Anterior, stress*

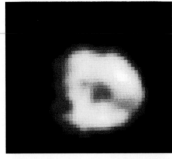

*b  Anterior, rest*

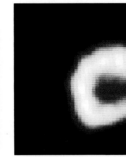

*c  LAO, stress*

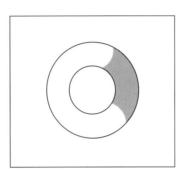

*d  LAO, rest*

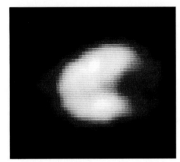

*e  Left lateral, stress*

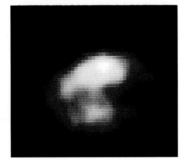

*f  Left lateral, rest*

**Fig. 6.72**

**(a–f)** ²⁰¹Tl *myocardial scan, showing lateral infarction.*
*The* LAO *view* **(c)** *shows a clear-cut absence of* ²⁰¹Tl *in the lateral wall. Note that this abnormality is not seen clearly on the other two views and that the redistribution image* **(d)** *shows the defect unchanged, which is typical of infarction.*

*Inferior infarction*

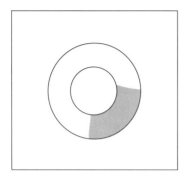

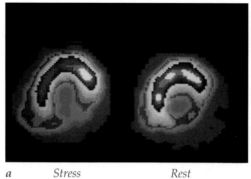

*a*      Stress          Rest

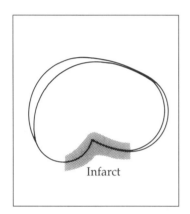

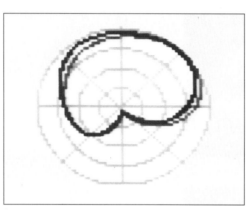

*b*

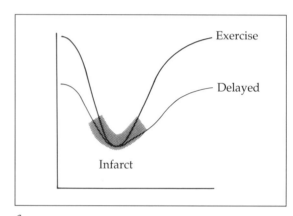

*c*

*Fig. 6.73*

$^{201}$Tl myocardial scan: **(a)** tomographic slices; **(b)** relative uptake outlines; **(c)** washout curves.

   The tomographic slices show the massive defect inferiorly caused by an inferior infarct in the territory of the right coronary artery or, possibly, a relatively dominant left circumflex artery.

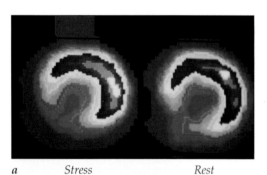

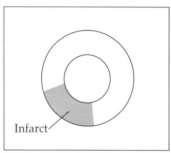

*a*      Stress        Rest        Exercise

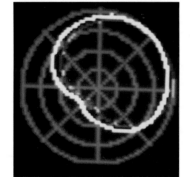

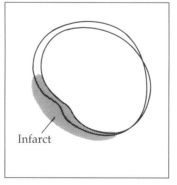

*b*

*Fig. 6.74*

$^{201}$Tl myocardial scan, showing inferior infarction due to occlusion of the right coronary artery: **(a)** tomographic slices; **(b)** relative uptake outlines.

   Infarcts in the distribution of the right coronary artery will depend on the dominance of the right coronary vessel and the branch involved. This is a tomographic section through the left ventricular cavity following a major infarct of the right coronary territory.

## Posterior infarction

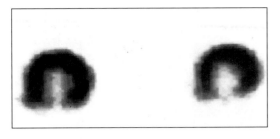

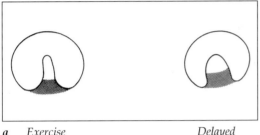

a  Exercise                    Delayed

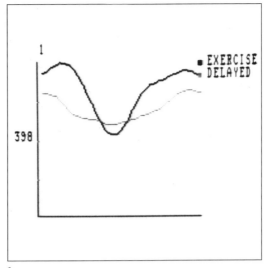

b

Fig. 6.75

$^{201}$Tl myocardial scan:
(a) tomographic images;
(b) washout curves.
 The small fixed inferior defect is typical of infarction caused by occlusion of the posterior descending branch of the right coronary artery.

## Ischaemia and infarction: planar imaging

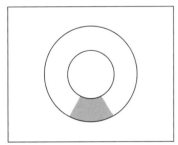

Anterior

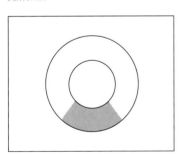

LAO 45°

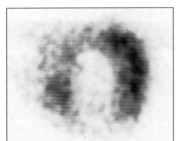

a  Anterior, stress

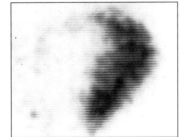

c  LAO 45°, stress

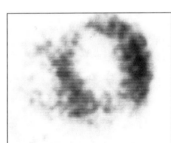

b  Anterior, rest

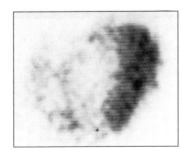

d  LAO 45°, rest

Fig. 6.76

(a–d) $^{201}$Tl myocardial scan, showing ischaemia and infarction.
 There is massive loss of $^{201}$Tl uptake in the septum and inferior wall. There is some reversible ischaemia seen inferiorly on the anterior view. These findings were due to a septal infarct with inferior ischaemia caused by a right coronary artery stenosis.

## CLINICAL APPLICATIONS

*Inferoposterior infarction*

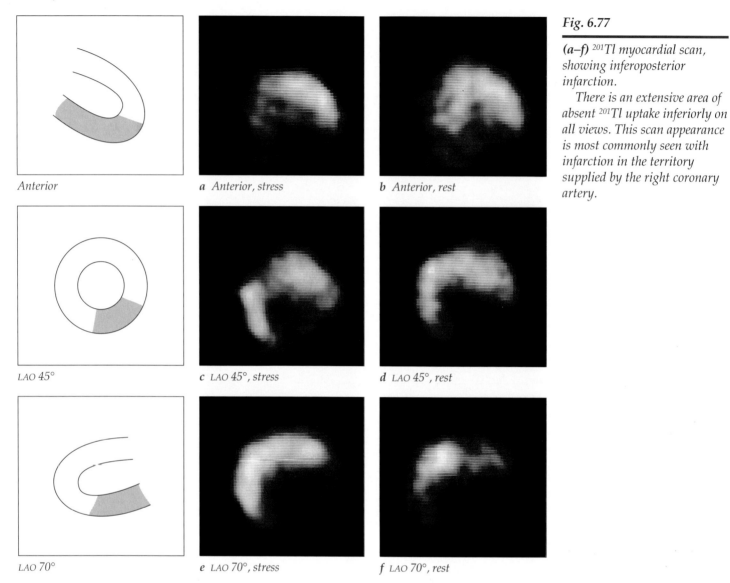

| Anterior | *a* Anterior, stress | *b* Anterior, rest |
| LAO 45° | *c* LAO 45°, stress | *d* LAO 45°, rest |
| LAO 70° | *e* LAO 70°, stress | *f* LAO 70°, rest |

**Fig. 6.77**

**(*a–f*)** $^{201}$*Tl myocardial scan, showing inferoposterior infarction.*

*There is an extensive area of absent* $^{201}$*Tl uptake inferiorly on all views. This scan appearance is most commonly seen with infarction in the territory supplied by the right coronary artery.*

## Posterolateral infarction

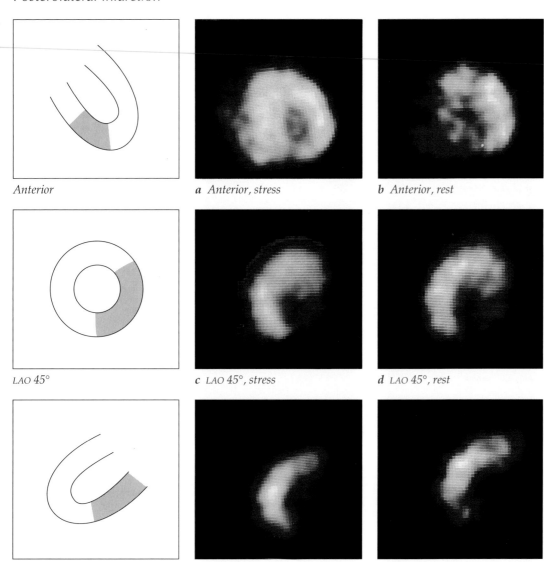

Anterior

a Anterior, stress

b Anterior, rest

LAO 45°

c LAO 45°, stress

d LAO 45°, rest

Left lateral

e Left lateral, stress

f Left lateral, rest

**Fig. 6.78**

*(a–f)* $^{201}$Tl *myocardial scan with absent uptake of* $^{201}$Tl *posterolaterally which does not improve on the rest views.*

*This scan appearance is typical of posterolateral infarction, and may be in the territory of the circumflex or posterior descending coronary artery. Note how this appearance may not be visible on the anterior view.*

## Multiple infarction

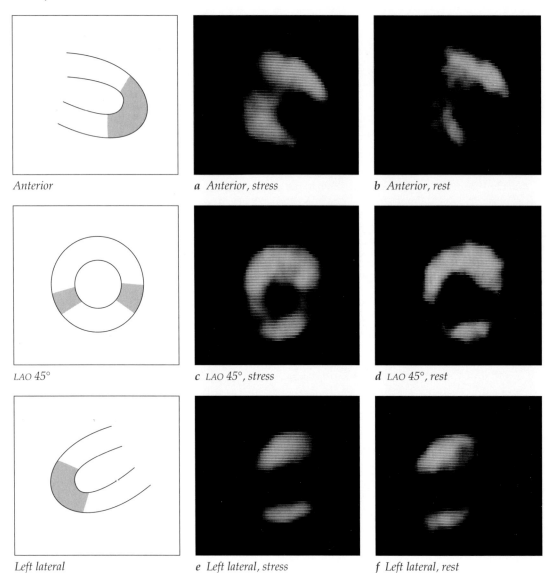

Anterior

*a* Anterior, stress

*b* Anterior, rest

LAO 45°

*c* LAO 45°, stress

*d* LAO 45°, rest

Left lateral

*e* Left lateral, stress

*f* Left lateral, rest

### Fig. 6.79

*(a–f)* [201]Tl myocardial scan, showing multiple infarction.
    There are two infarcts: an inferoseptal infarct (distribution of the right coronary artery) and a lateral infarct (circumflex territory).

*Extensive infarction with ischaemia: tomographic imaging with $^{201}Tl$*

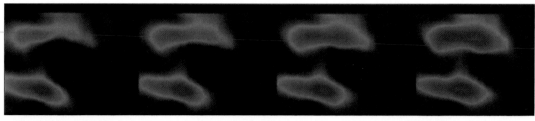

*a Vertical long axis, stress*

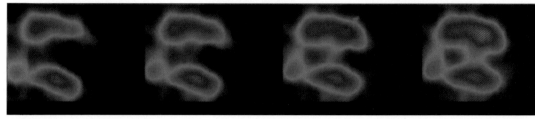

*b Vertical long axis, rest*

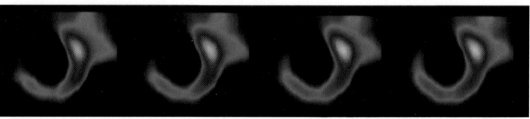

*c Short axis, stress*

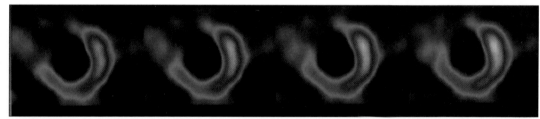

*d Short axis, rest*

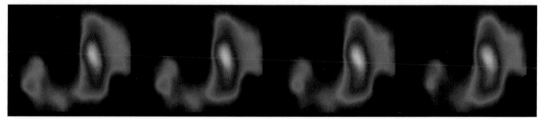

*e Horizontal long axis, stress*

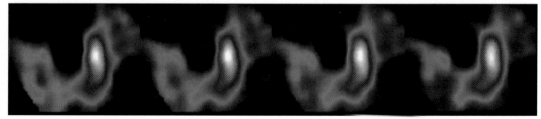

*f Horizontal long axis, rest*

**Fig. 6.80**

*A 63-year-old man with a 7-week history of severe but atypical chest pain. The ECG was difficult to interpret, since the patient had a pacemaker in situ.*

*The $^{201}Tl$ tomographic study (a–f) shows fixed perfusion defects in the anterior and inferior walls, septum and apex, diagnosing multiple infarcts. Reversibility is seen inferolaterally, consistent with ischaemia in the circumflex territory.*

## Presence of ischaemia after myocardial infarction

A major factor in deciding on further investigation with a view to intervention following myocardial infarction is the presence of more extensive ischaemia. This can best be evaluated using an exercise ²⁰¹Tl scan.

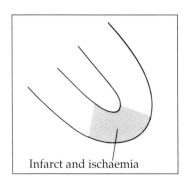

Infarct and ischaemia

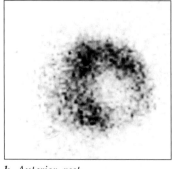
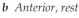

*a  Anterior, stress*

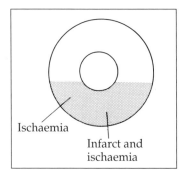

Ischaemia

Infarct and
ischaemia

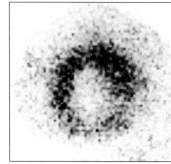

*c  LAO 45°, stress*

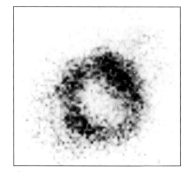

*b  Anterior, rest*

*d  LAO 45°, rest*

### Fig. 6.81

*(a–d)* ²⁰¹Tl *myocardial scan.*
*This exercise* ²⁰¹Tl *scan shows a focus of decreased uptake inferiorly. However, delayed views show some reversible changes, although the study remains abnormal. This patient has a full-thickness inferior myocardial infarct, and the clinical question was whether there was significant residual reversible ischaemia induced by exercise. This study clearly shows that this is so with changes present in the territory of the right coronary artery. Further invasive interventional studies are indicated, with a view to surgical correction.*

# CLINICAL APPLICATIONS

*Ischaemia and infarction: tomographic imaging with $^{201}$Tl*

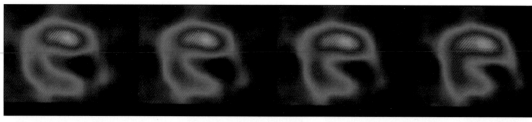

*a Vertical long axis, stress*

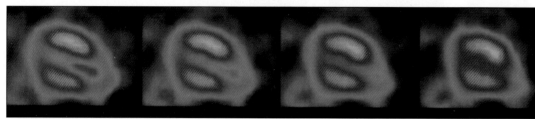

*b Vertical long axis, rest*

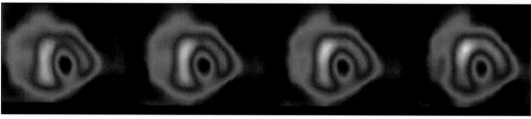

*c Short axis, stress*

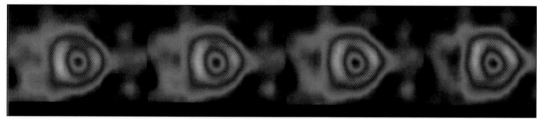

*d Short axis, rest*

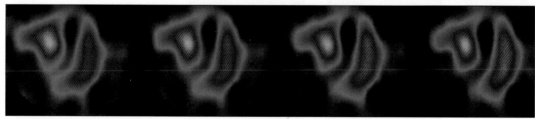

*e Horizontal long axis, stress*

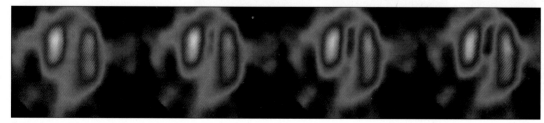

*f Horizontal long axis, rest*

**Fig. 6.82**

*A 74-year-old woman with a known apical infarct but persistent chest pain.*

*The $^{201}$Tl study (a–f) confirms an apical infarct but identifies good reversibility in the inferior wall. The patient proceeded to catheterization and angioplasty, with a good resolution of chest pain.*

## Ischaemia and infarction: tomographic imaging with $^{99m}$Tc isonitrile

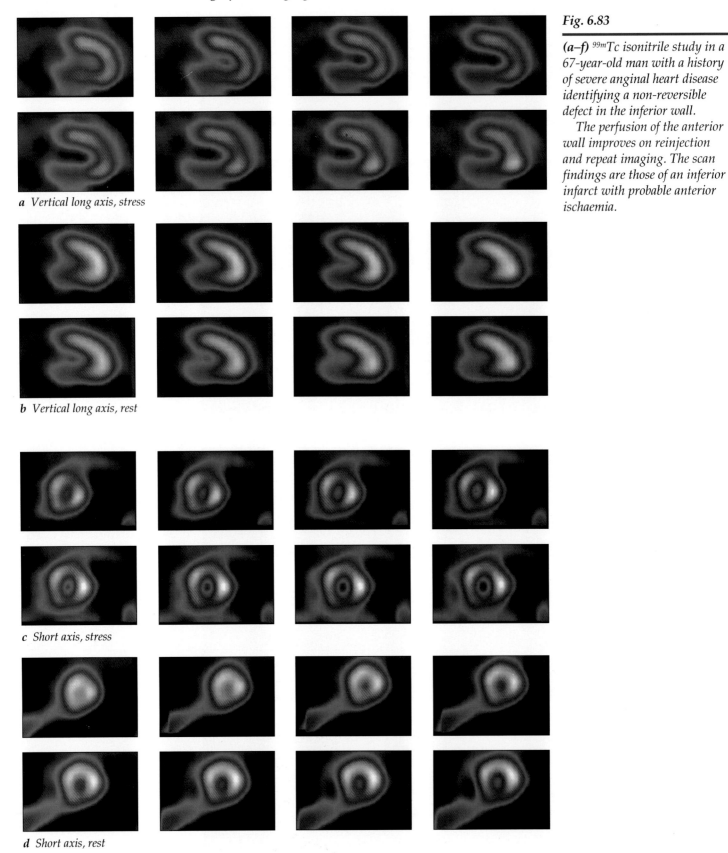

*a* Vertical long axis, stress

*b* Vertical long axis, rest

*c* Short axis, stress

*d* Short axis, rest

**Fig. 6.83**

**(a–f)** $^{99m}$Tc isonitrile study in a 67-year-old man with a history of severe anginal heart disease identifying a non-reversible defect in the inferior wall.

The perfusion of the anterior wall improves on reinjection and repeat imaging. The scan findings are those of an inferior infarct with probable anterior ischaemia.

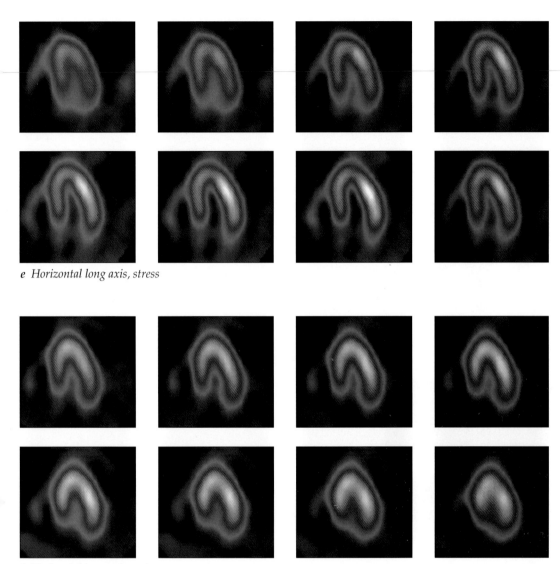

*e Horizontal long axis, stress*

*f Horizontal long axis, rest*

## Diagnosis and assessment of ventricular aneurysm

A ventricular aneurysm is an area of myocardium which moves paradoxically during ventricular systole. It is almost always caused by previous myocardial infarction. Clinically it presents with progressive impairment of ventricular function, occasionally with chest pain, and arrhythmias may be a feature. The ventricular function studies are needed to diagnose the presence of a localized aneurysm and to assess its extent, thereby determining its potential surgical operability.

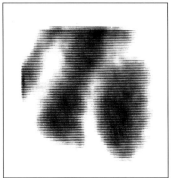

*a* LAO, diastolic

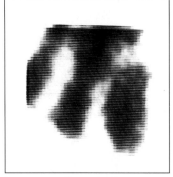

*b* LAO, systolic

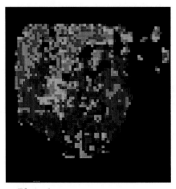

*c* Phase image

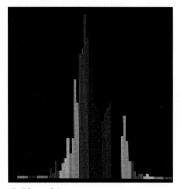

*d* Phase histogram

**Fig. 6.84**

*Gated cardiac study: **(a)** LAO diastolic image; **(b)** LAO systolic image; **(c)** phase image; **(d)** phase histogram.*

*This study shows generalized left ventricular dilatation, poor contraction (ejection fraction of 18%) and disorganized contraction seen on the phase image and confirmed with the histogram. This patient had suffered multiple previous myocardial infarcts, with progressive left ventricular dysfunction, and was referred for the evaluation of any possible aneurysm which could be treated surgically. The study clearly shows that there is generalized poor ventricular function and excludes a focal aneurysm.*

## CLINICAL APPLICATIONS

The earliest appearance of an aneurysm is a focal area of ventricular akinesis, which may contain an area within it which moves paradoxically with ventricular systole.

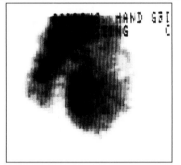

*a* LAO, diastolic

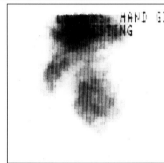

*b* LAO, systolic

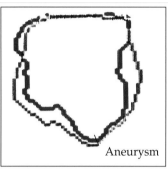

*c* Diastolic/systolic contours

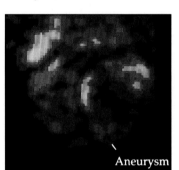

*d* Amplitude image

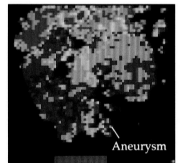

*e* Phase image

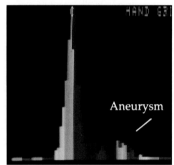

*f* Phase histogram

**Fig. 6.85**

*Gated cardiac study: (a) LAO diastolic image; (b) LAO systolic image; (c) diastolic/systolic contours, (d) amplitude image; (e) phase image; (f) phase histogram.*

This gated study shows a dilated left ventricle (ejection fraction of 35%) with inferoapical akinesis containing a small area which contracts paradoxically. This patient was referred for the assessment of a possible aneurysm. However, the very small area of paradoxical movement is not of functional significance, and surgery is unlikely to improve the ejection fraction significantly.

## Assessment after infarction

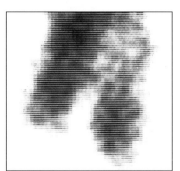

*a* LAO, diastolic

*b* LAO, systolic

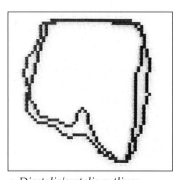

*c* Diastolic/systolic outlines

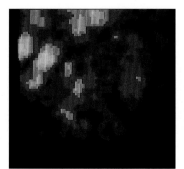

*d* Amplitude image

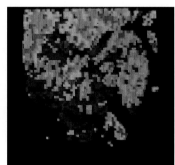

*e* Phase image

**Fig. 6.86**

*Gated cardiac study: (a) LAO diastolic image; (b) LAO systolic image; (c) diastolic/systolic outlines; (d) amplitude image; (e) phase image.*

This study was performed following a myocardial infarct to assess the extent of myocardial akinesis. A ventricular aneurysm is demonstrated. The amplitude and phase images demonstrate the area of wall that is moving paradoxically in time with the atria. Note that the area round the aneurysm is akinetic and therefore has no intensity on either the amplitude or the phase image.

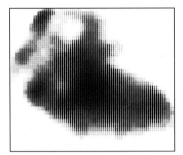

*a* Anterior, diastolic

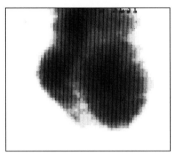

*b* LAO, diastolic

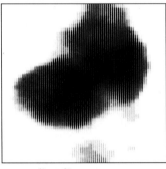

*c* LPO, diastolic

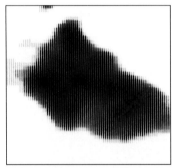

*d* RAO, diastolic

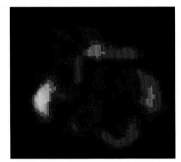

*e* Amplitude

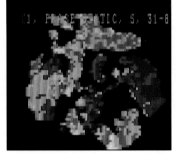

*f* Phase image

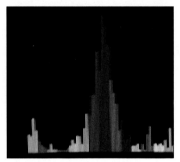

*g* Phase histogram

### Fig. 6.87

*Gated cardiac study: (a) anterior, (b) LAO, (c) LPO and (d) RAO diastolic images; (e) amplitude image; (f) phase image; (g) phase histogram.*

*This patient was a 56-year-old man who was being assessed after a myocardial infarct because of progressive dyspnoea and cardiomegaly. The study shows a large apicoinferior aneurysm which is well demonstrated by the combination of the amplitude and phase images as an area moving well but paradoxically, with a bimodal distribution on the phase histogram.*

**Four views are essential for a complete evaluation of an extensive wall motion abnormality, and occasionally small aneurysms can be missed entirely if only one view is used.**

## CLINICAL APPLICATIONS

## Appearance of an aneurysm

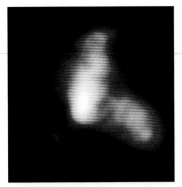

*a Anterior, diastolic*

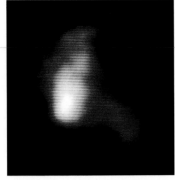

*b Anterior, systolic*

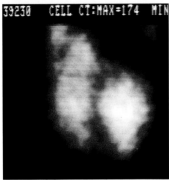

*c LAO, diastolic*

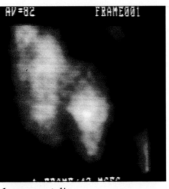

*d LAO, systolic*

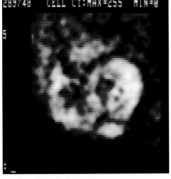

*e Amplitude image*

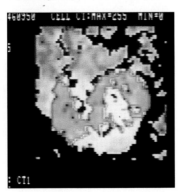

*f Phase image*

**Fig. 6.88**

*Gated blood pool study of a patient with a large left ventricular aneurysm: (a) anterior diastolic view: (b) anterior systolic view; (c) LAO diastolic view; (d) LAO systolic view; (e) amplitude image; (f) phase image.*

*The LAO view shows the aneurysm best, and there is a large area of paradoxical contraction identified on the LAO phase image. This area is shown to have good 'movement' on the amplitude image.*

## Follow-up after intervention

*Aims of coronary bypass grafting and angioplasty in the treatment of coronary artery disease*

• Cure angina by increasing the myocardial blood flow during exercise
• Improve ventricular function by increasing myocardial blood flow
• Decrease mortality from subsequent coronary occlusion.

Radionuclide studies provide ideal techniques for the follow-up of patients after intervention to assess the improvements in myocardial blood flow and ventricular function.

### $^{201}Tl$ myocardial imaging following bypass surgery

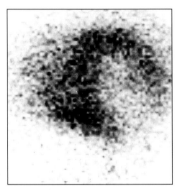 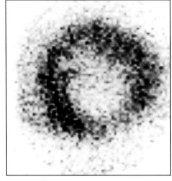 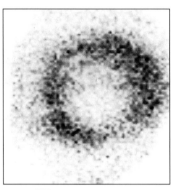 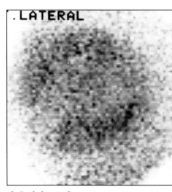

*a Anterior*      *b LAO 45°*      *c LAO 55°*      *d Left lateral*

**Fig. 6.89**

**(a–d)** *$^{201}Tl$ myocardial scan.*
*This patient had triple vessel bypass grafting carried out five years previously. He was referred for investigation of recurrent chest pain. The exercise $^{201}Tl$ scan shows a dilated left ventricle, with generalized patchy distribution of thallium uptake, and absent uptake inferior to the apex. The delayed views were identical, and the scan findings were attributed to a previous myocardial infarction. In this case there was no evidence of reversible myocardial ischaemia as a cause for the chest pain, and it was considered that deteriorating ventricular function was the main factor.*

# CLINICAL APPLICATIONS

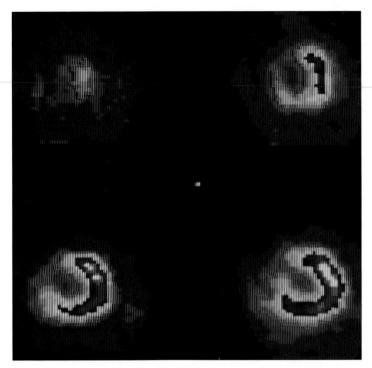

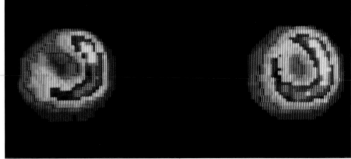

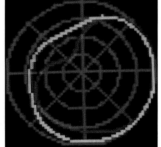

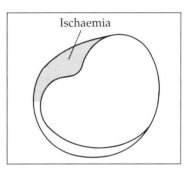

*a*

*b*

*c*

## Fig. 6.90

*²⁰¹Tl myocardial scan following coronary artery bypass grafting:
(a) exercise study; (b) single exercise/delayed slice; (c) relative
uptake outlines. The key to the tomographic images in (a) is as
follows:*

| Apex | Mid-cavity |
|------|------------|
| *Mid-cavity* | *Base* |

This tomographic study shows decreased ²⁰¹Tl uptake in the
proximal septum and anterior wall, which reverts to normal on the
delayed views. This patient had responded well to bypass grafting,
but several years later developed some recurrent chest pain, and
was being investigated for this. The study shows there is reversible
ischaemia which is caused by stenosis of the left anterior
descending artery graft.

## CLINICAL APPLICATIONS

### $^{201}$Tl myocardial imaging after angioplasty

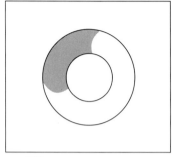

LAO 55°

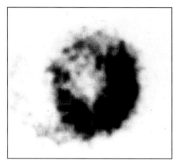

*a* LAO 55°, stress

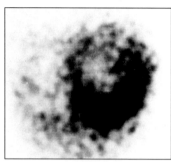

*b* LAO 55°, rest

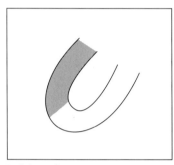

Left lateral

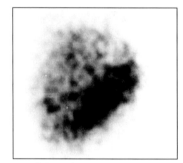

*c* Left lateral, stress

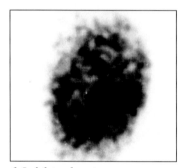

*d* Left lateral, rest

**Fig. 6.91**

*(a–d) $^{201}$Tl myocardial scan following angioplasty.*

*This patient was not assessed before angioplasty. However, he was subsequently referred for $^{201}$Tl scanning, since it was suspected that the angioplasty of the left anterior descending artery had not been successful. The study shows a markedly decreased uptake of $^{201}$Tl in the septum and anterior wall on the LAO 55° and left lateral views, clearly demonstrating that the angioplasty had not been completely successful. However, any possible improvement following angioplasty could not be evaluated because of the lack of a baseline study.*

### $^{201}$Tl myocardial imaging pre- and post-angioplasty

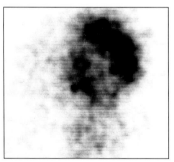

*a* Pre-angioplasty, anterior, stress

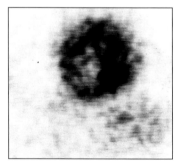

*b* Pre-angioplasty, LAO 45°, stress

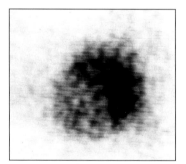

*c* Post-angioplasty, anterior, stress

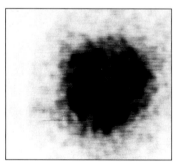

*d* Post-angioplasty, LAO 45°, stress

**Fig. 6.92**

*(a, b) Pre-angioplasty $^{201}$Tl study. (c, d) Post-angioplasty $^{201}$Tl study.*

*This patient developed angina and underwent investigations which showed double vessel disease (left anterior descending and right coronary arteries). Double vessel angioplasty was performed, but angina persisted; he was therefore referred for $^{201}$Tl scanning.*

*The pre-angioplasty anterior and LAO views demonstrate inferior and septal ischaemia. The post-angioplasty study shows that the septum is now normally perfused, but the inferior ischaemia persists, and may even be more marked, indicating successful angioplasty of the left anterior descending artery but a failure of angioplasty of the right coronary artery.*

## CLINICAL APPLICATIONS

*Pre-angioplasty: stress*

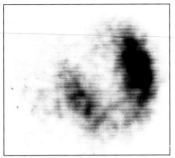

*a Anterior*

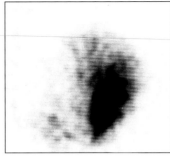

*b LAO*

*Pre-angioplasty: rest*

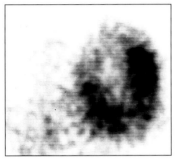

*c Anterior*

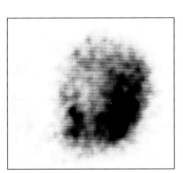

*d LAO 45°*

*Post-angioplasty: stress*

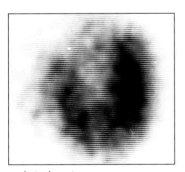

*e Anterior, stress*

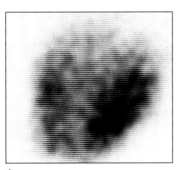

*f LAO*

**Fig. 6.93**

**(a–d)** *Pre-angioplasty* [201]*Tl study.* **(e, f)** *Post-angioplasty* [201]*Tl study.*

*The planar* [201]*Tl exercise study performed pre-angioplasty* **(a, b)** *shows the appearances of a severe lesion of the left anterior descending artery, with reversible ischaemia in the entire septum extending to the inferior wall (the right coronary artery was non-dominant). The delayed views* **(c, d)** *confirm the reversibility of these changes. Note also the left ventricular dilatation on the exercise study, which was not present on the delayed study. The study performed after the successful dilatation of the stenosis* **(e, f)** *shows a clear-cut improvement in thallium uptake in the septum at exercise, although this is not entirely normal.*

- In the case illustrated in Fig. 6.93 there was a marked improvement following successful angioplasty. However, without the baseline study, the degree of improvement could not have been assessed.
- A full assessment of the functional effect of an angioplasty can only be made if a pre-angioplasty study is also undertaken.

## Post-angioplasty infarction

### $^{99m}$Tc pyrophosphate

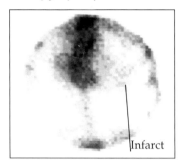

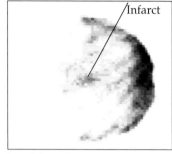

*a* Anterior

*b* Left lateral

### $^{201}$Tl

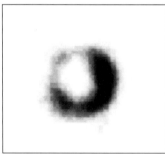

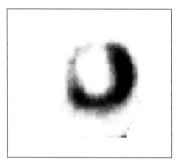

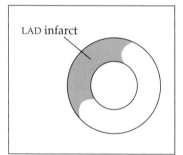

*c* Exercise

*d* Delayed

**Fig. 6.94**

*Radionuclide investigation of post-angioplasty infarct, taken 5 hours post-injection: (a, b) $^{99m}$Tc pyrophosphate study; (c, d) $^{201}$Tl exercise study.*

*In this case, following a long and difficult angioplasty of the left anterior descending artery there was a suspicion that myocardial infarction had occurred. A $^{99m}$Tc pyrophosphate study (a) shows positive uptake of tracer. The subsequent exercise $^{201}$Tl scan (b) shows a fixed defect typical of an infarct in the territory of the left anterior descending artery.*

## Presence of residual ischaemia after intervention

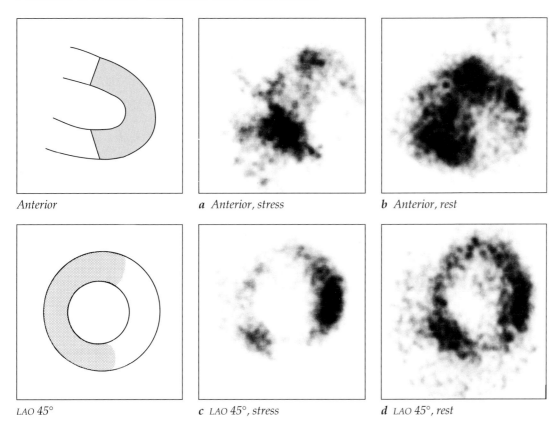

Anterior

*a* Anterior, stress

*b* Anterior, rest

LAO 45°

*c* LAO 45°, stress

*d* LAO 45°, rest

**Fig. 6.95**

**(a–d)** *$^{201}$Tl myocardial scan.*
*This planar $^{201}$Tl study shows a dilated left ventricular cavity, with gross diminution of $^{201}$Tl uptake in the anterior wall, the septum, and the inferior wall. The delayed views* **(b, d)** *show considerable normalization throughout, with the exception of the apex. This man had previously undergone a four-vessel coronary bypass graft, but subsequently had persistent impaired ventricular function and some atypical chest pain. The clinical question was whether, despite the grafting, residual ischaemia persisted. The $^{201}$Tl scan clearly answers this by showing the areas of reversible ischaemia in the upper septum, anterior wall and, to a lesser extent, inferiorly. Subsequent arteriography showed multiple graft occlusions.*

# 6.4.2 Assessment of cardiac function

The assessment of cardiac function is essential in the adequate management of many patients with a variety of diseases. The gated blood pool study is a simple, cheap and non-invasive direct method of assessing ventricular function. It may be helpful in the following situations:

• Assessment of ventricular function before coronary artery bypass grafting, as the prognosis is significantly worse with severely impaired function
• Assessment of ventricular function after myocardial infarction, since the degree of functional impairment is directly related to the long-term prognosis

• Follow-up of patients with myocarditis and cardiomyopathies
• Follow-up of patients after angioplasty
• Detection of deteriorating ventricular function in patients with valvular heart disease
• Assessment of ventricular function in patients receiving potentially cardiotoxic drugs
• Assessment of an aneurysm.

## *Gated blood pool studies*
*Normal gated rest study with global deterioration following haemodynamic stress*

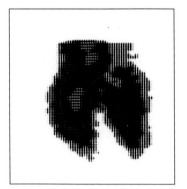 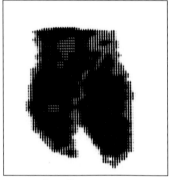 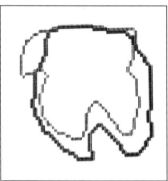 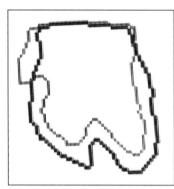

*a* LAO, *diastolic, rest*     *b* LAO, *diastolic, stress*     *c* *Isocount contours*     *d* *Isocount contours*

**Fig. 6.96**

*Resting* LAO *diastolic view* **(a)** *compared with the same view during isometric stress* **(b)**, *together with the corresponding isocount contours* **(c, d)**.

*The effect of afterload stress in this patient with ischaemic heart disease is to cause dilatation of the left ventricle and a drop in ejection fraction from 55% to 43%, but no focal wall abnormality.*

• **These changes with stress are non-specific, and may be seen in practically any myocardial disorder.**
• **Slight left ventricular dilatation is commonly seen in older patients. However, a significant drop in ejection fraction (>5%) does not normally accompany this.**

## CLINICAL APPLICATIONS

*Normal rest study with focal myocardial wall motion abnormality appearing with stress*

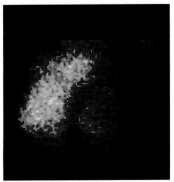 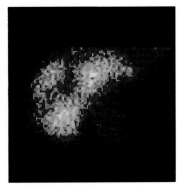 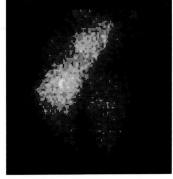 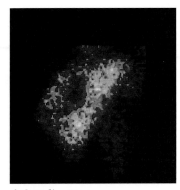

*a  Diastolic, rest*      *b  Systolic, rest*      *c  Diastolic, stress*      *d  Systolic, stress*

**Fig. 6.97**

*Gated blood pool study at rest: (a) diastolic; (b) systolic views. Gated blood pool study following haemodynamic stress: (c) diastolic; (d) systolic views.*

*In this case the diastolic volume can be seen to increase slightly following stress, but more significantly the apex of the left ventricle becomes totally akinetic. This is a typical example of a focal stress-induced wall motion abnormality caused by coronary artery disease.*

**Focal wall motion abnormalities are much more specific for coronary artery disease than generalized global deterioration with stress.**

*Focal wall motion abnormality at rest*

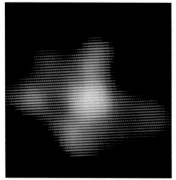

*a  Anterior, diastolic*

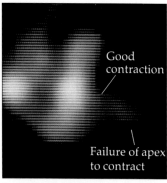

Good contraction

Failure of apex to contract

*b  Anterior, systolic*

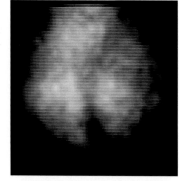

*c  LAO, diastolic*

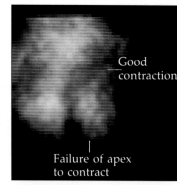

Good contraction

Failure of apex to contract

*d  LAO, systolic*

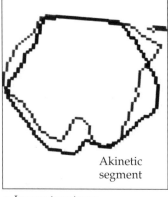

Akinetic segment

*e  Isocount contours*

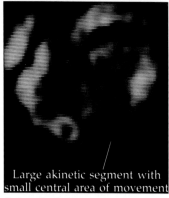

Large akinetic segment with small central area of movement

*f  Amplitude image*

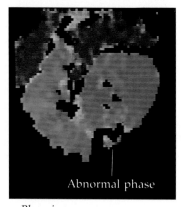

Abnormal phase

*g  Phase image*

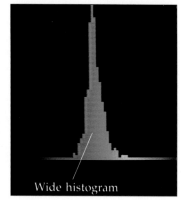

Wide histogram

*h  Phase histogram*

**Fig. 6.98**

*Gated blood pool study: (a) anterior diastolic image; (b) anterior systolic image; (c) LAO diastolic image; (d) LAO systolic image; (e) isocount contours; (f) amplitude image; (g) phase image; (h) phase histogram.*

*A patient with previous myocardial infarction. The anterior views show a failure of long axis shortening of the left ventricle during systole, and the oblique views clearly show the focal wall motion abnormality highlighted by the isocount contours. The amplitude image shows the area of absent contraction, whereas the phase image shows that there is a small focal area which is paradoxical within the akinetic segment. Note that the histogram of the left ventricle is broadened as a result of some generalized left ventricular impairment.*

• Although in the case shown in Fig. 6.98 all the methods of display demonstrate the abnormality, in general no one method is consistently reliable. It is therefore valuable to demonstrate ventricular function using a number of different display methods.

• A myocardial infarct will produce a focal wall motion abnormality at rest, either hypokinesia or akinesia, as opposed to an ischaemic area, which will only appear as a wall motion abnormality under conditions of haemodynamic stress.

## Assessment of ventricular function

### Diastole

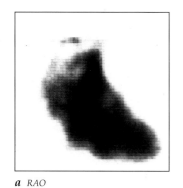

*a* RAO

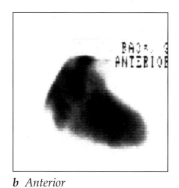

*b* Anterior

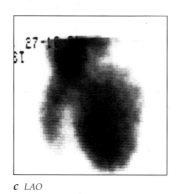

*c* LAO

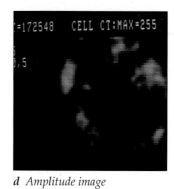

*d* Amplitude image

### Systole

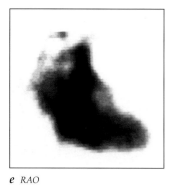

*e* RAO

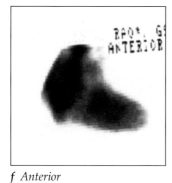

*f* Anterior

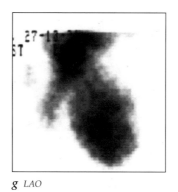

*g* LAO

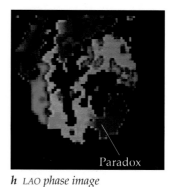

*h* LAO phase image

**Fig. 6.99**

*Gated blood pool study:* **(a–c, e–g)** *gated images;* **(d)** *amplitude image;* **(h)** LAO *phase image.*

This patient was known to have had a previous myocardial infarction, and was referred for functional assessment as a guide to prognosis. The left ventricle was seen to be grossly dilated, with complete akinesis of the septum and the inferior wall. There is only a small area of paradox, and no aneurysmal dilatation. The ejection fraction was only 20%. These findings make it unlikely that surgical treatment would be of value, and the prognosis is poor.

## *Follow-up of myocarditis*

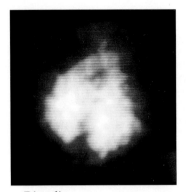

*a Diastolic*

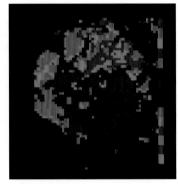

*b Systolic*

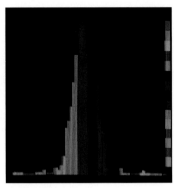

*c Phase image*

*d Phase histogram*

**Fig. 6.100**

*Gated blood pool study:* **(a)** *diastolic image;* **(b)** *systolic image;* **(c)** *phase image;* **(d)** *right and left ventricular phase histogram.*

   *This patient was a child with deteriorating cardiac function. This study was undertaken to exclude a shunt and to assess ventricular function. The first pass study (not shown) revealed no evidence of intracardiac shunting. The gated study shows good right ventricular function. The left ventricle shows moderate function, with an ejection fraction of 25%, but akinesis of the apex and the septum. Note the phase study shows early activation of the right ventricle because of the pacemaker, which had been placed in as an emergency. This child was subsequently shown to have a viral myocarditis, confirmed on myocardial biopsy, and responded well to immunosuppression and corticosteroids. The gated study was used to measure the ventricular function during the course of the recovery period.*

## Ischaemic cardiomyopathy

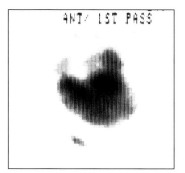

*a Anterior, diastolic*

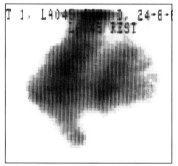

*b LAO, diastolic*

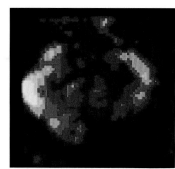

*c Amplitude image*

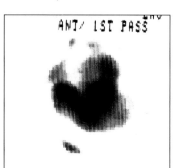

*d Anterior, systolic*

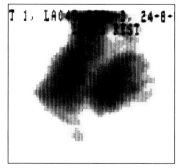

*e LAO, systolic*

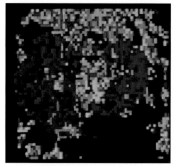

*f Phase image*

**Fig. 6.101**

*Gated blood pool study: (**a, b, d, e**) gated images; (**c**) amplitude image; (**f**) phase image.*

*This patient was referred for functional assessment. He was known to have end stage ischaemic cardiomyopathy and had failed all medical treatment. Conventional surgical treatment was not considered appropriate. The study was undertaken to document the ventricular function prior to referral for cardiac transplantation. The gated study can be seen to show extremely poor right and left ventricular contraction; the ejection fraction was 12%. The amplitude and phase images show complete disorganization of contraction, with very little measurable wall motion.*

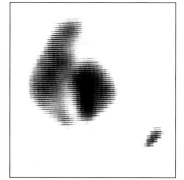

*a LAO, diastolic*

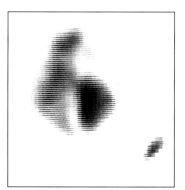

*b LAO, systolic*

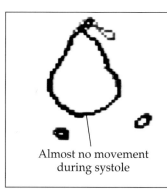

Almost no movement during systole

*c Isocount contours*

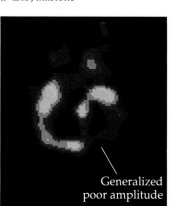

Generalized poor amplitude

*d Amplitude image*

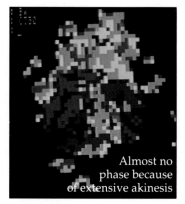

Almost no phase because of extensive akinesis

*e Phase image*

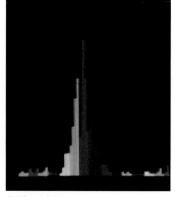

*f Phase histogram*

**Fig. 6.102**

*Gated blood pool study of a patient with advanced ischaemic cardiomyopathy: (**a**) LAO diastolic image; (**b**) LAO systolic image; (**c**) isocount contours; (**d**) amplitude image; (**e**) phase image; (**f**) phase histogram.*

*Note that the systolic and diastolic images are almost indistinguishable, and the isocount contours are unable to clearly demonstrate any area of wall motion. The amplitude image shows some contraction of the right ventricle and some contraction superolaterally in the left ventricle. There is marked broadening of the histogram on the phase image, but no localized aneurysm is demonstrated. These are typical appearances of severe generalized ischaemic cardiomyopathy. The ejection fraction was 17%.*

## CLINICAL APPLICATIONS

*Follow-up of cardiomyopathy*

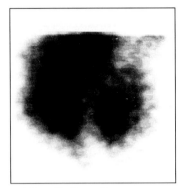

*a Diastolic, 0 months*

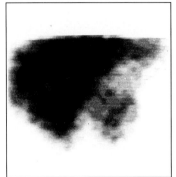

*b Systolic, 0 months*

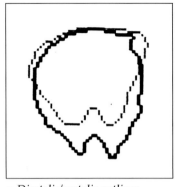

*c Diastolic/systolic outlines, 0 months*

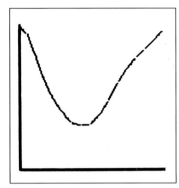

*d T/A curve, 0 months*

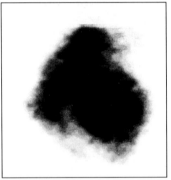

*e Diastolic, 3 months*

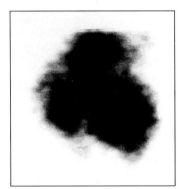

*f Systolic, 3 months*

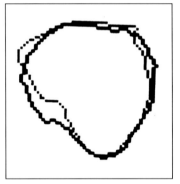

*g Diastolic/systolic outlines, 3 months*

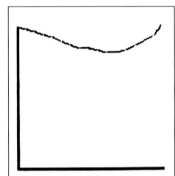

*h T/A curve, 3 months*

**Fig. 6.103**

*Initial gated blood pool study:* (**a**) *diastolic image;* (**b**) *systolic image;* (**c**) *diastolic/systolic outlines;* (**d**) *T/A volume curve of the left ventricle.* (**e–h**) *Repeat study, 3 months later.*

In this case of cardiomyopathy the initial study shows moderately good ventricular function, with a left ventricular ejection fraction of 68% and no regional wall motion abnormalities. However, as the disease progressed, in spite of treatment with steroids and immunosuppression, the left ventricle dilated and the ejection fraction gradually dropped to 11%. Note on the repeat study that the changes are global rather than focal.

## CLINICAL APPLICATIONS

*Quantitation in the assessment and follow-up of cardiomyopathy*

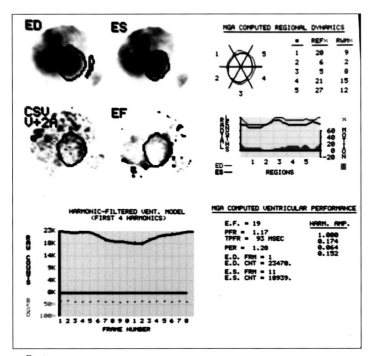

*a  Rest*

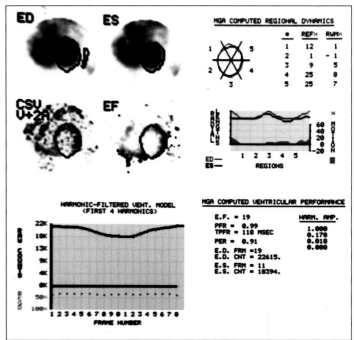

*b  Cold pressor*

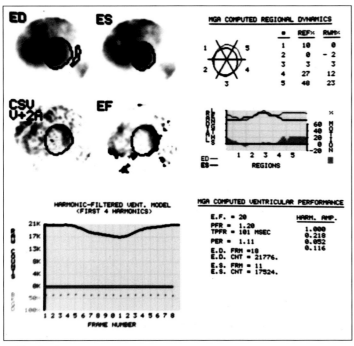

*c  Hand grip*

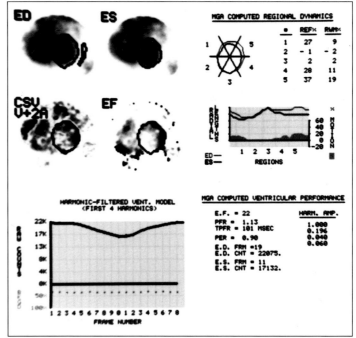

*d  Post-stress*

**Fig. 6.104**

**(a)** *Rest quantitation.* **(b)** *Cold pressor stress quantitation.* **(c)** *Hand-grip stress quantitation.* **(d)** *Post-stress quantitation.*

*This 70-year-old man presented with known ischaemic cardiomyopathy and severe left ventricular failure. A quantitation study (a–d) was performed prior to commencing captopril therapy. The left ventricular ejection fraction is significantly impaired (19%) and there is no significant change with stress. Regional ejection fraction values confirm global hypokinesia.*

## *Alcoholic cardiomyopathy*

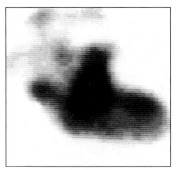

*a  Anterior, diastolic*

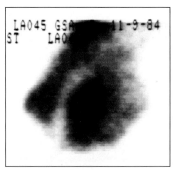

*b  LAO 45°, diastolic*

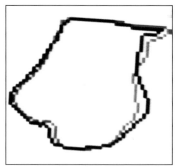

*c  Diastolic/systolic outlines*

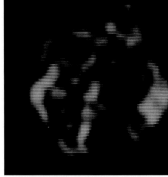

*d  Amplitude image*

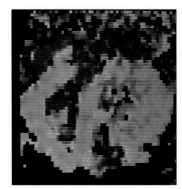

*e  Phase image*

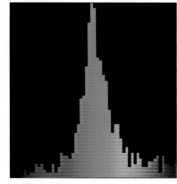

*f  Phase histogram*

**Fig. 6.105**

*Gated blood pool study: (a) anterior diastolic image; (b) LAO 45° diastolic image; (c) diastolic/systolic outlines; (d) amplitude image; (e) phase image; (f) phase histogram.*

*This patient had developed alcoholic cardiomyopathy, and the study was undertaken to provide a baseline for follow-up purposes. The gated study shows gross dilatation of the left ventricle, with an ejection fraction of only 21%. There was some ventricular dilatation, but no significant further deterioration in function with afterload stress.*

**With severe impairment of ventricular function, stress studies do not materially contribute to the assessment of the patient, and may be dangerous.**

## CLINICAL APPLICATIONS

## Valvular heart disease

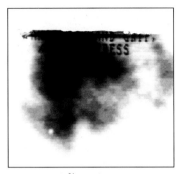

*a* LAO, systolic, rest

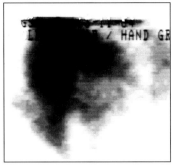

*b* LAO, diastolic, rest

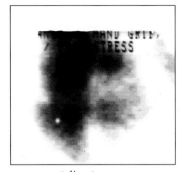

*c* LAO, systolic, stress

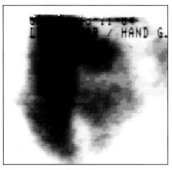

*d* LAO, diastolic, stress

**Fig. 6.106**

*(a–d) Gated blood pool study, LAO views.*

*In this patient with aortic valve disease at rest the ventricular function is slightly impaired, with an ejection fraction of 48%. With cold pressor stress, dilatation of the left ventricle can be seen, and the ejection fraction falls to 42%. There is therefore evidence of impaired ventricular function, which may be an indication that surgical treatment of this patient with aortic valve disease should be undertaken.*

• The ejection fraction may not rise in response to exercise in patients with aortic valve disease. A fall in ejection fraction, however, is abnormal and indicates early ventricular decompensation.
• Gated blood pool studies provide a non-invasive method of accurately following patients with aortic valve regurgitation, and assist in determining the optimum time for surgery.

## Potentially cardiotoxic drugs

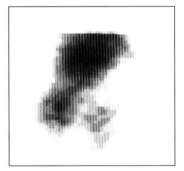

*a* Systolic, rest

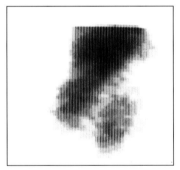

*b* Systolic, hand grip

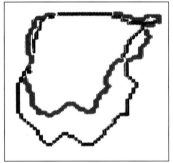

*c* Rest

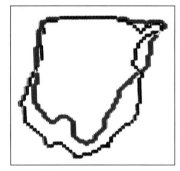

*d* Hand grip

**Fig. 6.107**

*Gated blood pool images: (a) systolic rest; (b) systolic hand grip. Diastolic/systolic outlines: (c) rest; (d) hand grip.*

*This patient had a lymphoma, and was undergoing treatment with cytotoxic drugs, which included Adriamycin. He had reached the level at which cardiotoxicity is known to occur, and was being assessed to see whether further treatment could be justified. The gated study shows normal ventricular function at rest, with an ejection fraction of 66%. With isometric hand grip, there is a clear dilatation of the left ventricle with hypokinesis around the apex, and the ejection fraction drops to 55%. As a consequence, further Adriamycin therapy was withheld.*

• A pretreatment assessment of ventricular function is required to identify pretreatment dysfunction.
• Cardiotoxic effects may be focal or global.

## CLINICAL APPLICATIONS

*Obstructive cardiomyopathy with a conduction defect*

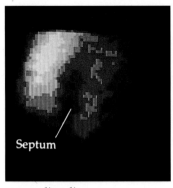
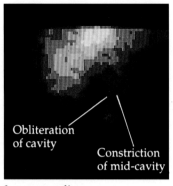
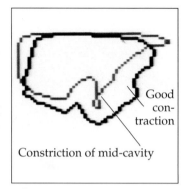
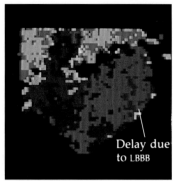

*a* LAO, diastolic      *b* LAO, systolic      *c* Isocount contours      *d* Phase image

**Fig. 6.108**

*Gated blood pool study: (**a**) LAO diastolic image; (**b**) LAO systolic image; (**c**) isocount contours; (**d**) phase image.*

*It is apparent on the blood pool images that the left ventricle shows very good contraction, with an ejection fraction of 79%. During contraction, however, there is constriction of the mid-left ventricular cavity typical of obstructive cardiomyopathy. This may isolate the distal left ventricular cavity and result in a severe drop in ejection fraction. Note also the thick hypertrophied septum, which is well visualized on the oblique views. The phase study demonstrates delayed contraction of the entire left ventricle, typical of a left bundle branch block pattern (LBBB).*

# 6.4.3   Congenital heart disorders

## *Classification of principal congenital heart disorders*

### *Acyanotic*

- Ventricular septal defect (VSD)
- Atrial septal defect (ASD):
     ostium secundum defect
     ostium primum defect
- Patent ductus arteriosus (PDA)
- Congenital aortic stenosis
- Coarctation of the aorta
- Pulmonary valve stenosis.

### *Cyanotic*

- Transposition of the great vessels (TGV)
- Fallot's tetralogy (VSD, over-riding aorta/pulmonary stenosis and right ventricular hypertrophy)
- Tricuspid atresia
- Single ventricle
- Atrioventricular canal defect.

## *Clinical uses of functional radionuclide investigation in congenital heart disorders*

- Measurement of the size of the left to right shunt
- Assessment of ventricular function
- Diagnosis of congenital heart disease when a murmur is picked up on a routine medical examination
- Assessment of the distribution of pulmonary blood flow.

## CLINICAL APPLICATIONS

### First pass studies

First pass studies are used to measure left to right shunts, right to left shunts and several congenital cardiac malformations. An understanding of the common abnormalities is essential for a correct interpretation of first pass studies.

### Diagnosis of intracardiac left to right shunting: VSD

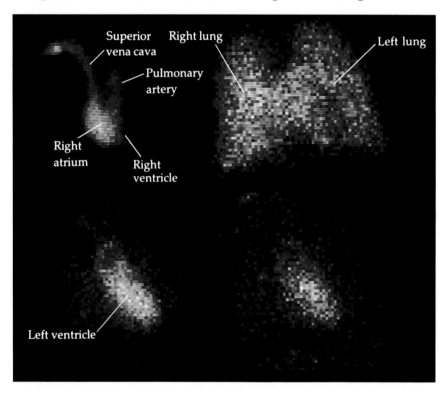
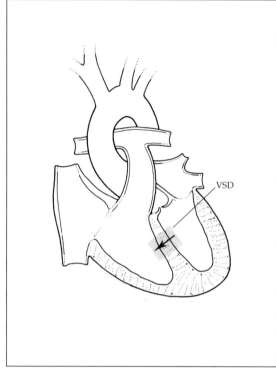

**Fig. 6.109**

VSD: *anterior view during the first passage of the bolus.*

*There is a right-sided injection, and tracer is seen to enter the right atrium through the superior vena cava and fill the right ventricle. As it enters the lungs, a clear negative left ventricle phase is seen. Blood returns to the left ventricle, but the level of activity seen in the lungs never completely clears because of continual recirculation. Changes are due to a simple VSD.*

 The absence of visualization of a negative left ventricle may be seen:

• With right to left shunting
• With a large right ventricle
• With a small left ventricle
• With children less than two years old, when the resolution may be inadequate to display the photon-deficient area occupied by the left ventricle.

## CLINICAL APPLICATIONS

*Quantitation of shunt*

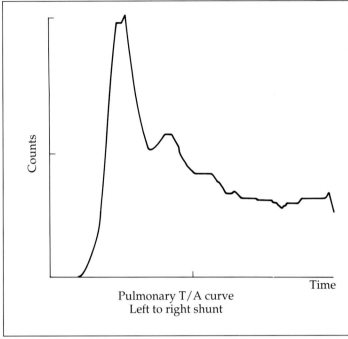

*a*

Pulmonary T/A curve
Left to right shunt

Time

Counts

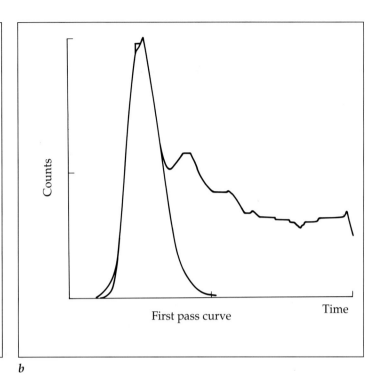

*b*

First pass curve

Time

Counts

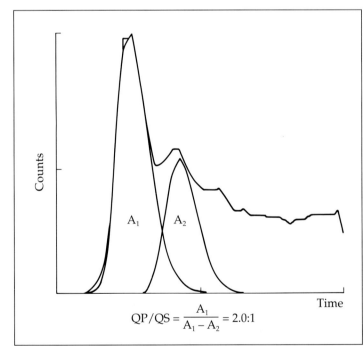

*c*

$$QP/QS = \frac{A_1}{A_1 - A_2} = 2.0:1$$

Counts

$A_1$    $A_2$

Time

### Fig. 6.110

**(a)** *T/A curve from the lung, showing a marked skew to the right caused by the intracardial left to right pulmonary recirculation.* **(b)** *A symmetrical curve is fitted by the computer from the ascending and initial descending portions of the real curve to represent the predicted curve with no shunt.* **(c)** *The predicted curve $A_1$ is subtracted from the real curve, and the difference representing the amount of blood recirculating through the lungs (ie size of left to right shunt) is plotted as a second curve, $A_2$.*

*ASD*

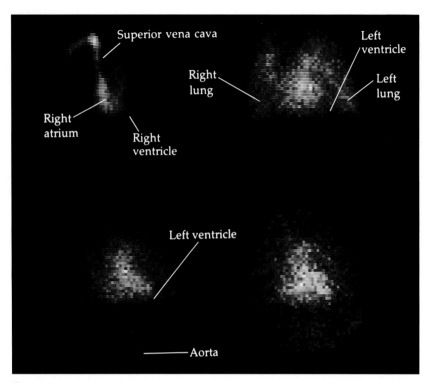

*a*

### Fig. 6.111

*(a) In this example of an ASD tracer can be seen entering the right atrium and right ventricle normally, with a negative left ventricle, indicating no right to left shunting. The lungs fill and there is subsequent systemic filling, but the activity in the lungs does not clear in the normal way, indicating pulmonary recirculation caused by the left to right shunting. The shunt calculation (b) confirms a left to right shunt. The gated study (Fig. 6.112) shows slight right ventricular dilatation only.*

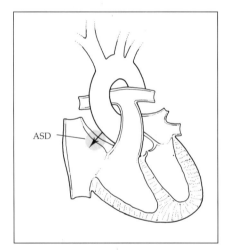
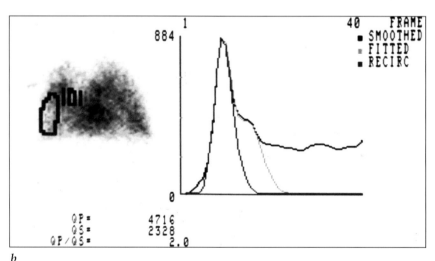

*b*

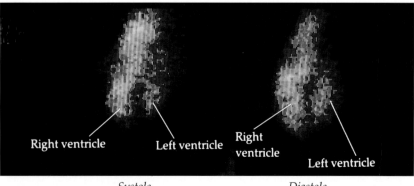

### Fig. 6.112

*The gated blood pool study shows right ventricular dilatation, typical of an ASD.*

## CLINICAL APPLICATIONS

*Comparison of the two common causes of left to right shunting:* ASD *and* VSD

When the shunt is small, ie below 2:1, it may be impossible to differentiate between a VSD and an ASD. However, with larger shunts there are a number of features which help in this differentiation: these are demonstrated in Fig. 6.113.

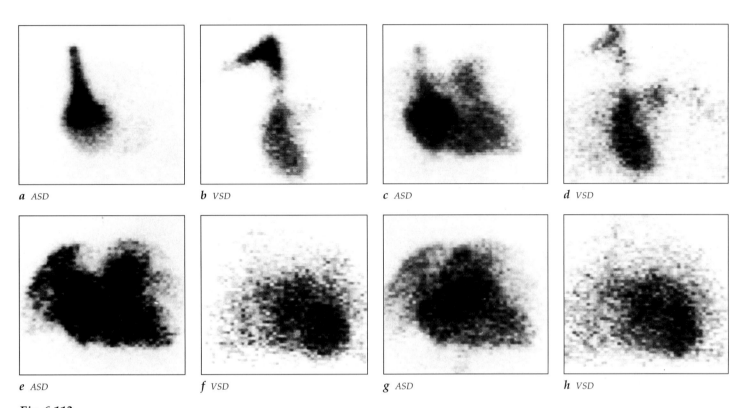

*a* ASD  *b* VSD  *c* ASD  *d* VSD

*e* ASD  *f* VSD  *g* ASD  *h* VSD

**Fig. 6.113**

*(a, b) As the tracer enters the right atrium, dilution of the bolus may be seen in the case of an* ASD. *(c, d) There is a very clearly seen negative left ventricle in the* VSD, *but it is not so clear in the case of an* ASD. *The reason for this lies in the relative volumes of the two ventricles. (e, f) As the tracer enters the left ventricle, a large globular left ventricle is seen in the case of an* VSD, *and only a small one in the case of an* ASD. *(g, h) In both instances there is a failure of clearance from the lungs caused by pulmonary recirculation. In addition, the aorta and great vessels to the neck are not clearly defined, because of the obscuring high lung background.*

## Intracardiac left to right shunt: gated cardiac study

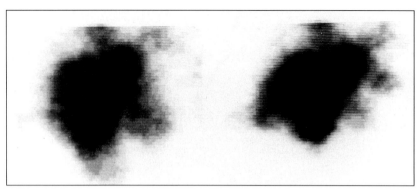

*a* ASD

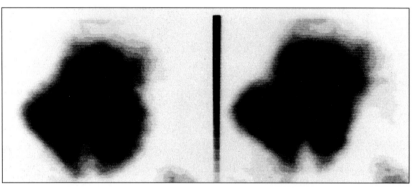

*b* VSD

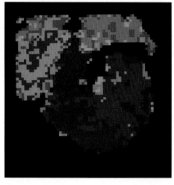

*c*

**Fig. 6.114**

**(a)** *Gated study* ASD *(diastole and systole).* **(b)** *Gated study* VSD *(diastole and systole). The gated studies clearly differentiate the relatively volume-overloaded right ventricle with a small-volume left ventricle in the* ASD, *and the volume-overloaded but well-contracting left ventricle in the case of the* VSD. *Occasionally, an additional feature is some right ventricular delay in the case of an* ASD, *seen on the phase image* **(c)**, *and this is secondary to either a conduction defect or the volume overload of the right ventricle.*

**Table 6.7   Differential features**

| ASD | VSD |
| --- | --- |
| Atrial dilution of bolus | — |
| Volume-overloaded right ventricle | — |
| — | Volume-overloaded left ventricle |
| Right ventricular phase delay | — |

## CLINICAL APPLICATIONS

*VSD*

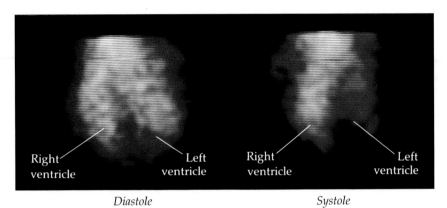

Diastole                    Systole

**Fig. 6.115**

*VSD LAO gated blood pool study, showing a dilated right ventricle and slight volume overload of the left ventricle, but with good contraction. The ejection fraction of the left ventricle was 64%, typical of VSD.*

*ASD*

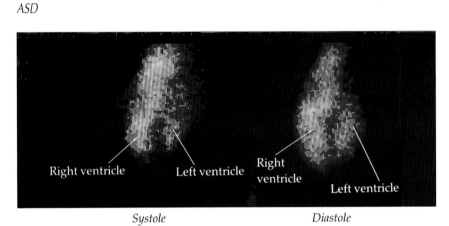

Systole                    Diastole

**Fig. 6.116**

*Gated blood pool study, showing slight right ventricular dilatation, typical of an ASD.*

## *Presentation with incidental murmur*

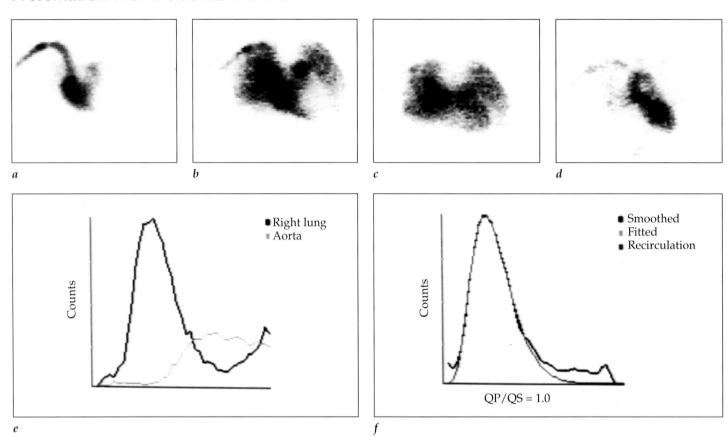

a          b                    c                  d

e                                        f

**Fig. 6.117**

*First pass study: (a) right atrium/right ventricle filling; (b) lungs filling/negative left ventricle; (c) left ventricle filling; (d) aorta and great vessels. (e) T/A curves from lung and aorta. (f) Left to right shunt calculation.*

This patient was a 10-year-old child who was detected as having a murmur on a routine medical examination at school. He was referred to the paediatric clinic and a first pass study was performed as an initial screening procedure. This study shows a normal sequence of chamber filling on the series of images, with no evidence of a right to left or a left to right shunt. The absence of intracardiac shunting is confirmed on the T/A curves of the lung and aorta and also on the deconvolved right lung QP/QS calculation. The subsequent gated study (not shown) confirmed normal ventricular function. This is a good example of how the first pass and gated study can be used as an initial screening test in the case of innocent murmurs detected on routine medical examination. Cardiac catheterization is not necessary in these circumstances, and thus only non-invasive investigation is required.

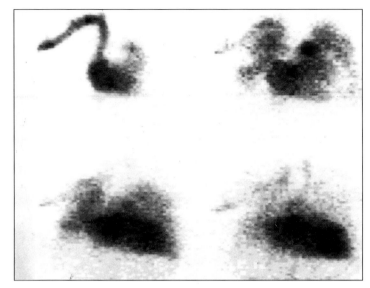

a

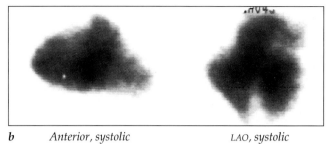

b     Anterior, systolic      LAO, systolic

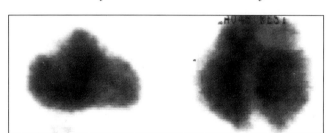

c     Anterior, diastolic      LAO, diastolic

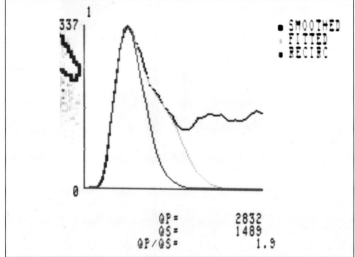

d

### Fig. 6.118

**(a)** First pass study, showing left ventricular dilatation and pulmonary recirculation. **(b, c)** Gated blood pool study. **(d)** Pulmonary T/A curve with left to right shunt calculation.

    This child was found on a routine school medical examination to have a murmur and progressive dyspnoea. The first pass study demonstrates a moderate left to right shunt, and the dilated left ventricle on the gated study indicates that the case is most probably a VSD.

## Transposition of the great vessels

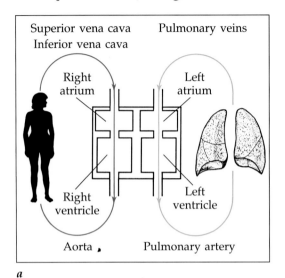 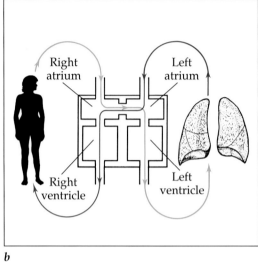

a   b

**Fig. 6.119**

**(a)** *Uncorrected transposition of the great vessels.*
**(b)** *Surgically corrected transposition with a 'baffle' in the atria to divert the blood.*

### Transposition: first pass study

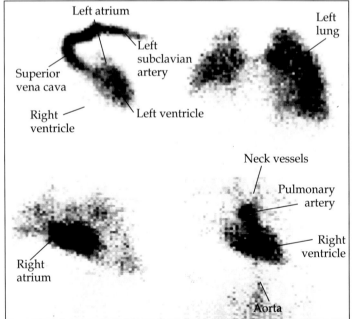

**Fig. 6.120**

*Series of first pass images, showing tracer injected from the left arm entering the superior vena cava and filling the left atrium and left ventricle. There is a negative right-sided ventricle, and the lungs fill before the right-sided ventricle fills. These are the typical scan appearances of a surgically corrected transposition, where the atrial baffle diverts systemic venous blood into the left atrium and left ventricle.*

### Transposition: gated cardiac study

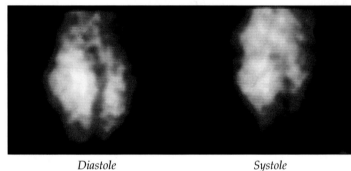

Diastole                    Systole

**Fig. 6.121**

*Gated study, showing that the left and right ventricles are contracting well, with only slight right ventricular dilatation.*

## CLINICAL APPLICATIONS

*Transposition: post-surgical assessment*

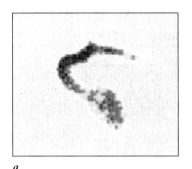 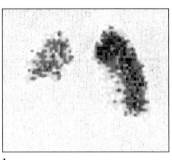 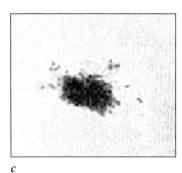 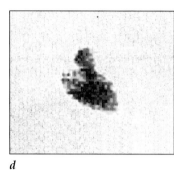

*a*            *b*            *c*            *d*

**Fig. 6.122**

*First pass study: **(a)** tracer entering the right atrium/left atrium and left ventricle with no 'hold up';*
***(b)** tracer entering both lungs; **(c)** tracer entering the right atrium and right ventricle; **(d)** tracer*
*filling the aorta from the right ventricle.*
   *This child had congenital transposition of the great vessels which had been corrected surgically by*
*an atrial baffle to divert blood from the right atrium to the left ventricle. This first pass study was*
*undertaken to see if the diversion was successful. The study shows complete diversion of tracer, with*
*no hold up at the atrial level.*

 **The main complications arising from surgical correction of transposition of
the great vessels are:**
    **• Obstruction to the venous return by the baffle**
**• Inadequate diversion of blood by the baffle**
**• Failure of the right ventricle, which is acting as the systemic ventricle.**

## *Tricuspid atresia with right to left shunt*

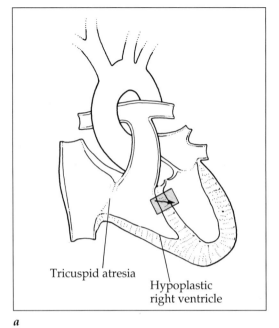

*a*

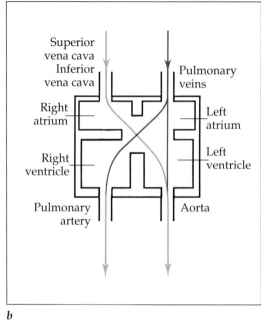

*b*

*Fig. 6.123*

*(a–f) Tricuspid atresia. The first pass study (c) shows tracer entering the superior vena cava and filling the right atrium. Immediately after this the left atrium and left ventricle fill through a patent ASD. Note the small amount of tracer refluxing down the inferior vena cava. Because of the single ventricle, the pulmonary curves (d) show the appearance of massive left to right shunting, and the aortic curve shows simultaneous filling with the lungs, indicating right to left shunting. Note the small empty triangular area between and below the left ventricle and the right atrium. This is occupied by the small redundant right ventricle. The gated study (e, f) shows a large, well contracting, somewhat volume-overloaded ventricle, and the small triangle between the atrium and ventricle is now filled because of tracer eventually reaching equilibrium in the small right ventricle.*

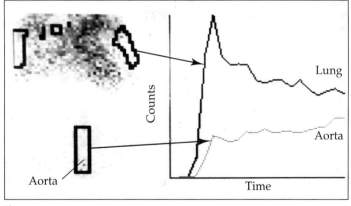

*c First pass study*

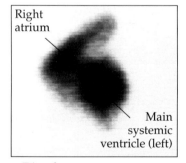

*e Diastole*

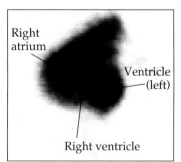

*f Systole*

*d*

## Tricuspid atresia presenting as cyanosis

### First pass study

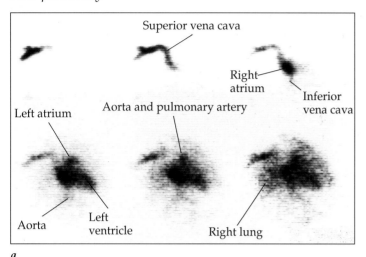

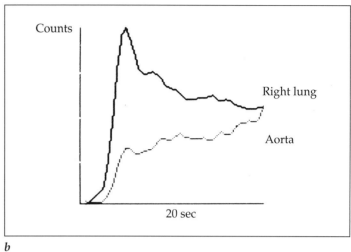

*a*

*b*

### Gated blood pool study

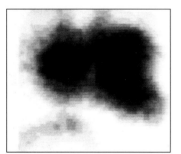

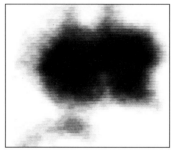

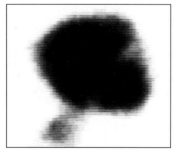

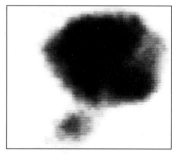

*c Anterior, diastolic*

*d Anterior, systolic*

*e* LAO, *diastolic*

*f* LAO, *systolic*

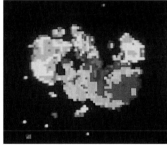

*g Phase image*

**Fig. 6.124**

*(a) First pass study, showing tracer entering the right atrium and filling the left ventricle and simultaneous lung and systemic vessel filling. (b) T/A curve from lung and aorta. (c–f) Gated blood pool study: (c, e) anterior and LAO diastolic images; (d, f) anterior and LAO systolic images. (g) Phase image.*

*This child was cyanosed, and the investigation was performed to assess the cause as well as the ventricular function. The first pass study shows the appearances of atresia of the tricuspid valve. The gated study confirms that there is only one functional ventricle, the right ventricle being hypoplastic.*

## CLINICAL APPLICATIONS

### *Patent ductus arteriosus (PDA)*

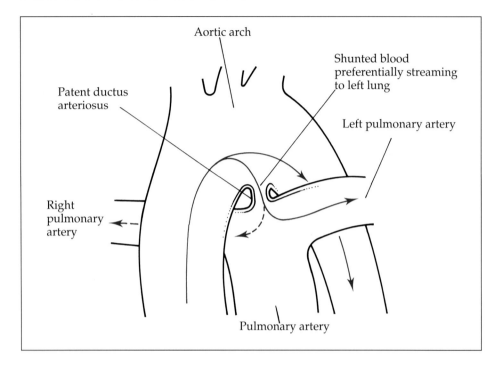

**Fig. 6.125**

*Diagrammatic representation of a patent ductus arteriosus.*

### *First pass study in PDA*

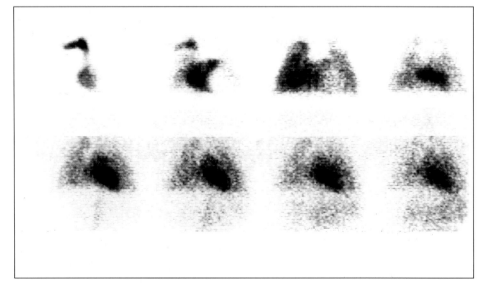

**Fig. 6.126**

**(a)** *First pass study of a child with a PDA. There is a normal sequence of chamber filling, but with persistent lung activity typical of left to right shunt. (Continued.)*

## CLINICAL APPLICATIONS

*Left lung analysis*

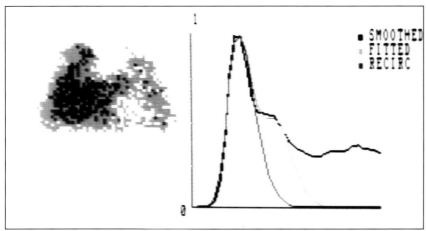

**b** *QP/QS = 1.8*

*Right lung analysis*

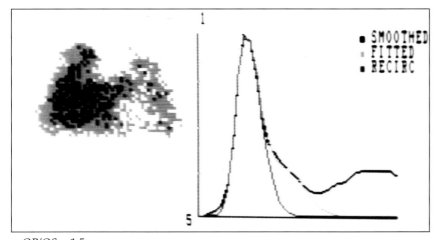

**c** *QP/QS = 1.5*

**Fig. 6.126** (Continued)

*(b, c) T/A curves.*

*It may be impossible to confidently diagnose a PDA. However, the left to right shunting is frequently directed mainly towards the left lung, as in this case, when only a small shunt can be calculated from the right lung curve (b), and a much larger shunt from the left lung curve (a). There may also tend to be some left ventricular volume overload, as in a VSD.*

## Measurement of intracardiac shunt size postoperatively

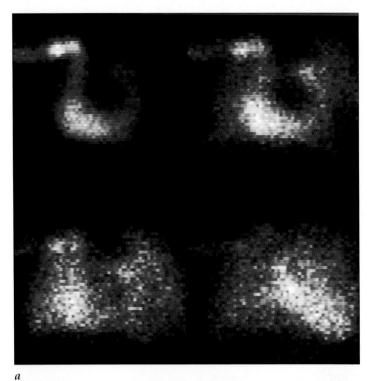

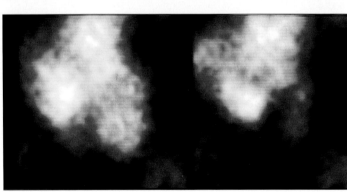

*a*

*b*

**Fig. 6.127**

**(a)** *First pass study, two frames per second.* **(b)** *Gated blood pool study,* LAO *diastolic/systolic image.* **(c)** *T/A curve with left to right shunt calculation.*

This child had Fallot's tetralogy, and was being assessed postoperatively for the size of the intracardiac shunt and ventricular function. The first pass study demonstrates pulmonary recirculation with a 1.5:1 left to right shunt, and the gated blood pool study shows a dilated left ventricle with good function (ejection fraction of 66%).

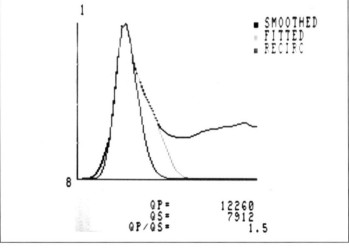

*c*

# 6.4.4 Assessment of pulmonary blood flow
## *Measurement of right to left shunt*

[99mTc]-labelled human albumin microspheres may be used to measure the size of a right to left shunt. In a normal person (Fig. 6.128, *left*) the size of the labelled microspheres ensures that they are all extracted by the pulmonary capillary bed. However, in the case of a right to left shunt the pulmonary capillary bed is partially bypassed (Fig. 6.128, *right*), and the micro-spheres will appear in the systemic circulation. The size of the shunt is directly proportional to the number of microspheres that reach the systemic circulation, and can be measured by whole-body scanning, measuring the ratio of pulmonary activity to the remainder of the body (pulmonary systemic flow ratio).

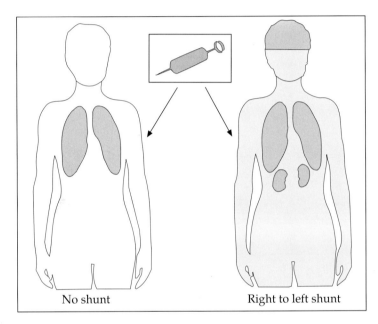

No shunt   Right to left shunt

**Fig. 6.128**

*Use of [99mTc]-labelled microspheres to measure a right to left shunt.*

## *Right to left shunt assessment: Fallot's tetralogy*

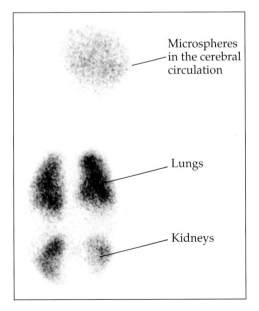

Microspheres in the cerebral circulation

Lungs

Kidneys

**Fig. 6.129**

*A case of right to left shunt with quantitation. [99mTc]-labelled microsphere study: posterior view.*

*This patient was a 7-year-old girl with Fallot's tetralogy. It is apparent that there is a large amount of tracer present in the systemic circulation, as demonstrated by the uptake in the brain and kidneys. This child had a large right to left shunt which measures 3:1.*

## Right to left shunt assessment: Blalock shunt

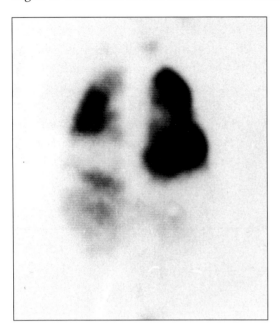

**Fig. 6.130**

*In this case a left Blalock shunt (left subclavian to left pulmonary artery anastomosis) was performed for pulmonary atresia. The whole-body scan following peripheral vein microsphere injection demonstrates the markedly increased left lung blood flow, compared with the right side, confirming that the Blalock shunt is patent and providing a good blood supply to the left lung. Note also the extrapulmonary microsphere distribution caused by the right to left shunting.*

## Right to left shunt assessment: post-arterial switch for RTA

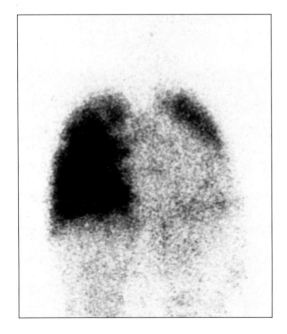

**Fig. 6.131**

*A 3-year-old girl following arterial switch for RTA with residual VSD and tricuspid regurgitation.*

*The study confirms a right to left shunt; cardiomegaly and a significant disparity in perfusion between the right and left lung. The right lung is receiving 80% of pulmonary artery blood flow.*

## Assessment of regional lung blood flow

It may be important in deciding on treatment in complex congenital heart disease to assess the regional blood flow and the feeding vessels of origin. Injection of microspheres may help in this evaluation, as in the case shown in Fig. 6.132 of a patient with pulmonary atresia, a VSD and multiple collateral pulmonary vessels arising from the aorta.

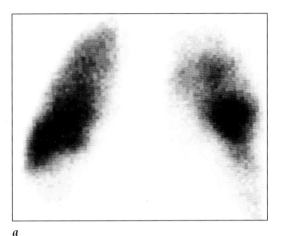

a

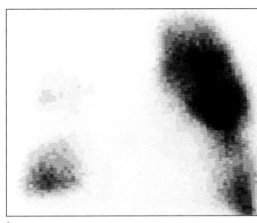

b

c

### Fig. 6.132

(a) Anterior lung scan image after a peripheral vein injection of microspheres. It demonstrates that there is approximately equal, although irregular, pulmonary perfusion, but does not identify whether it originates from the pulmonary artery or from the aortic collaterals. (b) The same anterior view after injection into the main pulmonary artery, demonstrating that most of the pulmonary arterial flow is going to the left lung, and therefore much of the right lung blood supply must be coming from aortic collaterals. (c) The same anterior view after injection into the collateral vessels, demonstrating that these predominantly supply the right lung. Because of the dependence of the right lung on collaterals, it was decided not to occlude them surgically.

## 6.4.5 Identification of thrombus

### *¹¹¹In–labelled platelets*

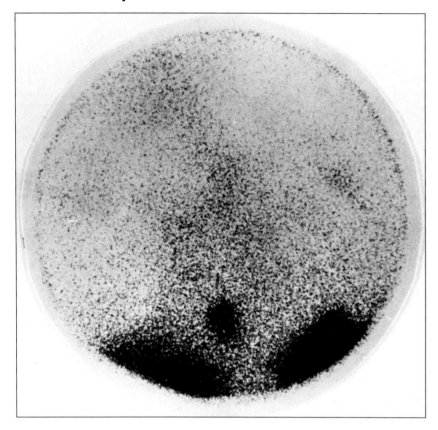

**Fig. 6.133**

*Anterior view of chest following the injection of ¹¹¹In-labelled autologous platelets.*

*Note the normal liver and spleen activity. There is a focus of platelet accumulation in the midline. This patient was being investigated to identify the source of recurrent systemic emboli following myocardial infarction. The labelled platelets identified thrombus in the left atrium. (Courtesy of Dr B Shepstone, Oxford, UK.)*

Although labelled platelet studies have not found a widespread clinical role, they are occasionally useful in difficult cases.

## CLINICAL APPLICATIONS

## *⁹⁹ᵐTc fibrin monoclonal antibody*

⁹⁹ᵐTc monoclonal antibodies to fibrin on platelets are now being developed to image thrombi on the lower limbs.

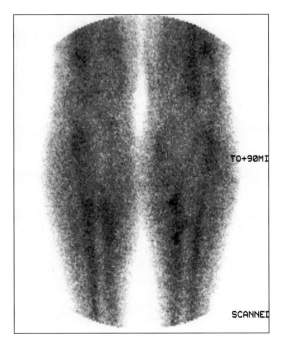

*a  Supine calves, 90 minutes*

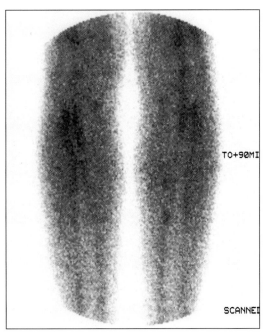

*b  Elevated calves, 90 minutes*

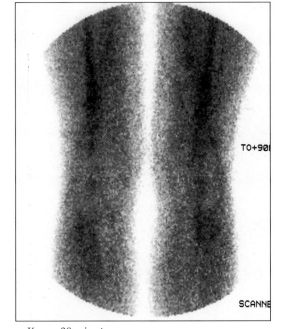

*c  Knees, 90 minutes*

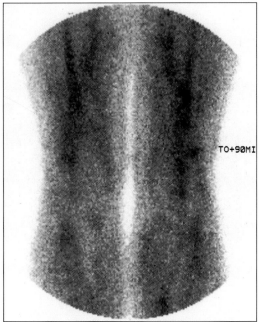

*d  Thighs, 90 minutes*

**Fig. 6.134**

*⁹⁹ᵐTc fibrin monoclonal antibody study: (a) supine calves; (b) elevated calves; (c) knees; (d) thighs.*

*This patient was a 62-year-old woman with pain in the left calf and slight swelling. The scan shows no focal uptake of tracer to suggest a* DVT.

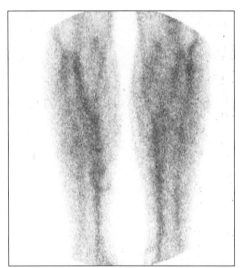

a  *Supine calves, 90 minutes*

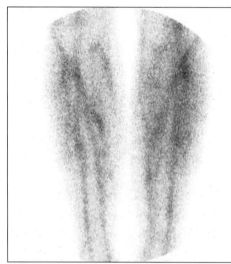

b  *Elevated calves, 90 minutes*

*Fig. 6.135*

$^{99m}$Tc fibrin monoclonal antibody study:
*(a, e)* supine calves; *(b, f)* elevated calves;
*(c)* knees; *(d)* thighs.

This patient was a 36-year-old woman
with pain and swelling of the left calf after
a sports accident. The images show blood
pool activity due, to varicosities, but
following leg elevation more focal uptake is
identified at sites of subsequently proven
thrombus (arrows, *f*).

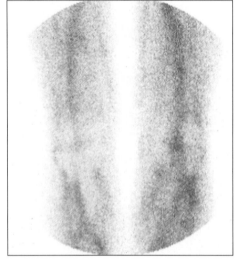

c  *Knees, 90 minutes*

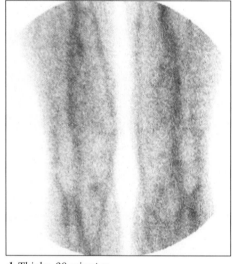

d  *Thighs, 90 minutes*

**Leg elevation assists in
the differentiation of
blood pool activity in**
**varicose veins from specific uptake
of tracer in a DVT.**

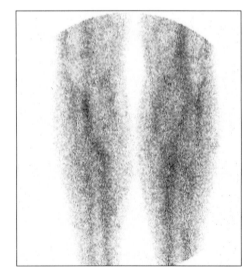

e  *Supine calves, 4 hours*

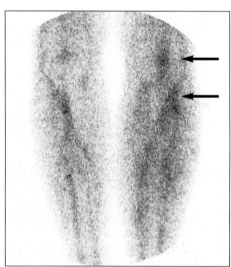

f  *Elevated calves, 4 hours*

# 6.4.6  Identification of cardiac tumour

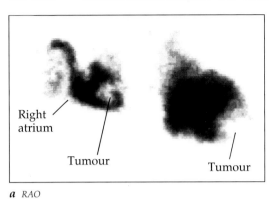

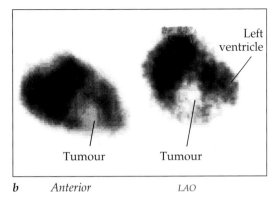

*a  RAO*                    *b        Anterior            LAO*

*Fig. 6.136*

*(a)* First pass study. *(b)* Gated blood pool study.

This child presented with weight loss, and was generally unwell with intermittent dyspnoea. Clinical investigation showed some cardiomegaly and a systolic murmur. Initial investigations included ultrasound and first pass and gated isotope angiograms. In this very unusual case the first pass study showed a space-occupying lesion in the apex of the right ventricle, which was confirmed on the gated study. Ultrasound examination also confirmed the finding. The lesion was subsequently discovered to be a fibrosarcoma of the right ventricle and was treated surgically.

# 6.4.7  Cardiac transplantation

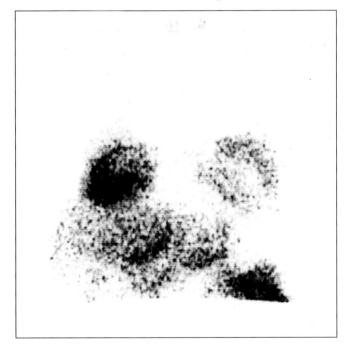

*Fig. 6.137*

$^{201}$Tl scan in a patient who has had a 'piggyback' cardiac transplantation.

The native heart is shown taking up $^{201}$Tl extremely poorly on the left side. The new transplant on the right side shows avid accumulation of $^{201}$Tl, confirming that it is well supplied with blood and is viable. *(Courtesy of Dr B Shepstone, Oxford, UK.)*

# CHAPTER 7

# LUNG

In the healthy individual there is a precise physiological balance between regional lung perfusion and regional alveolar ventilation, enabling the right-sided cardiac output to come into close proximity with alveolar gas and its oxygen load. Respiratory disease may lead to various imbalances between these two functions, which are often reflected by the lung scan. When both perfusion and ventilation images are obtained these are evaluated together to assess whether abnormalities are present and whether these are matched or mismatched.

Lung perfusion scanning may be assessed using technetium-99m ($^{99m}$Tc) labelled macroaggregates of albumin (MAA). These particles are injected intravenously, have an average size of between 10 and 40 μm, and pass into the pulmonary circulation, where they obstruct a small number of these vessels. The distribution throughout these vessels reflects regional lung perfusion, and imaging thus shows the relative distribution of pulmonary arterial blood flow through the lungs. As particles remain in the lungs, images can be obtained in multiple views.

Ventilation lung imaging provides a visual display of regional ventilation. In this case an isotope is mixed in air and is breathed by the patient. This study can provide either static images of ventilation in various views using krypton-81m ($^{81m}$Kr), which has a continual 'wash-in' phase because of its very short half-life, or else dynamic information representing the movement of the air into, and out of, various lung areas, using xenon-133 ($^{133}$Xe) for example. Each of these techniques has advantages and disadvantages, which are summarized in Table 7.2. Ventilation may also be assessed less accurately using aerosols or fine carbon particles labelled with $^{99m}$Tc. These agents have the advantage of availability.

In the case of suspected pulmonary thromboembolic disease (PTE), if there are segmental perfusion defects in both lungs and these areas are normally ventilated then the probability of disease is high, whereas if all defects are matched on both studies then the probability of PTE is low, and it is likely that parenchymal lung disease is present. Clearly, there is a greater need for combined ventilation and perfusion studies in the elderly since parenchymal lung disease is common among them. It should always be remembered, however, that abnormalities caused by parenchymal disease may be seen in the young on perfusion lung scans, particularly when acute bronchospasm is present. In all cases, when abnormalities are seen on the lung scan, a current chest x-ray should be available for comparison.

It should be noted that if a perfusion study only is obtained then this cannot be diagnostic for PTE. A normal study, however, will virtually exclude this diagnosis, and such information may be of great value.

## CHAPTER CONTENTS

# 7.1 ANATOMY

## Broncho-pulmonary segments

An understanding of the anatomical distribution of the broncho-pulmonary segments is necessary to obtain the most diagnostic information from the lung scan. It is also essential to increase confidence in differentiating between segmental and non-segmental perfusion defects, and to provide an indicator of the likely segmental vessels involved in those cases where arteriography is undertaken. Further, extending the diagnosis from simple pattern recognition to an anatomical basis provides greater credibility when reporting studies, and is of value in teaching.

The following illustrations (Figs 7.1a–f) are from casts of the broncho-pulmonary segments. Each segment has a pulmonary segmental artery, and provides the basis for segmental defects seen on subsequent lung scans. It should be noted that there is variation in site and position of the segments from individual to individual.

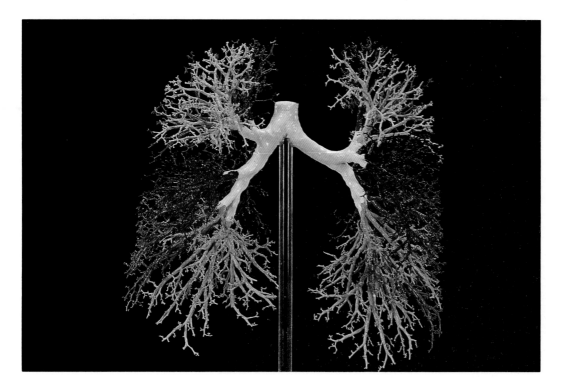

*Fig. 7.1*

*(a–f) Casts of the broncho-pulmonary segments. (Courtesy of Dr M. Hutchinson, London, UK.)*

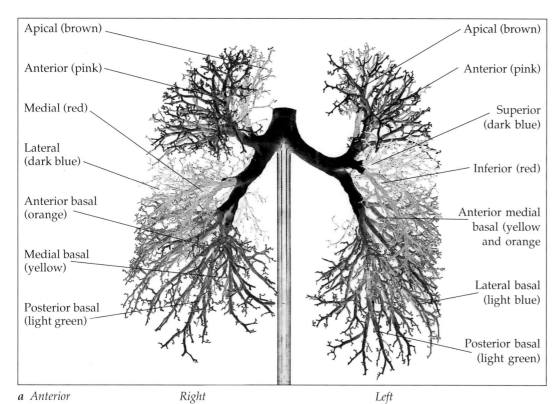

Apical (brown)

Anterior (pink)

Medial (red)

Lateral (dark blue)

Anterior basal (orange)

Medial basal (yellow)

Posterior basal (light green)

Apical (brown)

Anterior (pink)

Superior (dark blue)

Inferior (red)

Anterior medial basal (yellow and orange

Lateral basal (light blue)

Posterior basal (light green)

*a  Anterior*          Right                              Left

*continued*

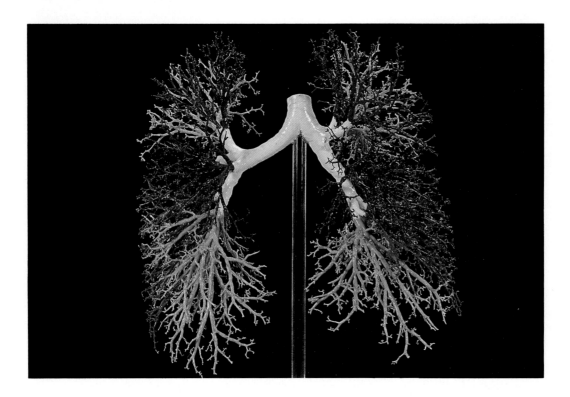

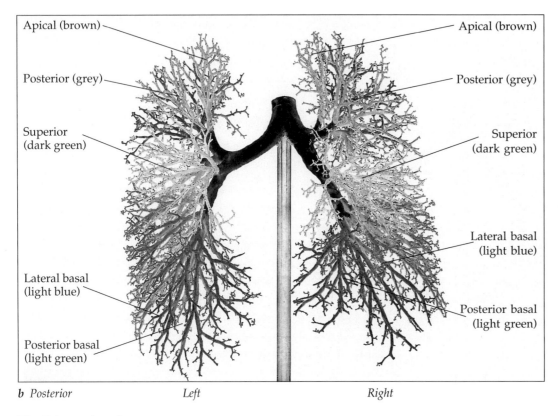

Apical (brown)

Posterior (grey)

Superior
(dark green)

Lateral basal
(light blue)

Posterior basal
(light green)

Apical (brown)

Posterior (grey)

Superior
(dark green)

Lateral basal
(light blue)

Posterior basal
(light green)

**b** *Posterior*                *Left*                        *Right*

*Fig. 7.1 continued*

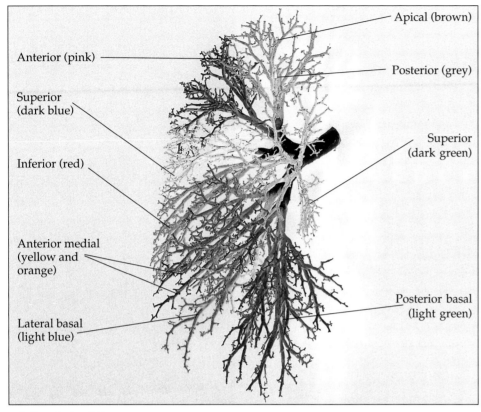
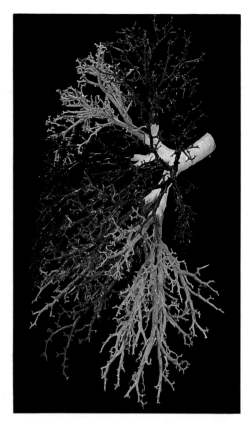

Apical (brown)

Anterior (pink)

Posterior (grey)

Superior
(dark blue)

Superior
(dark green)

Inferior (red)

Anterior medial
(yellow and
orange)

Posterior basal
(light green)

Lateral basal
(light blue)

*c  Left posterior oblique*

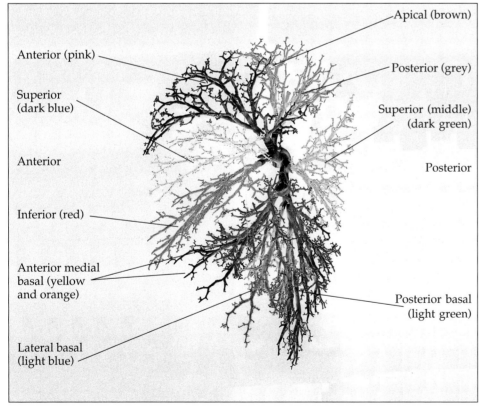
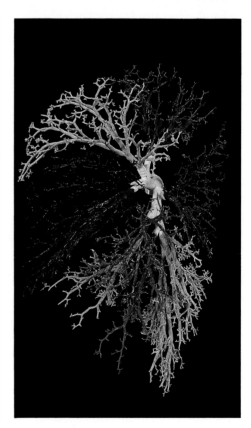

Apical (brown)

Anterior (pink)

Posterior (grey)

Superior
(dark blue)

Superior (middle)
(dark green)

Anterior

Posterior

Inferior (red)

Anterior medial
basal (yellow
and orange)

Posterior basal
(light green)

Lateral basal
(light blue)

*d  Left lateral*

**Fig. 7.1 continued**

*continued*

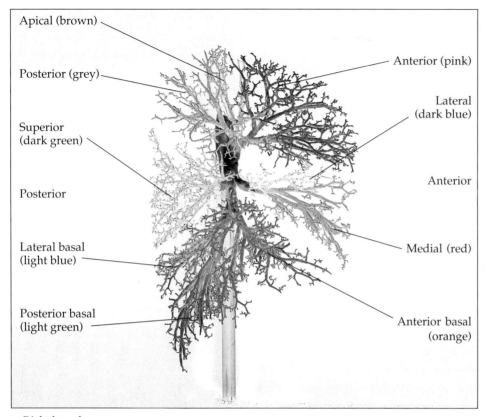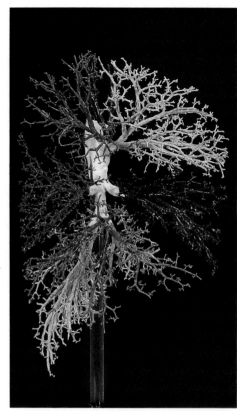

Apical (brown)

Posterior (grey)

Superior
(dark green)

Posterior

Lateral basal
(light blue)

Posterior basal
(light green)

Anterior (pink)

Lateral
(dark blue)

Anterior

Medial (red)

Anterior basal
(orange)

*e Right lateral*

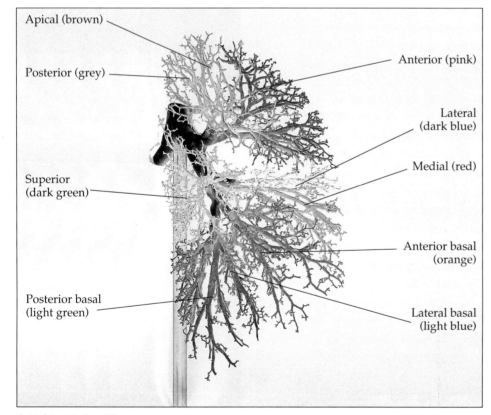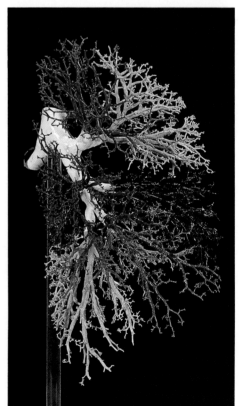

Apical (brown)

Posterior (grey)

Superior
(dark green)

Posterior basal
(light green)

Anterior (pink)

Lateral
(dark blue)

Medial (red)

Anterior basal
(orange)

Lateral basal
(light blue)

*f Right posterior oblique*

**Fig. 7.1 continued**

# 7.2 RADIOPHARMACEUTICALS

*Table 7.1 Radiopharmaceuticals for lung imaging*

| | Perfusion | | Ventilation | | | | |
|---|---|---|---|---|---|---|---|
| | $^{99m}$Tc MS | $^{99m}$Tc MAA | $^{133}$Xe | $^{127}$Xe | $^{81m}$Kr | $^{99m}$Tc DTPA aerosol | $^{99m}$Tc Technegas |
| Size | 20–45 µm | 10–60 µm | gas | gas | gas | 0.25–2.0 µm | carbon particles |
| Number | 100 000 | 400 000 | NA | NA | NA | NA | NA |
| $T_{1/2}$ | 6 hours | 6 hours | 5.25 days | 36.4 days | 13 sec | 6 hours | 6 hours |
| Origin | generator | generator | reactor | accelerator | generator | generator | generator |
| Energy (keV) | 140 | 140 | 80 | 375 (22%) 203 (65%) 172 (20%) | 190 | 140 | 140 |

NA, not applicable

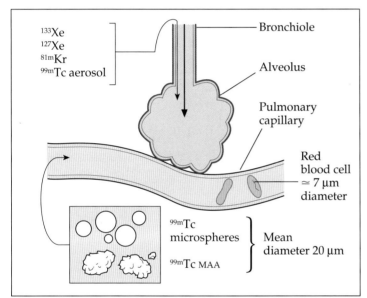

*a  Normal*

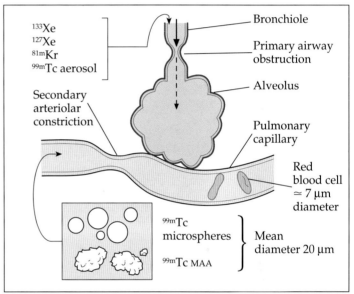

*b  Primary airway problem results in matched defect*

## Fig. 7.2

*Basic principles of perfusion/ventilation imaging.*

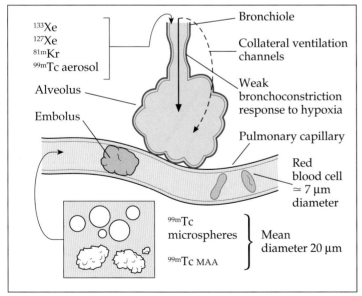

*c  Primary arteriolar problem (pulmonary embolus) results in unmatched defect*

# 7.3 NORMAL SCANS WITH VARIANTS AND ARTEFACTS

## 7.3.1 Normal perfusion lung scan

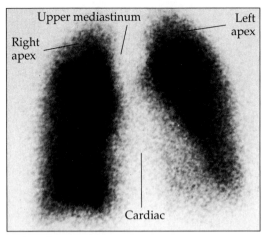

*a Anterior*

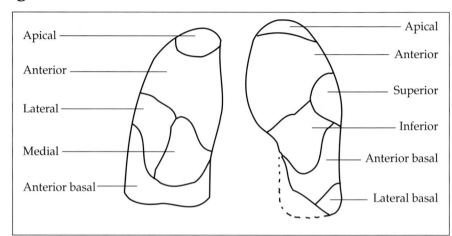

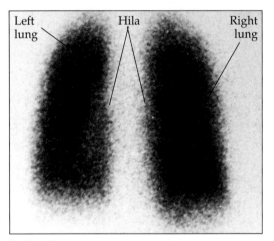

*b Posterior*

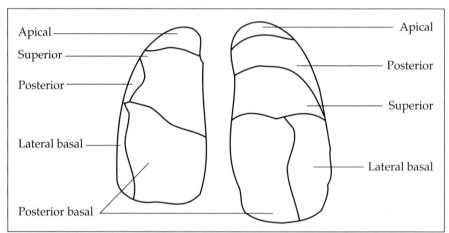

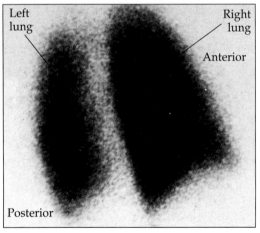

*c Right posterior oblique*

**Fig. 7.3**

*(a–f) A normal perfusion lung scan performed following the injection of $^{99m}$Tc MAA, showing the normal and even distribution of perfusion through both lung fields with the extrapulmonary impression from heart and great vessels.*

## NORMAL SCANS WITH VARIANTS AND ARTEFACTS

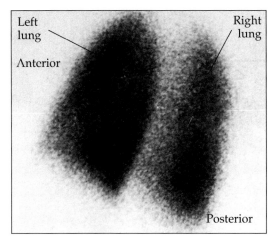
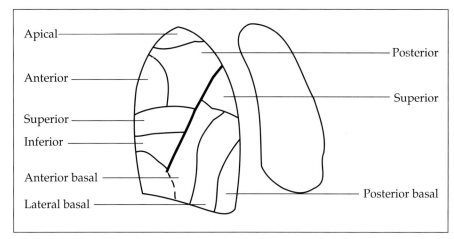

*d Left posterior oblique*

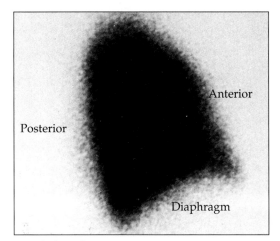
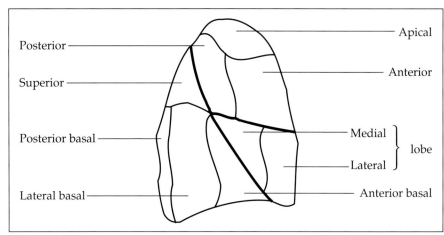

*e Right lateral*

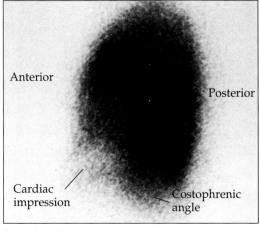
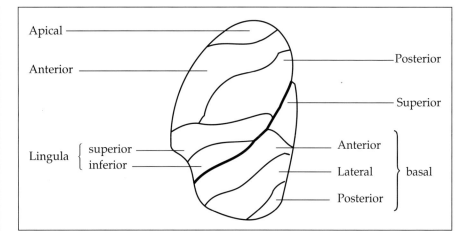

*f Left lateral*

## NORMAL SCANS WITH VARIANTS AND ARTEFACTS

*Table 7.2 Choice of ventilation method*

| Radiopharmaceutical | Advantages | Disadvantages |
|---|---|---|
| $^{81m}$Kr | Good images<br>Multiple views<br>Identical views can be obtained immediately after perfusion | Not available daily<br>Expensive<br>Ventilation only |
| $^{133}$Xe | Ventilation/volume/washout<br>Cheap | Single view only<br>Long half-life requires trapping equipment<br>Cannot be performed after perfusion study |
| $^{127}$Xe | Ventilation/volume/washout<br>Can be performed after perfusion | Expensive<br>Long half-life, requires trapping equipment<br>Not widely available |
| $^{99m}$Tc aerosol | Daily availability | Single view only<br>Technically difficult in patients with chronic obstructive airways disease<br>Cannot easily be performed after perfusion<br>Not true ventilation |
| $^{99m}$Tc Technegas | Daily availability | Not true ventilation<br>Cannot easily be performed after perfusion |

*Table 7.3 Comparison of functional information*

| Radiopharmaceutical | Ventilation | Volume | Washout |
|---|---|---|---|
| $^{81m}$Kr | yes | no | no |
| $^{133}$Xe | yes | yes | yes |
| $^{127}$Xe | yes | yes | yes |
| $^{99m}$Tc aerosol | approx | no | no |
| $^{99m}$Tc Technegas | approx | no | no |

## 7.3.2 Normal $^{81m}$Kr ventilation lung scan

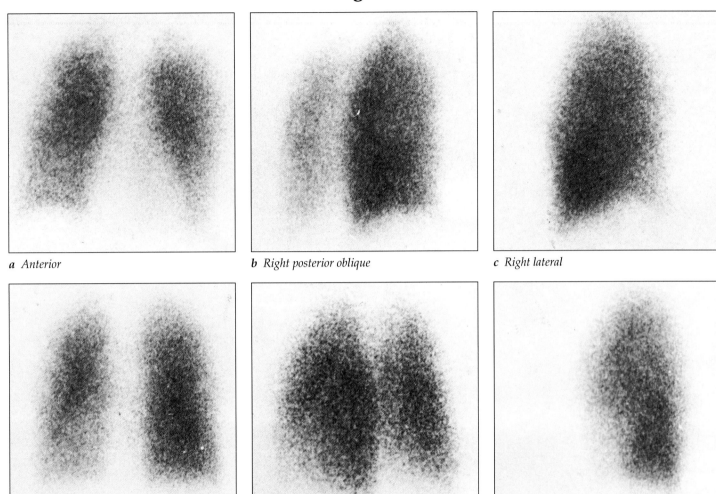

*a Anterior*

*b Right posterior oblique*

*c Right lateral*

*d Posterior*

*e Left posterior oblique*

*f Left lateral*

**Fig. 7.4**

*(a–f) A normal ventilation lung scan using $^{81m}$Kr immediately after the individual perfusion view.*

*Note the close matching of the distribution of blood flow and the distribution of ventilation.*

## 7.3.3    Normal $^{133}$Xe ventilation scan

The $^{133}$Xe ventilation scan shows three distinct phases. The initial phase is the wash-in or ventilation phase providing information about the rate of ventilation of different segments. This is comparable to the $^{81m}$Kr images. The second phase is the equilibrium phase representing the gas volume, which may be large (eg in a bulla, where the ventilation is poor). Finally, the wash-out phase, when the xenon has been disconnected, gives information about the possibility of any gas trapping, which may occur in obstructive airways disease.

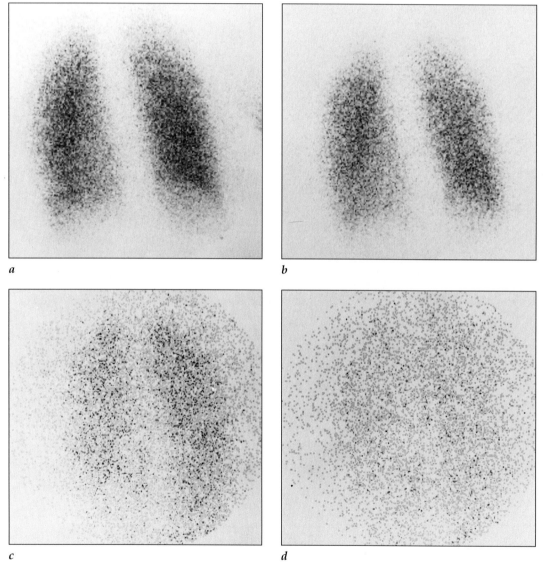

a

b

c

d

**Fig. 7.5**

Normal $^{133}$Xe ventilation scan, posterior view: **(a)** inspiratory wash-in phase; **(b)** equilibrium breath-hold phase; **(c,d)** washout phase. (Courtesy of Dr Tom Nunan, London, UK.)

**NORMAL SCANS WITH VARIANTS AND ARTEFACTS**

## 7.3.4    Normal ventilation study: ⁹⁹ᵐTc DTPA aerosol

*Fig. 7.6*

*(a–f) Normal ⁹⁹ᵐTc DTPA aerosol study.*

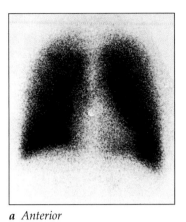

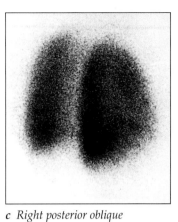

*a  Anterior*              *b  Posterior*              *c  Right posterior oblique*

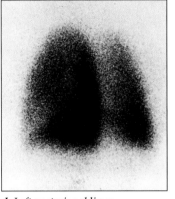

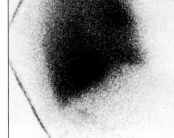

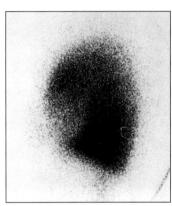

*d  Left posterior oblique*     *e  Right lateral*              *f  Left lateral*

## 7.3.5    Normal ventilation study: ⁹⁹ᵐTc Technegas

*Fig. 7.7*

*(a–c) Normal ⁹⁹ᵐTc Technegas study.*

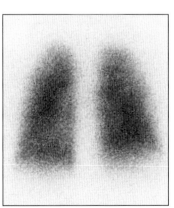

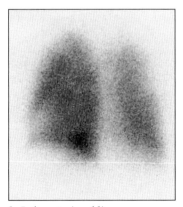

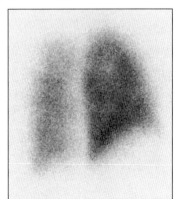

*a  Posterior*              *b  Left posterior oblique*      *c  Right posterior oblique*

## 7.3.6 Pulmonary permeability study

In addition to imaging with an aerosol, quantitation of the disappearance rate of tracer from regions of the lung can provide further information about lung permeability, eg smoking causes increased permeability and may degrade the ventilation images very rapidly (see page 575).

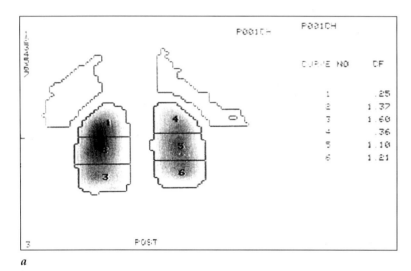

*a*

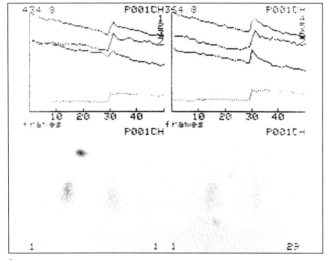

*b*

***Fig. 7.8***

*Normal pulmonary permeability study, based on $^{99m}$Tc DTPA aerosol study:*
*(a) regions of interest; (b) computer-generated curves; (c) results of pulmonary permeability from regions of interest (normal half-life greater than 60 minutes). (Courtesy of Drs P Wraight and L Smith, Cambridge, UK.)*

P001CH LUNG PERM

| CURVE NO | CF | HALF-LIFE | +/- MINS | R≠R |
|---|---|---|---|---|
| 1 | .25 | 104.9 | -4.5 | .95 |
| 2 | 1.37 | 89.6 | -4.1 | .95 |
| 3 | 1.60 | 120.0 | -18.9 | .59 |
| 4 | .36 | 94.0 | -4.3 | .95 |
| 5 | 1.10 | 94.6 | -3.5 | .96 |
| 6 | 1.21 | 81.2 | -7.2 | .82 |

*c*

# 7.3.7 Variants and artefacts

## ⁹⁹ᵐTc MAA: *thyroid visualization*

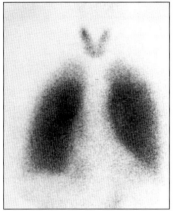

*Anterior*

**Fig. 7.9**

*⁹⁹ᵐTc MAA perfusion image, showing clear visualization of the thyroid gland and faint visualization of the stomach. These findings are due to free pertechnetate in the injection.*

## ⁸¹ᵐKr: *face mask*

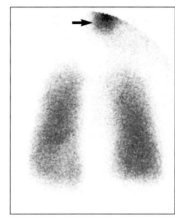

*Posterior*

**Fig. 7.10**

*Posterior ventilation image using ⁸¹ᵐKr. Activity from the face mask is seen at the upper edge of the image (arrow).*

## *Aerosol clumping*

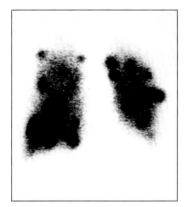

*a Anterior*

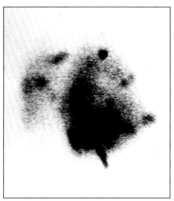

*b Right posterior oblique*

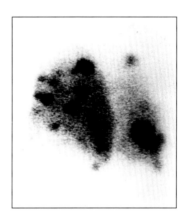

*c Left posterior oblique*

**Fig. 7.11**

*(a–c) ⁹⁹ᵐTc aerosol ventilation images, showing significant particle clumping due to chronic obstructive airways disease.*

## *Technegas particle clumping*

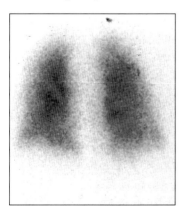

*a Posterior*

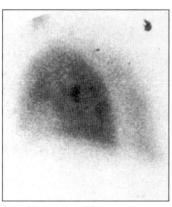

*b Left posterior oblique*

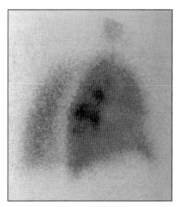

*c Right posterior oblique*

**Fig. 7.12**

*(a–c) Technegas ventilation images, showing particle clumping. This is caused by incorrect heating of carbon particles.*

## *Appearances typical of cardiomegaly*

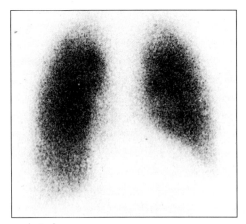

*a Anterior*

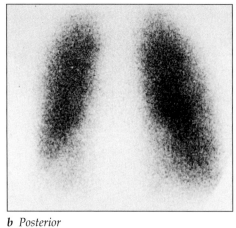

*b Posterior*

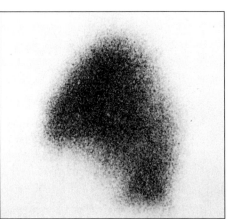

*c Left lateral*

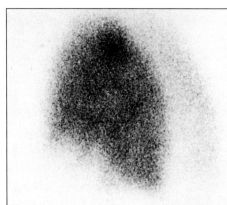

*d Left posterior oblique*

### Fig. 7.13

*(a–d) Perfusion lung scan in a 76-year-old man with cardiomegaly.*

The heart will always produce a perfusion/ ventilation 'defect'. This may be very pronounced when there is significant cardiomegaly, as in the case in Fig. 7.13.

## *Appearances typical of pleural effusion*

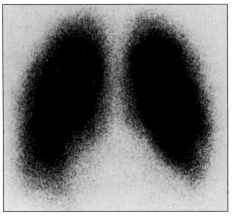
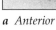

*a Anterior*

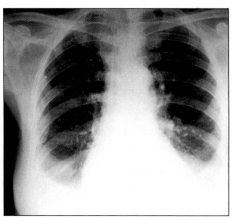

*b X-ray*

### Fig. 7.14

*(a) Perfusion lung scan, showing the typical loss of perfusion in both costophrenic regions. (b) Chest x-ray, showing the appearances of bilateral plural effusions.*

## NORMAL SCANS WITH VARIANTS AND ARTEFACTS

## *Appearances typical of pulmonary venous hypertension*

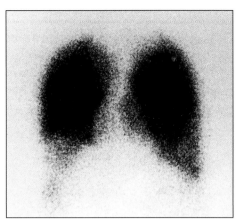

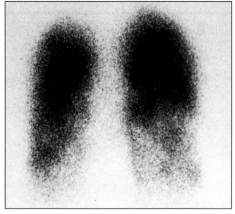

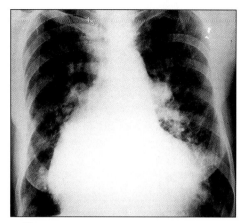

*a Anterior*

*b Posterior*

*c X-ray*

**Fig. 7.15**

*(a, b) Perfusion lung scan, demonstrating pulmonary venous hypertension. (c) Chest x-ray.*

*On the perfusion lung scan there is gross upper lobe diversion of tracer with irregular non-segmental perfusion defects in both lower lobes. Cardiomegaly is noted. The chest x-ray shows gross parenchymal lung disease. The scan appearances are those of pulmonary venous hypertension.*

**In patients with pulmonary venous hypertension the injection of microspheres should be given with the patient sitting upright to achieve distribution to the bases.**

## *Appearances typical of extrapulmonary structures*

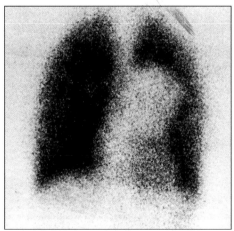

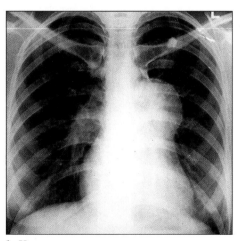

*a Anterior*

*b X-ray*

**Fig. 7.16**

*(a) Perfusion lung scan and (b) chest x-ray, demonstrating aneurysmal dilation of the pulmonary artery.*

*There is a gross area of decreased perfusion in the upper left hilum, which corresponds to the dilated pulmonary artery seen on the chest x-ray. The scan findings were attributable to aneurysmal dilation of the pulmonary artery.*

**The case in Fig. 7.16 again demonstrates the vital importance of evaluating the current chest x-ray for proper interpretation of the lung scan.**

# 7.4  CLINICAL APPLICATIONS

The clinical applications of perfusion/ventilation lung scanning are listed below, and examples of the various clinical problems are given on subsequent pages.

**7.4.1  Pulmonary embolism**
Assessment of functional patterns on the lung scan
Diagnosis of pulmonary embolism
Pulmonary embolism associated with chronic obstructive airways disease
Pulmonary embolism diagnosed in the presence of pleural effusion
Perfusion/ventilation lung scan in the management and follow-up of pulmonary embolism

**7.4.2  Parenchymal lung disease**
Single matched defect: emphysema
Matched defects caused by chronic obstructive airways disease
Matched subsegmental defect caused by a parenchymal lung lesion
Bilateral basal matched defects

**7.4.3  Differential diagnosis of massive loss of perfusion to one lung**
Causes of massive loss of perfusion
Pulmonary embolism
Bullous emphysema
Carcinoma of the bronchus

Pulmonary metastasis
Atresia of the right pulmonary artery
Pleural effusion

**7.4.4  Conditions simulating pulmonary embolism**
Asthma
Vasculitis
Pulmonary metastases
Tumour emboli
Emphysematous bulla
Fibrotic lung disease
Cardiac failure

**7.4.5  Chronic obstructive airways disease**
Patterns of abnormality with $^{133}$Xe ventilation
Patterns of abnormality with $^{99m}$Tc aerosol
Ventilation defects more severe than perfusion defects, caused by pneumonia
Ventilation/perfusion lung scan appearance of pneumonia

**7.4.6  Assessment of carcinoma of the bronchus**

**7.4.7  Inhaled foreign body**

**7.4.8  Assessment of lung permeability**

# 7.4.1    Pulmonary embolism

The main indication for radionuclide lung scanning is the identification of pulmonary emboli. History and clinical examination are often non-specific in this situation, and lung scanning and pulmonary angiography provide the only diagnostic investigations (see below). It should be realized that pulmonary embolization may, and usually does, occur without infarction. An embolus arises when a thrombus is dislodged, most often from a peripheral vein, enters the pulmonary artery and becomes impacted.

Infarction does not normally occur, since the viability of the lung is maintained by the systemic bronchial arteries. A pulmonary embolus, unaccompanied by infarction, does not cause changes on the chest x-ray.

It should be noted that all the above features are non-specific, and the only diagnostic tests are the lung scan and pulmonary angiography. The advantages and disadvantages of each are listed in Table 7.4.

*Table 7.4*

| Perfusion/ventilation lung scan | Pulmonary angiography |
| --- | --- |
| Simple to perform | Difficult to perform |
| Easy to repeat | Difficult to repeat |
| Safe | Occasional serious complications |
| No morbidity | Some morbidity |
| Sensitive | Less sensitive |
| Non-specific | Much more specific |

## *Assessment of functional patterns on the lung scan*

Perfusion defects may be:

- Subsegmental, ie lying within a segment but smaller than a whole segment (less than 25% of the segment)
- Segmental, ie outlining the anatomical vascular segment (greater than 75% of the segment)
- Non-segmental, ie not reflecting the anatomical limits defined by the vessels supplying the segment.

The ventilation may:

- Match the perfusion defect, ie show the same area of loss
- Be unmatched:
  (a) show normal ventilation or considerably less effect on ventilation, or much less commonly
  (b) show more ventilation abnormality, or ventilation abnormalities, where the perfusion is normal.

- **Emboli are most commonly segmental because they block the vascular supply to a segment.**
- **Parenchymal disease is not primarily vascular, and therefore is non-segmental.**
- **Subsegmental defects may be caused by either emboli or parenchymal lung disease.**

## Diagnosis of pulmonary embolism

A perfusion lung scan provides a sensitive method of assessing the presence of pulmonary pathology, but appearances are non-specific. A normal perfusion study can be reported as such without a chest x-ray being available. However, if there is any perfusion abnormality present, interpretation is not possible unless the findings are correlated with a high-quality chest x-ray obtained within 24 hours of the perfusion study. The majority of lesions, such as consolidation, effusion, collapse and bullae, which are visualized on x-ray, will produce both perfusion and ventilation defects. In the case of a pulmonary embolus the perfusion study will be abnormal as a result of the thrombus being impacted in a pulmonary artery or one of its branches, whereas the ventilation study will be normal. The chest x-ray will also be normal, unless pulmonary infarction has occurred.

*Table 7.5 Patterns of lung scan findings in the evaluation of pulmonary embolic disease*

| Lung scan finding | Interpretation |
|---|---|
| *Diagnostic (no PTE or PTE)* | |
| Normal perfusion lung scan and a normal chest x-ray | No PTE |
| Subsegmental perfusion defect or defects with matched ventilation defects and a normal chest x-ray | Low probability of PTE (less than 5%) |
| Segmental, lobar or large non-segmental perfusion defect with matched ventilation and a normal chest x-ray | Low probability of PTE (less than 5%) |
| Bilateral segmental perfusion defects with normal ventilation (ie unmatched defects) and a normal chest x-ray | High probability of PTE (greater than 95%) |
| One lung with matched ventilation/perfusion defect with corresponding abnormality on chest x-ray, and the other lung with multiple segmental perfusion defects and normal ventilation | High probability of PTE (greater than 95%) (Probable pulmonary infarct plus PTE) |
| *Probable PTE (50–70% probability)* | |
| Multisegmental perfusion defect in one lung only, with normal ventilation and a normal chest x-ray | |
| *Non-diagnostic for PTE (30–50% probability)* | |
| Any matched perfusion/ventilation abnormality associated with an abnormality on chest x-ray. (This is often seen with widespread parenchymal lung disease, consolidation or pleural effusion.) The lung scan is non-diagnostic and, if clinically relevant, pulmonary angiography is required to establish a diagnosis of PTE | |

## CLINICAL APPLICATIONS

### Perfusion

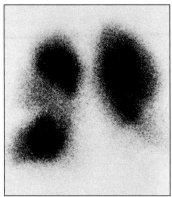
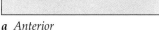

*a Anterior*

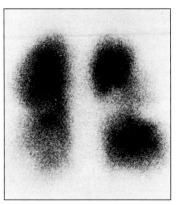

*b Posterior*

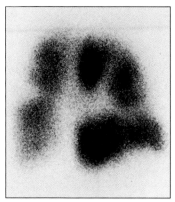

*c Right posterior oblique*

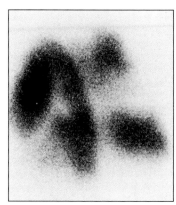

*d Left posterior oblique*

### Ventilation

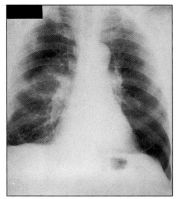

*e X-ray*

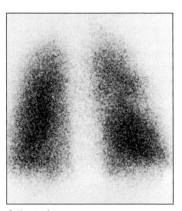

*f Posterior*

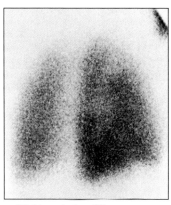

*g Right posterior oblique*

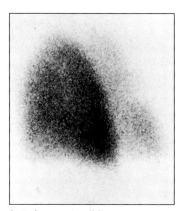

*h Left posterior oblique*

**Fig. 7.17**

*(a–d)* Perfusion lung scan in a 60-year-old man with pulmonary embolic disease. *(e)* Chest x-ray. *(f–h)* Ventilation lung scan.

Points to note from this case about pulmonary embolism are as follows. The perfusion defects are well demarcated and segmental. The ventilation scan using $^{81m}Kr$ shows normal ventilation in most of the areas that have perfusion defects, although the most profoundly abnormal perfusion areas do show a minor ventilation abnormality which is quite commonly seen in pulmonary embolism, and is often associated with some minor infarction. Pulmonary embolism is frequently multifocal. The chest x-ray, although showing some minor mid-zone abnormalities on the right where the more profound perfusion defects and the minor ventilation defect are seen, is quite normal in most of the other areas. Note that the chest x-ray corresponds more closely to ventilation scans than it does to perfusion scans.

- Over 90% of all lung scans are undertaken as part of the initial evaluation or follow-up of patients suspected or known to have pulmonary embolism.
- A normal perfusion lung study excludes PTE.
- The pattern of bilateral segmental perfusion defects which are normally ventilated is diagnostic of PTE.
- An abnormal perfusion scan showing multiple defects which changes over seven days raises the probability of PTE being present.
- The accurate diagnosis of PTE is important, since anti-coagulation is associated with a significant risk of major complications. However, therapeutic anticoagulation in the presence of PTE reduces the mortality fourfold.
- A pulmonary angiogram displays the anatomy of the pulmonary vascular bed, while a lung scan displays the distribution of ventilation and pulmonary blood flow.

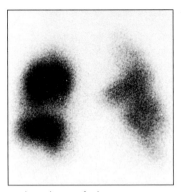

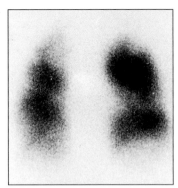

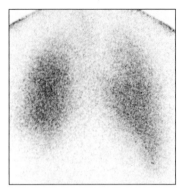

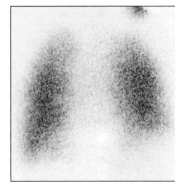

*a* Anterior, perfusion     *b* Posterior, perfusion     *c* Anterior, ventilation     *d* Posterior, ventilation

**Fig. 7.18**

*(a, b)* Perfusion lung scan in a 75-year-old man with PTE. *(c, d)* Ventilation lung scan.
   There are multiple segmental perfusion defects seen throughout both lung fields. The ventilation study, however, is essentially normal. There is a high right diaphragm present.

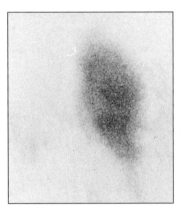

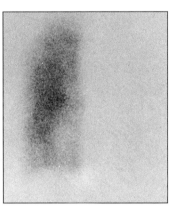

**Fig. 7.19**

*(a, b)* Perfusion lung scan in a 45-year-old woman with massive pulmonary embolism occluding the right pulmonary artery.
   Perfusion to the left lung is relatively normal, but there is no perfusion to the right lung.

*a* Anterior     *b* Posterior

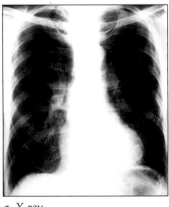

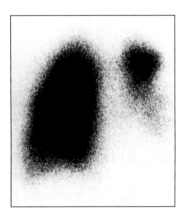

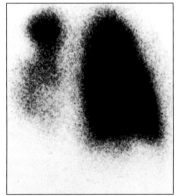

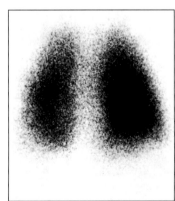

*a* X-ray     *b* Anterior, perfusion     *c* Posterior, perfusion     *d* Posterior, ventilation

**Fig. 7.20**

Perfusion/ventilation scan of a 61-year-old woman who presented postoperatively with chest pain. *(a)* Chest x-ray. *(b, c)* Perfusion lung scan. *(d)* Ventilation scan.
   The chest x-ray shows slight hypertranslucency of the left lung only, but the perfusion scan confirms that this is due to massive loss of perfusion to the left lung, which on the ventilation scan is essentially normal. This is an example of a massive unilateral left-sided pulmonary embolus.

## Diagnosis of pulmonary embolism using ¹³³Xe

### Ventilation

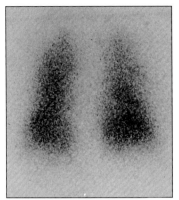 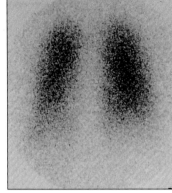 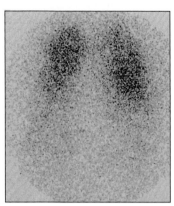 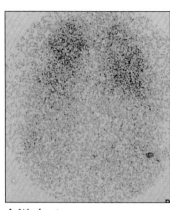

**a** Wash-in  **b** Equilibrium  **c** Washout  **d** Washout

### Perfusion

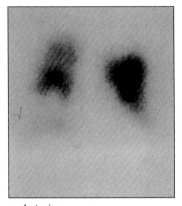 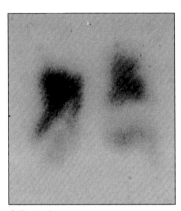 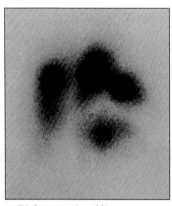 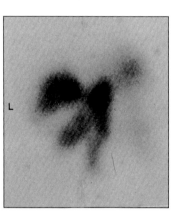

**e** Anterior  **f** Posterior  **g** Right posterior oblique  **h** Left posterior oblique

**Fig. 7.21**

*(a–d) The sequence of ¹³³Xe studies performed prior to the perfusion scan demonstrates almost normal ventilation. The perfusion images (e–h) show multiple segmental perfusion defects diagnostic of pulmonary emboli. (Courtesy of Dr Tom Nunan, London, UK.)*

The disadvantages of ¹³³Xe are that a single view only can be obtained and the need to perform the study prior to the perfusion scan; therefore the optimal view cannot be selected to demonstrate ventilation in a particular area of interest.

*Diagnosis of pulmonary embolism using $^{99m}Tc$ aerosol*

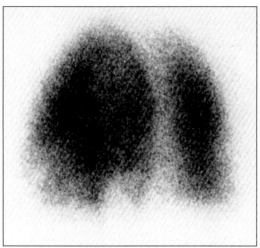

**a** Left posterior oblique

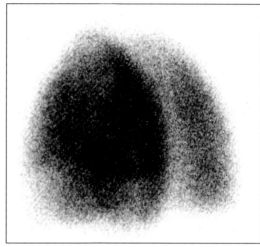

**b**

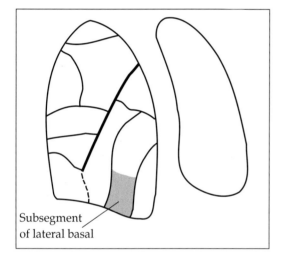

Subsegment
of lateral basal

*Fig. 7.22*

(a) *Perfusion lung scan.*
(b) *Aerosol image.*

*A subsegmental perfusion defect is seen involving the lateral basal segment of the left lung. This is ventilated. It should be noted that this pattern is not in itself diagnostic of pulmonary embolic disease.*

*Nevertheless, this study illustrates well how the aerosol ventilation method can provide additional information following a perfusion study, if $^{81m}Kr$ or $^{127}Xe$ are not available.*

**Subtraction of perfusion from a subsequent ventilation image may assist in difficult cases when both radiopharmaceuticals are $^{99m}Tc$-labelled.**

## CLINICAL APPLICATIONS

*Diagnosis of pulmonary embolism using $^{99m}$Tc Technegas*

*Perfusion*

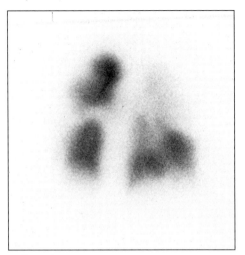

*a Posterior*

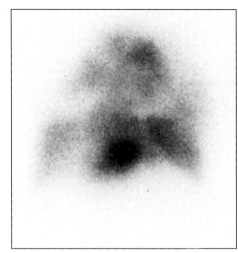

*b Left posterior oblique*

*c Right posterior oblique*

*Technegas*

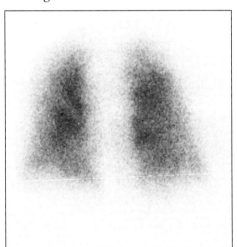

*d Posterior*

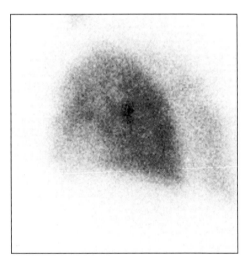

*e Left posterior oblique*

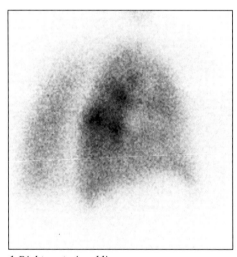

*f Right posterior oblique*

**Fig. 7.23**

*This patient is a 63-year-old female with a 10-day history of chest pain and a normal chest x-ray. The perfusion images (a–c) show multiple perfusion defects and the Technegas images (d–f) show relatively normal ventilation, although deposition of activity in the central airways is noted.*

## Pulmonary embolism associated with chronic obstructive airways disease

Although it is necessary to be aware that chronic obstructive lung disease will cause perfusion defects, pulmonary embolism may still be diagnosed in the presence of chronic obstructive airways disease.

*Perfusion*

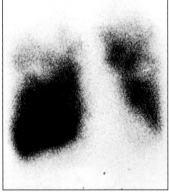 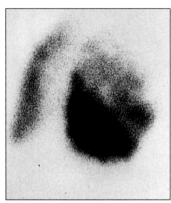 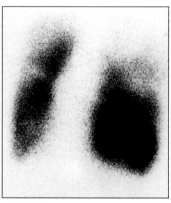 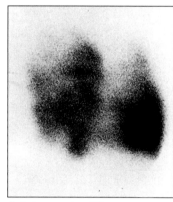

*a Anterior*   *b Right posterior oblique*   *c Posterior*   *d Left posterior oblique*

*Ventilation*

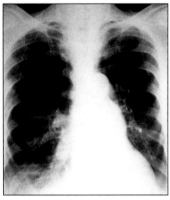 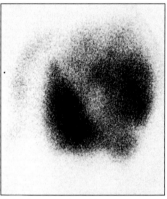 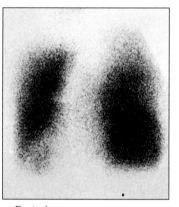 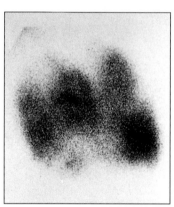

*e X-ray*   *f Right posterior oblique*   *g Posterior*   *h Left posterior oblique*

**Fig. 7.24**

*(a–d) Perfusion lung scan. (e) Chest x-ray. (f–h) Ventilation lung scan.*

*This elderly man, who was known to have chronic obstructive airways disease, developed clinical features suggestive of pulmonary embolism, which included calf-swelling, haemoptysis and pleuritic pain. The lung scan shows non-segmental perfusion defects, many of which are matched by ventilation defects. There are, in addition, ventilation defects which are more severe than perfusion abnormalities, eg at the left base, best seen on the left posterior oblique view (h).*

*Furthermore, there are segmental defects at the right apex and mid-zone, which have relatively normal ventilation, caused by pulmonary embolic disease. This is best demonstrated on the posterior (g) and right posterior oblique (f) views.*

 **The presence of parenchymal lung disease is not a contraindication to performing a perfusion lung scan, but it must be assessed with the ventilation scan with extreme care.**

## CLINICAL APPLICATIONS

### *Pulmonary embolism diagnosed in the presence of pleural effusion*

*Perfusion*

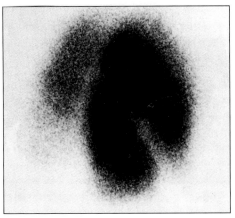

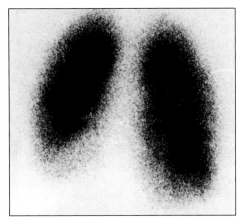

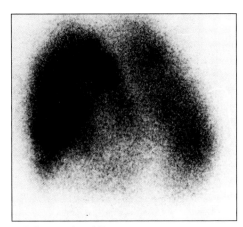

*a Right posterior oblique*

*b Posterior*

*c Left posterior oblique*

*Ventilation*

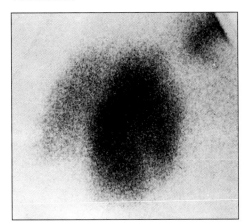

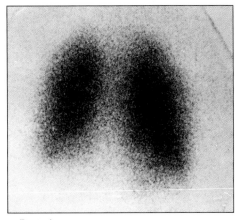

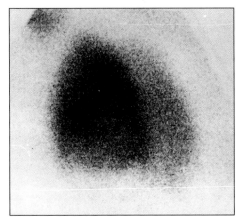

*d Right posterior oblique*

*e Posterior*

*f Left posterior oblique*

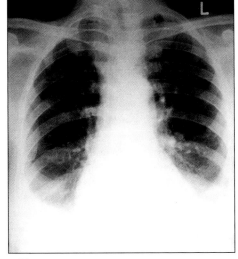

*g X-ray*

**Fig. 7.25**

*(a–c)* Perfusion lung scan. *(d–f)* Ventilation lung scan. *(g)* Chest x-ray.

On the perfusion study there is some non-homogeneity of tracer uptake throughout both lung fields, with a large segmental defect occupying most of the lower left lobe, seen best in the left posterior oblique view *(c)*. In addition, subsegmental defects are seen in the right base, and there is a defect in the region of the interlobar fissure. The ventilation study shows good ventilation to the left lower lobe, with the other defects matched. The scan findings at both bases were in keeping with known pleural effusions *(g)*, and the defect in the interlobar fissure reflected fluid at that site. However, there is a huge area of mismatch occupying the left lower lobe, and the scan findings were due to a pulmonary embolus.

Careful analysis of perfusion/ventilation lung scans may allow the diagnosis of pulmonary embolic disease, even in the presence of pleural effusion.

## *Perfusion/ventilation lung scan in the management and follow-up of pulmonary embolism*

Serial lung scans may be of value in the management of patients with pulmonary embolic disease, to help decide when anticoagulant therapy should be discontinued. From such studies, it is now recognized that pulmonary emboli may clear as early as 24 hours, or residual defects may persist indefinitely. If a patient is developing new lesions despite adequate anticoagulation then this might influence a decision with regard to more invasive therapy, such as insertion of a filter into the inferior vena cava. Following a pulmonary embolus, a lung scan will also establish a new baseline, in order that further episodes may be distinguished from residual defects. The clearing of perfusion defects may be of assistance in itself in establishing a diagnosis of pulmonary embolic disease, when this was only initially suspected but not proven.

### *Situations likely to delay the clearing of pulmonary emboli*

- Elderly patient
- Underlying chronic lung disease
- Underlying heart failure
- Very extensive infarction.

### *Follow-up of pulmonary emboli*

- Partial resolution
- Complete resolution
- Persistent defects
- New abnormalities.

 If an embolus is going to clear, it will do so by three months. What is left after three months will persist indefinitely.

## Partial resolution of emboli

### Initial scan

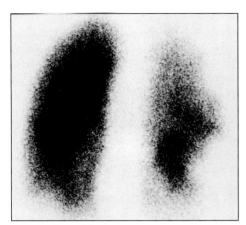

*a* Posterior, perfusion

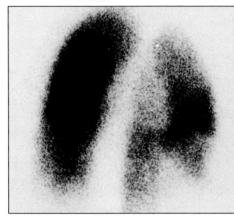

*b* Right posterior oblique, perfusion

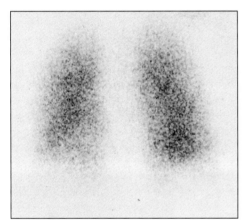

*c* Posterior, ventilation

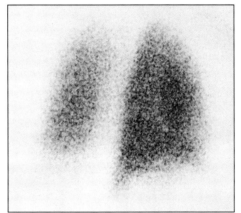

*d* Right posterior oblique, ventilation

### Four days later on heparin

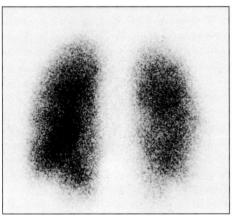

*e* Posterior, perfusion

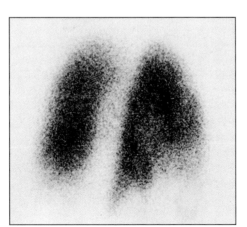

*f* Right posterior oblique, perfusion

**Fig. 7.26**

**(a, b)** Initial perfusion lung scan.
**(c, d)** Initial ventilation lung scan.
**(e–f)** Repeat perfusion lung scan.

This elderly patient developed dyspnoea postoperatively and was thought to have had a pulmonary embolus. The initial perfusion lung scan shows widespread segmental defects, mainly affecting the right lung. The ventilation study is normal, confirming the diagnosis of pulmonary embolic disease. After only 4 days on subcutaneous heparin, it can be seen from the repeat perfusion scan that there has been significant partial resolution in the right lung, although there are small defects persisting at the base.

## Partial resolution of segmental defects

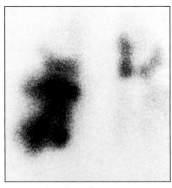
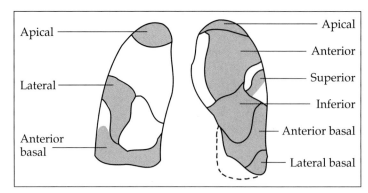

*a  Anterior, 0 weeks*

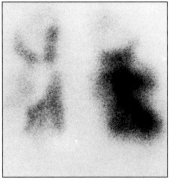
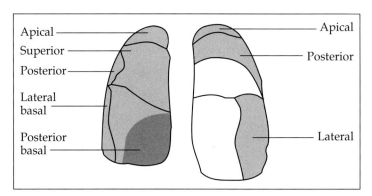

*b  Posterior, 0 weeks*

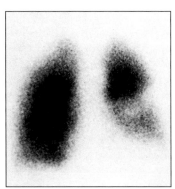
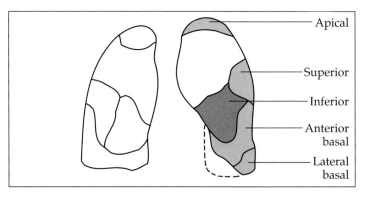

*c  Anterior, 3 weeks*

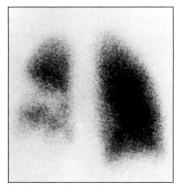
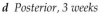
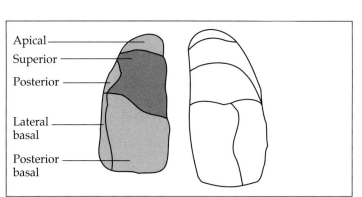

*d  Posterior, 3 weeks*

***Fig. 7.27***

***(a, b)** Perfusion lung scan.* ***(c, d)** Repeat study 3 weeks later.*

*On the original study there are very extensive clear-cut segmental perfusion defects involving both lung fields, affecting the left lung more severely than the right. The ventilation study was normal, and the scan findings were therefore classically those of extensive pulmonary embolic disease. The repeat study 3 weeks later shows the right lung to be completely normal. The left lung shows marked improvement, but there are still perfusion defects at the left base. There has therefore been clear evidence of partial resolution of former pulmonary embolic disease, with no evidence of new lesions occurring.*

## CLINICAL APPLICATIONS

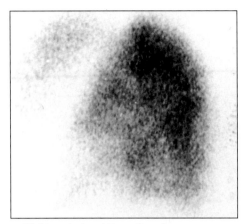

*a  Right posterior oblique, 0 weeks*

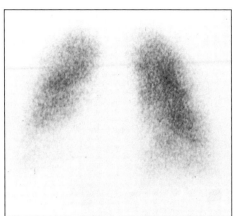

*b  Anterior, 0 weeks*

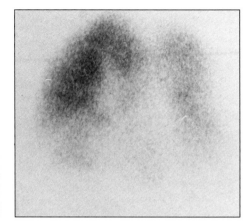

*c  Left posterior oblique, 0 weeks*

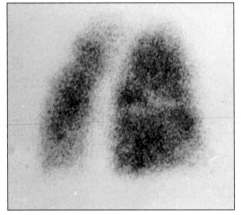

*d  Right posterior oblique, 3 months*

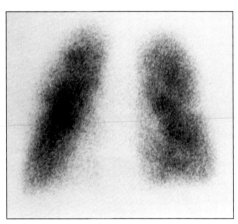

*e  Anterior, 3 months*

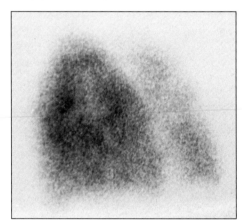

*f  Left posterior oblique, 3 months*

**Fig. 7.28**

*(a–c) Initial perfusion lung scan. (d–f) Repeat study 3 months later.*

*   In this further case of pulmonary embolic disease the original perfusion study shows
large segmental defects at both bases. The ventilation study was normal. On the repeat
study 3 months later there is essentially resolution of these defects. It should be noted,
however, that there are multiple minor subsegmental defects present throughout the lung
fields, of uncertain significance.*

## Complete resolution of pulmonary emboli

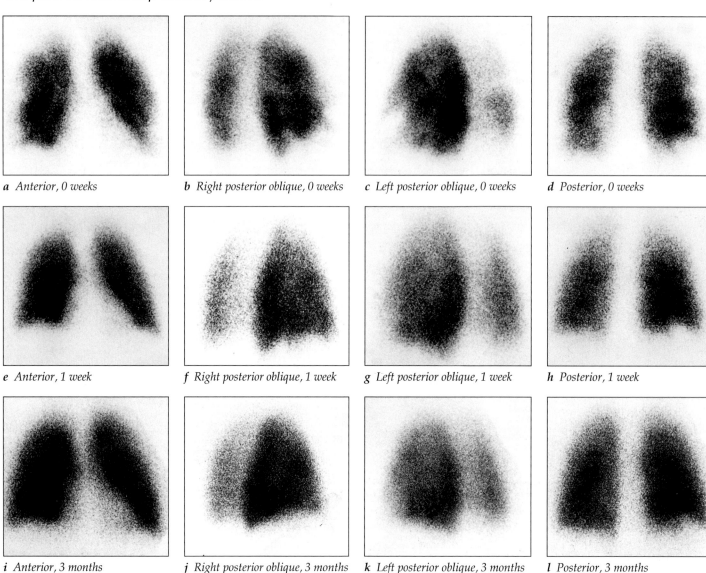

*a  Anterior, 0 weeks*    *b  Right posterior oblique, 0 weeks*    *c  Left posterior oblique, 0 weeks*    *d  Posterior, 0 weeks*

*e  Anterior, 1 week*    *f  Right posterior oblique, 1 week*    *g  Left posterior oblique, 1 week*    *h  Posterior, 1 week*

*i  Anterior, 3 months*    *j  Right posterior oblique, 3 months*    *k  Left posterior oblique, 3 months*    *l  Posterior, 3 months*

**Fig. 7.29**

**(a–d)** *Initial perfusion lung scan.* **(e–h)** *Repeat study 1 week later.* **(i–l)** *Repeat study 3 months later.*
 *A 38-year-old man with* PTE. *On the initial perfusion study there is non-homogeneity of tracer uptake throughout both lung fields, with multiple segmental defects seen, particularly at both bases and the right mid-zone. The ventilation study was normal, confirming the diagnosis of pulmonary embolic disease. The repeat perfusion study 1 week later shows subsegmental perfusion defects at both bases, but overall there has been marked resolution of the previously noted pulmonary emboli. The further repeat study at 3 months is essentially normal.*

## CLINICAL APPLICATIONS

### Persistent segmental perfusion defect

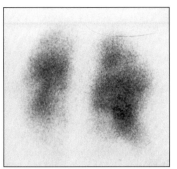

*a  Posterior, 0 months*

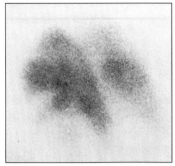

*b  Left posterior oblique, 0 months*

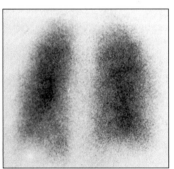

*c  Posterior, 6 months*

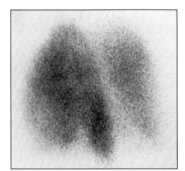

*d  Left posterior oblique, 6 months*

**Fig. 7.30**

*(a, b) Initial perfusion lung scan. (c, d) Repeat study 6 months later.*

*In this case of pulmonary embolic disease the original perfusion lung scan shows multiple segmental defects throughout both lung fields. The repeat study 6 months later shows resolution of the majority of defects, although there is a clear segmental defect still present at the left base. This is best seen on the left posterior oblique view (d), and it should be noted that this defect is smaller than previously.*

**A persistent perfusion defect with normal ventilation can occur without infarction because the nutritional requirements are met by an adequate bronchial blood supply.**

### Persistent defects after six months

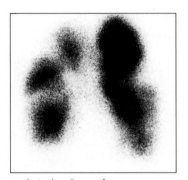

*a  Anterior, 0 months*

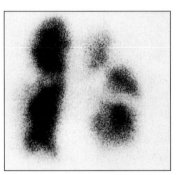

*b  Posterior, 0 months*

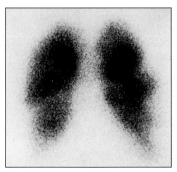

*c  Anterior, 6 months*

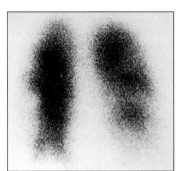

*d  Posterior, 6 months*

**Fig. 7.31**

*An 82-year-old man with pulmonary embolic disease. (a, b) Initial perfusion lung scan. (c, d) Repeat perfusion scan 6 months later.*

*On the original perfusion study there are multiple segmental defects present, which were normally ventilated. This pattern is therefore diagnostic of pulmonary embolic disease. On the repeat study 6 months later considerable resolution has occurred, but there are persistent segmental abnormalities present at both bases.*

## Unchanged perfusion defects

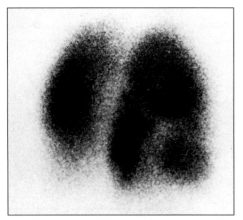

*a Right posterior oblique, perfusion, 0 months*

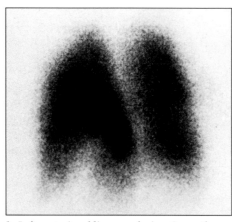

*b Left posterior oblique, perfusion, 0 months*

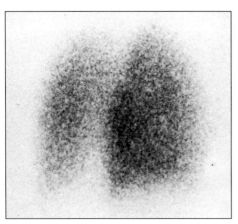

*c Right posterior oblique, ventilation, 0 months*

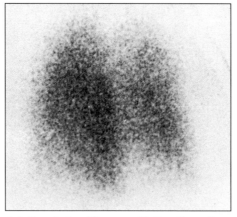

*d Left posterior oblique, ventilation, 0 months*

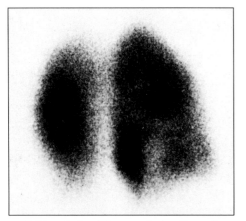

*e Right posterior oblique, perfusion, 3 months*

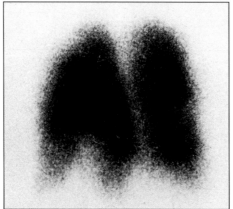

*f Left posterior oblique, perfusion, 3 months*

**Fig. 7.32**

*A 28-year-old woman with deep vein thrombosis and pulmonary emboli related to the contraceptive pill. Failure of pulmonary emboli to resolve. (a, b) Initial perfusion scan. (c, d) Ventilation lung scan. (e, f) Repeat perfusion scan 3 months later.*

*On the original study perfusion defects are seen in the basal segments of both lungs. These areas are seen to ventilate and there is therefore mismatch, in keeping with multiple pulmonary emboli. On the repeat study 3 months later there has essentially been no change in the scan appearances, and the findings presumably represent old pulmonary emboli which have failed to resolve.*

## CLINICAL APPLICATIONS

## Non-resolving defects

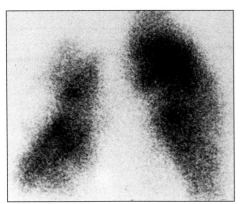

*a  Anterior, 0 months*

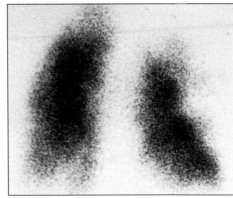

*b  Posterior, 0 months*

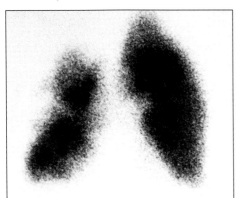

*c  Anterior, 3 months*

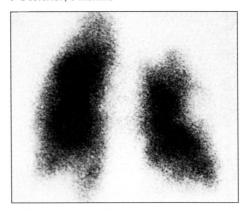

*d  Posterior, 3 months*

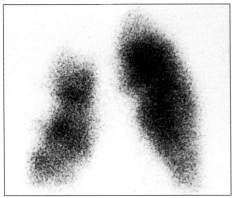

*e  Anterior, 8 months*

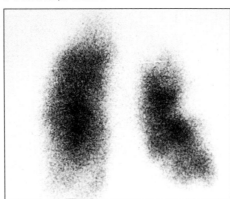

*f  Posterior, 8 months*

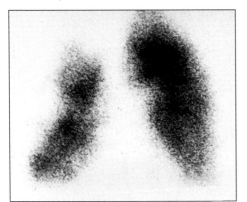

*g  Anterior, 3 years*

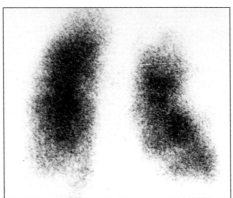

*h  Posterior, 3 years*

**Fig. 7.33**

*(a, b) Initial perfusion lung scan. Repeat perfusion scans: (c, d) after 3 months; (e, f) after 8 months; (g, h) after 3 years.*

*The initial perfusion lung scan shows extensive segmental perfusion defects throughout both lung fields. The ventilation study was absolutely normal. The scan findings are classically those of widespread multiple pulmonary emboli. However, over the next 3 years, the scan findings were essentially unchanged and were attributable to continuing non-resolution of old pulmonary emboli. These defects, which were initially diagnosed as pulmonary embolism, have shown no change over a period of 3 years. It is highly probable that they were old lesions when the initial scan was performed. This sequence of scans shows that it is impossible to date the timing of an embolus with absolute certainty.*

**In spite of the classical features of pulmonary embolism, the date of a pulmonary embolus cannot be ascertained with certainty.**

## Resolution of defects with the onset of new lesions

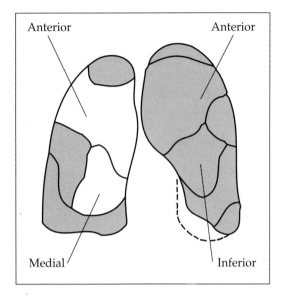

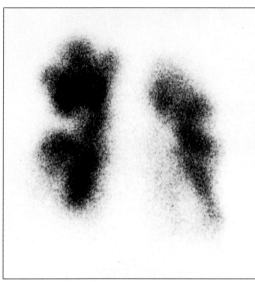

*a  Anterior, 0 weeks*

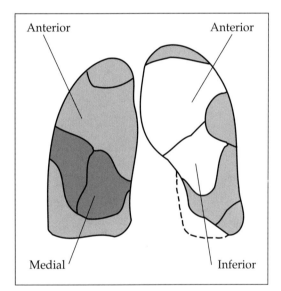

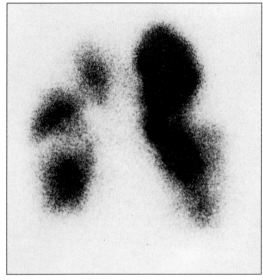

*b  Anterior 1 week*

**Fig. 7.34**

*PTE with some evidence of resolution but with new lesions. (a) Initial perfusion lung scan. (b) Repeat study 1 week later.*

*On the original study there are multiple segmental defects throughout both lung fields. The ventilation study was normal, and there was therefore a high probability of widespread pulmonary embolic disease. On the repeat study 1 week later there is evidence of resolution of many of the segmental perfusion defects, but there are new defects present in the anterior segment of the right upper lobe and the medial segment of the right middle lobe. The ventilation scan was again normal. Once again the lung scan indicates pulmonary embolic disease. While there is evidence of resolution, there is also evidence of new segmental emboli occurring, which may be an indication for surgical insertion of an IVC filter.*

• **Resolution of perfusion defects after pulmonary emboli is very variable. Defects may resolve completely, partially, or remain unchanged.**
• **A perfusion/ventilation scan should be performed prior to discontinuing anticoagulant therapy to assess residual defects.**

## CLINICAL APPLICATIONS

*Progression of pulmonary embolic disease following discontinuation of anticoagulant therapy*

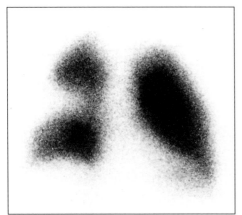

*a  Anterior, 0 months*

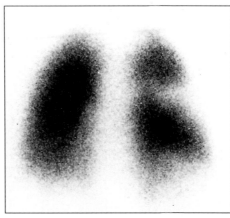

*b  Posterior, 0 months*

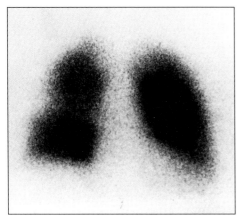

*c  Anterior, 8 months*

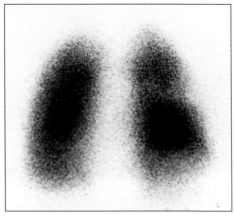

*d  Posterior, 8 months*

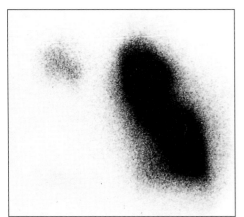

*e  Anterior, 10 months*

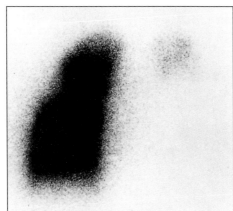

*f  Posterior, 10 months*

### Fig. 7.35

*(a, b)* Initial perfusion scan. Repeat studies: *(c, d)* after 8 months; *(e, f)* after 10 months.

On the original perfusion study there is a large segmental defect seen in the right mid-zone, with further smaller defects present at the left base. A ventilation study showed mismatch, in keeping with pulmonary embolic disease. A repeat perfusion study 8 months later revealed that the segmental defect in the right mid-zone was much less prominent, suggesting partial resolution of disease. Several weeks later the patient was seen for review and was found to be clinically well; anticoagulation therapy was discontinued. However, shortly thereafter the patient again became progressively dyspnoeic. A further perfusion study revealed virtually no perfusion to the right lung, with only a small amount of uptake at the apex. In addition, a segmental defect was visualized in the mid-zone of the left lung. The scan findings were those of a massive pulmonary embolus blocking the right main pulmonary artery, with further emboli in the left lung. The chest x-ray at that time showed a large right pulmonary artery. It is apparent that there has been dramatic deterioration in the scan findings when compared with previous studies.

## 7.4.2 Parenchymal lung disease

### *Single matched defect: emphysema*

*Perfusion*

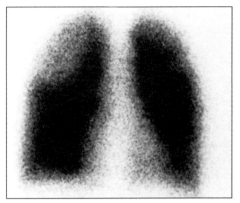

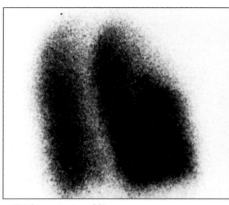

*a Anterior*     *b Posterior*     *c Right posterior oblique*

*Ventilation*

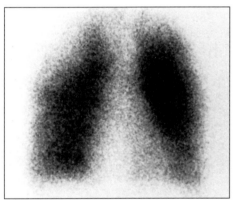 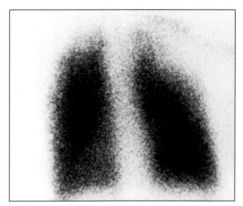 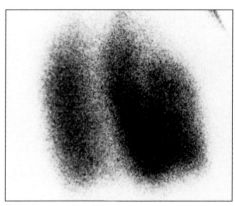

*d Anterior*     *e Posterior*     *f Right posterior oblique*

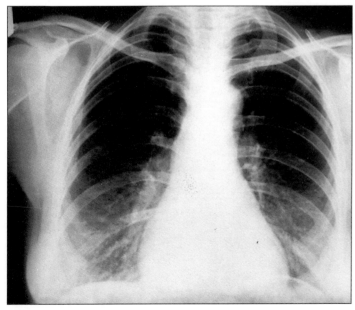

*g X-ray*

**Fig. 7.36**

*A 52-year-old woman with right apical bulla. (**a–c**) Perfusion lung scan. (**d–f**) Ventilation studies. (**g**) Chest x-ray.*

*This study confirms the presence of a matched ventilation/perfusion defect in the right upper zone, which corresponds to the radiographic diagnosis of an apical bulla.*

## *Matched defects caused by chronic obstructive airways disease*

*Perfusion*

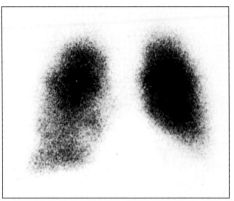
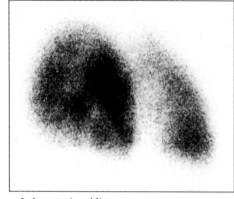

*a Anterior*      *b Right posterior oblique*      *c Left posterior oblique*

*Ventilation*

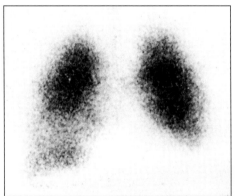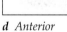
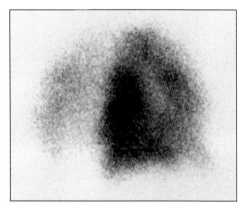
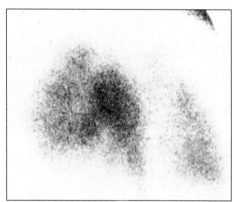

*d Anterior*      *e Right posterior oblique*      *f Left posterior oblique*

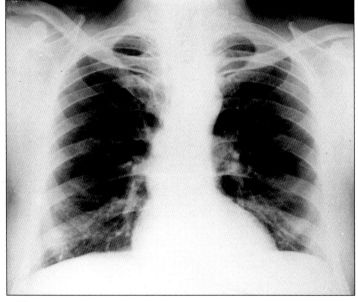

*g X-ray*

### *Fig. 7.37*

*A 70-year-old man with obstructive airways disease and suspected pulmonary embolism. (a–c) Perfusion lung scan. (d–f) Ventilation scan. (g) Chest x-ray.*

*On the perfusion lung scan there is marked non-homogeneity of tracer uptake, which is present in both lung fields. It is apparent that defects extend across normal segmental boundaries. Appearances are essentially the same in the ventilation study. The scan findings are typical of parenchymal lung disease and illustrate well the appearance of non-segmental and subsegmental perfusion abnormalities, which are bilateral and matched on the ventilation study.*

## *Matched subsegmental defect caused by a parenchymal lung lesion*

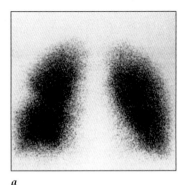

*a*

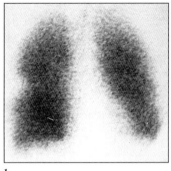

*b*

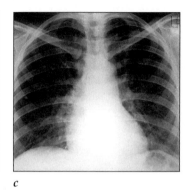

*c*

**Fig. 7.38**

*On the anterior perfusion lung scan (a) there is a subsegmental defect in the lateral segment of the right middle lobe. No other abnormality is seen. The ventilation study (b) shows a matched pattern. The chest x-ray (c) shows evidence of a previous small primary tubercular focus at that site.*

 Previous tuberculosis may lead to disproportionately large perfusion defects on the lung scan when compared with radiological findings.

## *Bilateral basal matched defects*

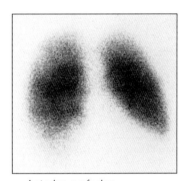

*a Anterior, perfusion*

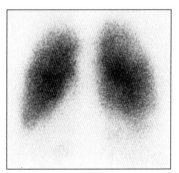

*b Posterior, perfusion*

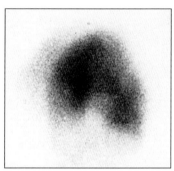

*c Right posterior oblique, perfusion*

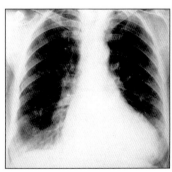

*d X-ray*

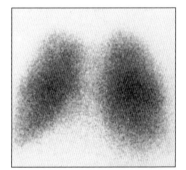

*e Posterior, ventilation*

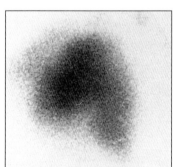

*f Right posterior oblique, ventilation*

**Fig. 7.39**

*(a–c) Perfusion lung scan.
(d) Chest x-ray.
(e, f) Ventilation lung scan.*

*There is reduced perfusion to both lower zones, with non-homogeneity of tracer uptake throughout the remainder of the lung fields. The ventilation study shows a matched pattern. There is virtually no perfusion and ventilation to both lower lobes. Scan findings are those of gross parenchymal lung disease.*

# 7.4.3 Differential diagnosis of massive loss of perfusion to one lung

## *Causes of massive loss of perfusion*

- Pulmonary embolism
- Bullous emphysema
- Carcinoma of the lung
- Metastases

- Atresia of a pulmonary artery
- Pneumonectomy
- Pleural effusion

## *Pulmonary embolism*

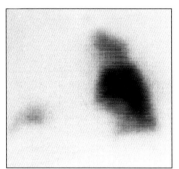 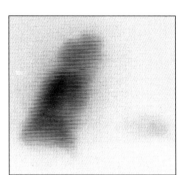 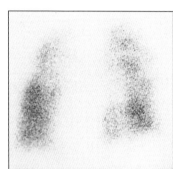

*a Anterior, perfusion*     *b Posterior, perfusion*     *c Posterior, ventilation*

*Fig. 7.40*

*Massive pulmonary embolus. (a, b) Perfusion lung scan. (c) ventilation study.*

*There is practically no perfusion to the right lung, apart from a small segment at the base. The left lung shows segmental perfusion defects. The ventilation study shows reasonably good ventilation throughout both lung fields, although there is a somewhat non-homogeneous distribution of tracer. The scan findings were due to a massive right-sided pulmonary embolus, with multiple smaller pulmonary emboli involving the left lung.*

Although massive pulmonary embolism is well recognized, it is not commonly visualized on a lung scan, because the embolus has usually broken up and migrated distally, causing multiple segmental defects. It is important to appreciate some of the other causes of massive loss of perfusion.

## *Bullous emphysema*

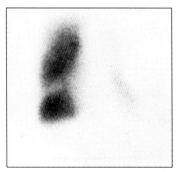 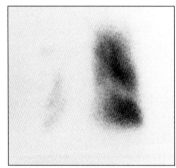 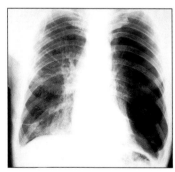 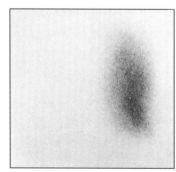

*a Anterior, perfusion*     *b Posterior, perfusion*     *c X-ray*     *d Posterior, ventilation*

*Fig. 7.41*

*Bullous emphysema. (a, b) Perfusion lung scan. (c) Chest x-ray. (d) Ventilation lung scan.*

*The perfusion study shows only a small amount of perfusion to the left base. There is moderately good perfusion to the right lung, with multiple, non-segmental perfusion defects present. While the right lung is moderately well ventilated, there is no ventilation demonstrated in the left lung. The absent ventilation of the left lung is attributable to the bullous emphysema seen on the chest x-ray. Nevertheless, it should be noted that there is a small amount of residual perfusion. The non-segmental perfusion defects in the right lung are attributable to parenchymal lung disease.*

## *Carcinoma of the bronchus*

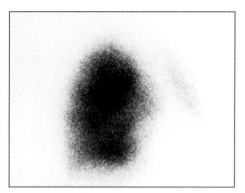

*a  Anterior, perfusion*

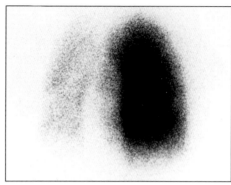

*b  Posterior, perfusion*

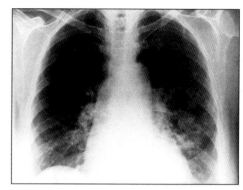

*c  X-ray*

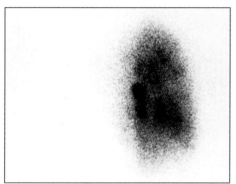

*d  Posterior, ventilation*

**Fig. 7.42**

*Reduced perfusion caused by carcinoma of the lung. (**a, b**) Perfusion lung scan. (**c**) Chest x-ray. (**d**) Ventilation lung scan.*

*The perfusion study shows strikingly reduced perfusion to the whole of the left lung. There is virtually no ventilation seen to the left lung. This 63-year-old woman had carcinoma of the left lung, and the scan findings were due to obstruction of the left main pulmonary artery and bronchus.*

## *Pulmonary metastasis*

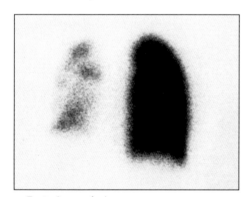

*a  Posterior, perfusion*

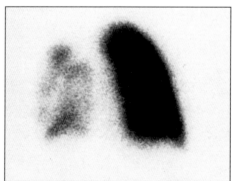

*b  Left posterior oblique, perfusion*

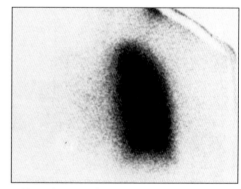

*c  Posterior, ventilation*

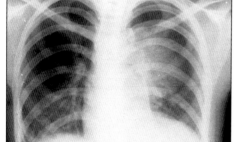

*d  X-ray*

**Fig. 7.43**

*Absent perfusion caused by an obstructive lesion. (**a, b**) Perfusion lung scan. (**c**) Ventilation lung scan. (**d**) Chest x-ray.*

*On the perfusion study there is markedly reduced perfusion throughout the left lung, with a large photon-deficient area centrally. There is no ventilation to the left lung. The scan findings are not those of pulmonary embolus, and are compatible with a large central obstructive lesion. A large left mediastinal mass is seen on the chest x-ray, caused by a metastasis from a primary osteosarcoma.*

## CLINICAL APPLICATIONS

## *Atresia of the right pulmonary artery*

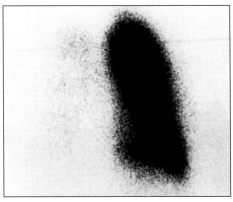
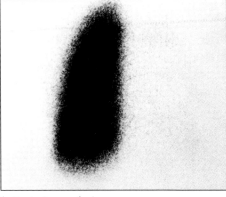
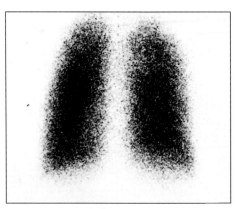

*a  Anterior, perfusion*  *b  Posterior, perfusion*  *c  Posterior, ventilation*

**Fig 7.44**

*A 43-year-old woman with congenital atresia of the right pulmonary artery.
(a, b) Perfusion lung scan. (c) Ventilation lung scan.*
    *There is virtually a complete absence of perfusion to the whole of the right lung. The left
lung appears normal. The ventilation scan shows normal ventilation to both lungs. This
patient had congenital atresia of the right pulmonary artery.*

## *Pleural effusion*

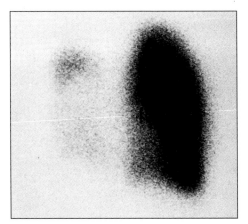
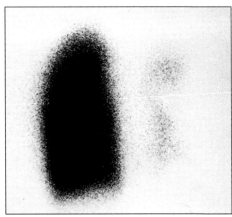
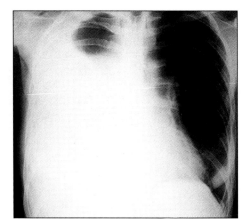

*a  Anterior, perfusion*  *b  Posterior, perfusion*  *c  X-ray*

**Fig. 7.45**

*Massive perfusion defect caused by a pleural effusion. (a, b) Perfusion study. (c) Chest
x-ray. (d) Ventilation lung scan.*
    *There is a major defect in both ventilation and perfusion involving the right lung. The
scan findings were due to a massive pleural effusion causing collapse of the right lung,
with essentially matched impairment of perfusion and ventilation.*

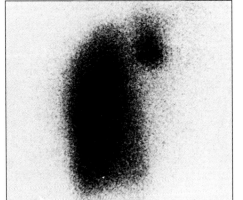

*d  Posterior, ventilation*

## 7.4.4 Conditions simulating pulmonary embolism

### Asthma

Asthma is one of the commonest causes of an incorrect diagnosis of pulmonary embolism. On the perfusion study there may be widespread, clearly segmental perfusion defects, and the appearances may be indis-tinguishable from multiple pulmonary emboli. However, if a ventilation scan is obtained, an exactly matched pattern will be found.

*Before bronchodilator therapy*

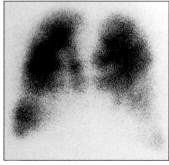 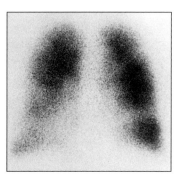 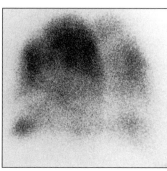

*a Anterior*    *b Posterior*    *c Left posterior oblique*

*After bronchodilator therapy*

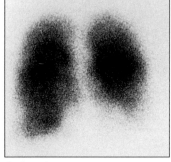 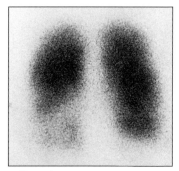 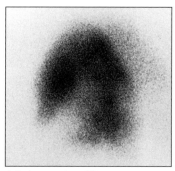

*d Anterior*    *e Posterior*    *f Left posterior oblique*

**Fig. 7.46**

*(a–c) Initial perfusion lung scan. (d–f) Perfusion lung scan after bronchodilator therapy.*

*This is the scan of a young woman presenting with dyspnoea shortly after discharge from hospital following a gynaeological operation. The clinical diagnosis was considered to be pulmonary embolism, and the first perfusion study shows multiple small, segmental defects throughout both lung fields. A ventilation study was not obtained. However, it was noted that the patient had bronchospasm, and the study was repeated after bronchodilators had been administered. The repeat scan shows resolution of the perfusion abnormalities.*

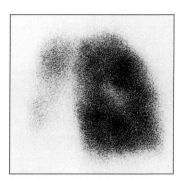

*a Right posterior oblique, 0 days*    *b Right posterior oblique, 2 days*

**Fig. 7.47**

*(a) Initial perfusion scan. (b) Repeat scan 2 days later.*

*This perfusion scan is an excellent example of how acute bronchospasm can cause a segmental defect during the acute episode, which resolves with the treatment of bronchospasm. The scan appearance clearly simulates an acute pulmonary embolus at the right base.*

• It is essential to assess whether a patient having a lung scan has acute bronchospasm at the time that the study is performed.
• It is essential to obtain a ventilation study whenever perfusion defects are found.

## CLINICAL APPLICATIONS

## *Vasculitis*

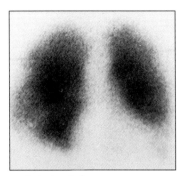
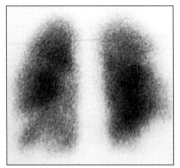
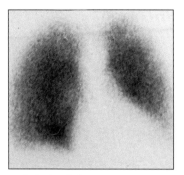
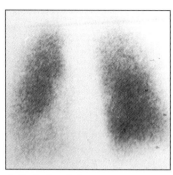

*a  Anterior, 0 days*     *b  Posterior, 0 days*     *c  Anterior, 8 days*     *d  Posterior, 8 days*

### Fig. 7.48

*(a, b) Initial perfusion lung scan. (c, d) Repeat study 8 days later.*
   *This is a 38-year-old woman with systemic lupus erythematosus and nephrotic syndrome. The original study shows segmental perfusion defects present at both bases and mid-zones. 8 days later, following a course of steroid therapy, resolution of perfusion defects was seen. The original defects were due to vasculitis, which responded to steroid therapy.*

**Vasculitis caused by polyarteritis nodosa, systemic lupus erythematosus or other collagen disorders is physiologically indistinguishable from pulmonary emboli and will cause unmatched perfusion/ventilation defects.**

## *Pulmonary metastases*

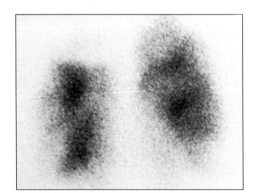
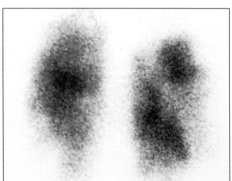
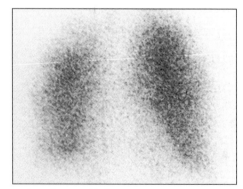

*a  Anterior, perfusion*     *b  Posterior, perfusion*     *c  Anterior, ventilation*

### Fig. 7.49

*Pulmonary metastases simulating pulmonary embolic disease. (a, b) Perfusion lung scan. (c) Ventilation lung scan.*
   *The perfusion study shows marked non-homogeneity of tracer uptake throughout both lung fields, with more segmental defects present. Note the absent perfusion at the right apex, with a horizontal lower border. The ventilation study is completely normal. This patient had carcinoma of the breast with widespread pulmonary metastases. There was no evidence, on extensive investigation, for a diagnosis of pulmonary embolism. This patient, in addition, had previous radiotherapy to the right breast. The above scan findings indicate widespread pulmonary arterial lesions, which are most probably due to metastases. Changes at the right apex may be due to previous radiotherapy.*

- **Metastases are an uncommon cause of pulmonary arterial lesions.**
- **The typical findings on lung scans following radiation are greater diminution of perfusion than of ventilation in the irradiated area. Furthermore, radiation fields will rarely correspond to bronchopulmonary segments.**

## CLINICAL APPLICATIONS

## *Tumour emboli*

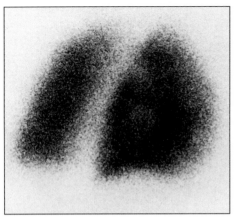

*a Right posterior oblique, perfusion*

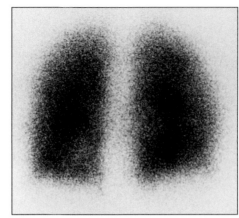

*b Posterior, perfusion*

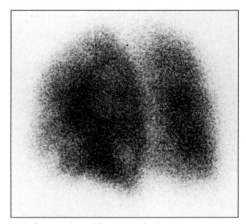

*c Left posterior oblique, perfusion*

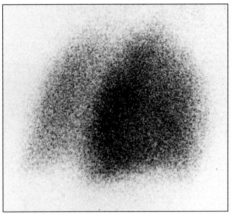

*d Right posterior oblique, ventilation*

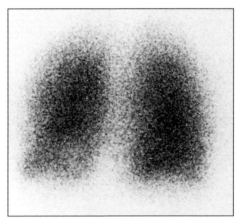

*e Posterior, ventilation*

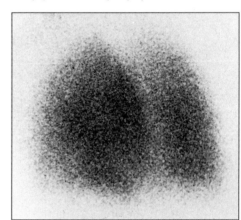

*f Left posterior oblique, ventilation*

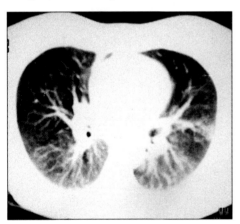

*g CT*

**Fig. 7.50**

*(a–c) Perfusion lung scan. (d–f) Ventilation lung scan. (g) CT scan of the chest.*

*This patient with carcinoma of the breast presented with dyspnoea. The chest x-ray was normal. The perfusion scan shows multiple subsegmental perfusion defects, and the ventilation study is normal. As part of the staging process prior to chemotherapy, a pulmonary CT scan was performed, which shows multiple small metastases. The diagnosis here is likely to be multiple small tumour emboli. It should be noted that the scan findings are those of subsegmental perfusion defects, and, while there is a mismatch on the ventilation study, the findings are not typical of pulmonary embolic disease.*

**Subsegmental perfusion defects with normal ventilation may be seen with both tumour and fat emboli.**

## CLINICAL APPLICATIONS

### *Emphysematous bulla*

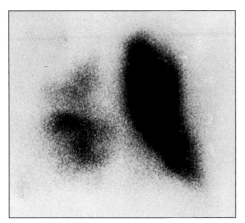

*a  Anterior, perfusion*

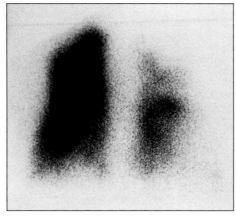

*b  Posterior, perfusion*

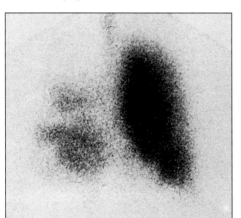

*c  Anterior, ventilation*

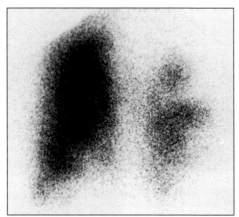

*d  Posterior, ventilation*

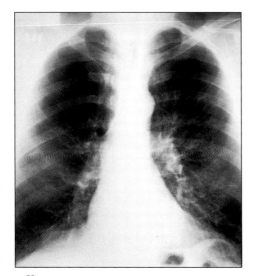

*e  X-ray*

*Fig. 7.51*

*(a, b) Perfusion lung scan.*
*(c, d) Ventilation lung scan.*
*(e) Chest x-ray.*

   *On the perfusion study there is marked non-homogeneity of tracer uptake throughout the right lung, with clearly segmental defects present. There is, in addition, some non-homogeneity of tracer uptake throughout the left lung, but this appears 'relatively' normal. The ventilation study shows an exactly matched pattern. The scan findings are those of obstructive airways disease, with the presence of bullae in the right lung. This is confirmed on the chest x-ray.*

• The presence of obstructive airways disease should not cause diagnostic problems on a perfusion lung scan, when a ventilation study is also obtained.
• When there is extensive parenchymal lung disease with major perfusion defects, the presence of coexistent pulmonary embolic disease cannot be absolutely excluded.

## Fibrotic lung disease

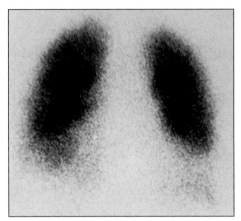

a Anterior, perfusion

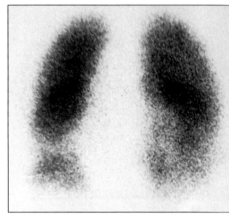

b Posterior, perfusion

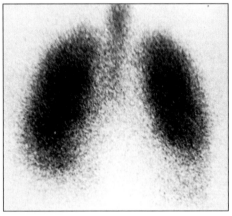

c Anterior, ventilation

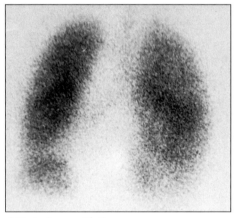

d Posterior, ventilation

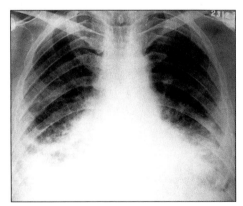

e X-ray

**Fig. 7.52**

Asbestosis. **(a, b)** Perfusion lung scan. **(c, d)** Ventilation lung scan. **(e)** Chest x-ray.

The perfusion lung scan shows non-homogeneity of tracer uptake throughout both lung fields, with major defects present at both bases. The ventilation study shows an exactly matched pattern. The chest x-ray showed features in keeping with asbestosis.

## Cardiac failure

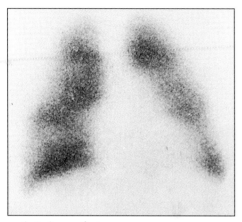

*a* Anterior, perfusion

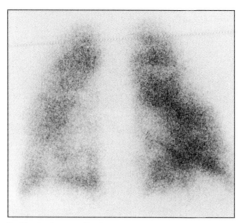

*b* Posterior, perfusion

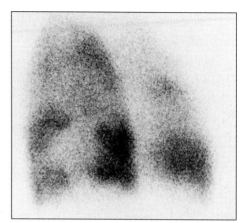

*c* Left posterior oblique, perfusion

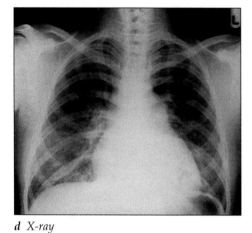

*d* X-ray

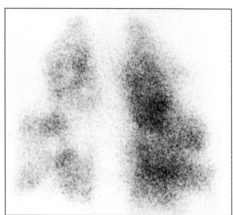

*e* Posterior, ventilation

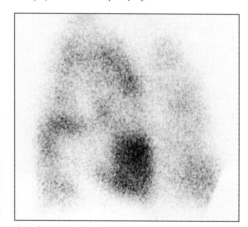

*f* Left posterior oblique, ventilation

**Fig. 7.53**

**(a–c)** *Perfusion lung scan.* **(d)** *Chest x-ray.* **(e, f)** *Ventilation lung scan.*

This 35-year-old male presented with drug overdose. On examination he was acutely dyspnoeic and in cardiac failure. The possibility of pulmonary embolic disease being present was raised. The perfusion lung scan shows extensive defects throughout both lung fields. However, while segmental defects are present, the majority of lesions are non-segmental, and the ventilation study shows an exactly matched pattern. The findings were due to gross cardiac failure with pulmonary oedema.

## 7.4.5 Chronic obstructive airways disease

### *Patterns of abnormality with ¹³³Xe ventilation*

*Ventilation*

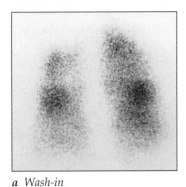 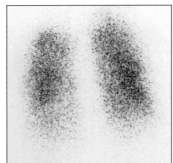 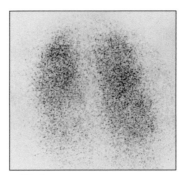 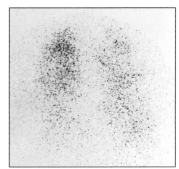

*a* Wash-in     *b* Equilibrium     *c* Washout     *d* Washout

*Perfusion*

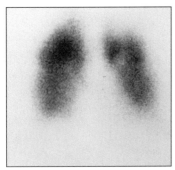 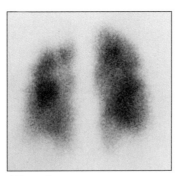 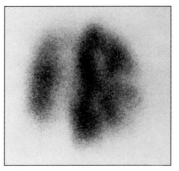 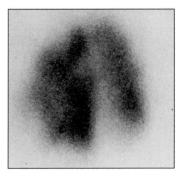

*e* Anterior     *f* Posterior     *g* Right oblique     *h* Left oblique

**Fig. 7.54**

*(a–d) Ventilation study with ¹³³Xe. (e–h) Perfusion lung scan.*

*This middle-aged man presented with recent onset of shortness of breath. There was no history of smoking or previous lung disease. The perfusion lung scan shows multiple small, mainly subsegmental defects, but with a clear segmental defect present at the right upper zone. The chest x-ray was normal, and, in view of the clinical history, the perfusion lung scan in isolation would raise the suspicion of pulmonary embolic disease being present. However, the ventilation study showed some decreased ventilation at the right apex and delayed washout generally, with irregular trapping of tracer. The scan findings are matched, and the overall appearances are typical of chronic obstructive lung disease, which in this case had not previously been diagnosed. (Courtesy of Dr Ton Nunan, London, UK.)*

 **The delayed washout on a xenon study** can provide useful additional information in the diagnosis of chronic obstructive airways disease.

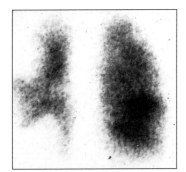 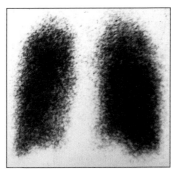

*b* Before     *c* After

**Fig. 7.55**

*Posterior ventilation study (a) before and (b) following physiotherapy. The original study shows an irregular pattern of ventilation in both lung fields, but with large defects present throughout the left lung. Following physiotherapy, these defects have essentially resolved.*

 **Patients with chronic lung disease may demonstrate temporary ventilation defects as a result of mucous plugging of the bronchi.**

## CLINICAL APPLICATIONS

### Ventilation

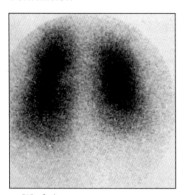

*a Wash-in*

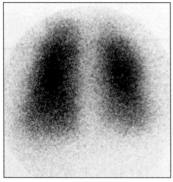

*b Equilibrium*

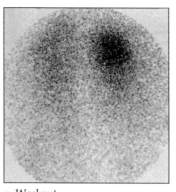

*c Washout*

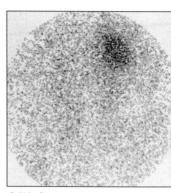

*d Washout*

### Perfusion

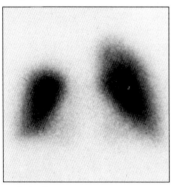

*e Anterior*

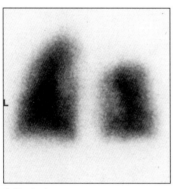

*f Posterior*

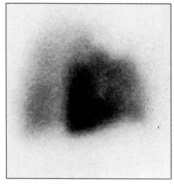

*g Right oblique*

**Fig. 7.56**

**(a–d)** [133]Xe ventilation lung scan, posterior view. **(e–g)** Perfusion lung scan.

On the perfusion study there is a large, irregular, non-segmental perfusion defect at the right upper zone. The ventilation study obtained with [133]Xe shows somewhat decreased ventilation in the wash-in image. There is, however, relatively normal equilibrium, but during the washout phase there is marked trapping of tracer at the right apex. Thus the perfusion defect is matched by significant ventilation abnormalities typical of chronic obstructive airways disease, and the findings were due to an emphysematous bulla. (Courtesy of Dr Ton Nunan, London, UK.)

## Patterns of abnormality with ⁹⁹ᵐTc aerosol

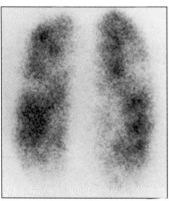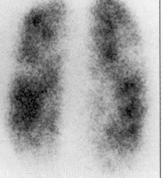

*a Posterior, perfusion*

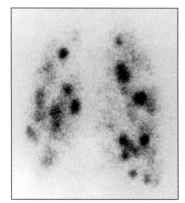

*b Posterior, aerosol*

**Fig. 7.57**

**(a)** Perfusion lung scan. **(b)** Aerosol study with ⁹⁹ᵐTc DTPA.

The perfusion image shows non-homogeneity of tracer uptake throughout both lung fields, in keeping with known parenchymal lung disease. The ventilation study with ⁹⁹ᵐTc DTPA aerosol shows non-homogeneity which is more pronounced, with multiple, more focal areas of markedly increased tracer uptake. This case illustrates one of the problems that may be seen with aerosol studies in patients with severe parenchymal lung disease, ie 'clumping' of tracer in the main bronchi and their major branches, which may lead to artificial mismatching.

## *Ventilation defects more severe than perfusion defects, caused by pneumonia*

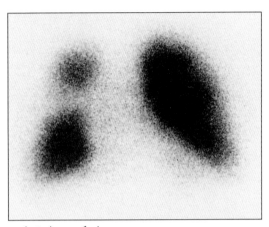

*a  Anterior, perfusion*

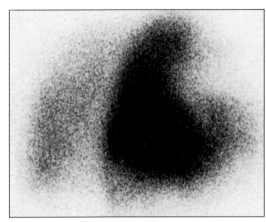

*b  Right posterior oblique, perfusion*

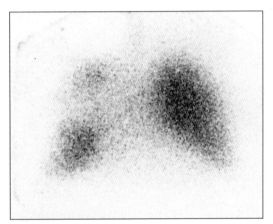

*c  Anterior, ventilation*

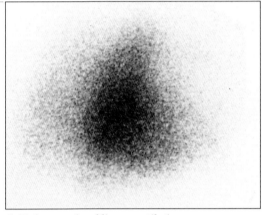

*d  Right posterior oblique, ventilation*

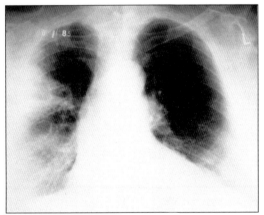

*e  X-ray*

*Fig. 7.58*

*Mismatched perfusion/ventilation defect caused by consolidation.*
*(a, b) Perfusion lung scan.*
*(c, d) Ventilation study.*
*(e) Chest x-ray.*

*The perfusion study shows a large defect in the right upper lobe anteriorly, with further subsegmental defects present at the right base. The ventilation study shows more extensive defects. The scan findings were due to parenchymal lung disease, with the large defect corresponding to an area of consolidation seen on the chest x-ray.*

 Mismatched defects, where the ventilation is affected but the perfusion changes are insignificant or less marked, may occasionally be seen in acute pneumonia. However, usually the perfusion is similarly affected.

**CLINICAL APPLICATIONS**

## *Ventilation/perfusion lung scan appearance of pneumonia*

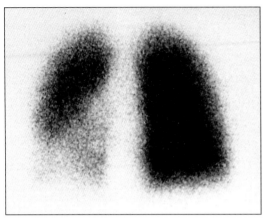

*a Posterior, perfusion*

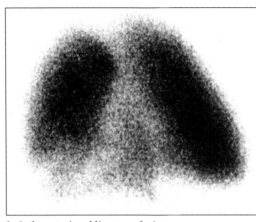

*b Left posterior oblique, perfusion*

**Fig. 7.59**

*(a, b) Perfusion lung scan.*
*(c–d) Ventilation study.*
  *This patient had pneumonic consolidation involving the left lower lobe. The perfusion lung scan shows some loss of perfusion to the left lower lobe. Ventilation defects, however, are more marked than perfusion changes. The scan findings were attributable to the known pneumonia.*

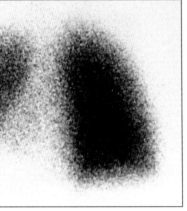

*c Posterior, ventilation*

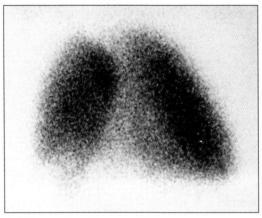

*d Left posterior oblique, ventilation*

**Mismatch usually means better ventilation than perfusion. However, it may be the reverse, as in the case of pneumonia shown in Fig. 7.59, when the alveolar disturbance is more affected than the blood flow.**

# 7.4.6  Assessment of carcinoma of the bronchus

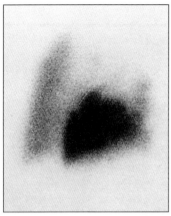

*a  Right posterior oblique, perfusion*

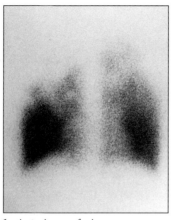

*b  Anterior, perfusion*

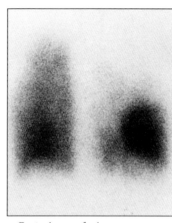

*c  Posterior, perfusion*

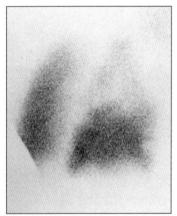

*d  Right posterior oblique, ventilation*

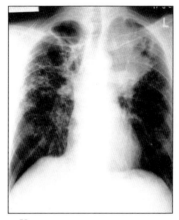

*e  X-ray*

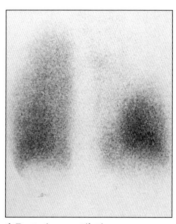

*f  Posterior, ventilation*

*Fig. 7.60*

*(a–c) Perfusion lung scan.*
*(d, f) Ventilation lung scan.*
*(e) Chest x-ray.*
*A 43-year-old male heavy smoker with carcinoma of the lung as shown on the chest x-ray (e).*

*The perfusion study shows almost complete absence of perfusion to the right upper zone, and this area has an irregular lower margin. There is also some irregularity of perfusion throughout the remainder of the lung fields. On the ventilation study there is a similar pattern, but with perhaps slightly improved ventilation. This patient was being considered for a left pneumonectomy, but this study provided valuable additional information, in as much as it was recognized that there would be a very poor residual function in the remaining right lung. This patient had a past history of tuberculosis and obstructive airways disease.*

# 7.4.7  Inhaled foreign body

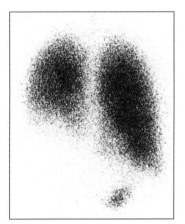

*a  Anterior*

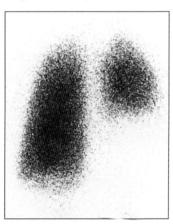

*b  Posterior*

*Fig. 7.61*

*(a, b) Ventilation lung scan with ⁸¹ᵐKr.*

*It was thought that this child had swallowed a toy building brick, although there was the suspicion that he might have inhaled it. A chest x-ray was normal. The ventilation study, however, is grossly abnormal, indicating blocked ventilation to the right lower lobe.*

**A mass lesion in the lung, particularly at the hilum, will cause a massive perfusion defect, and usually a matching ventilation abnormality. Occasionally, it may involve the pulmonary artery only and spare the bronchus, in which case there may be a mismatch defect.**

CLINICAL APPLICATIONS

# 7.4.8 Assessment of lung permeability

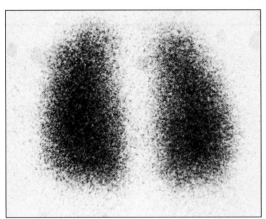

*a  Posterior, 0 hours*

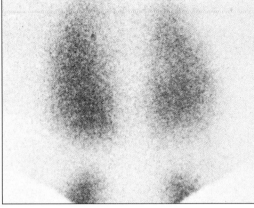

*b  Posterior, 1 hour*

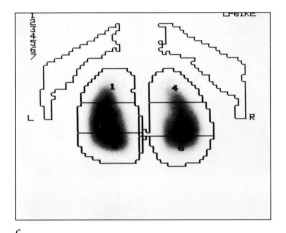

*c*

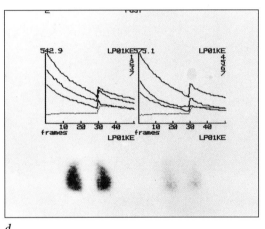

*d*

**Fig. 7.62**

*Pulmonary permeability study in a case of sarcoidosis. Lung permeability study with $^{99m}$Tc DTPA aerosol: (a) posterior lung scan, immediate view and (b) 1 hour later; (c) regions of interest and (d) computer-generated curves.*

*It is apparent in this case that there is rapid washout of tracer from the lungs, with markedly shortened results for pulmonary permeability (half-life in the region of 15 minutes). This patient had sarcoidosis, which accounted for the increased lung permeability. (Courtesy of Drs P Wraight and L Smith, Cambridge, UK.)*

> Increased lung permeability is non-specific and may be seen in many conditions. The commonest situation to cause increased permeability is cigarette smoking. Usually the change of permeability is not significant clinically; however, if it is very rapid, it may be impossible to achieve a satisfactory ventilation study with aerosols.

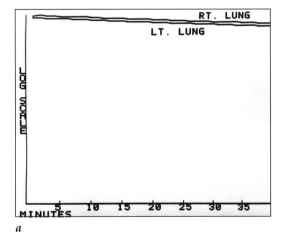

*a*

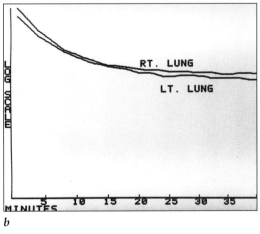

*b*

**Fig. 7.63**

*Aerosol permeability curves from two patients who were HIV-positive haemophiliacs. (a) Normal slow clearance of aerosol from both lungs in an asymptomatic patient. (b) Rapid clearance from both lungs in a symptomatic breathless patient who was subsequently proved to have pneumocystis carinii. (Courtesy of Dr M O'Doherty, London, UK.)*

# CHAPTER 8

# LIVER AND SPLEEN

## Liver/spleen colloid imaging

Although ultrasound of the liver has largely replaced liver/spleen colloid imaging in the detection of metastatic disease, colloid imaging using technetium-99m ($^{99m}$Tc) sulphur colloid (SC) continues to offer an accurate and easily performed method of investigating the liver and spleen. It is operator-independent and reproducible, and is particularly useful for monitoring progression or regression of liver metastases. Liver/spleen colloid imaging assesses the integrity of the reticuloendothelial system (RES) within the liver and spleen. Following the injection of the radioactive colloid, the particles (approximately 0.01 μm in size) become trapped in the endothelial lining Kupffer cells of the liver and in the macrophages of the spleen. There is also slight uptake of radiocolloid in the RES cells of the bone marrow, but this is generally not seen in a normal subject since most of the $^{99m}$Tc SC is incorporated in the liver and spleen. However, when diffuse hepatic disease such as cirrhosis exists, less radiocolloid will be taken up by the liver, and more is 'diverted' and thus available for other RES sites such as the spleen and bone marrow. When space-occupying lesions such as metastases are present, these completely replace the RES cells and therefore appear as photon-deficient areas on the scan.

## Hepatobiliary imaging

Hepatobiliary imaging is nowadays performed with one of the $^{99m}$Tc iminodiacetic acid (IDA) derivatives. These compounds are known collectively as HIDA (hepatic IDA). $^{99m}$Tc HIDA is taken up and excreted by the hepatocytes, and is therefore used for imaging the gall bladder and visualizing the major ducts in the biliary tree. In the normal subject the liver, common bile duct, gall bladder and duodenum should be visualized within 1–1½ hours after injection, but if any of these structures is not visualized then delayed views for up to 4 hours should be obtained. The study may be discontinued earlier if there is no remaining hepatic activity, but bowel activity has to be excluded from the field of view with lead shielding to assess this adequately. Absence of gall bladder visualization indicates cystic duct obstruction and supports the diagnosis of acute cholecystitis. Occasionally, the gall bladder is not visualized when chronic disease is present, but it will then usually be seen on the delayed images. The technique may provide evidence of obstruction in the biliary tree when this is present.

Good biliary visualization can be consistently achieved when bilirubin levels are normal or else slightly elevated, but as hepatic function deteriorates and bilirubin levels progressively rise, a greater proportion of $^{99m}$Tc HIDA is excreted via the kidneys (normally less than 15%) and less via the hepatobiliary route. $^{99m}$Tc di-isopropyl IDA (DISIDA) is of use in patients with raised bilirubin levels.

## CHAPTER CONTENTS

# 8.1 ANATOMY/PHYSIOLOGY

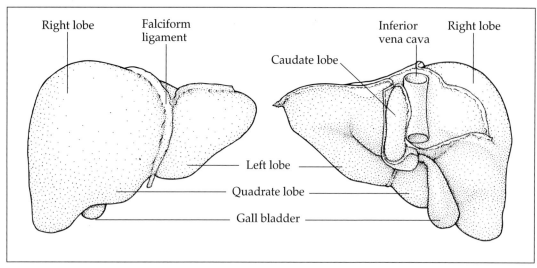

Right lobe

Falciform ligament

Inferior vena cava

Right lobe

Caudate lobe

Left lobe

Quadrate lobe

Gall bladder

*Anterior view*

*Posterior view*

**Fig. 8.1**

*Anatomy of the liver.*

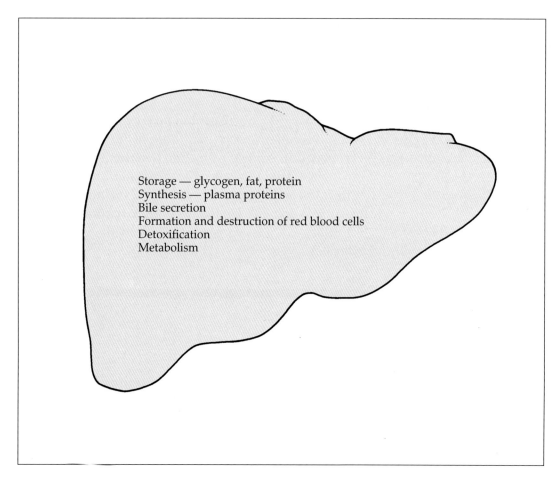

Storage — glycogen, fat, protein
Synthesis — plasma proteins
Bile secretion
Formation and destruction of red blood cells
Detoxification
Metabolism

**Fig. 8.2**

*Functions of the liver.*

# 8.2 RADIOPHARMACEUTICALS

*Table 8.1 Radiopharmaceuticals for liver and spleen imaging*

| | Radiopharmaceutical | Site of accumulation | Main use | Comment |
|---|---|---|---|---|
| Liver and spleen | 99mTc sulphur colloid<br>99mTc tin colloid<br>99mTc albumin minimicrospheres | Reticuloendothelial system (RES) (Kupffer cells and macrophages) | Routine liver spleen scanning | Particle size will determine the distribution throughout the RES |
| | 99mTc-labelled red blood cells | Vascular spaces | Identification of vascular space-occupying lesions | Used in conjunction with 99mTc colloid scan |
| Liver only | 99mTc HIDA and derivatives | Hepatocytes and excretion via biliary system | Functional assessment of hepatocytes and biliary excretion. Separation of liver and splenic tissue | Cholecystokinin (CCK) infusion or other gall bladder stimulants may be used in addition to empty the gall bladder |
| | 67Ga citrate | Hepatocytes and malignant, inflammatory or infective lesions | Diagnosis of hepatoma and other malignant or infective lesions in and around the liver | 99mTc colloid scan must be used in conjunction with 67Ga |
| Spleen only | Heat or chemically denatured 99mTc-labelled red cells | Macrophages in RES of the spleen | Delineation of splenic lesions, splenic function, separation of liver and spleen | Usually performed after a 99mTc colloid scan |

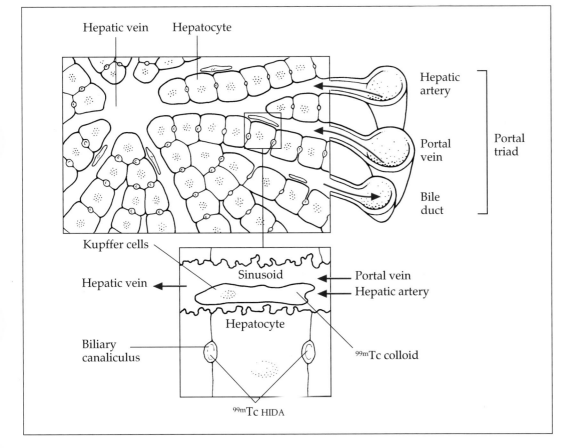

*Fig. 8.3*

*Radiopharmaceutical localization.*

# 8.3 NORMAL SCANS WITH VARIANTS AND ARTEFACTS

## 8.3.1 Normal colloid liver/spleen scan

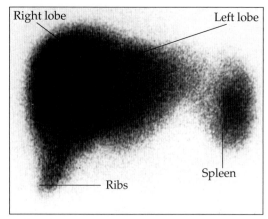

*a* Anterior

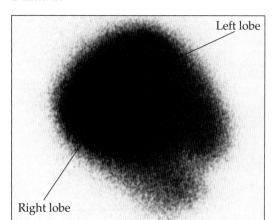

*c* Right lateral

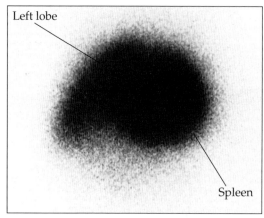

*b* Posterior

*d* Left lateral

### Fig. 8.4

*(a–d)* Normal colloid liver/spleen scan.

# NORMAL SCANS WITH VARIANTS AND ARTEFACTS

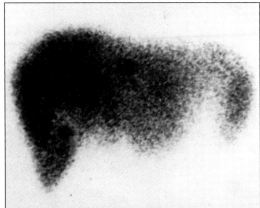

a  Anterior

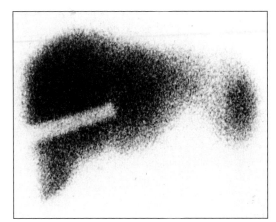

b  Anterior

*Fig. 8.5*

*(a,b)  A 10 cm lead marker has been placed on the costal margin to identify the position of the liver and to measure its size.*

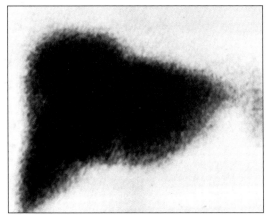

a  Anterior

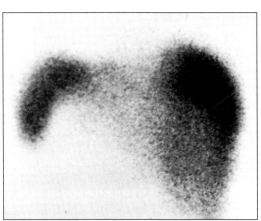

b  Posterior

*Fig. 8.6*

*(a,b)  The right kidney causes a variable-sized impression on the posterior liver view.*

**It is important to be aware of the normal anatomical impressions and not confuse these with space-occupying lesions.**

## Normal variants of the lobes of the liver

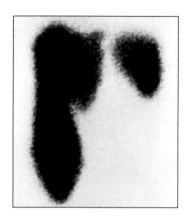

**Fig. 8.7**

*Extreme prolongation of the right lobe (Riedel's lobe) is present, with an almost absent left lobe.*

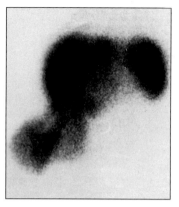

**Fig. 8.8**

*A prominent Riedel's lobe is present in this patient with a very flaccid abdominal wall.*

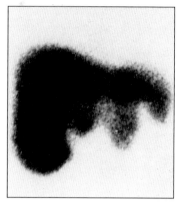

**Fig. 8.9**

*An example of a prominent quadrate lobe.*

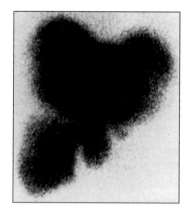

**Fig. 8.10**

*A patient with prominent Riedel's and quadrate lobes. Note also the deep rib indentation in the right lobe.*

## Floating lobe of the liver

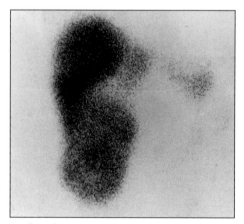

*a  Anterior*

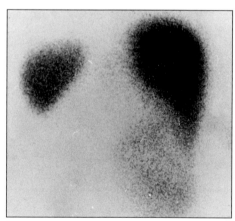

*b  Posterior*

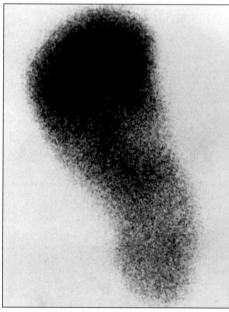

*c  Right lateral*

**Fig. 8.11**

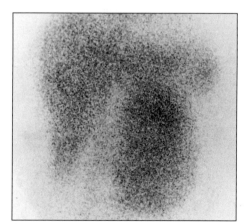

*d  Anterior HIDA*

*(a–c)* Colloid liver/spleen scan. *(d)* HIDA liver scan.

*There is a large mass of functional liver tissue lying below the right lobe of the liver. When the study was repeated with HIDA, the previously seen mass was lying to the left side of the abdomen. The scan findings were due to a 'floating' left lobe of the liver. Although uncommon, this is a normal variant.*

## NORMAL SCANS WITH VARIANTS AND ARTEFACTS

## *Confusion between the left lobe of the liver and the spleen*

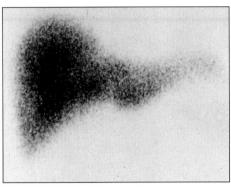 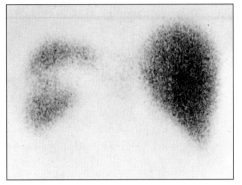 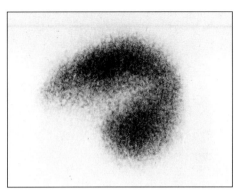

*a Anterior*　　　　　　　　*b Posterior*　　　　　　　　*c Left lateral*

**Fig. 8.12**

*(a–c)* Liver scan.

This is a normal study, but there is an elongated thin left lobe which extends right over into the left of the abdomen. Unless the clinician is aware of this appearance, the posterior view in particular could be confused with a space-occupying lesion in the spleen.

## *Left lobe of the liver mimicking the spleen*

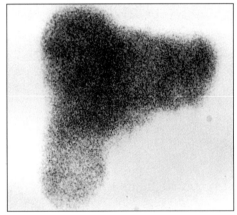 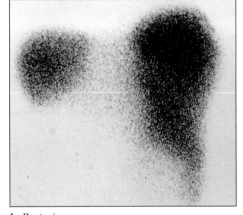 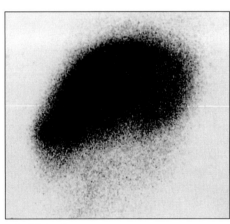

*a Anterior*　　　　　　　　*b Posterior*　　　　　　　　*c Left lateral*

**Fig. 8.13**

*(a–c)* Liver scan.

This patient has had a previous splenectomy. On the anterior and posterior views the appearances would be compatible with a poorly functioning spleen, but are in fact due to the left lobe of the liver. It should be noted that the spleen cannot be identified on the left lateral view.

## 8.3.2    Normal hepatobiliary liver scan

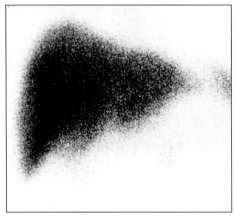

*a  Anterior, 5 minutes*

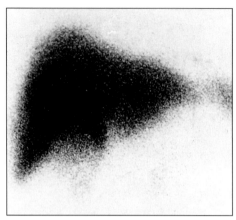

*b  Anterior, 10 minutes*

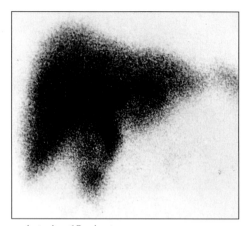

*c  Anterior, 15 minutes*

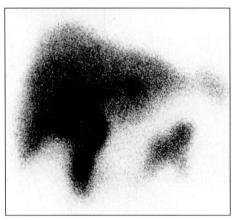

*d  Anterior, 25 minutes*

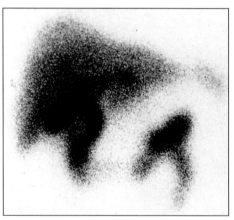

*e  Anterior, 30 minutes*

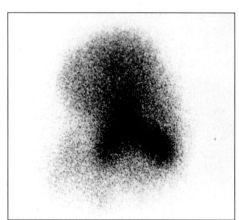

*f  Right lateral*

**Fig. 8.14**

**(a–e)** *Views of the liver following injection of* $^{99m}$Tc HIDA. **(f)** *Right lateral view to show the anterior position of the gall bladder.*

There is homogeneous distribution of tracer throughout the liver before biliary visualization occurs. Note that in this case the left lobe of the liver extends across the abdomen under the left diaphragm. Note also that the collecting systems of both kidneys are just visualized. In a normal study tracer should enter the common bile duct, and soon after this (approximately 20–25 minutes) the gall bladder and duodenum should be visualized. The gall bladder should continue to fill, while the common bile duct is draining.

## NORMAL SCANS WITH VARIANTS AND ARTEFACTS

### *Some normal variants of gall bladder appearance on HIDA scan*

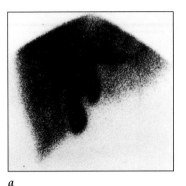 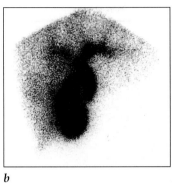 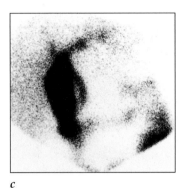 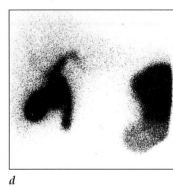

*a*        *b*        *c*        *d*

**Fig. 8.15**

*(a–d)* Normal $^{99m}$Tc HIDA hepatobiliary scan images.

    Note that the gall bladder may vary considerably in shape, position and size. It can usually be identified by the time at which it is first visualized and its position on the anterior and right lateral views.

### *Simulation of gall bladder by renal collecting system*

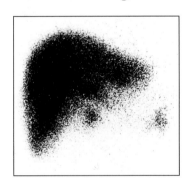 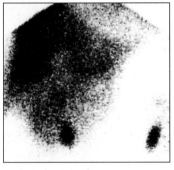 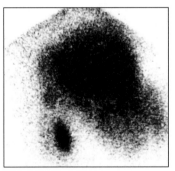

*Anterior, 5 minutes*     *a Anterior, 10 minutes*     *b Right lateral, 10 minutes*

**Fig. 8.16**        **Fig. 8.17**

$^{99m}$Tc HIDA image, showing prominent renal pelves.

*(a,b)* On these $^{99m}$Tc HIDA images, once again, prominent renal pelves are present, and on the lateral view it is apparent that activity is lying posteriorly.

The right renal pelvis simulating a functioning gall bladder is a common misinterpretation of scan findings. It can be differentiated by:

• The time of filling—it fills much earlier and empties much earlier than a normal gall bladder
• Position—the right lateral view demonstrates that it lies posteriorly when compared with the anterior position of a gall bladder.

## 8.3.3 Normal denatured red cell scan of the spleen

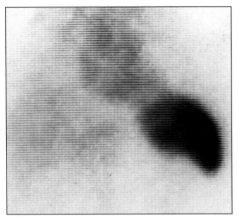 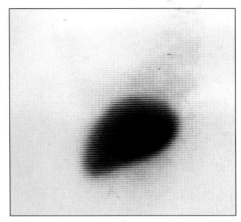

*Fig. 8.18*

*(a,b)* Normal denatured red blood cell scan
of the spleen.

*a Anterior*          *b Posterior*

## 8.3.4 Combined liver/spleen and lung imaging

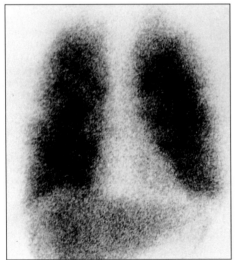 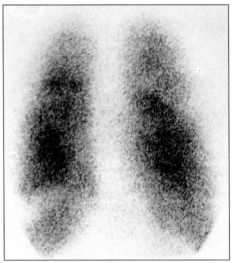 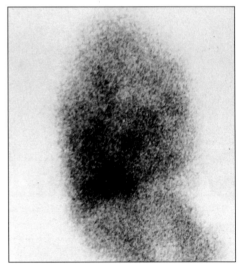

*a Anterior*          *b Posterior*          *c Right lateral*

*Fig. 8.19*

*(a–c)* Normal liver/lung scan, demonstrating normal relationship of the right lung to the
right lobe of the liver, with no space normally visualized between these two organs.

## 8.3.5 External pressure effects on the liver

The liver is a large soft organ, and it takes up the shape of surrounding structures. Because of this, it may show many different appearances, depending on external pressure effects.

### Common examples

- Diaphragmatic effects:
  pleural effusion
  respiration
  overinflated lungs
- Subphrenic effects:
  subphrenic abscess
  subphrenic masses
  interposed colon

- Effect of ribs and xiphisternum
- Cardiac effects
- Renal masses
- Epigastric masses

## *Diaphragmatic effects*

*Pleural effusion*

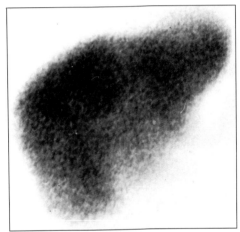

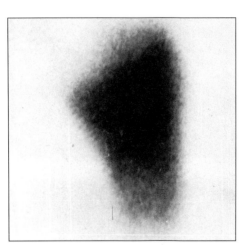

*a  Anterior*

*b  Right lateral*

**Fig. 8.20**

**(a,b)** *Liver/spleen scan.*
*An area of reduced tracer uptake is seen at the upper lateral border of the right lobe of the liver. This is due to a pleural effusion causing compression of the liver.*

*Bilateral pleural effusions*

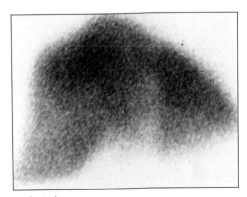

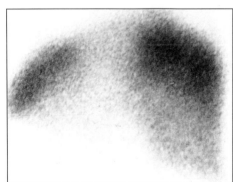

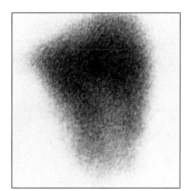

*a  Anterior*

*b  Posterior*

*c  Right lateral*

**Fig. 8.21**

**(a–c)** *Liver/spleen scan.*
*In this case there is evidence of bilateral pleural effusions. It should be noted that a left-sided effusion has to be large before it becomes apparent on such a study.*

## NORMAL SCANS WITH VARIANTS AND ARTEFACTS

### Respiration

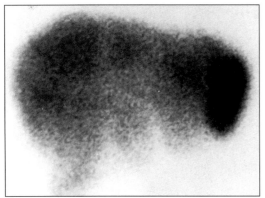

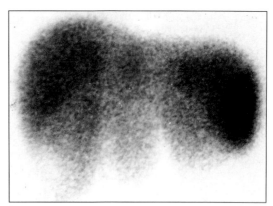

*a Anterior*

*b Anterior*

**Fig. 8.22**

*Liver/spleen scan:*
*(a) inspiration; (b) expiration.*
*Flattening of the upper aspect of the right lobe is seen on full inspiration. This patient had parenchymal liver disease, and it should also be noted that there is a prominent costal impression.*

### Overinflated lungs

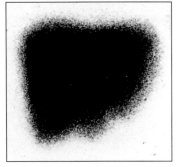

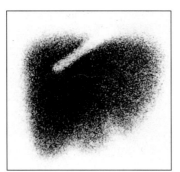

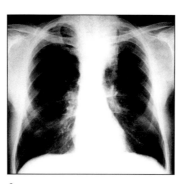

*a Anterior*

*b Anterior*

*c*

**Fig. 8.23**

*(a,b) Liver scan; (b) with costal marker. (c) Chest x-ray.*
*The liver is slightly enlarged, but low-lying in position. The chest x-ray shows hyperinflated (emphysematous) lungs.*

### The effect of the diaphragm on splenic position following pneumonectomy

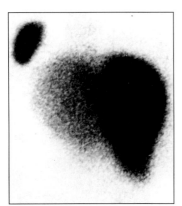

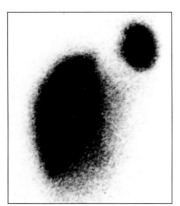

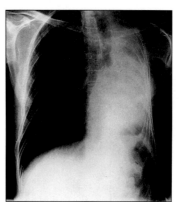

*a Posterior*

*b Left lateral*

*c*

**Fig. 8.24**

*(a,b) Liver/spleen scan.*
*(c) Chest x-ray.*
*It is apparent on the liver/spleen scan that the position of the spleen is very high. This patient had a previous left pneumonectomy, and the chest x-ray shows the elevated left hemidiaphragm.*

**Both the liver and spleen are mobile and soft. Therefore their appearance and position are highly dependent on the surrounding organs and the position of the diaphragm.**

## NORMAL SCANS WITH VARIANTS AND ARTEFACTS

### Subphrenic effects

*A subphrenic abscess showing impression on the upper portion of the right lobe of the liver*

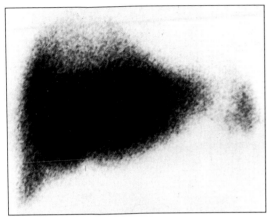

*a Anterior*

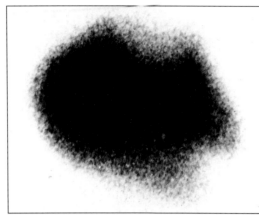

*b Right lateral*

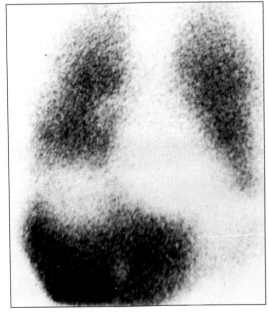

*c Anterior*

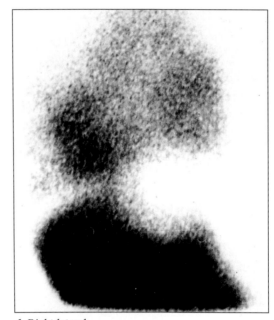

*d Right lateral*

**Fig. 8.25**

**(a,b)** *Liver/spleen scan.*
**(c,d)** *Combined liver/spleen and* $^{99m}Tc$ *microsphere lung scan.*

*This patient developed a right subphrenic abscess following abdominal surgery. Note the concave impression at the upper right lobe of the liver, as compared with the flat impression of a pleural effusion.*

*The use of simultaneous liver/spleen scan and lung imaging may occasionally help to define a subphrenic abscess, but ultrasound is the recommended investigation of choice.*

## NORMAL SCANS WITH VARIANTS AND ARTEFACTS

### Subphrenic mass

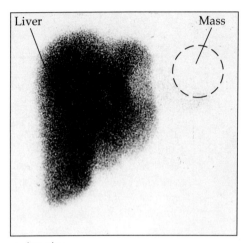

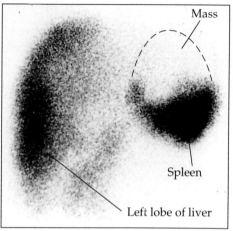

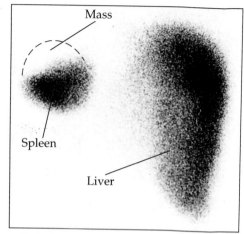

*a* Anterior      *b* Left lateral      *c* Posterior

**Fig. 8.26**

**(a–c)** *Liver/spleen scan.*

   *The spleen is depressed in position and has an irregular outline. The left lobe of the liver is slightly distorted and the overall size appears to be increased. It was suggested that the scan appearances were more likely to be due to a subphrenic mass, either arising from the spleen, or, more likely, distorting the spleen from above. A mass in the left hypochondrium was confirmed by ultrasound.*

### Interposed colon

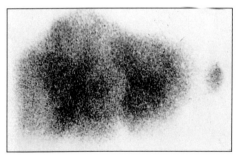

*a* Anterior

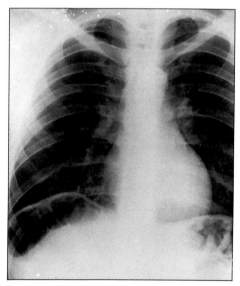

*b*

**Fig. 8.27**

**(a)** *Liver scan.* **(b)** *Chest x-ray.*

   *The liver is enlarged and there is markedly irregular distribution of colloid. There is a large focal defect seen at the upper lateral border of the right lobe. The scan appearances are in keeping with parenchymal liver disease. The defect in the upper right lobe simulates the appearances seen with a large pleural effusion or subphrenic abscess. In this case it was due to the colon lying under the diaphragm, as seen on the chest x-ray.*

## NORMAL SCANS WITH VARIANTS AND ARTEFACTS

## *Costal impression on the liver*

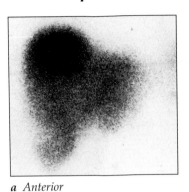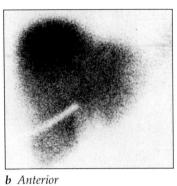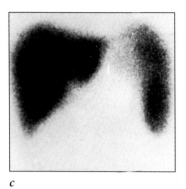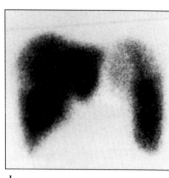

*a Anterior*          *b Anterior*          *c*          *d*

### Fig. 8.28

**(a)** *Liver/spleen scan;* **(b)** *with costal marker. In this patient the normal costal margin is seen to cause an indentation.*

*If there is any doubt as to whether this is a true lesion, views erect **(c)** and supine **(d)** or in inspiration and expiration will help differentiation (as seen in another patient). An extrinsic pressure effect will change its position relative to the liver, while an intrinsic liver lesion will not change its position.*

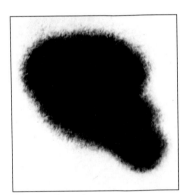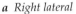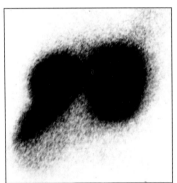

### Fig. 8.29

**(a,b)** *Liver scan.*

*The ribs may also cause impressions on the lateral views, as shown in these two examples.*

*a Right lateral*          *b Right lateral*

## *Cardiac impression on the liver*

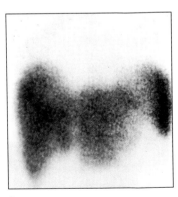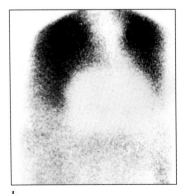

### Fig. 8.30

**(a)** *Liver/spleen scan.* **(b)** *Liver/spleen scan combined with* $^{99m}Tc$ *microsphere lung scan.*

*On the original study it was noted that there was a depression at the upper border of the central area of the liver. This was due to gross cardiomegaly, which is well demonstrated on the combined liver/spleen and lung scan.*

*a*          *b*

## NORMAL SCANS WITH VARIANTS AND ARTEFACTS

### *Costal impression secondary to scoliosis*

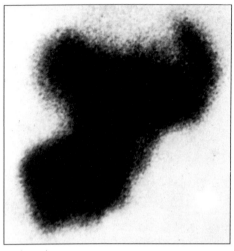

*a Anterior*

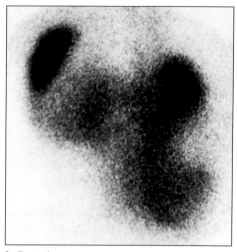

*b Posterior*

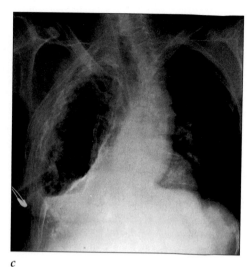

*c*

**Fig. 8.31**

*(a,b) Liver/spleen scan. (c) Chest x-ray.*

*On the liver/spleen scan there is a massive right costal margin impression, and it is noted that the spleen is lying high in position. The chest x-ray illustrates scoliosis and the gross distortion of anatomy.*

 **The shape of the liver will be affected by the surrounding structures, and scan interpretation will be dependent on clinical examination of the patient.**

### *Hot cross bun liver*

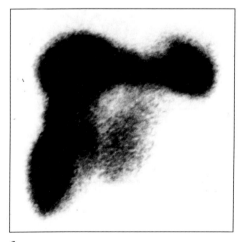

*a*

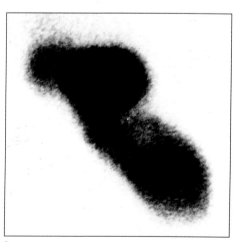

*b*

**Fig. 8.32**

*Compression by heart, costal margin and xiphisternum may combine to cause the 'hot cross bun liver'. This is a normal variant, but is frequently misinterpreted by inexperienced observers.*

## NORMAL SCANS WITH VARIANTS AND ARTEFACTS

### *Renal cyst causing liver compression*

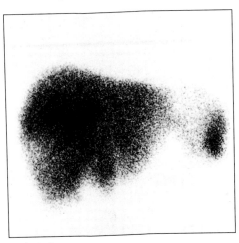 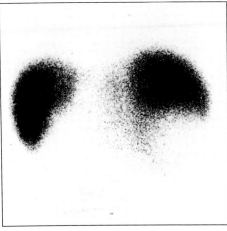 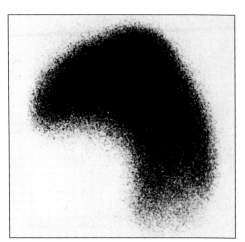

*a  Anterior*          *b  Posterior*          *c  Right lateral*

**Fig. 8.33**

*(a–c) Liver scan.*
  *The liver is diffusely enlarged and there is a massive area of absent colloid accumulation lying posteriorly in the right lobe. This was due to a large renal cyst.*

 Note the difference in shape of abnormal renal compression from normal renal compression shown on page 581.

### *Extrinsic pressure from epigastric mass*

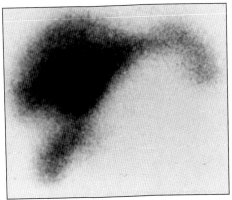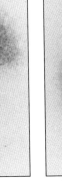 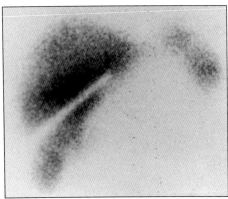

*a  Anterior*          *b  Anterior*

**Fig. 8.34**

*(a,b) Liver/spleen scan; (b) with costal marker.*
  *This patient was known to have a huge epigastric mass. Compression of the border of the left lobe is apparent. A prominent costal impression is also seen.*

## 8.3.6 Artefacts

### Coin artefacts

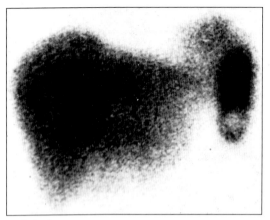 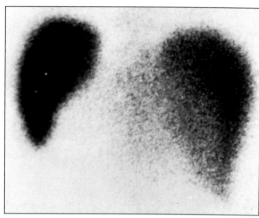

*a* Anterior

*b* Posterior

**Fig. 8.35**

*(a,b) Liver/spleen scan.*
*There is a focal defect seen in the lower pole of the spleen, caused by a coin in this patient's pyjama pocket. Note that no lesion is present on the posterior view, emphasizing the importance of visualizing lesions in two views whenever possible.*

### Photomultiplier tube defect

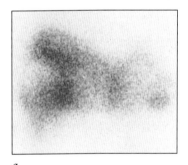 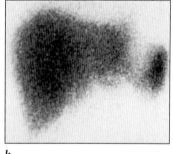

*a*

*b*

**Fig. 8.36**

*Liver/spleen scan: (a) and (b) repeat study.*
*On the original study (a), large focal defects are seen in the right lobe of the liver and the spleen. These were caused by photo-multiplier tube defects. The repeat study is essentially normal, with no space-occupying lesions present.*

### Breast absorption artefact

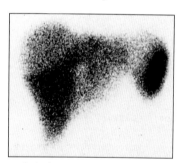 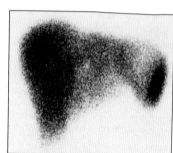

*a* Anterior

*b* Anterior

**Fig. 8.37**

*(a,b) Liver scan; (b) with breast elevated.*
*On the initial scan there is a large area of reduced tracer uptake present at the upper pole of the right lobe of the liver. This disappears once the breast is elevated.*

 The liver/spleen scan is highly susceptible to absorption artefacts from overlying tissue and other objects. An attempt should always be made to identify 'lesions' in more than one view.

 Routine elevation of the breasts during anterior imaging is an advisable precaution. However, gold rings on the patient's fingers may cause further artefacts!

# 8.4 CLINICAL APPLICATIONS

The clinical applications of liver/spleen imaging are listed below, and examples of the various clinical problems are given on subsequent pages.

**8.4.1 Metastatic disease**
Detection of metastatic disease
Monitoring of changes in metastatic disease after chemotherapy

**8.4.2 Parenchymal disease**
Assessment of parenchymal disease
Assessment of hepatomegaly

**8.4.3 Splenic disease**
Assessment of splenomegaly
Investigation of splenic function

**8.4.4 Trauma**
Liver/spleen scan in the investigation of trauma
Denatured red cells to demonstrate splenic trauma
Hepatic trauma
Investigation of suspected biliary leak

**8.4.5 Investigation of abnormal liver function tests**
Alcoholic liver disease
Metastatic liver disease

**8.4.6 Investigation of upper abdominal pain**
Unsuspected metastatic disease
Gall bladder mucocele
Splenic infarct

Investigation of acute cholecystitis
Chronic cholecystitis
Gastric reflux of bile as a cause of upper abdominal pain

**8.4.7 Investigation of jaundice**
Hepatic jaundice: acute
Hepatic jaundice: chronic
Investigation of intermittent jaundice
Cholestatic jaundice: intrahepatic
Cholestatic jaundice: extrahepatic

**8.4.8 Investigation of hepatic infection**
Amoebic abscess
Hydatid cyst
Pyogenic abscess

**8.4.9 Evaluation of response to interventional therapy**
Intrahepatic arterial cytotoxic perfusion therapy
Embolic therapy
Liver scanning prior to biopsy
Assessment of shunt for ascites
Hepatic damage caused by radiation therapy
Hepatic infarction caused by external radiation

# 8.4.1 Metastatic disease

## *Detection of metastatic disease*

The radionuclide colloid liver/spleen scan was the first technique for non-invasive imaging of the liver and metastases within it. In spite of advances in ultrasound, CT etc., there is still a role for this investigation in the staging of patients with known cancer. It remains a cheap, accurate screening investigation, which is less operator-dependent than ultrasound and provides information about the function of the liver. It is probably better than all the other modalities for serial imaging in evaluating rapidly the extent, progress or regression of metastatic disease. Finally, it remains the best imaging modality for non-expert clinicians, enabling them to understand the images as they are presented.

## *Solitary metastasis*

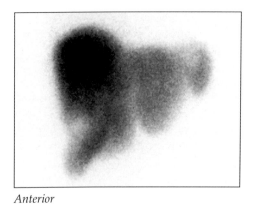

*Anterior*

**Fig. 8.38**

*Liver colloid image, showing a single photon-deficient area in the lateral aspect of right lobe.*

## *Multiple metastasis*

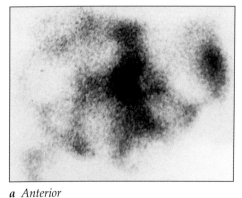

*a Anterior*

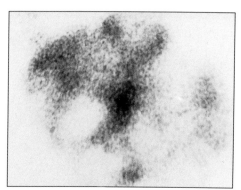

*b Right lateral*

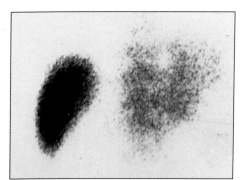

*c Posterior*

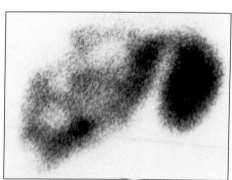

*d Left lateral*

**Fig. 8.39**

*(a–d) Liver/spleen scan.*
*The liver is enlarged and there are multiple focal defects throughout the organ. This is a typical example of multiple liver metastases in a patient with carcinoma of the colon.*

## CLINICAL APPLICATIONS

*Two further examples of multiple liver metastases*

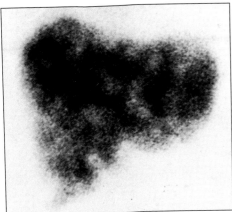

*a  Anterior*

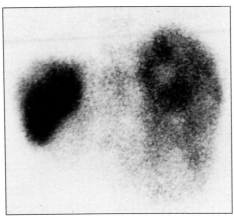
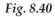

*b  Posterior*

***Fig. 8.40***

*(**a,b**) Liver/spleen scan.*
  *A patient presenting with lung cancer and liver metastases.*

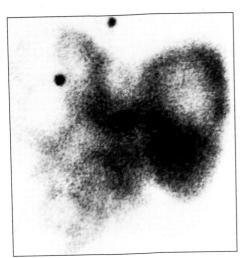

*a  Anterior*

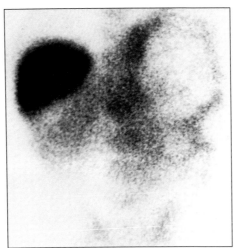
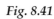

*b  Posterior*

***Fig. 8.41***

*(**a,b**) Liver/spleen scan.*
  *A patient presenting with gastric carcinoma and marked hepatomegaly caused by metastases.*

**Although exceptions occur, metastases to the liver from breast and lung cancer are small, while those from gastrointestinal carcinoma are large and clear-cut.**

*Liver metastases best demonstrated on lateral view*

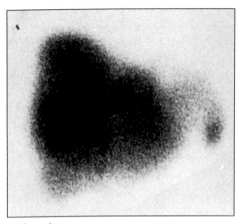

*a Anterior*

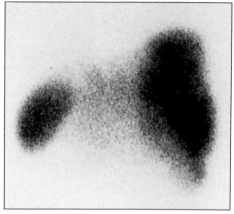

*b Posterior*

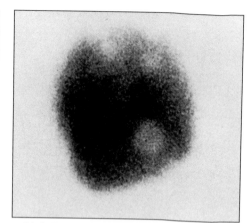

*c Right lateral*

### Fig. 8.42

**(a–c)** *Liver scan in a 60-year-old woman with carcinoma of the breast, with liver metastases.*

*The liver is enlarged and shows multiple focal abnormalities, particularly in the right lobe, which are best seen on the lateral view. The scan appearances are typical of metastatic disease involving the liver.*

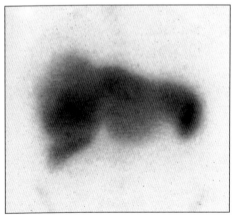

*a Anterior*

*b Posterior*

*c Right lateral*

### Fig. 8.43

**(a–c)** *Liver scan in a 58-year-old woman with liver metastases.*

*The liver is slightly enlarged and shows focal abnormalities throughout. The lesions are, however, best seen on the posterior view. The scan appearances are those of multiple metastases involving the liver.*

 These two cases demonstrate the **importance of multiple views.**

## CLINICAL APPLICATIONS

### Hepatic cysts mimicking metastases

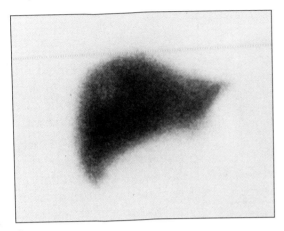

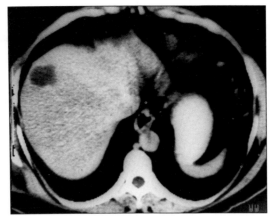

a              b

**Fig. 8.44**

*(a)* Liver/spleen scan. *(b)* CT scan.

   *The single photon-deficient area in the right lobe was caused by a cyst, which is shown well on the accompanying CT scan.*

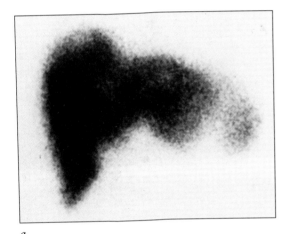

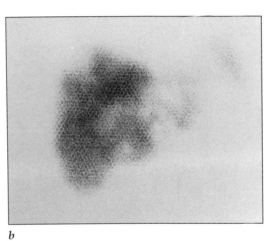

a              b

**Fig. 8.45**

*(a,b) Two patients who were being investigated for lung cancer. The multiple focal lesions are due to liver cysts and not metastatic deposits.*

It is important to remember that the finding of a focal lesion on the liver/spleen scan is non-specific. Simple cysts appear identical to metastases, and it could clearly affect patient management profoundly if metastases are assumed.

### An example of a solitary space-occupying lesion: hepatic cyst

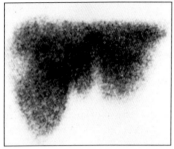
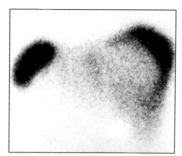
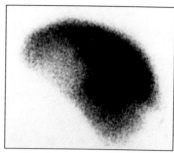

*a* Anterior    *b* Posterior    *c* Right lateral

**Fig. 8.46**

*(a–c) Liver/spleen scan.*
  *A large focal defect is present in the posterior aspect of the right lobe. This was due to a hepatic cyst.*

It may be impossible to differentiate a renal mass from an intra-hepatic mass, as in the case of the hepatic cyst shown in Fig. 8.46. When a rim of functioning liver tissue is present, this will confirm the intrahepatic position of the lesion. Ultrasound must be used to distinguish a solid lesion from a cyst.

### Tumour infiltration of the left lobe

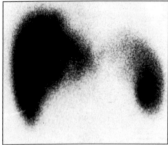
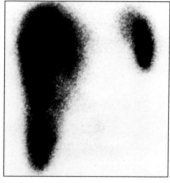
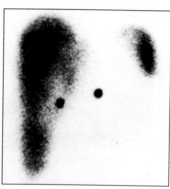

Anterior

**Fig. 8.47**

*a* Anterior    *b* Anterior

**Fig. 8.48**

*Liver/spleen scan.*
  *The right lobe of the liver appears normal. The left lobe of the liver is represented by a photon-deficient area with somewhat irregular borders. The scan findings indicate infiltration and replacement of the left lobe by tumour.*

*(a,b) Liver/spleen scan; (b) with marker on palpable mass.*
  *The original liver scan shows an absent left lobe, which could be a normal variant. However, the markers on the palpable mass confirm tumour infiltration of the left lobe.*

The abdomen must always be palpated for adequate liver scan reporting, with markers being placed on upper abdominal masses.

### Appearance of metastases in the left lobe of the liver

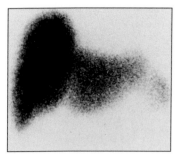
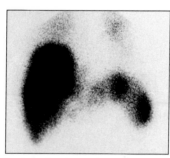

*a* Anterior, 0 months    *b* Anterior, 4 months

**Fig. 8.49**

*(a,b) Liver/spleen scan in a 63-year-old woman with carcinoma of the breast, with metastases involving the left lobe of the liver.*
  *The initial study shows slight hepatomegaly, but no focal defects are seen. A repeat study was requested because of deteriorating liver function. Once again, the liver is slightly enlarged, but on this occasion the left lobe is not visualized. Slight uptake of tracer is noted over the lungs. This is a non-specific finding, indicating increased phagocytic activity within the lungs, which is most commonly seen in association with either septicaemia or malignant effusion.*

*Unexpected tumour involvement of the left lobe of the liver*

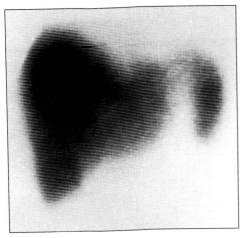

*a Anterior*

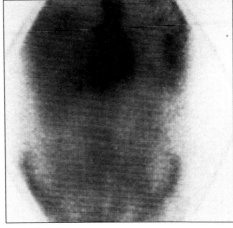

*b Anterior*

**Fig. 8.50**

*(a) Liver/spleen scan. (b) ⁶⁷Ga study of the abdomen.*

This patient was being staged for Hodgkin's disease. The liver scan appears essentially normal and shows only the frequently seen thinning of the left lobe. The ⁶⁷Ga scan, however, shows relatively increased tracer accumulation in the left lobe, indicating that the 'thinning' was, in fact, tumour replacement.

*Progressive metastatic disease predominantly involving the left lobe of the liver*

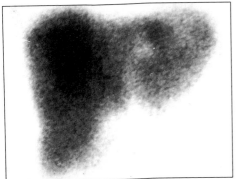

*a 0 months*

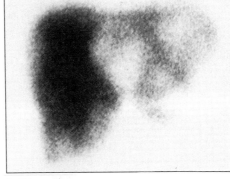

*b 12 months*

**Fig. 8.51**

*(a,b) Liver scan.*

On the original study, the liver is slightly enlarged, with irregularity of tracer uptake in the left lobe; the appearances are suggestive of focal involvement. The repeat study 1 year later shows dramatic progression of disease, with multiple focal defects present. This patient had carcinoma of the breast.

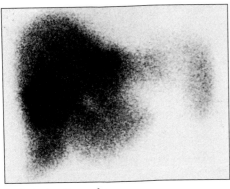

*a Anterior, 0 months*

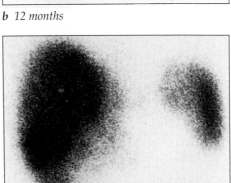

*b Anterior, 6 months*

**Fig. 8.52**

*(a,b) Liver/spleen scan in a 43-year-old woman with carcinoma of the breast and liver metastases.*

On the original study the left lobe of the liver is enlarged with focal lesions present caused by metastases. The subsequent study shows progression of disease, with virtually complete replacement of the left lobe by tumour.

- In many ways the second study (Fig. 8.52) appears more 'normal' than the first (Fig. 8.51), since no focal lesions are seen. However, this pattern should always alert the clinician to the possibility that the left lobe has been replaced by tumour.
- Occasionally, diffuse metastatic deposits from carcinoma of the breast will show only as slight inhomogeneities on the scan, and very rarely the only scan evidence will be hepatomegaly with homogeneous tracer distribution.

## Monitoring of changes in metastatic disease after chemotherapy

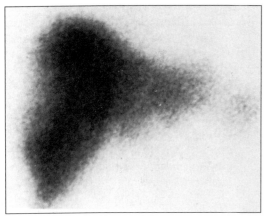

*a Anterior, before*

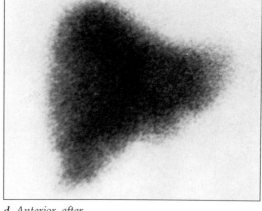

*d Anterior, after*

### Fig. 8.53

*Partial resolution of hepatic metastasis. Liver scan: (a–c) before and (d–f) after a course of chemotherapy.*

   *On the original study there is a large area of reduced colloid accumulation in the posterior portion of the right lobe. Following 5 months' chemotherapy, the lesion is again seen but is much smaller.*

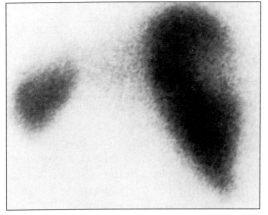

*b Posterior, before*

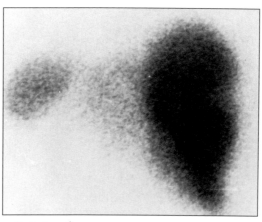

*e Posterior, after*

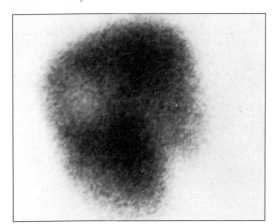

*c Right lateral, before*

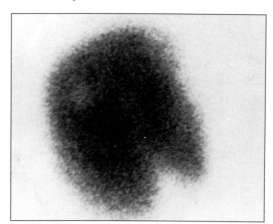

*f Right lateral, after*

Although ultrasound and CT demonstrate mass lesions in the liver extremely well, the radionuclide liver/spleen scan may be the best and simplest method to follow the progress or resolution of metastases. To be effective, however, it is vital that the magnification and intensity of the image, and the position of the patient, stay constant.

A further case of resolution of metastases after chemotherapy

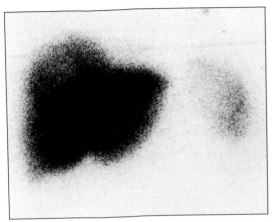

*a* Anterior, before

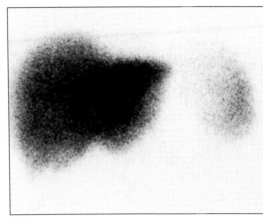

*d* Anterior, after

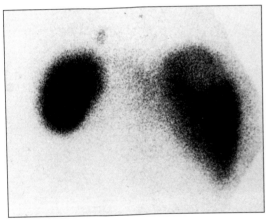

*b* Posterior, before

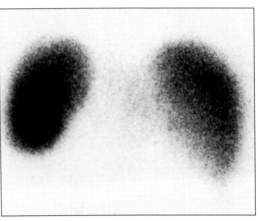

*e* Posterior, after

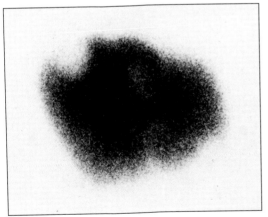

*c* Right lateral, before

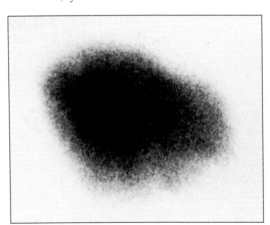

*f* Right lateral, after

**Fig. 8.54**

*A 64-year-old man with carcinoma of the lung. Liver scan: (**a–c**) before and (**d–f**) 4 months after a course of chemotherapy.*

*On the original study multiple focal defects are seen throughout the liver. Following chemotherapy, there is a dramatic improvement in the scan appearance. However, there is still a focal defect present in the posterior aspect of the upper right lobe, best seen on the right lateral view.*

## A shrinking liver may indicate resolution of metastases

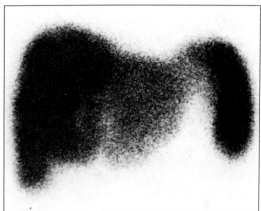

*a  Anterior, 0 months*

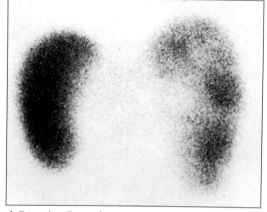

*b  Posterior, 0 months*

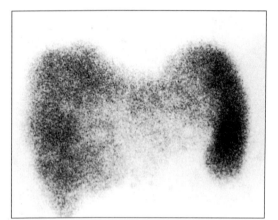

*c  Anterior, 5 months*

*d  Posterior, 5 months*

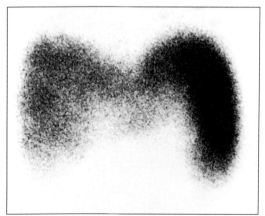

*e  Anterior, 8 months*

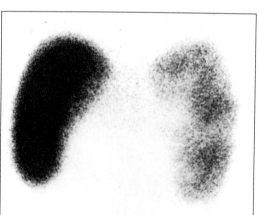

*f  Posterior, 8 months*

*Fig. 8.55*

*(a–f) Liver scan.*
   *On the original study the liver is slightly enlarged with evidence of tumour involvement. The spleen is also slightly enlarged. On subsequent images the liver becomes progressively smaller, with grossly irregular tracer uptake. The spleen has shown progressive enlargement over the three studies. Further, there is markedly increased uptake of tracer in the spleen relative to the liver. Although in this case the contracting liver with increasing splenomegaly is due to resolution of metastases, the finding is rare and most often seen with progressive parenchymal disease such as cirrhosis.*

## CLINICAL APPLICATIONS

*Three cases showing progressive metastatic disease*

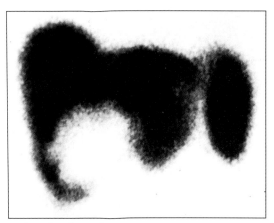

*a  Anterior, 0 months*

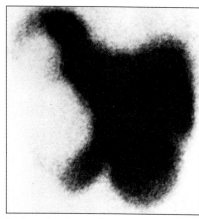

*b  Anterior, 3 months*

***Fig. 8.56***

***(a,b)*** *Liver/spleen scan.*
  This patient was known to have colonic carcinoma, and the original study showed massive metastases in the right lobe. A repeat study was requested to assess response to chemotherapy, but it is apparent that there has been gross extension of disease.

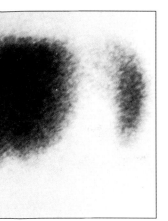

*a  0 months*

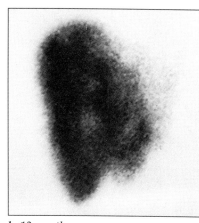

*b  12 months*

***Fig. 8.57***

***(a,b)*** *Liver/spleen scan.*
  In this case of Hodgkin's disease the original study was normal. However, 1 year later there is evidence of multiple deposits in the right lobe of the liver and replacement of the left lobe by tumour.

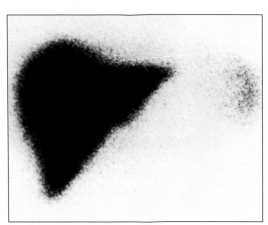

*a  Anterior, 0 months*

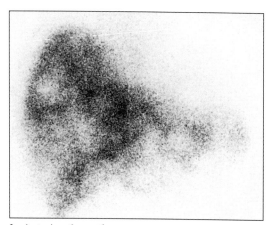

*b  Anterior, 6 months*

***Fig. 8.58***

***(a,b)*** *Liver/spleen scan.*
  The original study from this patient with carcinoma of the breast was normal. However, this patient subsequently developed hepatomegaly and had abnormal liver function tests. The repeat liver/spleen scan confirms widespread metastatic disease.

*Importance of a baseline study for serial examinations*

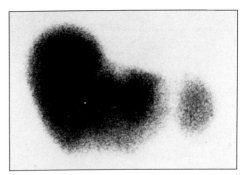

*a Anterior, 0 months*

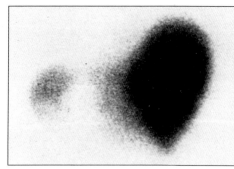

*b Posterior, 0 months*

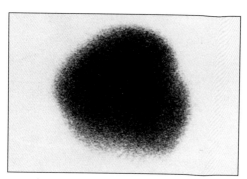

*c Right lateral, 0 months*

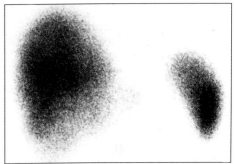

*d Anterior, 12 months*

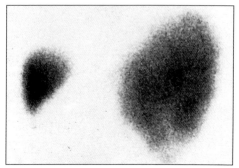

*e Posterior, 12 months*

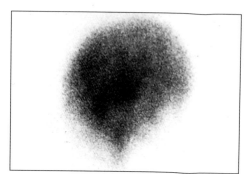

*f Right lateral, 12 months*

**Fig. 8.59**

A 68-year-old woman with hepatic metastases from carcinoma of the breast. Liver/spleen scan: *(a–c)* initial study; *(d–f)* 1 year later.

The initial study is normal. On the repeat study, the liver appears normal in size but there is non-homogeneity of tracer uptake with presence of focal abnormality in the right lower lobe posteriorly. In addition, the left lobe is no longer visualized. The scan appearances represent metastatic involvement, and abnormalities are much more obvious when related to the original study.

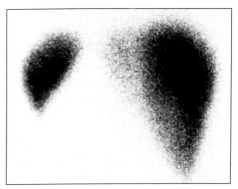

*a Posterior, 0 months*

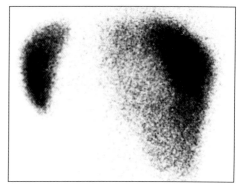

*b Posterior, 2 months*

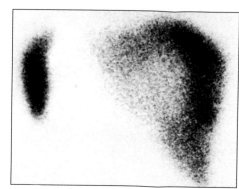

*c Posterior, 3 months*

**Fig. 8.60**

*(a–c)* Liver/spleen scan.

This series of studies shows the appearance and progression of a solitary metastatic deposit from carcinoma of the lung. Note how difficult the diagnosis of a metastatic deposit would be on study *(b)* without the baseline to compare it with.

**Review liver scans in comparison with previous studies to avoid errors of interpretation.**

## Metastatic deposits in the spleen

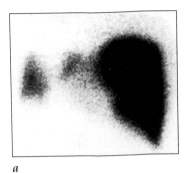 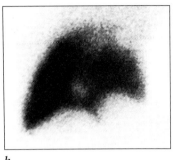 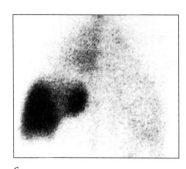 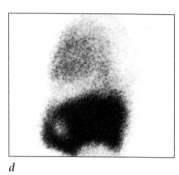

*a*  *b*  *c*  *d*

**Fig. 8.61**

*(a) Posterior colloid liver/spleen scan, showing abnormal appearances on the left side. (b) Left lateral colloid scan; the liver and spleen cannot be separated. (c) Posterior denatured red cell scan, showing the outline of the spleen and tumour infiltration. (d) Left lateral denatured red cell scan, clearly demonstrating a large spleen with space-occupying lesions. This patient was found to have tumour deposits in the spleen during the investigation and staging of breast cancer.*

Metastatic deposits in the spleen are rare. The splenic notch and position of the spleen and its relation to the left lobe may simulate metastases. It is always advisable to confirm metastases with a denatured red cell splenic scan.

## Lymphomatous deposit in the spleen

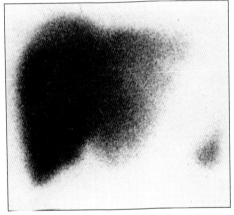  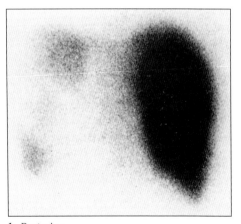 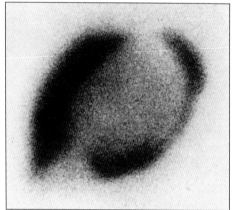 

*a  Anterior*  *b  Posterior*  *c  Left lateral*

**Fig. 8.62**

*Lymphoma of the spleen. (a–c) Liver scan.*
*The liver appears normal. The spleen is enlarged and there is a huge focal defect present. Indeed, there is only a rim of normal tissue visible surrounding the defect. The scan findings are those of a large space-occupying lesion and, in this case, were due to lymphoma.*

The presence of space-occupying lesions in the spleen should always raise the possibility of lymphoma rather than metastatic carcinoma.

*Multiple metastases demonstrated by SPECT*

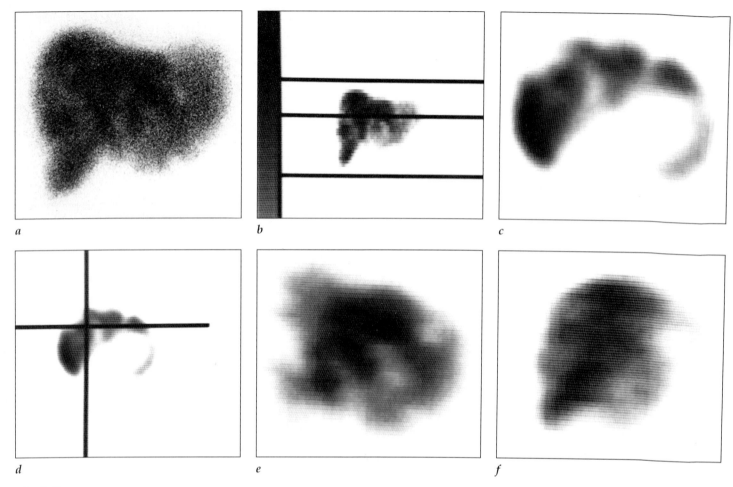

a  b  c

d  e  f

**Fig. 8.63**

*With SPECT imaging, sections in a variety of planes can be obtained, usually with clearer identification of individual lesions. (a) Anterior colloid planar section, showing multiple metastases. (b) Anterior projection, identifying level of transaxial section (central line) demonstrated in (c). (d) Transaxial section, identifying levels of coronal section (horizontal line) demonstrated in (e) and of sagittal section (vertical line) demonstrated in (f).*

*Sagittal*

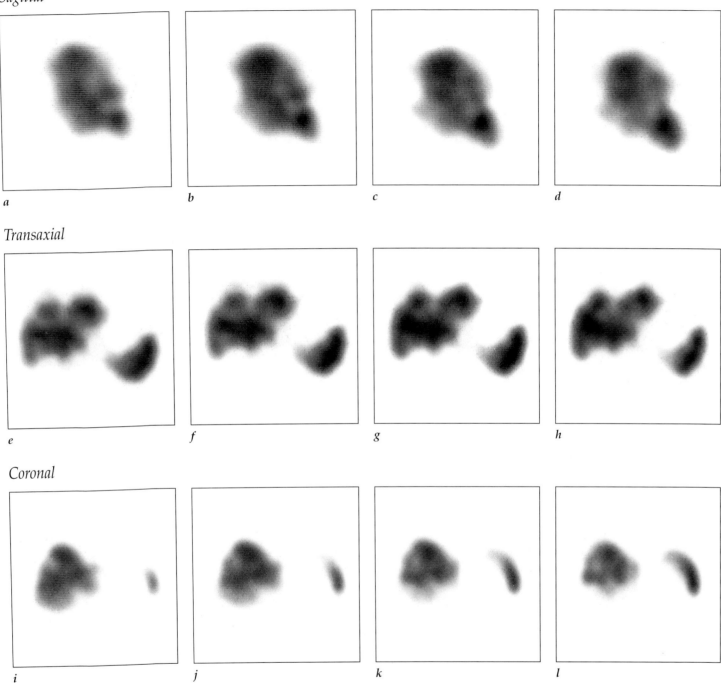

*Transaxial*

*Coronal*

**Fig. 8.64**

*A series of* SPECT *slices in the sagittal* **(a–d)**, *transaxial* **(e–h)** *and coronal* **(i–l)** *planes, showing multiple metastases.*

## 8.4.2 Parenchymal disease

### *Assessment of parenchymal disease*

*Features of parenchymal liver disease*

*Liver size*
- Early disease: left lobe hypertrophies
- Later disease: diffuse hepatomegaly occurs
- Advanced disease: small liver.

*Distribution of tracer*
- Liver inhomogeneities
- Increased splenic uptake with longstanding disease
- Increased bone marrow uptake.

*Early parenchymal liver disease*

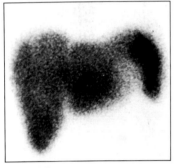
*a Anterior*

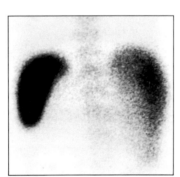
*b Posterior*

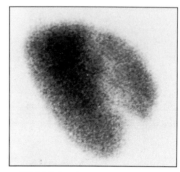
*c Right lateral*

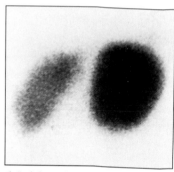
*d Left lateral*

**Fig. 8.65**

Assessment of parenchymal disease. (*a–d*) Liver/spleen scan.
  *This patient has moderate alcohol-related liver disease. Note that slight hepatomegaly is present on the scan. Further, there is non-homogeneity of tracer uptake. The spleen is somewhat enlarged and shows increased tracer uptake relative to the liver. Tracer uptake in bone marrow is also present.*

- **Increased activity in the spleen and bone marrow is seen because as progressive impairment of liver function occurs the high extraction efficiency of the liver for colloid diminishes, more colloid becoming available for uptake by the rest of the RES.**
- **The spleen lies posteriorly and should not normally appear 'hotter' than the liver on the anterior view.**

*A more advanced case of diffuse parenchymal liver disease*

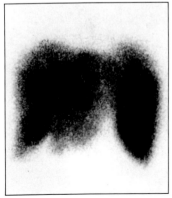
*a Anterior*

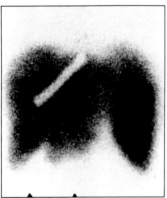
*b Anterior*

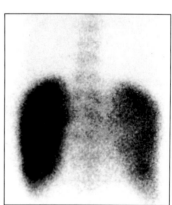
*c Posterior*

**Fig. 8.66**

(*a–c*) Liver scan; costal marker on (*b*).
  *The liver is enlarged and shows non-homogeneity of tracer uptake. No discrete focal abnormalities are seen. The spleen is enlarged and shows high uptake of tracer relative to the liver. Uptake of tracer by bone marrow is also seen. The scan appearances are those of significant parenchymal liver disease with portal hypertension and a degree of hepatic failure.*

## Severe parenchymal liver disease

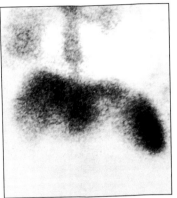
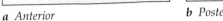
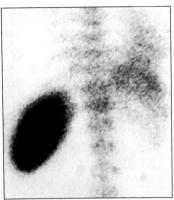

*a* Anterior
*b* Posterior

**Fig. 8.67**

*(a,b)* Liver/spleen scan.

Note that there is a small shrunken liver and an enlarged spleen. There is visualization of bone marrow. Tracer uptake by the lung is seen and this is of uncertain significance.

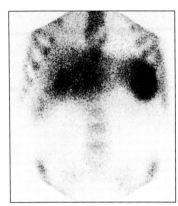
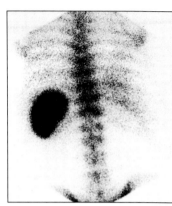

*a* Anterior
*b* Posterior

**Fig. 8.68**

*(a,b)* Liver/spleen scan.

In this case the uptake in the liver is extremely poor and the organ is hardly visualized on the posterior view.

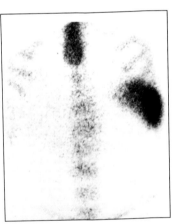
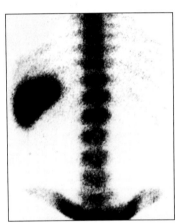

*a* Anterior
*b* Posterior

**Fig. 8.69**

*(a,b)* Liver/spleen scan.

This is a case of advanced cirrhosis. The liver/spleen scan was obtained during an acute exacerbation, with superimposed alcoholic hepatitis. Note the complete absence of tracer uptake in the liver.

• When the uptake is very poor, it may not be possible to visualize the liver sufficiently well to exclude a hepatoma.

• A second anterior view for a longer time and with the intensity turned up to saturate the spleen and bone marrow may help to visualize the liver.

## Effect of ascites

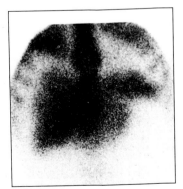

Anterior

**Fig. 8.70**

Liver/spleen scan.

This is a patient with advanced liver disease. Note that the presence of ascites causes a photon-deficient area around the liver and spleen. This is apparent because of the increased tracer uptake by marrow in the ribs.

## CLINICAL APPLICATIONS

### *Alcoholic hepatitis*

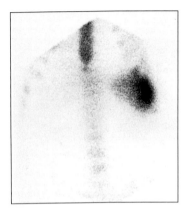
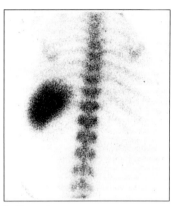

*a  Anterior*  *b  Posterior*

**Fig. 8.71**

*A 44-year-old woman with alcoholic hepatitis. (a,b) Views of the abdomen.*

*There is almost no uptake of colloid in the liver, but there is marked uptake in the bone marrow and spleen. The spleen is at the upper limit of normal in size. These scan appearances are typical of alcoholic hepatitis.*

**Absent uptake in the liver is probably due to a toxic effect on the Kupffer cells and is strongly suggestive of acute alcoholic hepatitis.**

### *Primary biliary cirrhosis*

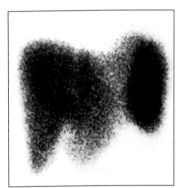
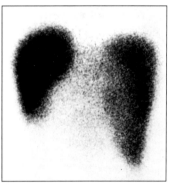

*a  Anterior*  *b  Posterior*  *Posterior*

**Fig. 8.72**

**Fig. 8.73**

*(a,b) Liver/spleen scan.*

*This is a middle-aged woman with moderately severe primary biliary cirrhosis. The liver is slightly enlarged, with some non-homogeneity of tracer uptake. Note, however, the large spleen with increased uptake of tracer, but very little uptake present in the bone marrow. Early bone marrow uptake of tracer is more commonly seen with alcoholic cirrhosis.*

*Liver/spleen scan.*

*This is a man with mild liver disease and an associated bleeding ulcer causing blood loss, anaemia and hyperactive bone marrow. Note the high uptake in the bone marrow, but without associated increased uptake in the spleen.*

**Although increased tracer uptake into bone marrow in association with impaired liver function is usually associated with increased uptake in the spleen, this is not always the case. For example, if there is splenic hypofunction (eg coeliac disease) associated with the liver disease, there will be increased uptake in the marrow without increased uptake in the spleen. Increased uptake in the marrow alone may be due either to marrow hyperactivity, eg in association with anaemia caused by blood loss or chronic haemolysis, or to primary marrow hyperactivity, as seen in polycythaemia rubra vera.**

## CLINICAL APPLICATIONS

*Budd–Chiari syndrome due to hepatic vein occlusion*

*Clinical features*

- Hepatomegaly
- Abdominal pain
- Ascites.

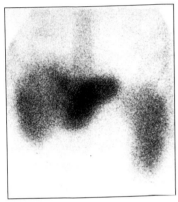
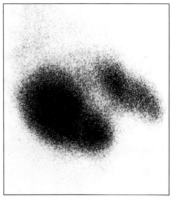
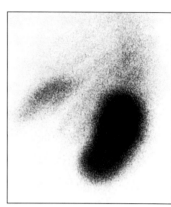

*a  Anterior*      *b  Posterior*      *c  Right lateral*      *d  Left lateral*

**Fig. 8.74**

**(a–d)** *Liver scan in 73-year-old man with parenchymal liver disease and Budd–Chiari syndrome.*
*The liver is relatively normal in size. There is striking non-homogeneity of tracer uptake throughout the liver, with marked reduction of tracer uptake in most of the right lobe. There is, however, relatively increased uptake in the region of the caudate lobe, which is hypertrophied. The spleen is enlarged, with high uptake of tracer, and there is also tracer uptake by bone marrow. The scan findings are in keeping with Budd–Chiari syndrome, parenchymal liver disease with portal hypertension and a degree of hepatic failure.*

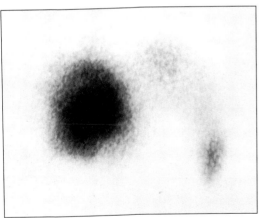
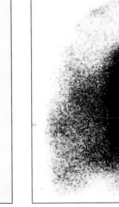

*a  Patient 1*      *b  Patient 2*

**Fig. 8.75**

**(a,b)** *Two further examples of anterior liver/spleen scans in patients with Budd–Chiari syndrome.*

- Tracer uptake is seen in the hypertrophied caudate lobe, since this has a different venous drainage which may be spared in the obstructive process.
- A hepatoma replacing the right lobe of the liver should not be misdiagnosed as Budd–Chiari syndrome.

## CLINICAL APPLICATIONS

### Multiple focal defects on the liver scan associated with appearances of diffuse parenchymal disease

#### Causes
- Diffuse liver disease with irregular scarring or with nodular regeneration
- Multiple metastases with secondary increased uptake in marrow due to hyperactivity from blood loss
- Multiple metastases in a patient with diffuse liver disease
- Diffuse parenchymal liver disease with superimposed multifocal hepatoma.

### Advanced cirrhosis with focal lesions in the liver due to fibrous scars

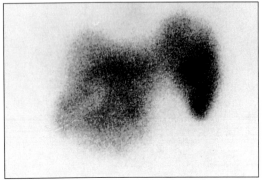 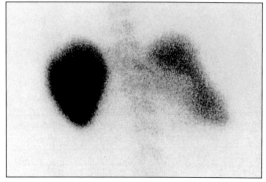

*a Anterior*

*b Posterior*

**Fig. 8.76**

*(a,b) Liver/spleen scan.*
   *The scan appearances show the typical features of parenchymal liver disease. While there is non-homogeneity of tracer uptake throughout the liver, more focal defects are also present. These were due to fibrous scars.*

### Parenchymal liver disease with multiple focal defects in the liver due to multifocal hepatoma

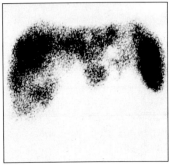  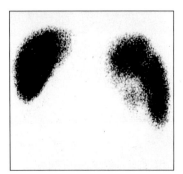 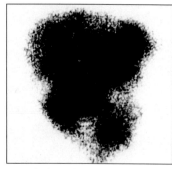

*a Anterior*

*b Posterior*

*c Right lateral*

**Fig. 8.77**

*(a–c) Liver/spleen scan.*
   *The liver is slightly enlarged, with multiple focal defects throughout. The spleen is significantly enlarged, with increased tracer uptake relative to the liver. The scan appearances are those of multiple space-occupying lesions in the liver, which were due to multifocal hepatoma.*

### Multiple metastases with some scan features of diffuse parenchymal liver disease

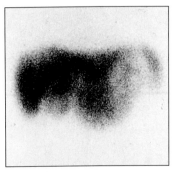 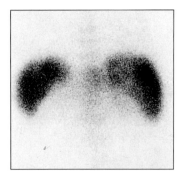 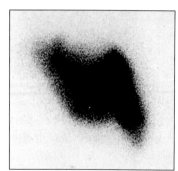

*a Anterior*

*b Posterior*

*c Right lateral*

**Fig. 8.78**

*(a–c) Liver/spleen scan.*
   *The liver is enlarged, mainly as the result of left lobe hypertrophy. There is striking non-homogeneity of tracer uptake, with multiple focal abnormalities throughout. The spleen appears normal.*

## CLINICAL APPLICATIONS

### $^{67}$Ga in the diagnosis of hepatoma

*Clinical indications for a $^{67}$Ga scan in cirrhosis*
- Sudden deterioration in liver function
- Sudden development of ascites
- Liver/spleen scan showing a significant focal defect
- High titre of serum alpha-fetoprotein (positive alpha-fetoprotein has a 60% sensitivity for hepatoma).

### Hepatoma

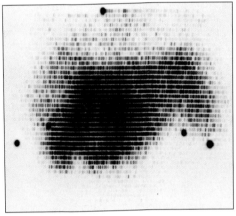

*a Anterior*

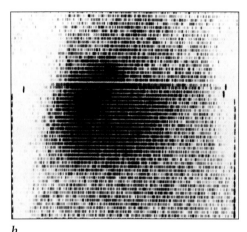

*b*

**Fig. 8.79**

*Hepatoma. **(a)** Rectilinear scan, liver/spleen scan. **(b)** $^{67}$Ga scan.*
   *On the colloid study a large focal defect is seen in the right lobe of the liver. However, the $^{67}$Ga scan of the same patient shows intense uptake at that site, strongly supporting the diagnosis of hepatoma.*

### A further case of hepatoma

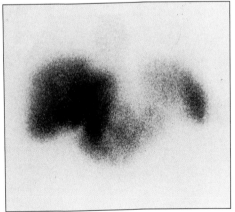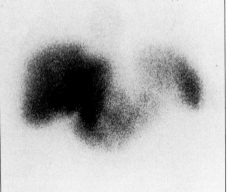

*a Anterior*

*b Anterior*

*c Anterior (subtraction)*

**Fig. 8.80**

*(a) Liver/spleen scan. (b) $^{67}$Ga. (c) Subtraction image ($^{67}$Ga – SC).*
   *The liver is enlarged. There is non-homogeneity of tracer uptake, with a huge focal abnormality involving much of the left lobe. This patient was known to have parenchymal liver disease, and the presence of a focal defect was suggestive of hepatoma. The $^{67}$Ga scan showed tracer uptake in the left lobe, and focal accumulation was confirmed on the subtraction image ($^{67}$Ga minus colloid scan).*

 **Carefully obtained subtraction images of colloid from a $^{67}$Ga study will increase the sensitivity for detection of mismatched lesions which are indicative of a hepatoma.**

## *Assessment of hepatomegaly*

### *Causes of hepatomegaly*

- Neoplasms:
  primary and secondary
- Cirrhosis
- Venous congestion (congestive cardiac failure, inferior vena cava obstruction, etc.)
- Infiltration, eg fatty liver (alcohol and diabetes), lymphoma, amyloid, glycogen storage

- Infections:
  focal, eg abscess
  diffuse, eg viral hepatitis
- Wilson's disease
- Haemachromatosis.

### *Apparent hepatomegaly*

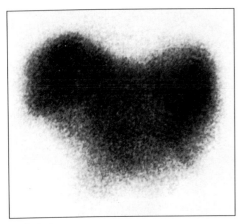

*a Anterior*

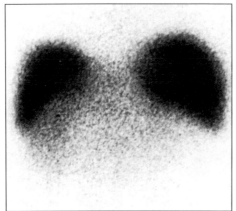

*b Posterior*

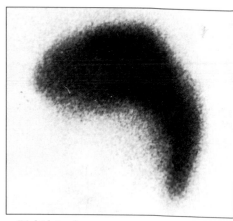

*c Right lateral*

**Fig. 8.81**

*(a–c) Liver scan.*

*This patient presented with a mass in the right hypochondrium, suspected of being caused by hepatomegaly. There is a massive area of absent colloid accumulation at the lower pole of the right lobe of the liver. In this case the abnormality was due to an extrinsic liver mass from hypernephroma.*

### *Hepatomegaly due to metastases*

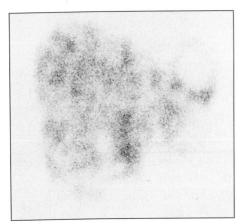

*Anterior*

**Fig. 8.82**

*Liver/spleen scan.*

*This young woman presented with hepatomegaly of unknown cause. The liver scan clearly demonstrates the presence of multiple focal lesions, which were subsequently shown to be due to metastases from carcinoma of the breast.*

## CLINICAL APPLICATIONS

*Infiltration*

*Cirrhosis*

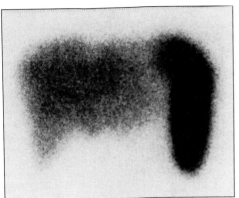

*a* Anterior

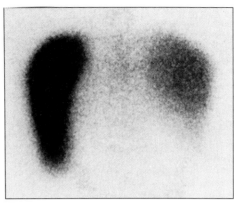

*b* Posterior

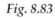

**Fig. 8.83**

*(a,b)* Liver/spleen scan.

The liver is diffusely enlarged. The spleen is markedly enlarged and shows increased colloid avidity. There is some tracer uptake seen in the bone marrow. The scan appearances are those of moderately severe parenchymal liver disease with portal hypertension.

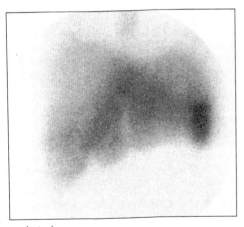

*a* Anterior

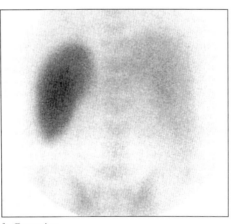

*b* Posterior

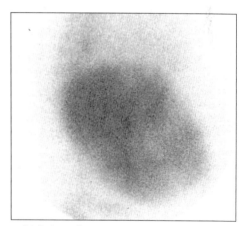

*c* Right lateral

**Fig. 8.84**

*(a–c)* Grossly enlarged liver with reduced patchy uptake secondary to fatty infiltrate and reduced function due to alcoholic liver disease. Note bone marrow uptake and large spleen.

*Hepatosplenomegaly due to amyloidosis*

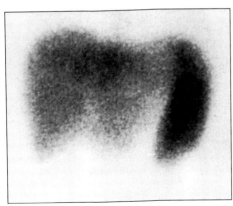

*Anterior*

**Fig. 8.85**

The liver and spleen are both enlarged. The scan appearances are in keeping with diffuse parenchymal liver disease. However, in this case the patient had amyloid associated with familial Mediterranean fever.

## 8.4.3   Splenic disease

### *Assessment of splenomegaly*

*Important causes of splenomegaly*

*With increased splenic colloid uptake*
- Cirrhosis
- Acute infections
- Haemolytic anaemias
- Hypersplenism.

*With decreased splenic uptake of colloid*
- Myelofibrosis
- Lymphoma and leukaemia
- Metastases
- Amyloid and storage diseases
- Cysts
- Haemorrhage.

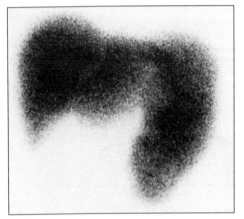

*a  Anterior*

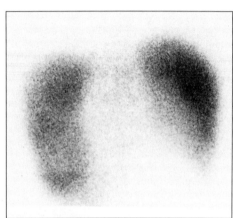

*b  Posterior*

### Fig. 8.86

*(a,b) Liver/spleen scan.*
*There is striking splenomegaly present. The abnormality in this case was due to myelofibrosis, which is one of the causes of massive splenomegaly without increased tracer uptake in the spleen and with absent marrow uptake.*

### *Investigation of incidental splenomegaly*

*Three cases of lymphoma of the spleen presenting as an incidental finding of left hypochondrial mass*

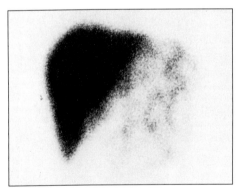

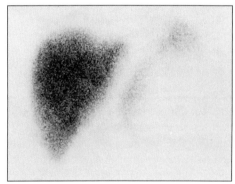

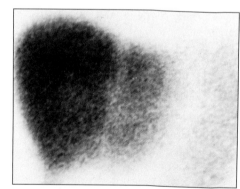

### Fig. 8.87

*The spleen is massively enlarged, with multiple focal abnormalities throughout.*

### Fig. 8.88

*There is a large space-occupying lesion involving much of the spleen.*

### Fig. 8.89

*In this case the spleen is markedly enlarged, with diffusely reduced uptake of tracer relative to the liver.*

## CLINICAL APPLICATIONS

## Two cases of massive splenomegaly due to benign causes

### Fibrous splenic cyst

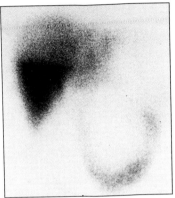 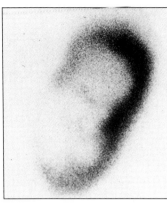

*a Anterior*  *b Posterior*  *c Left lateral*

**Fig. 8.90**

*(a–c) Liver/spleen scan.*
  *The liver appears normal. The spleen is massively enlarged by a large area of decreased uptake centrally. This patient had a splenectomy. The spleen was found to contain a fibrous wall. There was no evidence of malignancy.*

### Haemorrhagic cyst of spleen

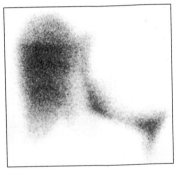 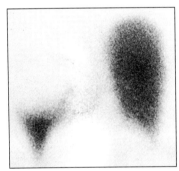

*a Anterior*  *b Posterior*

**Fig. 8.91**

*(a,b) Liver/spleen scan.*
  *The liver appears normal, although there is some distortion of the left lobe. The spleen is massively enlarged, with a huge focal defect present. There is a large space-occupying lesion involving the spleen; this was shown to be a simple haemorrhagic cyst.*

## Use of denatured red cells in the investigation of splenomegaly

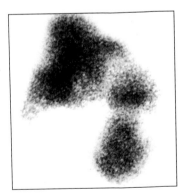 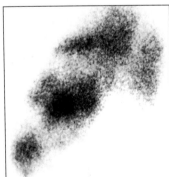 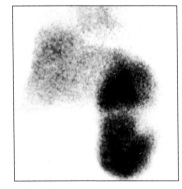 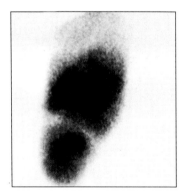

*a Anterior*  *b Left lateral*  *c Anterior*  *d Left lateral*

**Fig. 8.92**

*(a,b) Liver/spleen scan. (c,d) Denatured cell study.*
  *This patient was being investigated for splenomegaly. The liver/spleen scan shows the difficulty, if not the impossibility, of defining what is liver and what is spleen in the left hypochondrium. The denatured red cell study clearly identifies the spleen, and the anterior and left lateral views elegantly demonstrate the space-occupying lesion caused by lymphoma.*

# Investigation of splenic function

## Splenunculus

*a Anterior*

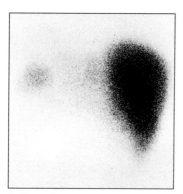

*b Posterior*

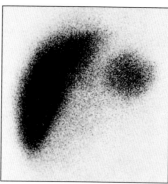
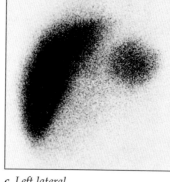

*c Left lateral*

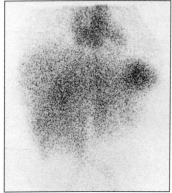

*d Anterior*

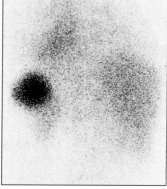

*e Posterior*

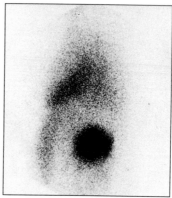

*f Left lateral*

**Fig. 8.93**

*(a–c) Liver/spleen scan.*
*(d–f) Denatured red cell study.*
This middle-aged man had a past history of splenectomy, but on a liver/spleen scan splenic tissue appeared to be present. Note that this was not visualized on the anterior view. The denatured red cell study confirmed the presence of functional splenic tissue (splenunculus).

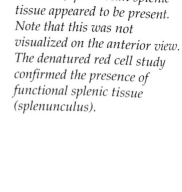

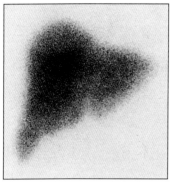

*a Anterior*

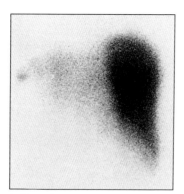

*b Posterior*

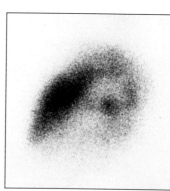

*c Left lateral*

**Fig. 8.94**

*(a–c) Liver/spleen scan.*
This patient had a previous splenectomy. However, a small focus of splenic activity is present in the left hypochondrium, best seen on the posterior and left lateral views. The scan findings represent a hypertrophied accessory spleen following previous splenectomy.

## CLINICAL APPLICATIONS

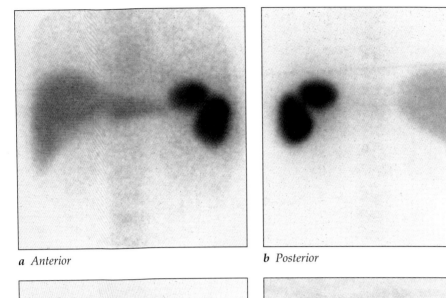
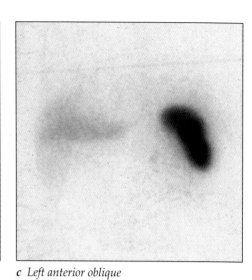

*a* Anterior

*b* Posterior

*c* Left anterior oblique

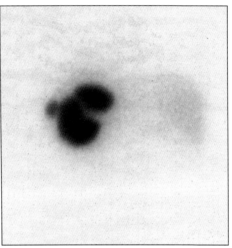

*d* Left lateral

*e* Left posterior oblique

*Fig. 8.95*

**(a–e)** Denatured red cell study.

This 52-year-old male was found to have a 'blush' in the left upper quadrant of the abdomen seen on angiography for haematemesis. The denatured red blood cell imaging of the spleen confirms that the 'blush' is due to a bilobe spleen with a small splenunculus.

## CLINICAL APPLICATIONS

## Hyposplenism

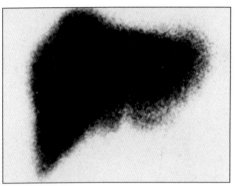

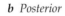
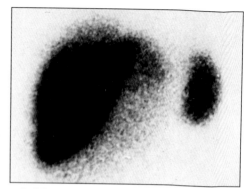

*a Anterior*

*b Posterior*

*c Left lateral*

**Fig. 8.96**

*(a–c) Liver/spleen scan.*
   Note that there is a small, poorly functioning spleen. This patient had coeliac disease, with associated hyposplenism.

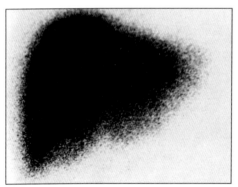
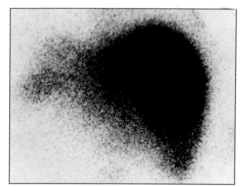
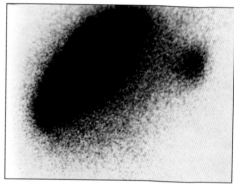

*a Anterior*

*b Posterior*

*c Left lateral*

**Fig. 8.97**

*(a–c) Liver/spleen scan.*
   In this case the spleen is very small and shows reduced uptake of colloid. This patient had splenic hypoplasia associated with ulcerative colitis.

## Functional asplenia

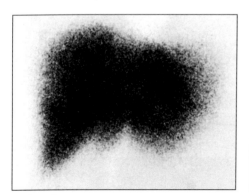
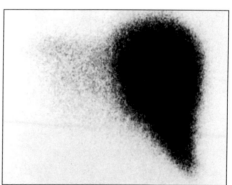

*a Anterior*

*b Posterior*

**Fig. 8.98**

*(a,b) Liver/spleen scan.*
   There is no evidence of functioning splenic tissue present. This is a case of functional asplenia in association with coeliac disease.

## CLINICAL APPLICATIONS

### Alterations in splenic function with time

#### Splenic hypofunction due to inflammatory bowel disease

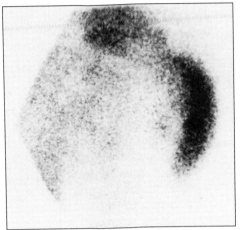 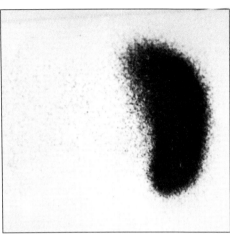

*a  Anterior, 0 months*　　　　*b  Anterior, 6 months*

*Fig. 8.99*

*(a,b)* Denatured red cell study.

　This patient was known to have severe Crohn's disease. On the original study there is poor splenic accumulation of the denatured red cells. Six months later, after a successful course of anti-inflammatory therapy, the scan shows the normal high concentration of red cells.

### Splenic infarction

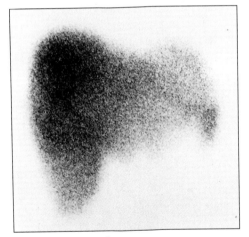 

*a  Anterior, 0 months*　　　　*b  Anterior, 12 months*

*Fig. 8.100*

*(a,b)* Liver/spleen scan.

　On the original study the spleen is clearly seen. On the subsequent study there is no visualization of the spleen and apparently reduced uptake in the left lobe of the liver. This patient was known to have carcinoma of the breast and had complained of left-sided abdominal pain. The clinical history, taken together with previous visualization of the spleen, gives a high probability of acute splenic infarction. The scan appearances also raised the possibility of metastatic involvement of the left lobe of the liver. Ultrasound confirmed the presence of a spleen, increasing the probability of infarction.

 **The absolute uptake of denatured red cells and the rate of uptake into the spleen can both be used as quantitative measures of splenic function.**

## Asplenia associated with situs inversus

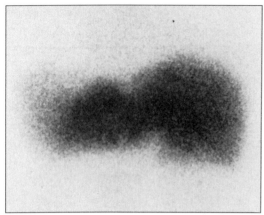

*a* Anterior

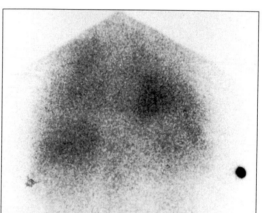

*b* Posterior

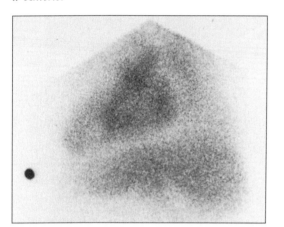

*c* Anterior

*d* Posterior

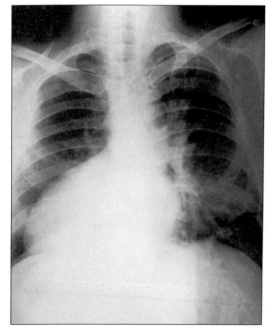

*e*

**Fig. 8.101**

*A 26-year-old man with situs inversus. (**a,b**) Liver scan. (**c,d**) $^{99m}$Tc-labelled denatured red cell study. (**e**) Chest x-ray.*

*On the liver scan it is noted that the liver is lying in the left of the abdomen, in keeping with the patient's known situs inversus. The liver is of somewhat unusual shape. Ultrasound examination had indicated a probable absence of spleen. The liver study did not clarify this issue. Further, this patient had a past history of subacute bacterial endocarditis and the spleen, if present, could have been hypofunctional. A denatured red cell study was performed which showed no accumulation at the site where the spleen would be expected.*

## CLINICAL APPLICATIONS

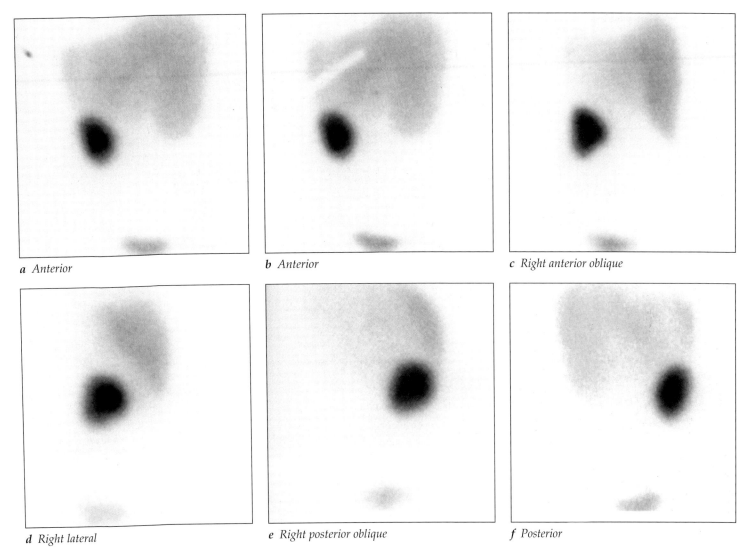

*a* Anterior

*b* Anterior

*c* Right anterior oblique

*d* Right lateral

*e* Right posterior oblique

*f* Posterior

**Fig. 8.102**

*(a–f) Denatured red cell scan; (b) with costal margin marker.*
*This patient was a 6-year-old child with Fallot's tetralogy and known situs inversus.*
*The denatured red cell scan was performed to determine whether a spleen was present. The*
*spleen was clearly visualized at the right side, in keeping with the known situs inversus.*
*A large liver was noted secondary to congenital heart disease and pulmonary hypertension.*

## 8.4.4 Trauma

### Liver/spleen scan in the investigation of trauma

#### Splenic rupture

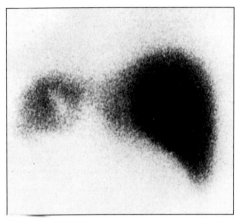

Posterior

**Fig. 8.103**

*Liver/spleen scan.*
   *This 14-year-old child suffered abdominal trauma. A focal defect is seen in the lower two-thirds of the spleen.*

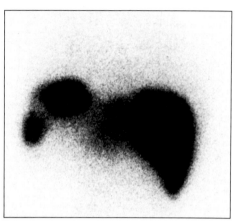

Posterior

**Fig. 8.104**

*Liver/spleen scan.*
   *This 30-year-old male complained of severe left-sided abdominal pain following a road traffic accident. A photon-deficient area is seen in the spleen due to splenic rupture.*

#### Splenic puncture

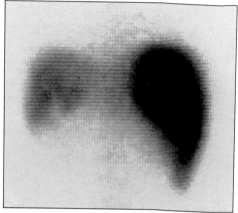

Posterior

**Fig. 8.105**

*Liver/spleen scan.*
   *A focal defect is seen in the inferior margin of the spleen caused by a laceration from a penetrating knife wound.*

#### Splenic haematoma

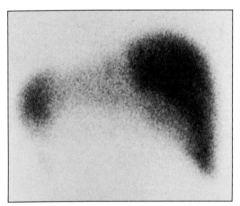

*a Posterior, analogue*

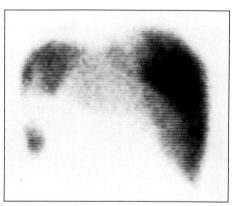

*b Posterior, digital*

**Fig. 8.106**

*Liver/spleen scan: (a) analogue and (b) digital studies.*
   *This patient was injured in a road traffic accident and had subsequent left-sided loin pain and haematuria. The analogue image shows a photon-deficient area in the middle of the spleen, but this is more clearly demonstrated on the digital image with increased intensity, and the tip of the spleen is now clearly visualized. This was subsequently confirmed to be a haematoma.*

## CLINICAL APPLICATIONS

### *Importance of oblique views*

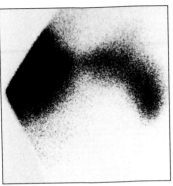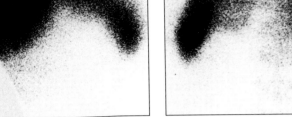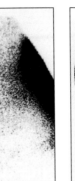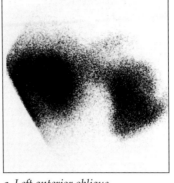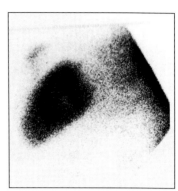

*a Anterior*  *b Posterior*  *c Left anterior oblique*  *d Left posterior oblique*

**Fig. 8.107**

*(a–d) Liver/spleen scan.*
*This patient was admitted with upper abdominal pain and swelling following blunt trauma. Note that on the anterior and posterior views there is only a faint suggestion of a lateral lesion in the spleen. The oblique views, however, both clearly show the rupture and a haematoma in the lateral portion of the spleen.*

A radionuclide colloid liver/spleen scan is the simplest, most rapid and accurate investigation for suspected liver/spleen trauma. This study can often be performed immediately after the patient has been seen in the accident department.

### **Denatured red cells to demonstrate splenic trauma**

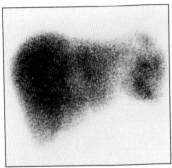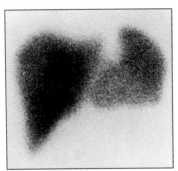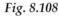

*a Anterior*  *b Left anterior oblique*

**Fig. 8.108**

*(a,b) Liver/spleen scan. (c,d) Denatured red cell study.*
*This patient sustained abdominal trauma. The colloid study shows the spleen to be of a somewhat unusual shape, but no discrete focal defect is identified. On the denatured red cell study, it is apparent that a focal defect is present in the anterior surface of the spleen, caused by a haematoma.*

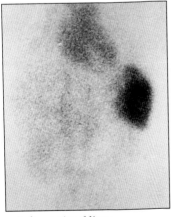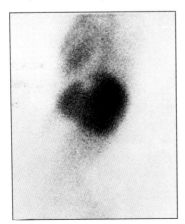

*c Left anterior oblique*  *d Left posterior oblique*

When the liver and spleen are difficult to separate on the colloid scan, a radio-pharmaceutical which localizes in one organ and not the other can be used. This may be a hepato-biliary agent for the liver, or denatured red cells for the spleen.

## Hepatic trauma

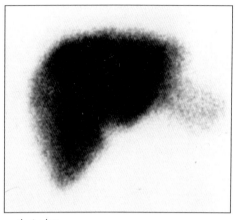 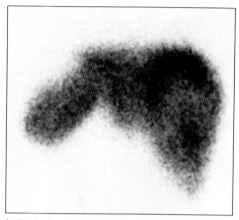 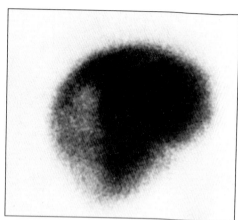

*a* Anterior       *b* Posterior       *c* Right lateral

**Fig. 8.109**

*(a–c) Liver/spleen scan.*
   *There is a large focal defect lying posteriorly in the right lobe of the liver. This represented a large subcapsular haematoma following trauma. The patient is a 4-year-old girl.*

## Demonstration of hepatic trauma by a hepatobiliary agent

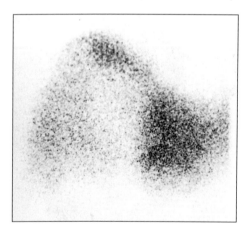 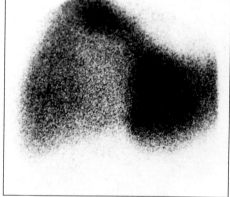 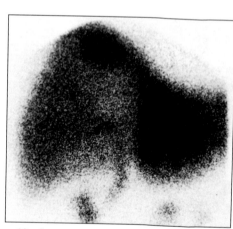

*a* 2 minutes       *b* 5 minutes       *c* 10 minutes

**Fig. 8.110**

*(a–c) $^{99m}Tc$ HIDA scan.*
   *In the initial functional stages there is markedly decreased hepatocyte function of the entire right lobe. Subsequently, there is rapid transit of tracer from the left lobe into the common bile duct, and normal transit into the duodenum. There is a focal area of absent function between the left and right lobes. The patient is a 20-year-old male who received a stab wound causing a large hepatic haematoma. On the delayed images there was no evidence of a biliary leak.*

## CLINICAL APPLICATIONS

## *Investigation of suspected biliary leak*

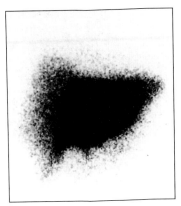 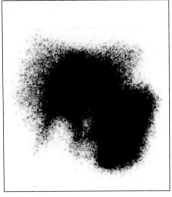 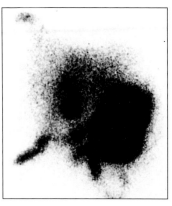 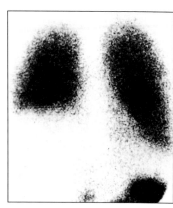

*a 5 minutes*  *b 20 minutes*  *c 45 minutes*  *d*

**Fig. 8.111**

*(a–c)* ⁹⁹ᵐTc HIDA *scan.* *(d) Image obtained following injection of* ⁹⁹ᵐTc-labelled microspheres.
   This patient developed pain in the abdomen following cholecystectomy. The hepatobiliary scan at 5 minutes shows some decreased uptake in the right side of the liver. At 20 minutes there is an apparently normal common bile duct and entry of tracer into the duodenum, At 45 minutes a clear track of labelled bile is noted below the right lobe of the liver, with some tracer appearing above the liver under the diaphragm. Labelled microspheres given immediately after this show a large, photon-deficient area below the right diaphragm caused by a bile collection.

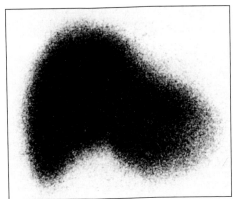 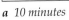 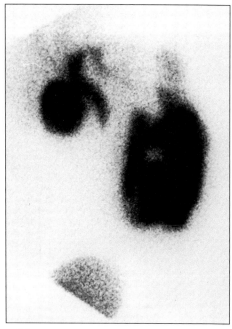

*a 10 minutes*  *b 1 hour*

**Fig. 8.112**

*(a–c)* ⁹⁹ᵐTc HIDA *scan.*
   This patient with a past history of renal transplant and recent cholecystectomy became generally unwell with abdominal pain. The hepatobiliary study *(a)* shows a homogeneous pattern of tracer uptake throughout the liver. On later images, the common bile duct is clearly seen, with free passage of tracer into the bowel. However, there is a large focus of tracer accumulation seen at the junction of the common bile duct and the right hepatic duct (arrow, *b*). This enlarges with time and represents a significant biliary leak.

*c 2 hours*

 If a bile leak is suspected, delaying imaging for up to 2 hours may be necessary to demonstrate the leak adequately.

## CLINICAL APPLICATIONS

### Postoperative damage to the bile duct causing a chronic stricture and partial intermittent obstruction

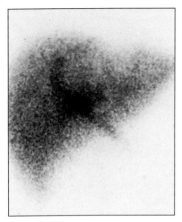 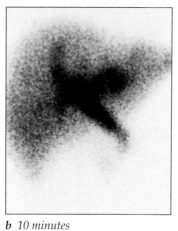 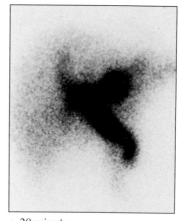 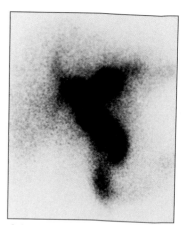

*a* 5 minutes      *b* 10 minutes      *c* 20 minutes      *d* 30 minutes

*Fig. 8.113*

*(a–d)* ⁹⁹ᵐTc HIDA *scan.*

*This elderly man had a previous cholecystectomy performed. The hepatobiliary study shows rapid uptake of tracer into the hepatic parenchyma. There is subsequently rapid transit of tracer into a normal common bile duct and right hepatic duct. The left hepatic duct is dilated and there is some delay in transit. There does, however, appear to be some drainage at 30 minutes, and the bile duct, therefore, is not completely obstructed. The scan findings were due to chronic stricture of the left hepatic duct, with partial intermittent obstruction.*

### Gallstones causing intermittent obstruction to common bile duct

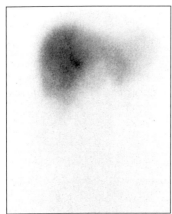 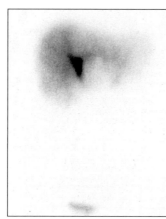 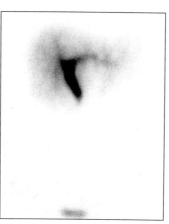 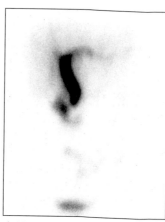

*a* 5 minutes      *b* 10 minutes      *c* 20 minutes      *d* 45 minutes

*Fig. 8.114*

*(a–d)* ⁹⁹ᵐTc HIDA *scan.*

*This patient is an elderly woman with a history of gallstones and intermittent jaundice. The hepatobiliary study shows good uptake of HIDA by the parenchyma with delayed transit of tracer through a dilated common bile duct. The gall bladder is non-functioning.*

# 8.4.5 Investigation of abnormal liver function tests

## *Alcoholic liver disease*

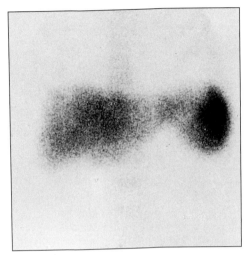

*a Anterior*

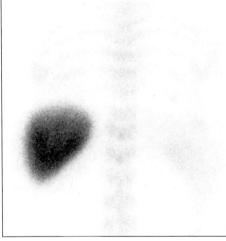

*b Posterior*

### Fig. 8.115

*(a–e) Liver/spleen scans.*

In these two cases abnormal liver function tests were noted on routine screening. The liver/spleen scans show typical appearances of parenchymal disease, which was subsequently shown to be related to alcohol abuse.

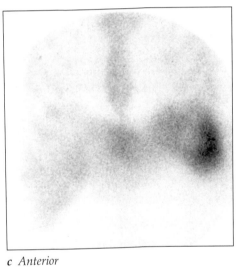

*c Anterior*

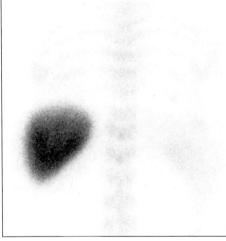

*d Posterior*

*e Right lateral*

## *Metastatic liver disease*

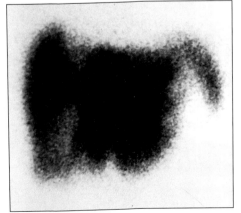

*a Anterior*

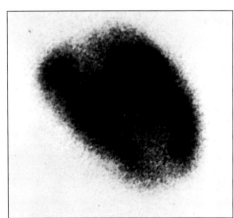

*b Right lateral*

### Fig. 8.116

*(a,b) Liver/spleen scan.*

In this case abnormal liver function tests were again noted on routine screening. However, the study demonstrates multiple focal lesions which were due to metastases from an unknown primary malignancy.

# 8.4.6   Investigation of upper abdominal pain

## *Unsuspected metastatic disease*

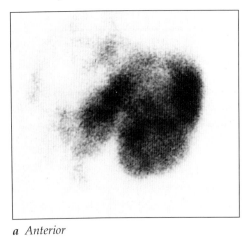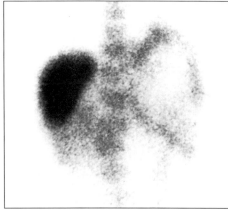

*a Anterior*          *b Posterior*

**Fig. 8.117**

*(a,b) Liver/spleen scan in a patient presenting with upper abdominal pain.*

*There is massive replacement of the right lobe and, to a lesser extent, of the left lobe of the liver, with metastatic deposits.*

## *Gall bladder mucocele*

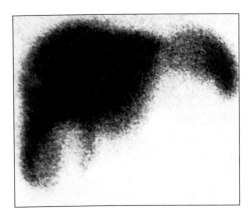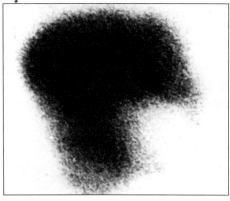

*a Anterior*          *b Right lateral*

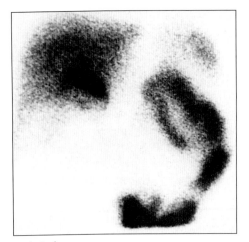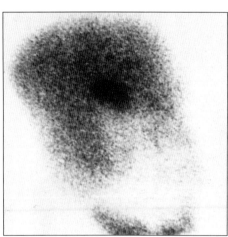

*a Anterior*          *b Lateral*

**Fig. 8.118**

*(a,b) Liver/spleen scan. (c,d) $^{99m}Tc$ HIDA scan.*

*This middle-aged woman had upper abdominal pain due to a gall bladder mucocele. On examination, there was a tender ballotable swelling below the costal margin. The anterior colloid scan (a) shows a focal lesion at the site of the gall bladder, which is more clearly seen on the lateral view (b). The anterior and lateral hepatobiliary scan views (c,d) show that this defect does not accumulate tracer. These are the typical clinical and scintigraphic appearances of a gall bladder mucocele.*

## Splenic infarct

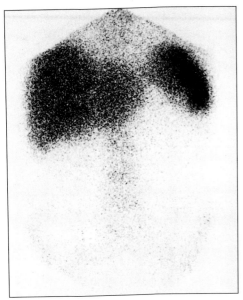

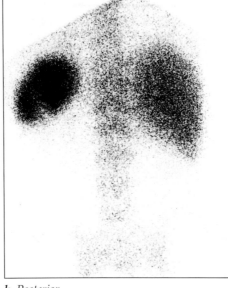

*a* Anterior

*b* Posterior

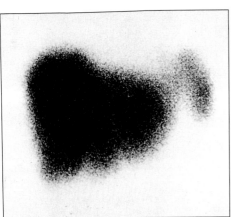

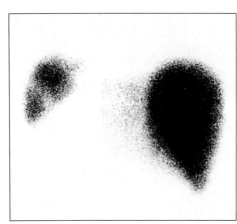

*a* Anterior

*b* Posterior

**Fig. 8.119**

*A 60-year-old man with known rheumatic heart disease and subacute bacterial endocarditis. (a,b) [111]In-labelled white cell scan of the abdomen. (c,d) [99m]Tc SC liver scan.*

*This patient was extremely ill with left loin pain. It was suspected that he had metastatic abscesses, and so an [111]In white cell scan was requested. The study did not show any abnormal site of localization either in the heart or elsewhere. The spleen showed normal uptake of autologous white cells, with a wedge-shaped defect within the organ, best seen on the posterior view (b). A liver/spleen scan was subsequently performed. The liver was normal. The spleen appears normal in size but shows multiple focal defects, one corresponding to the linear change seen in the previous white cell study with probably two further focal lesions in the upper pole. There are thus multiple splenic lesions which are attributable to multiple infarcts.*

## *Investigation of acute cholecystitis*

Acute cholecystitis is associated with obstruction of the cystic duct, with the exception of a very few cases of non-calculous acute cholecystitis. The use of a hepatobiliary agent has been accepted as the most sensitive method for the detection of cystic duct patency and therefore for the investigation of acute cholecystitis. If acute cholecystitis is suspected as a cause of right upper quadrant pain, visualization of the gall bladder will very rapidly rule out this possibility and allow the clinician to concentrate on other causes, and possibly prevent unnecessary surgery.

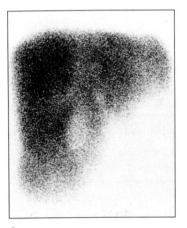
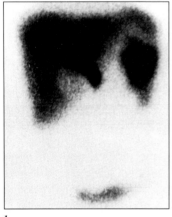

*a*  *b*

**Fig. 8.120**

*(a) Liver/spleen scan. (b) ⁹⁹ᵐTc HIDA 30-minute image.*
   *This patient presented with upper abdominal pain. The colloid liver scan shows slight enlargement of the right lobe of the liver, with a focal defect in the region of the gall bladder. The HIDA study confirms non-visualization of the gall bladder. The upper abdominal pain was believed to be due to recurrent episodes of acute cholecystitis.*

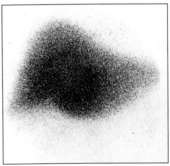
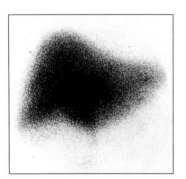

*a 2 minutes*  *b 10 minutes*

**Fig. 8.121**

*(a–e) ⁹⁹ᵐTc HIDA scan.*
   *There is homogeneous uptake of tracer throughout the liver. Prompt excretion of the hepatobiliary agent occurs via the common bile duct into the gut. The gall bladder, however, is not visualized. The scan findings are those of cystic duct obstruction, and were due to acute cholecystitis.*

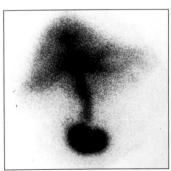
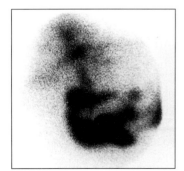
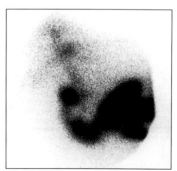

*c 30 minutes*  *d 45 minutes*  *e 60 minutes*

# CLINICAL APPLICATIONS

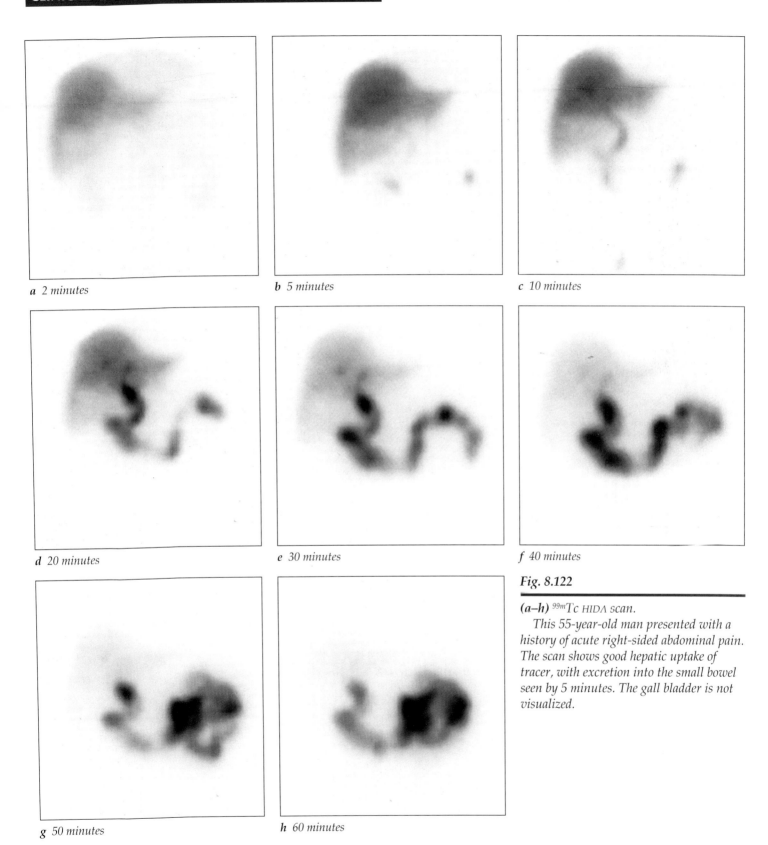

*a* 2 minutes

*b* 5 minutes

*c* 10 minutes

*d* 20 minutes

*e* 30 minutes

*f* 40 minutes

*g* 50 minutes

*h* 60 minutes

**Fig. 8.122**

(*a–h*) $^{99m}$Tc HIDA scan.

This 55-year-old man presented with a history of acute right-sided abdominal pain. The scan shows good hepatic uptake of tracer, with excretion into the small bowel seen by 5 minutes. The gall bladder is not visualized.

**CLINICAL APPLICATIONS**

## *Chronic cholecystitis*

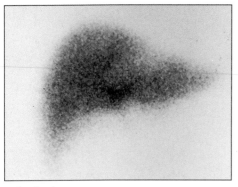

*a  1 minute*

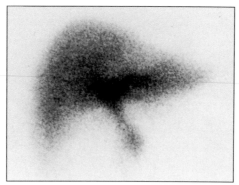

*b  15 minutes*

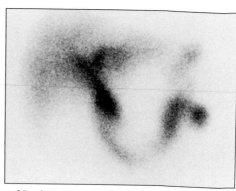

*c  30 minutes*

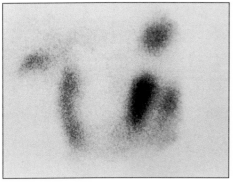

*d  1 hour*

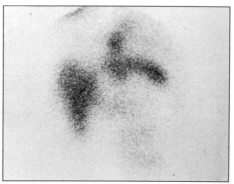

*e  Right lateral, 1 hour*

**Fig. 8.123**

*(a–e)* $^{99m}$Tc HIDA *scan.*

*This middle-aged man had a recurrent illness associated with upper abdominal pain. Radiological investigations of the gall bladder were normal. The HIDA scan images at 1, 15 and 30 minutes show no filling of the gall bladder. However, on the delayed view at 1 hour it can be seen that there is a small amount of tracer entering the gall bladder. This confirms that the function is poor, but the cystic duct is patent. The scan findings are typical of chronic cholecystitis. Note that gastric reflux of bile is seen (see Fig. 8.124).*

## *Gastric reflux of bile as a cause of upper abdominal pain*

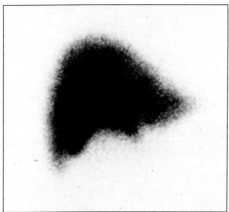
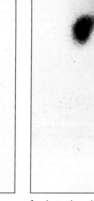

*a  Anterior, 30 minutes*

*b  Anterior, 40 minutes*

**Fig. 8.124**

*(a,b)* $^{99m}$Tc HIDA *scan in a 74-year-old man who complained of pain in the upper abdomen following an operation for peptic ulcer.*

*The gall bladder is clearly visualized, but at a somewhat delayed time of 30 minutes. Subsequently, tracer flows freely into the bowel. Note that there is bile in the region of the stomach. There is no evidence of cystic duct obstruction, but the scan appearances indicate biliary reflux into the stomach.*

# 8.4.7    Investigation of jaundice

Liver/spleen scanning with both sc and hepatobiliary agents is often helpful in evaluating patients with jaundice. The following cases illustrate some of the ways in which liver/spleen scans may indicate the diagnosis simply and rapidly. However, with the introduction of ultrasound, liver/spleen scanning is no longer the first investigation to ascertain the cause or site of obstructive jaundice, although it may be helpful in some of the more difficult cases.

**Table 8.2**  *Classification of types of jaundice and their scan appearances*

| Classification of jaundice | | Scan appearances |
|---|---|---|
| Prehepatic | Haemolytic<br>Congenital, eg Gilbert's disease | Normal colloid and HIDA |
| Hepatic | Acute, eg viral, toxic, alcoholic<br>Chronic, eg cirrhosis, metastases, chronic active heptatitis | Decreased uptake of colloid and HIDA; delayed excretion of HIDA |
| Cholestatic | Non-dilated bile duct—drugs<br>(intrahepatic)       sclerosing cholangitis<br>         benign recurrent viral<br>         cholangiocarcinoma | Decreased uptake of both agents. HIDA uptake is progressive with no excretion. Cholangiocarcinoma will have bile ducts showing as photon-deficient areas |
| | Dilated bile ducts—stones<br>(extrahepatic)     carcinoma of head of<br>         pancreas | Colloid scan shows multiple 'space-occupying lesions' caused by dilated ducts. HIDA shows delay or absent gut visualization |

## Hepatic jaundice: acute

*Jaundice caused by acute alcoholic hepatitis*

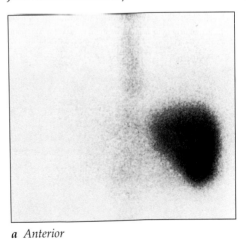
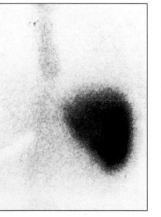
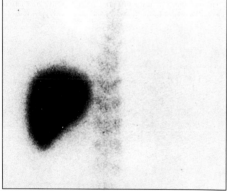

*a Anterior*          *b Anterior*          *c Posterior*

**Fig. 8.125**

*A 30-year-old woman presenting with jaundice. (**a–c**) Liver/spleen scan; (**b**) costal marker.*
   *The liver is essentially not visualized, while the spleen is enlarged, with high uptake of tracer. There is also considerable uptake of tracer by bone marrow. The scan appearances are those of acute alcoholic hepatitis.*

## Hepatic jaundice: chronic

Metastases as a cause of jaundice

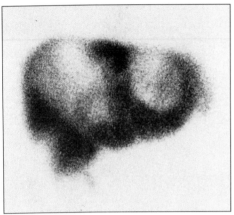

Anterior

**Fig. 8.126**

*Liver/spleen scan.*
   *This elderly man presented with jaundice. The liver scan shows massive focal lesions throughout the liver which were due to metastases.*

Metastases as a cause of jaundice detected on HIDA scan

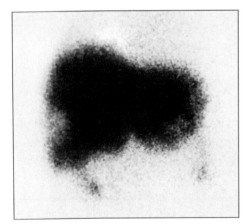

*a 5 minutes*

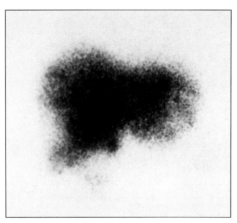

*b 15 minutes*

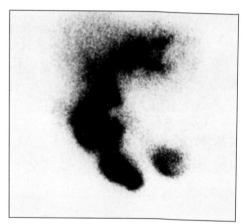

*c 30 minutes*

**Fig. 8.127**

*(a–c) $^{99m}$Tc HIDA scan.*
   *This patient presented with jaundice, which was thought initially to be due to bile duct obstruction. The hepatobiliary scan shows metastases in the parenchymal phase, and the later image shows that there is no obstruction of the common bile duct.*

The early parenchymal phases of the hepatobiliary scan are as sensitive as the colloid scan for detection of metastases, if performed carefully. The information obtained from the parenchymal phase should always be used, even when investigating the bile duct drainage system.

## CLINICAL APPLICATIONS

## Investigation of intermittent jaundice

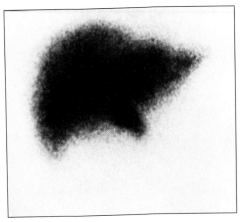
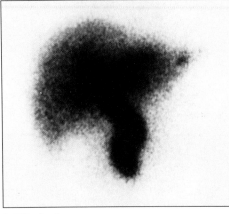
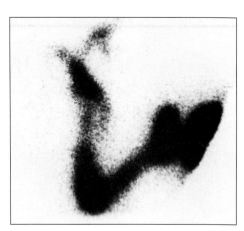

*a  5 minutes*

*b  15 minutes*

*c  30 minutes*

### Fig. 8.128

**(a–c)** $^{99m}$Tc HIDA scan.

    This patient developed intermittent jaundice following cholecystectomy. The hepatobiliary scan was performed to exclude obstruction. It is apparent that there is rapid entry of tracer into the common bile duct, with free passage into the duodenum. There is normal drainage from the common bile duct, thus excluding any functionally significant obstruction.

## Intermittent jaundice caused by partial obstruction of the common bile duct

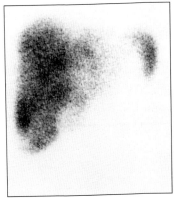
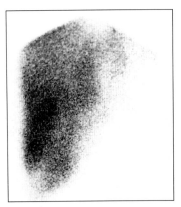
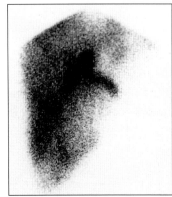
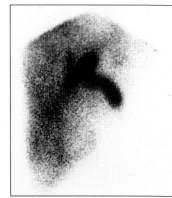

*a  Anterior*

*b  2 minutes*

*c  15 minutes*

*d  20 minutes*

### Fig. 8.129

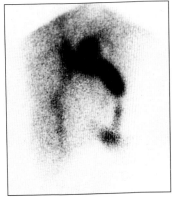

*e  30 minutes*

**(a)** Liver/spleen scan. **(b–e)** $^{99m}$Tc HIDA scan.

    On the colloid study the liver is enlarged, with irregular uptake of tracer throughout. The HIDA study confirms non-homogeneity of tracer uptake on the 2-minute image. By 15 minutes, the hepatic ducts and common bile ducts are visualized. The common bile duct subsequently appears slightly dilated, but tracer passes through into the duodenum. At no stage is the gall bladder visualized. Ultrasound in this case showed only slight dilatation of the intrahepatic bile ducts, but there was significant dilatation of the common bile duct with the suggestion of a calculus at its lower end. The gall bladder was contracted, with multiple calculi.

## *Cholestatic jaundice: intrahepatic*

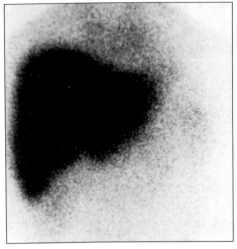 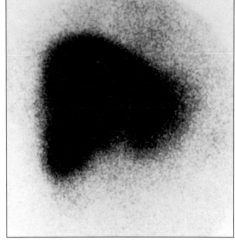 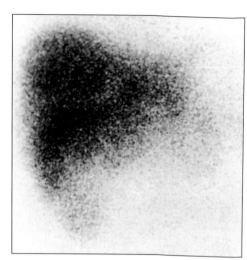

*a  2 hours*        *b  5 hours*        *c  22 hours*

**Fig. 8.130**

*(a–c)* $^{99m}Tc$ HIDA *scan.*
*There is good uptake of* HIDA *into the liver, but no evidence of transport into the hepatic ducts or gut over 22 hours. These findings indicated intrahepatic cholestasis.*

## *Cholestatic jaundice: extrahepatic*

*Two cases of extrahepatic bile duct obstruction*

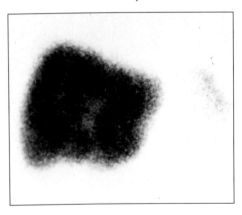 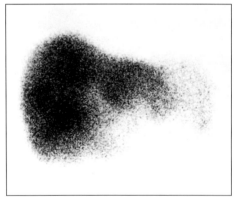

*Anterior*

 **The focal defects from long-standing bile duct obstruction may simulate multiple metastases.**

**Fig. 8.131**            **Fig. 8.132**

*Liver/spleen scan.*
*The liver is slightly enlarged as the result of left lobe hypertrophy. There is decreased colloid accumulation at the porta hepatis, with linear areas of reduced uptake spreading out from there.*

*Liver/spleen scan.*
*In this case there is also decreased colloid accumulation at the porta hepatis, spreading into the right and left lobes. The defects correspond to the position of the major bile ducts, which were dilated.*

# 8.4.8 Investigation of hepatic infection

## Amoebic abscess

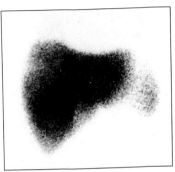 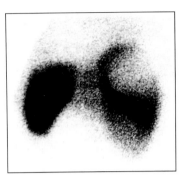 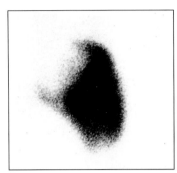

*a Anterior*          *b Posterior*          *c Right lateral*

**Fig. 8.133**

*(a–c) Liver scan in a 33-year-old man with amoebic abscess.*

*The liver is enlarged and there is a massive area of absent colloid accumulation in the upper half of the right lobe posteriorly. The spleen is slightly enlarged. The scan findings are those of a large space-occupying lesion in the liver, and in this case were due to an amoebic abscess.*

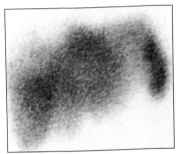 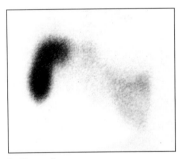 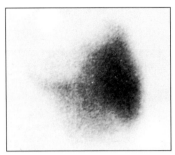

*a Anterior*          *b Posterior*          *c Right lateral*

**Fig. 8.134**

*(a–c) Liver/spleen scan.*

*The liver is enlarged, with a massive focal defect present in the right upper lobe posteriorly. The spleen is also enlarged and shows increased tracer uptake relative to the liver. This is a further case of amoebic liver abscess.*

## Hydatid cyst

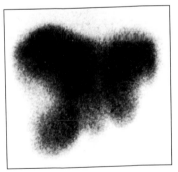 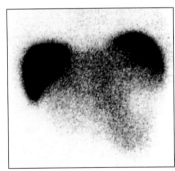

*a Anterior*          *b Posterior*

**Fig. 8.135**

*(a,b) Liver/spleen scan*

*The liver is enlarged, with a single focal defect present in the right mid-lobe. The scan findings were due to a hydatid cyst.*

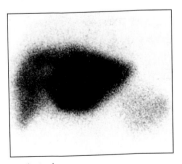 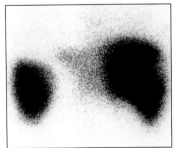 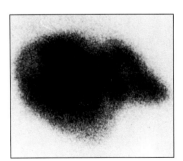

*a Anterior*          *b Posterior*          *c Right lateral*

**Fig. 8.136**

*(a–c) Liver scan.*

*On the liver scan, multiple focal defects were present, representing hydatid cysts.*

## CLINICAL APPLICATIONS

# *Pyogenic abscess*

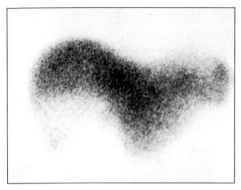

*a Anterior*

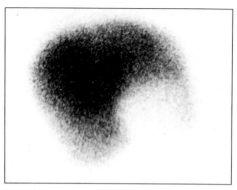

*b Right lateral*

**Fig. 8.137**

*(a,b) Liver/spleen scan.*
   *The liver is enlarged and there is a massive area of decreased colloid accumulation in the right lobe. The scan findings were due to an intrahepatic abscess.*

## Use of $^{67}$Ga to demonstrate pyogenic abscess

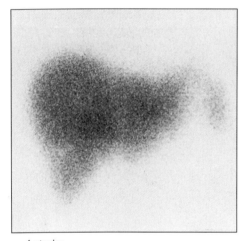

*a Anterior*

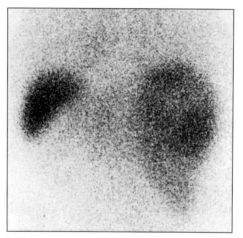

*b Posterior*

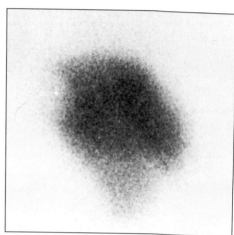

*c Right lateral*

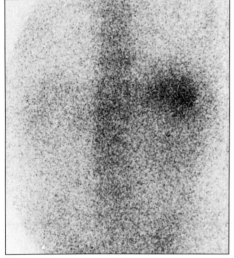

*d Posterior*

**Fig. 8.138**

*(a–c) Colloid liver/spleen scan. (d) $^{67}$Ga scan.*
   *On the colloid scan there is a focal area of reduced tracer uptake in the posterior upper right lobe of the liver. The scan appearances are those of a space-occupying lesion. The $^{67}$Ga scan shows avid tracer uptake corresponding to the focal defect on the liver scan. This patient had a liver abscess.*

 Because $^{67}$Ga is taken up into normal hepatic tissue as well as inflammatory or tumour tissue, abnormalities may be obscured on a $^{67}$Ga scan only. However, when compared with the $^{99m}$Tc liver colloid scan, there will be a mismatch between the uptake of the two isotopes, and therefore a colloid liver scan is an essential part of every $^{67}$Ga investigation when the liver may be abnormal.

# 8.4.9 Evaluation of response to interventional therapy

## Intrahepatic arterial cytotoxic perfusion therapy

In patients with hepatic malignancy selective intra-arterial chemotherapy may be of value. However, to achieve optimal results, the chemotherapeutic agent has to be reliably distributed to all affected regions, and the tip of the intra-arterial catheter has to be accurately positioned. While several methods have been proposed for evaluation, the use of $^{99m}$Tc macroaggregated albumin (MAA) particles most closely reproduces the pattern of the chemotherapy infusion.

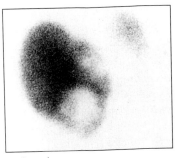

*a Anterior*

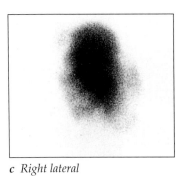

*b Posterior*

*c Right lateral*

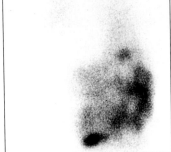

*d Anterior*

*e Posterior*

*f Right lateral*

**Fig. 8.139**

*A patient with liver metastases from carcinoma of the bowel. (a–c) $^{99m}$Tc SC liver scan. (d–f) $^{99m}$Tc MAA scan via infusaid pump.*

*The SC liver scan shows large focal defects, particularly in the left lobe, in keeping with metastases. Direct intra-arterial infusion of $^{99m}$Tc MAA shows high uptake in the region of the metastases. Note also tracer uptake by the lungs (e), indicating a degree of arteriovenous shunting. Tracer can be seen in the abdomen at the site of the injection and catheter (d).*

## Embolic therapy

### Splenic infarction

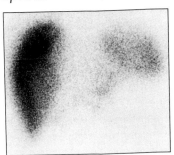

*a Anterior*

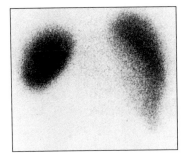

*b Posterior*

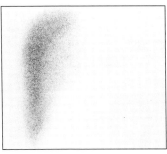

*c Anterior*

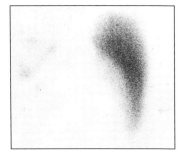

*d Posterior*

**Fig. 8.140**

*Liver/spleen scan (a,b) before and (c,d) following embolization.*

*On the original study it is apparent that the left lobe of the liver is replaced by tumour. Arterial embolization of the tumour was attempted. However, on the subsequent study it is apparent that the spleen shows diminished tracer uptake, with a large central focal defect. The scan findings were due to associated infarction of the spleen at the time of embolization.*

## Liver scanning prior to biopsy

### Haemangioma of the liver

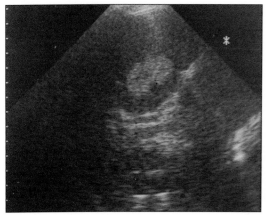

*a Ultrasound*

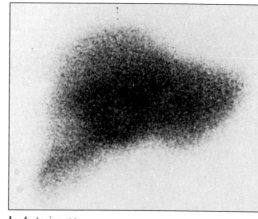

*b Anterior, SC*

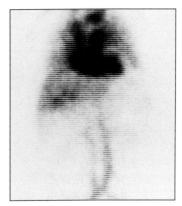

*c Anterior, RBC*

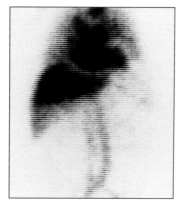

*d RBC with SC*

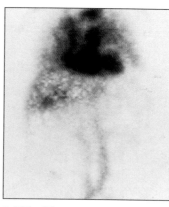

*e RBC − SC*

**Fig. 8.141**

*A 63-year-old man with haemangioma of the liver. (a) Ultrasound. (b) ⁹⁹ᵐTc SC liver scan. (c) ⁹⁹ᵐTc-labelled red cell scan. (d) ⁹⁹ᵐTc-labelled red cell scan with sulphur colloid. (e) Subtraction image (RBC–SC).*

*A solitary nodule in the liver was noted on ultrasound (a), and the possibility of a haemangioma was raised. The SC scan (b) was unremarkable, but there appeared to be a relative lack of colloid at that site. The red cell study (c) shows an apparent area of increased red cell accumulation in the right lobe of the liver which is confirmed on the subtraction image (e). These findings increase the probability that the hepatic lesion has a high blood volume.*

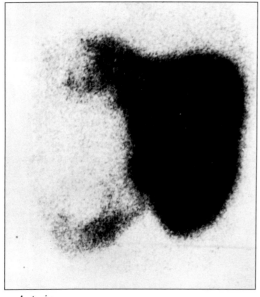

*a Anterior*

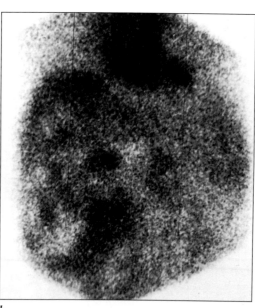

*b*

**Fig. 8.142**

*(a) Liver/spleen scan. (b) ⁹⁹ᵐTc-labelled red cell study.*

*This patient was investigated for hepatomegaly. The colloid scan shows a massive tumour in the right lobe of the liver. The red cell study performed after the colloid scan shows the appearance of a massive haemangioma. Previous biopsy had been performed, and resulted in massive haemorrhage.*

## CLINICAL APPLICATIONS

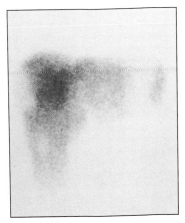

*a  Anterior*

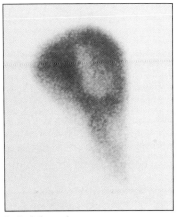

*b  Left lateral*

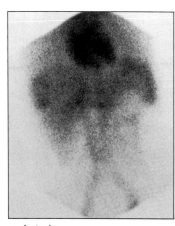

*c  Anterior*

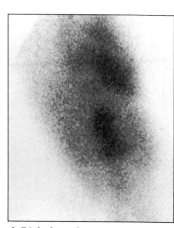

*d  Right lateral*

**Fig. 8.143**

*(a,b)* SC *liver/spleen scan.* *(c,d)* ⁹⁹ᵐTc RBC *study.*

   *The standard liver scan shows a space-occupying lesion in the upper right lobe, best seen on the lateral view. Dynamic studies (not shown) did not reveal increased blood flow. The labelled red cell study shows accumulation of red cells in the right lobe of the liver at the site of a known space-occupying lesion. This patient had a biopsy-proven haemangioma, and the above studies show the high blood volume associated with low blood flow that may be seen in haemangioma.*

**As colloid never reaches equilibrium in the blood (because extraction is so rapid), dynamic studies with colloid may misleadingly suggest a relatively avascular lesion.**

## Avascular tumour

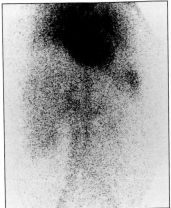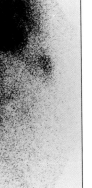

*a  0–40 seconds*

*b  2 minutes*

**Fig. 8.144**

*(a,b)* ⁹⁹ᵐTc-*labelled red cell vascular study of liver.*

   *This patient had a 3 cm by 5 cm lesion of the liver identified on ultrasound, and the possibility of haemangioma was raised. The blood pool study shows a moderately large, relatively avascular lesion in the region of the left lobe.*

## Metastases

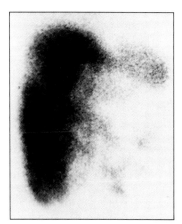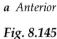

*a  Anterior*

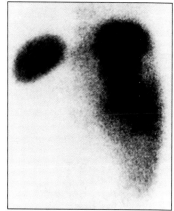

*b  Posterior*

**Fig. 8.145**

*(a,b) Liver/spleen scan.*

   *In this case of hepatic metastases a biopsy in the conventional axillary line would have produced normal liver. The biopsy was therefore taken from the left lobe, which was replaced by tumour.*

## Assessment of shunt for ascites

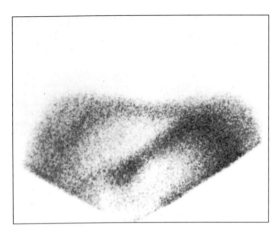

**Fig. 8.146**

*Anterior view of the abdomen following injection of $^{99m}$Tc colloid into the peritoneal cavity.*

*This patient with massive ascites had been treated with a LaVeen shunt. Recurrence of the ascites suggested that the shunt was blocked. The colloid is shown below the diaphragm. It failed to drain, thus confirming that the shunt was blocked.*

## Hepatic damage caused by radiation therapy

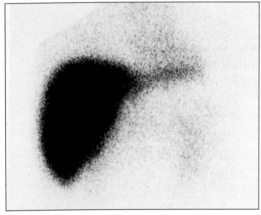

*Anterior*

**Fig. 8.147**

*Liver/spleen scan.*

*There is loss of hepatic uptake in the left lobe, which corresponds to the area of previous radiotherapy. Note the linearity of the hepatic borders in that area.*

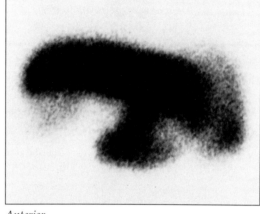

*Anterior*

**Fig. 8.148**

*Liver/spleen scan.*

*There is a large defect in the right lobe of the liver, with a linear horizontal upper margin. This was due to previous radiotherapy.*

The inclusion of the liver in the radiotherapy field may cause liver damage. The Kupffer cells, which take up colloid particles, may be permanently functionally impaired. The clue on the scan to possible radiation damage is almost always the geometric appearance of the defect.

## CLINICAL APPLICATIONS

# Hepatic infarction caused by radiation therapy

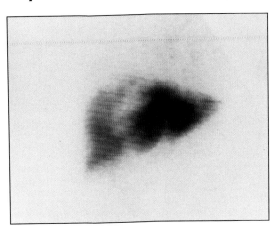

**Fig. 8.149**

*Hepatobiliary scan.*

*A huge mass of non-functioning liver tissue is seen in the upper portion of the right lobe. At post-mortem it was found that this patient had a large infarction in the liver and thrombosis of the intrahepatic artery, possibly secondary to radiotherapy.*

# CHAPTER 9

# GASTROINTESTINAL STUDIES

The gastrointestinal tract extends from the mouth to the anus, and is affected by various pathologies. Nuclear medicine studies provide information on the function of the various components of the gastrointestinal tract, and are therefore complementary to x-ray studies and ultrasound, which yield information on structure.

The functional information yielded by nuclear medicine approximates most accurately to normal physiology, since the agents used resemble normal meals (eg dual-phase gastric emptying study) when compared with non-physiological barium. No drugs are required to diminish gut activity, which is particularly relevant when disorders of gut motility are being studied. The complementary nature of nuclear medicine studies and radiology studies is shown in Table 9.1.

Similarly, the function of the salivary glands may be studied without the non-physiological requirement to cannulate the salivary ducts.

Table 9.1  *Complementary investigative studies of the gastrointestinal tract*

| Radiology | Nuclear medicine |
|---|---|
| Contrast sialography to show salivary ducts | $^{99m}$Tc pertechnetate salivary gland uptake and excretion for salivary gland function |
| Barium swallow studies for oesophageal disorders | Radionuclide oesophageal transit studies for physiological oesophageal measurement |
| Barium meal studies for gastric oesophageal reflux | $^{99m}$Tc pertechnetate studies, which demonstrate reflux quantitatively |
| Barium meal studies for gastric size and structure | Solid and liquid quantitative gastric emptying studies |
| Barium meal and follow through studies for post-gastrectomy assessment of anatomy | Bile reflux studies, showing the dynamics of bile flow |
| Barium follow-through studies for identifying Meckel's diverticulum | $^{99m}$Tc pertechnetate studies to demonstrate functioning gastric mucosa |
| Barium follow-through and enema studies to show abnormalities in inflammatory bowel disease | $^{111}$In white cell and $^{99m}$Tc WBC scans to demonstrate the sites of active inflammation |
| Mesenteric angiography for gastrointestinal bleeding localization | $^{99m}$Tc red cell study to identify the time and site of bleeding to optimize the use of angiography |

# CHAPTER CONTENTS

## 9.1 SALIVARY GLAND SCANNING: ANATOMY/RADIOPHARMACEUTICALS

Since technetium-99m pertechnetate ($^{99m}TcO_4$) is taken up by salivary glands and secreted by the ductal epithelium, a salivary gland scan can provide physiological information about the ability of the salivary glands to take up tracer, and the drainage of saliva.

Following intravenous injection of $^{99m}TcO_4$, rapid sequential images are obtained which show progressive concentration of activity within the salivary glands and the mouth. The thyroid is included in the field of view, and intensity of activity is generally similar to that in the salivary glands. After 10 minutes, the patient is given a sialogogue (ie lemon drops, ascorbic acid or lemon juice) which causes prompt salivation and drainage of the glands when the salivary ducts are patent.

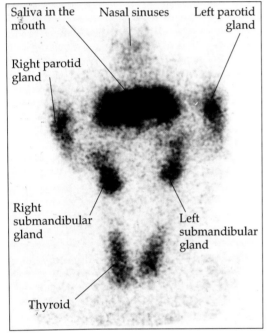

a Anterior

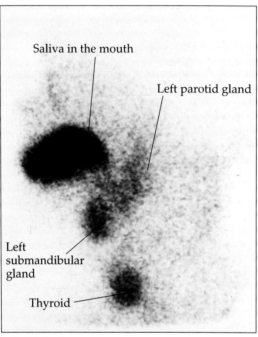

b Left lateral

Fig. 9.1

(a) Anterior view of face and neck. (b) Left lateral view of face and neck.

Normal salivary gland image at 15 minutes after injection.

## 9.2   SALIVARY GLAND SCANNING: NORMAL SCANS

# Normal salivary gland study

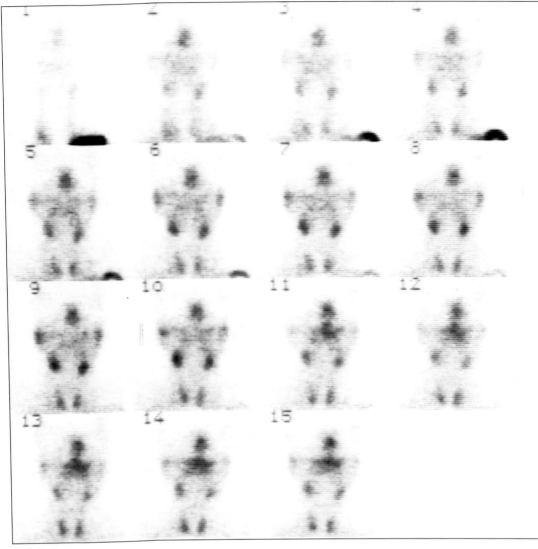

*a  Anterior*

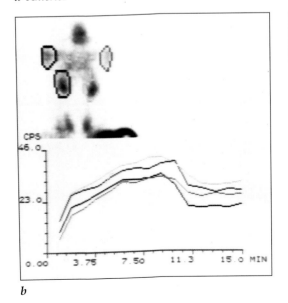

*b*

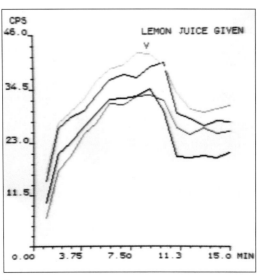

*c*

**Fig. 9.2**

**(a)** *One-minute images of face and neck following iv injection of $^{99m}TcO_4$, showing progressive accumulation in the salivary glands to 9 minutes. A sialogogue given at 10 minutes releases tracer from the salivary glands into the mouth.*
**(b)** *Areas of interest over the parotid and submandibular glands.* **(c)** *Time/activity (T/A) curves from the submandibular and parotid glands, with release at 10 minutes following the sialogogue.*

# 9.3 SALIVARY GLAND SCANNING: CLINICAL APPLICATIONS

The clinical applications of salivary gland imaging are
listed below, and examples of the various clinical
problems are given on subsequent pages.

**9.3.1 Recurrent salivary gland swelling**
Salivary duct obstruction
Recurrent parotitis

**9.3.2 Dry mouth**

**9.3.3 Function of a salivary gland mass**
Functioning tumour
Non-functioning tumour

# 9.3.1 Recurrent salivary gland swelling

## Salivary duct obstruction

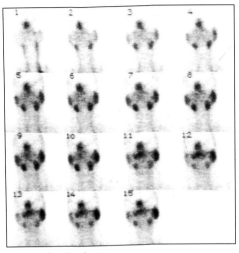

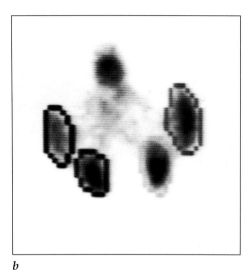

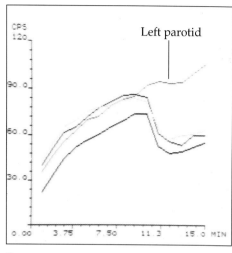

a *Anterior, 1 minute*

b

c

**Fig. 9.3**

*(a) Anterior view 1-minute images of face and neck, showing progressive uptake in all four salivary glands. A sialogogue at 10 minutes releases tracer from all glands, with the exception of the left parotid. Note the absence of thyroid uptake. (b)Areas of interest over the parotid and submandibular glands. (c) T/A curves from the salivary glands, showing the normal rise in tracer uptake until the sialogogue is given. This is followed by a rapid fall in activity in the normal glands, but continued rise in the obstructed left parotid gland.*

*The patient was a young man who had been treated for a differentiated thyroid cancer (hence the lack of thyroid uptake). He complained of intermittent swelling around the left jaw. The study is diagnostic of a left-sided parotid obstruction. A stone was subsequently removed surgically from the parotid duct.*

## Recurrent parotitis

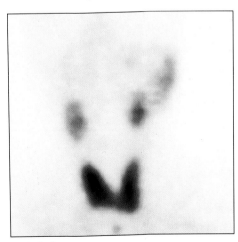

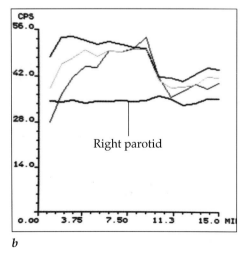

a *Anterior*

b

**Fig. 9.4**

*(a) Anterior view of face and neck 15 minutes after iv injection of $^{99m}TcO_4$, showing activity in the left parotid and submandibular glands but absent activity in the right parotid. (b) T/A curve, showing no accumulation in the right parotid gland.*

*The patient was a middle-aged woman who presented with intermittent, painful right parotid swelling. The study excludes obstruction as a cause of recurrent swelling because there is no function present. A diagnosis of recurrent parotitis is more likely. She was treated by right parotidectomy, and the diagnosis was confirmed histologically.*

**Longstanding obstruction will lead to a non-functioning gland.**

# 9.3.2    Dry mouth

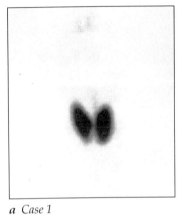

*a  Case 1*

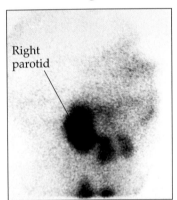

*b  Case 2*

**Fig. 9.5**

*(a) This patient with rheumatoid arthritis complained of a dry mouth. The salivary gland study shows complete failure of any of the glands to accumulate tracer. This scan appearance is typical of Sjögren's syndrome. (b) This patient had dry eyes, and the study was undertaken to investigate the likely involvement of other glands. There is very poor function of all glands demonstrated.*

# 9.3.3    Function of a salivary gland mass

## *Functioning tumour*

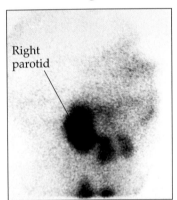

Right parotid

*a  Right lateral*

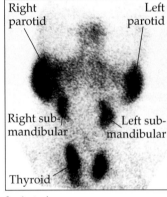

Right parotid

Left parotid

Right sub-mandibular

Left sub-mandibular

Thyroid

*b  Anterior*

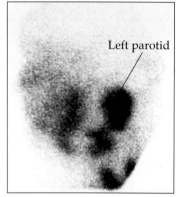

Left parotid

*c  Left lateral*

**Fig. 9.6**

*(a–c) Salivary gland scan.*

*This patient presented with a swelling of the right parotid gland which was shown on the study to be a functioning mass. This was subsequently removed, confirming a benign oxyphilic adenoma.*

 Functioning salivary gland tumours (eg Warthin's tumour and oxyphilic adenomas) are always benign.

## *Non-functioning tumour*

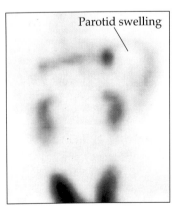

Parotid swelling

*Left anterior oblique*

**Fig. 9.7**

*Salivary gland scan.*

*The patient was a 50-year-old man who presented with a left-sided swelling. The study shows a non-functioning mass in the left parotid. Histologically, this was a mixed parotid tumour.*

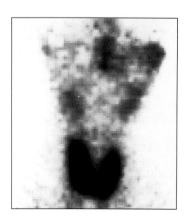

**Fig. 9.8**

*Salivary gland scan.*

*This patient had a right-sided tumour which arose from the parotid gland and had completely replaced it. There is no uptake of $^{99m}TcO_4$ seen.*

# 9.4 GASTROINTESTINAL TRACT STUDIES: ANATOMY/RADIOPHARMACEUTICALS

**Table 9.2** *Radiopharmaceuticals for gastrointestinal tract function studies*

| | |
|---|---|
| Oesophageal transit study | $^{99m}$Tc sulphur colloid in 10 ml water |
| Gastrointestinal reflux study | $^{99m}$Tc sulphur colloid in 200 ml acidified orange juice pH 6 |
| Bile reflux | $^{99m}$Tc HIDA iv<br>$^{111}$In DTPA orally in fatty meal to outline stomach |
| Gastric emptying | Solid phase: $^{99m}$Tc bran/Dowex<br>Liquid phase: $^{111}$In DTPA in orange juice |
| Investigation of inflammatory bowel disease | $^{111}$In WBC<br>$^{99m}$Tc HMPAO WBC |
| Detection of intra-abdominal sepsis | $^{111}$In WBC<br>$^{67}$Ga citrate |

HIDA, hepatic $^{99m}$Tc iminodiacetic acid; DTPA, diethylenetriamine pentaacetic acid; HMPAO, hexamethylenepropylamine oxine

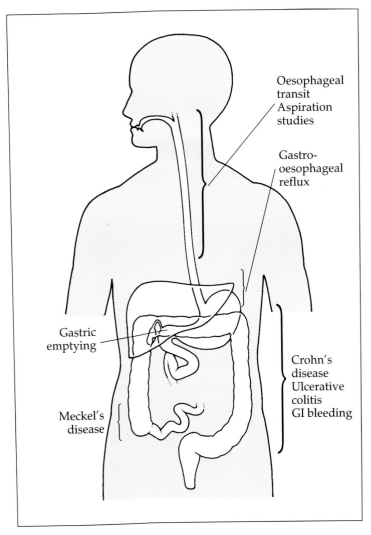

Oesophageal transit Aspiration studies

Gastro-oesophageal reflux

Gastric emptying

Meckel's disease

Crohn's disease Ulcerative colitis GI bleeding

**Fig. 9.9**

*Anatomy and pathology of the gastrointestinal tract.*

# 9.5 GASTROINTESTINAL TRACT STUDIES: CLINICAL APPLICATIONS

The clinical applications of gastrointestinal tract studies are listed below, and examples of the various clinical problems are given on subsequent pages.

**9.5.1    Gastrointestinal transit and reflux studies**
Oesophageal transit studies
Gastro-oesophageal reflux studies
Pulmonary aspiration studies
Bile reflux studies
Gastric emptying studies

**9.5.2    Gastrointestinal tract infection and inflammation studies**
Inflammatory bowel disease
Abdominal infection
Investigation of pyrexia of unknown origin (PUO)
Infected abdominal viscera

**9.5.3    Gastrointestinal tract bleeding studies**
Normal gastrointestinal tract bleeding study
Acute gastrointestinal bleeding
Timing of studies
False localization of site of bleeding
Incidental finding

**9.5.4    Ectopic gastric mucosa studies**
Detection of ectopic gastric mucosa

# GASTROINTESTINAL TRACT STUDIES: CLINICAL APPLICATIONS

## 9.5.1 Gastrointestinal transit and reflux studies

### Oesophageal transit studies

Radionuclide studies may be used to assess oesophageal function by measuring the rate at which a swallowed bolus passes through the oesophagus.

The fasted patient is positioned supine under a gamma camera linked to a microprocessor, so that the oropharynx, the whole oesophagus and gastric fundus are included in the same field. The patient swallows in a single swallow technetium-99m ($^{99m}$Tc) sulphur colloid in water through a straw and then swallows at 30-second intervals for 5 minutes. A computer analysis uses the marker view to define the oesophageal area of interest (Fig. 9.10). The count rate in this area determines the rate of oesophageal transit using the formula:

$$C_t = \frac{(E_{max} - E_t) \times 100}{E_{max}}$$

$C_t$ is the percentage clearance after time $t$, $E_{max}$ is the maximum count in the oesophagus and $E_t$ is the count in the oesophagus after time $t$.

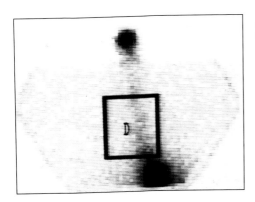

**Fig. 9.10**

*The use of the marker view to define the oesophageal area of interest.*

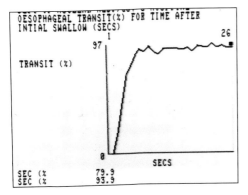

**Fig. 9.11**

*Normal tracing, where over 90% of the activity in the oesophagus has been cleared 15 seconds after swallowing the technetium.*

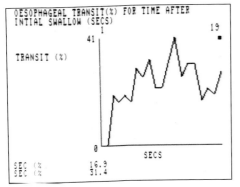

**Fig. 9.12**

*Tracing from a patient with diffuse oesophageal spasm, showing less than 40% clearance after 15 seconds. After 2 minutes the clearance has reached the normal range of over 90%.*

## Gastro-oesophageal reflux studies

The presence of gastro-oesophageal reflux may be demonstrated semiquantitatively with isotopes by imaging the abdomen and lower thorax while increasing pressures are applied to the abdomen using an abdominal binder.

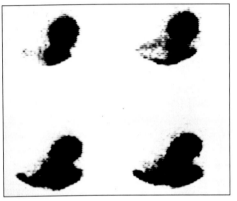

*a* Normal     *b* Abnormal

**Fig. 9.13**

**(a)** *This normal study clearly shows the fundus of the stomach with no reflux occurring at any pressure level.* **(b)** *This abnormal study also clearly identifies the fundus of the stomach, with no reflux occurring at 40 mmHg, but reflux is clearly present at 80 mmHg, and has increased at 120 mmHg. Key to images:*

| *0 pressure* | *40 mmHg* |
|--------------|-----------|
| *80 mmHg* | *120 mmHg* |

### Low pressure reflux

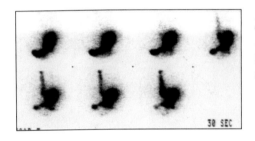

30 SEC

**Fig. 9.14**

*Reflux has occurred at 60 mmHg, and is increasing throughout the study to the maximum pressure of 120 mmHg.*

### High pressure reflux

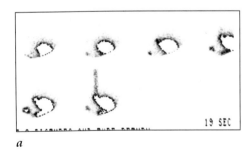

*a*

19 SEC

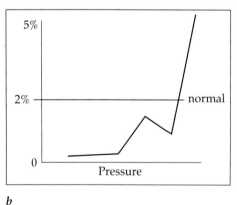

*b*

**Fig. 9.15**

**(a)** *Reflux is occurring at only the highest pressure (120 mmHg).* **(b)** *T/A curve, showing the time at which reflux occurs and the percentage of the gastric contents which enter the oesophagus.*

### Comparison of radionuclide and barium techniques to assess reflux

*Radionuclide reflux*
- Simple and quick as a screening test
- Quantitative information
- More reproducible

*Barium reflux*
- Permits simultaneous assessment of anatomical abnormalities.

## GASTROINTESTINAL TRACT STUDIES: CLINICAL APPLICATIONS

### *Pulmonary aspiration studies*

Pulmonary aspiration of gastric contents may occur in infants and in debilitated patients. Reflux in children may cause:

- Failure to thrive
- Aspiration pneumonia
- Oesophagitis
- Stricture.

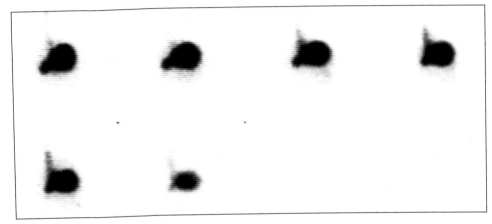
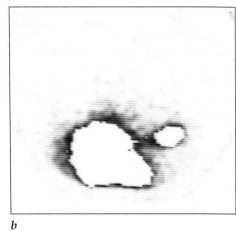

*a  30 seconds*

b

### Fig. 9.16

*(a) 30-second images obtained after ingestion of $^{99m}$Tc colloid in a milk feed. No abdominal pressure has been applied. Note that reflux is occurring intermittently and spontaneously.*
*(b) Enhanced image of lung fields to facilitate detection of small amounts of tracer in the lungs.*
*   The patient was a baby with recurrent chest infection. The lungs were scanned the next morning to ascertain whether tracer was present in the lung fields. In this instance imaging of the lungs was negative. However, this is a relatively insensitive test for pulmonary aspiration.*

## GASTROINTESTINAL TRACT STUDIES: CLINICAL APPLICATIONS

### *Bile reflux studies*
#### *Duodenogastric bile reflux*

Reflux of bile into the stomach is most frequently found as a complication of previous gastric surgery, but may occur spontaneously. It is often associated with painful gastritis and occasionally with bile vomiting, when gastro-oesophageal reflux is present.

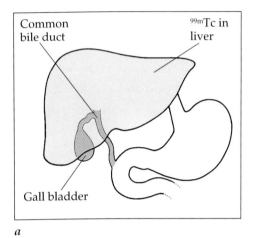 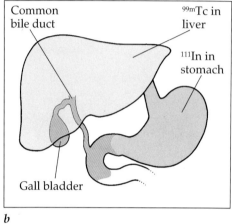 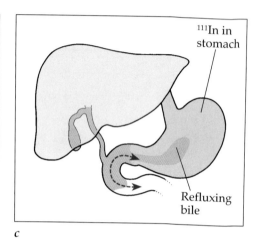

*a*  *b*  *c*

**Fig. 9.17**

*(a) Approximately 15–20 minutes after iv injection of* $^{99m}$*Tc* HIDA *there is labelled bile in the gall bladder and common bile duct but none in the duodenum. (b) At this time the* $^{111}$*In-labelled fatty meal is given to outline the stomach and stimulate gall bladder contraction. (c) Stomach is emptying contents; bile enters the duodenum and may reflux into the stomach.*

#### *Simultaneous dual isotope imaging*

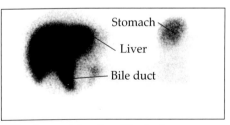 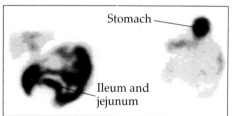

*a  Normal, 20 minutes*  *b  Normal, 30 minutes*

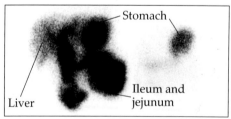

*c  Duodenogastric reflux, 20 minutes*  *d  Duodenogastric reflux, 30 minutes*

**Fig. 9.18**

*Case 1 (a, b) Tracer rapidly enters the duodenum and small gut. No tracer enters the stomach.*

*Case 2 (c, d) There is marked tracer accumulation in the stomach.*

*In both these cases the patients had previous cholecystectomies. Note that the gall bladders are not visualized.*

# GASTROINTESTINAL TRACT STUDIES: CLINICAL APPLICATIONS

*Two further cases of gastric reflux of bile*

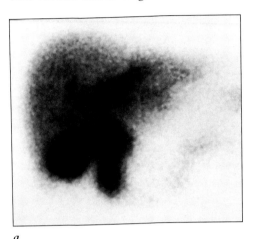 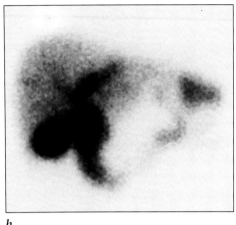 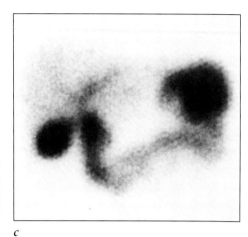

*a*            *b*            *c*

**Fig. 9.19**

*(a)* 20 minutes after iv injection of $^{99m}$Tc HIDA, showing gall bladder and common bile duct. *(b)* 5 minutes after fatty meal, showing early gastric reflux. *(c)* 10 minutes after fatty meal, showing massive gastric reflux.

The patient was a 52-year-old woman who presented with recurrent abdominal pain. A barium meal was normal. The radionuclide study clearly demonstrates reflux of bile, which was the cause of her symptoms.

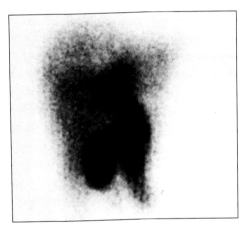 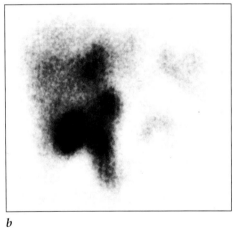 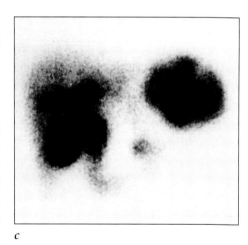

*a*            *b*            *c*

**Fig. 9.20**

*(a)* 20 minutes after iv injection of $^{99m}$Tc HIDA. *(b)* 5 minutes after fatty meal, showing early gastric reflux. *(c)* 15 minutes after fatty meal, showing filling of the stomach with labelled bile.

The patient was a 64-year-old man who had recurrent abdominal pain and vomiting following a Pólya gastrectomy for peptic ulcer. The study shows massive bile reflux. A Roux-en-Y diversion prevented the reflux and corrected the patient's symptoms.

- When there is massive bile reflux, it will be apparent on a $^{99m}$Tc HIDA study alone, although dual isotope imaging is always advisable to outline the stomach.
- Following Pólya gastrectomy, some bile reflux into the stomach is inevitable.

## Duodenal/gastric/oesophageal reflux of bile

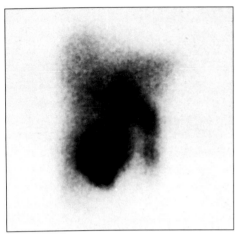

*a  30 minutes*

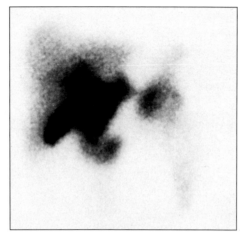

*b  40 minutes*

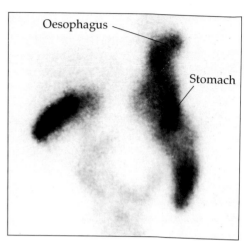

*c  60 minutes*

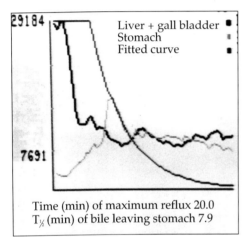

*d  T/A curve*

Time (min) of maximum reflux 20.0
T½ (min) of bile leaving stomach 7.9

**Fig. 9.21**

*(a)* 30 minutes after iv injection of $^{99m}Tc$ HIDA, showing bile in the gall bladder and common bile duct. *(b)* 40-minute image, showing the gall bladder contracting and tracer entering the duodenum. *(c)* 60-minute image. Tracer has entered the stomach and oesophagus. *(d)* T/A curve, demonstrating gastric reflux of bile with subsequent rapid emptying.

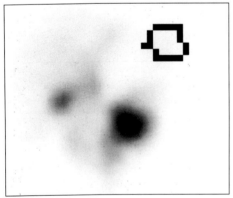

*a  $^{99m}Tc$ HIDA*

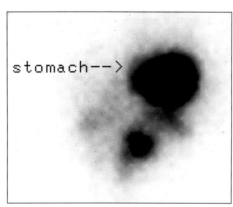

*b  $^{111}In$ milk*

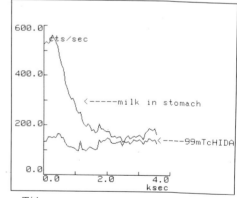

*c  T/A curve*

**Fig. 9.22**

*(a)* $^{99m}Tc$ HIDA image. *(b)* $^{111}In$ milk image, *(c)* T/A curve from the ROI over the fundus of the stomach, confirming the presence of $^{111}In$ milk in the stomach but showing no reflux of $^{99m}Tc$ HIDA into the stomach. This was therefore a negative reflux study. Note the absent gall bladder.

This patient presented with symptoms of nausea and occasional vomiting after a Pólya gastrectomy followed by revision.

## Gastric emptying studies

Depending on the clinical problem, a liquid labelled meal, a solid labelled meal or both simultaneously can be used to measure the rate of gastric emptying.

### Normal gastric emptying study

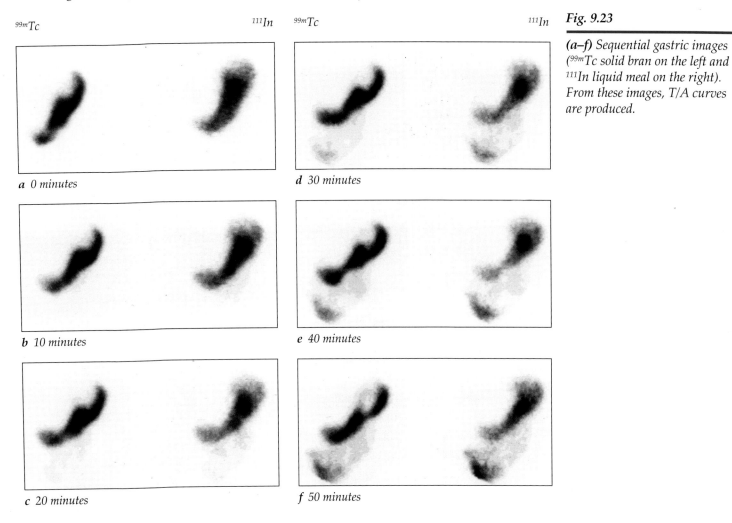

$^{99m}Tc$         $^{111}In$    $^{99m}Tc$         $^{111}In$

*a  0 minutes*

*b  10 minutes*

*c  20 minutes*

*d  30 minutes*

*e  40 minutes*

*f  50 minutes*

**Fig. 9.23**

*(a–f) Sequential gastric images ($^{99m}Tc$ solid bran on the left and $^{111}In$ liquid meal on the right). From these images, T/A curves are produced.*

# GASTROINTESTINAL TRACT STUDIES: CLINICAL APPLICATIONS

Serial imaging of drainage from the stomach will provide qualitative information about the rate of drainage; however, like many other radionuclide studies, the strength of nuclear medicine lies in its ability to measure physiological function.

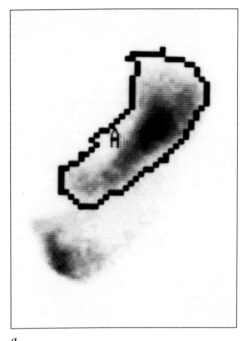

*a*

*b*

## Fig. 9.24

*A region of interest is drawn around the stomach **(a)**, and T/A curves for the liquid and solid phases are constructed. **(b)** Using an exponential curve-fitting technique, the $T_{1/2}$ for solid and liquid emptying may be calculated.*

- There is no 'absolute' rate for gastric emptying. The rate will depend on a number of factors, which include:

(a) volume of meal
(b) osmolarity of meal
(c) carbohydrate/fat content of meal
(d) solid/liquid components
(e) psychological factors.

- Emptying rates will therefore provide a rough guide to true gastric emptying but are of most value in assessing the response to intervention, eg with drugs, using the patient as his or her own control.

# GASTROINTESTINAL TRACT STUDIES: CLINICAL APPLICATIONS

## Rapid gastric emptying

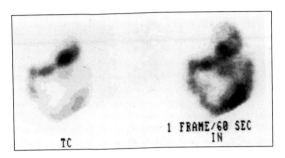

*a*

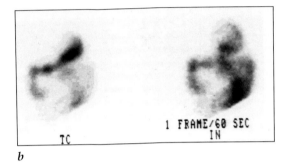

*b*

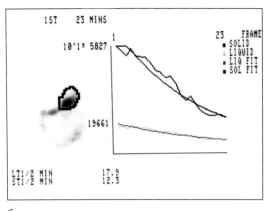

*c*

**Fig. 9.25**

*(a–c) Solid and liquid gastric emptying study.*

*Note the very rapid emptying of both components (liquid 17.9 minutes, solid 12.3 minutes). When gastric emptying is very fast, as in this case, there may be some emptying occurring before the measurements can be started. This patient had a partial gastrectomy and was suffering postprandial symptoms of feeling bloated.*

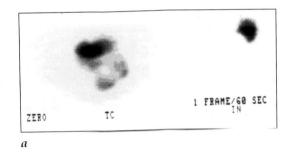

*a*

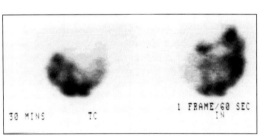

*b*

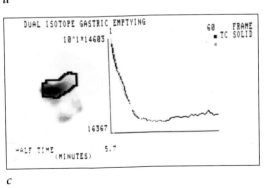

*c*

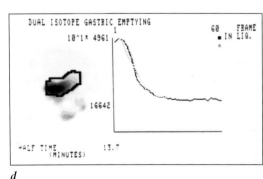

*d*

**Fig. 9.26**

*(a–d) Solid and liquid gastric emptying study.*

*This patient had abdominal pain and sweating suggestive of a dumping syndrome. The rapid emptying (liquid 13.7 minutes, solid 5.7 minutes) confirmed that this was probably the cause of her symptoms.*

## Delayed gastric emptying

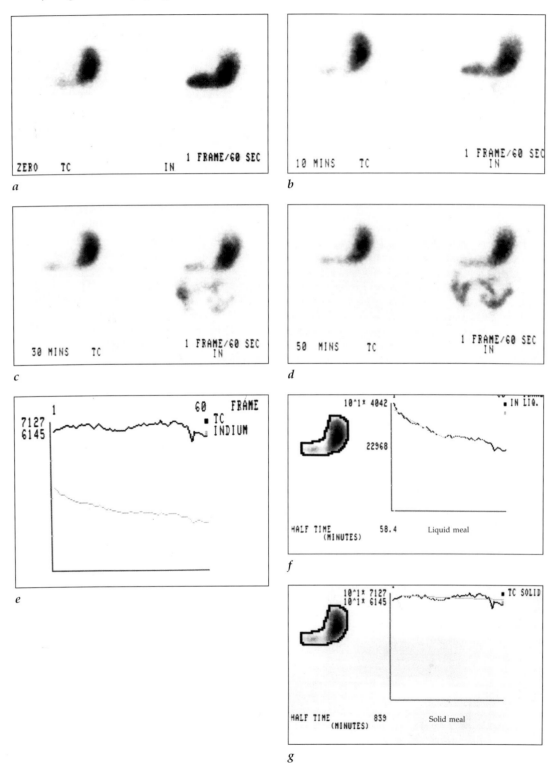

a

b

c

d

e

f

g

*Fig. 9.27*

*(a–d) Series of images from a dual phase (solid and liquid) gastric emptying study, showing the solid meal on the left and the liquid meal on the right. (e–g) T/A curves and calculated half-time measurements, showing the liquid emptying with a relatively normal rate (58 minutes), while the solid empties with a very prolonged (839 minutes) delay.*

## 9.5.2 Gastrointestinal tract infection and inflammation studies

### Inflammatory bowel disease

Indium-111 ($^{111}$In) and technetium-99m ($^{99m}$Tc) leucocytes are taken up into sites of bowel wall inflammation. Positive studies are found in:

- Active Crohn's disease
- Ulcerative colitis
- Infective colitis.

*Table 9.3   Comparison of $^{111}$In WBC and $^{99m}$Tc WBC in inflammatory bowel disease*

|  | Advantages | Disadvantages |
|---|---|---|
| $^{111}$In | No non-specific activity in bowel at 24 hours<br>Availability of $^{111}$In | Inferior image quality |
| $^{99m}$Tc | Availability of $^{99m}$Tc<br>Good quality images | Non-specific bowel activity at 24 hours |

### Normal $^{111}$In WBC images

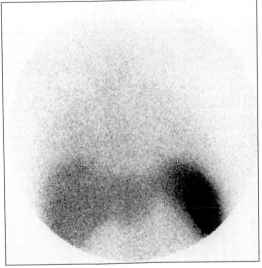

a  *Anterior chest, 3 hours*

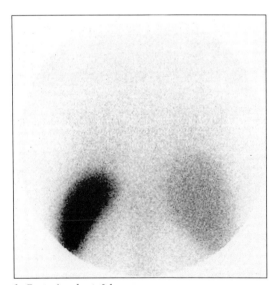

b  *Posterior chest, 3 hours*

**Fig. 9.28**

*Normal $^{111}$In WBC study:*
*(a, b) chest, 3 hours;*
*(c, d) abdomen, 3 hours;*
*(e, f) chest, 24 hours;*
*(g, h) abdomen, 24 hours.*
    *The scans demonstrate normal biodistribution in the bone marrow, liver and spleen. Note the intense activity in the spleen.*

*continued*

*Fig. 9.28 continued*

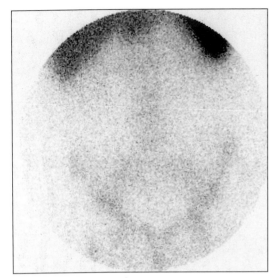

*c* Anterior abdomen, 3 hours

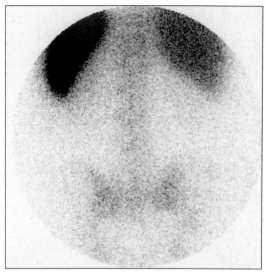

*d* Posterior abdomen, 3 hours

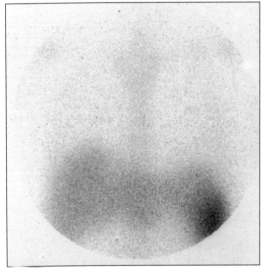

*e* Anterior chest, 24 hours

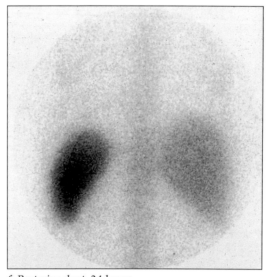

*f* Posterior chest, 24 hours

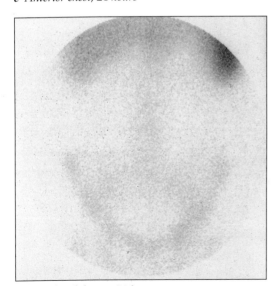

*g* Anterior abdomen, 24 hours

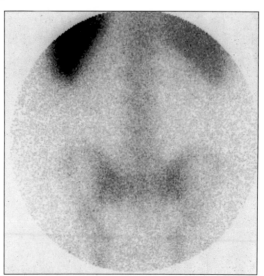

*h* Posterior abdomen, 24 hours

# GASTROINTESTINAL TRACT STUDIES: CLINICAL APPLICATIONS

## Potential pitfalls in imaging with $^{111}$In WBC
### Importance of early imaging

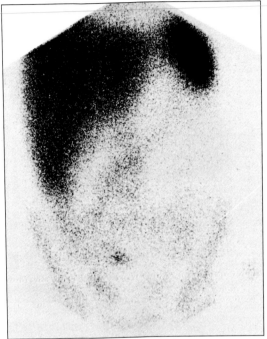

*a Anterior, 2 hours*

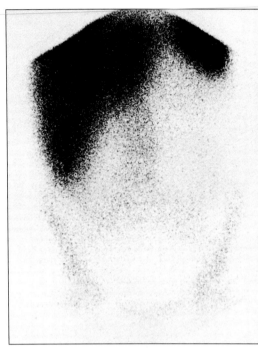

*b Anterior, 24 hours*

**Fig. 9.29**

**Case 1 (a)** *Anterior view of abdomen at 2 hours. There is tracer uptake in the small bowel, but note also the small focus on the right side of the pelvis.* **(b)** *Anterior view at 24 hours, which is normal.*

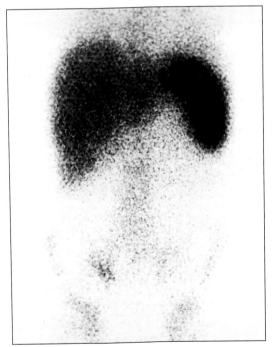

*c Anterior, 2 hours*

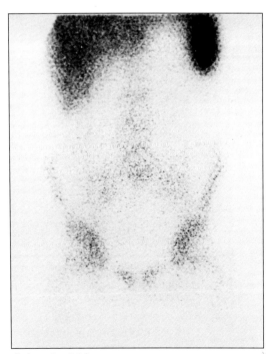

*d Anterior, 24 hours*

**Case 2 (c)** *Anterior view of abdomen at 2 hours, showing a small focus of tracer uptake on the right side of the pelvis.* **(d)** *Anterior view at 24 hours. This is now normal.*

*These two cases of inflammatory bowel disease show the importance of early imaging. The small collections of white cells in the inflamed bowel wall at 2 hours have migrated and dispersed by 24 hours. Thus there would have been false negative studies if imaging had been delayed.*

*False localization from delayed images: normal gut transit of activity*

*a Anterior, 2 hours*

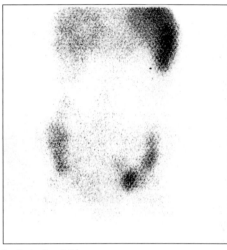

*b Anterior, 24 hours*

**Fig. 9.30**

*(a, b)* $^{111}$In WBC *of abdomen.*

*Tracer uptake is seen in the region of the terminal ileum and caecum. However, on the delayed image there is increased white cell accumulation in the ascending colon, descending colon and sigmoid. The $^{111}$In scan findings are those of inflammatory bowel disease. Note, however, that the pattern of initial tracer uptake is different from that later seen, which is a typically large bowel pattern. While disease is present in the ileum, the subsequent images were due to exudation of white cells into the bowel lumen. Imaging later would have resulted in a positive study, but false localization of disease.*

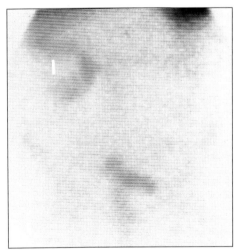

*a Anterior, 2 hours*

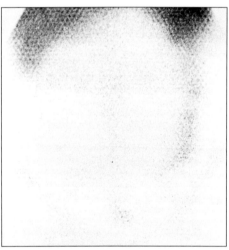

*b Anterior, 24 hours*

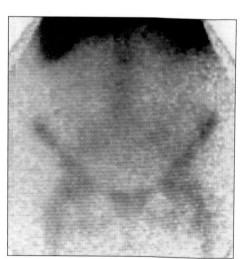

*c Anterior, 48 hours*

**Fig. 9.31**

*(a–c)* $^{111}$In WBC *scan of abdomen.*

*On the 2-hour image there is white cell localization in the right flank, most probably in the region of the ileocolic anastomosis. There is also significant tracer uptake in the rectosigmoid region. By 24 hours, the descending colon contains white cells. The 48-hour image is normal. Scan findings were due to active Crohn's disease involving the ileum and rectosigmoid junction. Once again, imaging at 24 hours would have resulted in a positive study, but false localization. Imaging at 48 hours would have resulted in a false negative study.*

**In inflammatory bowel disease, causing white cell migration into the lumen, delay in imaging may result in:**
- **a false negative scan**
- **false localization of disease.**

# GASTROINTESTINAL TRACT STUDIES: CLINICAL APPLICATIONS

## Normal $^{99m}$Tc WBC *images*

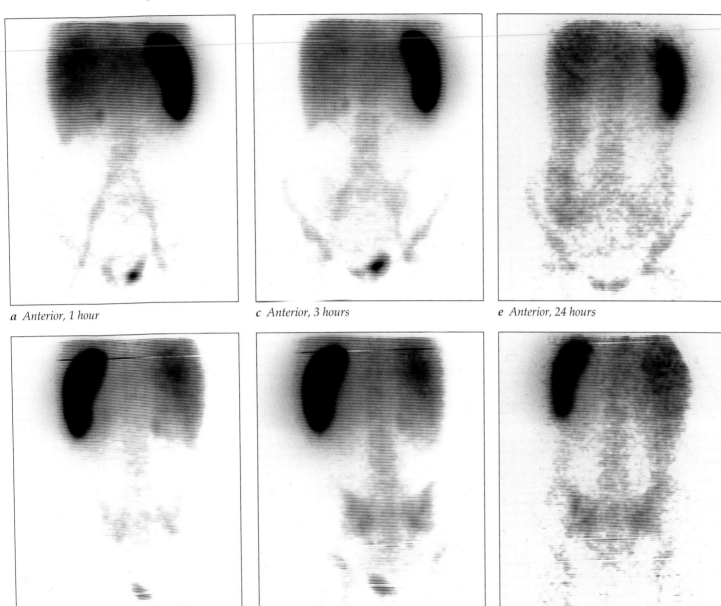

*a* Anterior, 1 hour

*c* Anterior, 3 hours

*e* Anterior, 24 hours

*b* Posterior, 1 hour

*d* Posterior, 3 hours

*f* Posterior, 24 hours

**Fig. 9.32**

Normal $^{99m}$Tc WBC abdominal study.

Note the normal biodistribution in the liver, spleen, renal collecting system and bladder, at 1 hour (*a*, *b*), 3 hours (*c*, *d*) and 24 hours (*e*, *f*), when enterohepatic secretion of $^{99m}$Tc HMPAO results in visualization of the large bowel.

## GASTROINTESTINAL TRACT STUDIES: CLINICAL APPLICATIONS

*Potential pitfalls in imaging with $^{99m}$Tc WBC*

*Accumulation of tracer in dilated renal collecting systems*

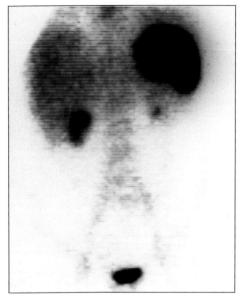

*a  Anterior, 1 hour*

*b  Anterior, 3 hours*

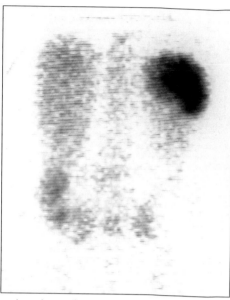

*c  Anterior, 24 hours*

**Fig. 9.33**

*(a) The $^{99m}$Tc WBC image at 1 hour shows two foci of activity below the liver and the spleen. These are less clearly seen at 3 hours (b) and have disappeared by 24 hours (c). These foci are due to dilation of the renal pelves and are not caused by inflammatory bowel disease or infected foci. Note also the non-specific bowel activity at 24 hours (c).*

*Diagnosis of an abnormality in the abdomen*

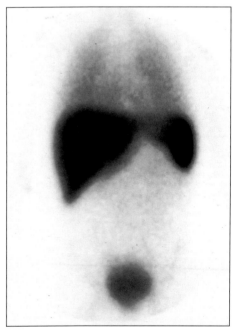

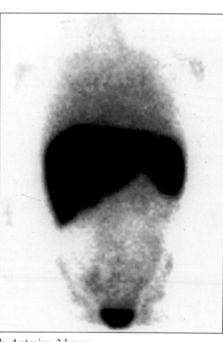

*a  Anterior, 1 hour*

*b  Anterior, 3 hours*

**Fig. 9.34**

*Normal $^{99m}$Tc HMPAO WBC study of abdomen.*

*No activity is seen on the 1-hour image (a), although activity is seen in the abdomen at 3 hours (b). Rapid appearance of activity in the bowel may occur, but if the 1-hour image is negative, the findings are not significant.*

**Both 1- and 3-hour images must be positive if an abnormality in the abdomen is to be diagnosed.**

# GASTROINTESTINAL TRACT STUDIES: CLINICAL APPLICATIONS

## Crohn's disease
### $^{111}$In study

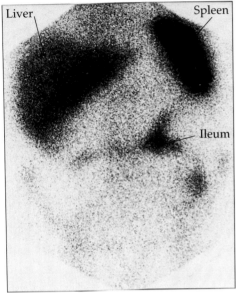

*a Anterior, 2 hours*

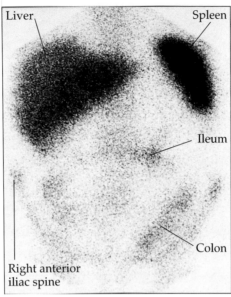

*b Anterior, 24 hours*

*Fig. 9.35*

*(a, b) $^{111}$In WBC scan of abdomen.*

*This is a case of Crohn's disease. The clinical problem was whether disease was active and, if so, where was the active site of bowel involvement. The 2-hour image shows tracer uptake in the ileum, identifying active disease. The 24-hour image shows less uptake in the inflammatory site in the ileum, and tracer is now visualized in the lumen of the colon.*

- In inflammatory bowel disease white cells migrate through the wall into the lumen of the gut during the time course of the study (2–24 hours).
- The typical $^{111}$In WBC scan appearance in inflammatory bowel disease is positive uptake at 2 hours, with either a normal or very much less prominent study at 24 hours.

$^{99m}Tc$ WBC *study*

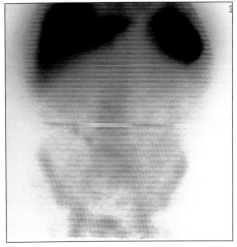

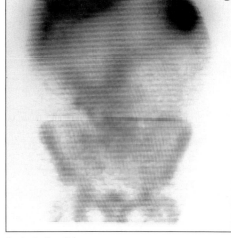

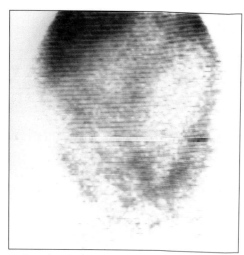

*a  Anterior, 1 hour*

*b  Anterior, 3 hours*

*c  Anterior, 24 hours*

**Fig. 9.36**

$^{99m}Tc$ WBC *study.*

In this case of Crohn's disease activity is seen in the small bowel at 1 hour **(a)**. By 3 hours **(b)** activity is also seen in the transverse colon but is non-specific transit of $^{99m}Tc$ WBC. At 24 hours **(c)** activity is seen throughout the large bowel.

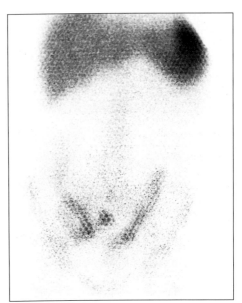

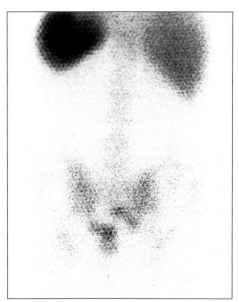

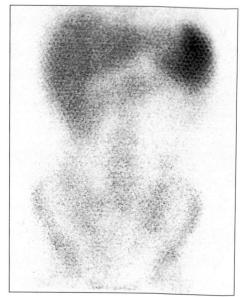

*a  Anterior*

*b  Posterior*

*c  Anterior*

**Fig. 9.37**

$^{99m}Tc$ WBC *scan.*

This patient was a 30-year-old woman with known Crohn's disease and a recent exacebation of symptoms. The anterior scan at 3 hours **(a)** shows uptake in the distal ileum, and the anterior and descending colon. The posterior view **(b)** also identifies rectal disease. At 24 hours **(c)** the pattern of bowel activity has changed with WBC migration.

**The typical $^{99m}Tc$ WBC scan appearance in inflammatory bowel disease is positive uptake at 1 and 3 hours. Non-specific bowel activity may be seen at 24 hours.**

# GASTROINTESTINAL TRACT STUDIES: CLINICAL APPLICATIONS

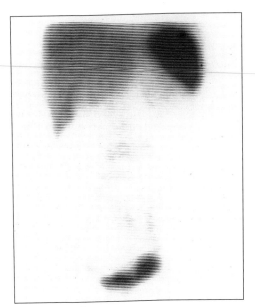

*a Anterior, 1 hour*

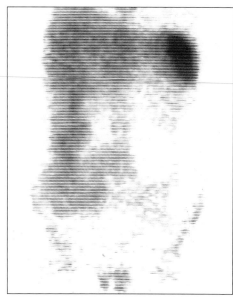

*c Anterior, 3 hours*

*e Anterior, 24 hours*

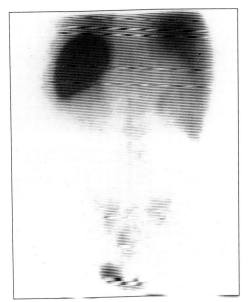

*b Posterior, 1 hour*

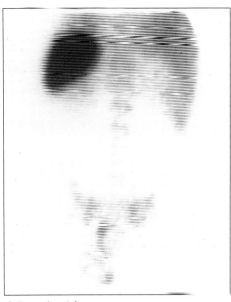

*d Posterior, 3 hours*

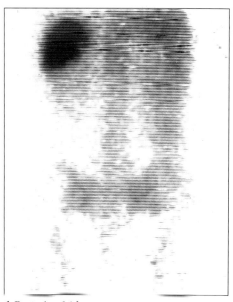

*f Posterior, 24 hours*

## Fig. 9.38

$^{99m}Tc$ WBC scan.

This patient was a woman with symptoms of bloody diarrhoea. The 1-hour scan (**a**) shows faint uptake in the left pelvis. Rectal activity is seen more clearly on the posterior view (**b**). At 3 hours activity is more clearly visualized, confirming Crohn's disease confined to the distal large bowel only (**c, d**). At 24 hours non-specific activity only is seen (**e, f**).

**A posterior view is vital to assess the rectum in patients with Crohn's disease (see page 672). A squat view may occasionally be helpful.**

## Ulcerative colitis: colon

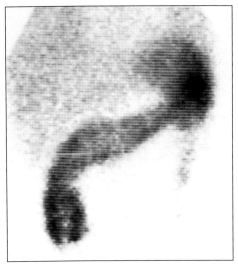

*a* Anterior, 2 hours

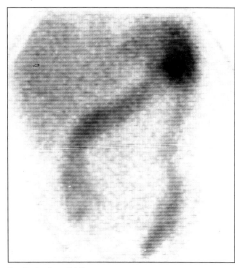

*b* Anterior, 24 hours

### Fig. 9.39

**(a, b)** [111]In WBC *scan of abdomen.*

The patient was a 56-year-old man with known ulcerative colitis, admitted during an acute exacerbation of inflammatory colitis. There is increased tracer uptake associated with the ascending and transverse colon. Note that the bowel is dilated. At 24 hours white cells are in the bowel lumen and visualization of the descending colon is now apparent.

## Proctitis

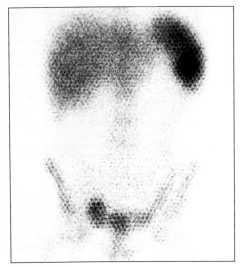

Anterior, 3 hours

### Fig. 9.40

[111]In WBC *scan of abdomen.*

This study shows tracer localized in the pelvis in a patient with acute ulcerative proctitis.

## Pseudomembranous colitis

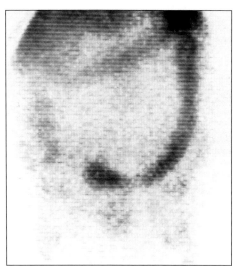

Anterior, 2 hours

### Fig. 9.41

[111]In WBC *scan of abdomen.*

The patient was a 70-year-old man with end-stage renal failure who had been treated by haemodialysis for 5 years. Over the previous 3 months he had septic arthritis. There is abnormal white cell accumulation involving rectum and entire colon. The scan appearances suggest infective colitis, but in the clinical context these appearances were almost certainly due to pseudomembranous colitis.

# GASTROINTESTINAL TRACT STUDIES: CLINICAL APPLICATIONS

## Response to therapy

The $^{111}$In WBC/$^{99m}$Tc WBC scan provides a useful method of following the response to therapy, as illustrated by the case below.

### Initial study

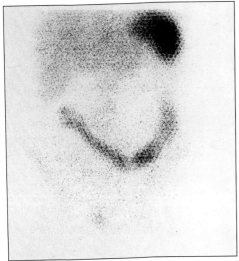

*a Anterior, 2 hours*

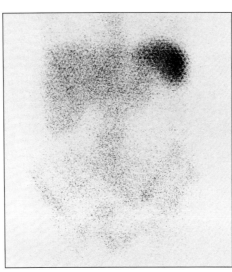

*b Anterior, 24 hours*

### Study 2 months later

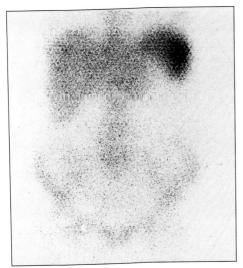

*c Anterior, 2 hours*

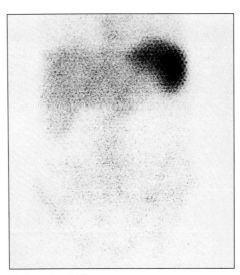

*d Anterior, 24 hours*

**Fig. 9.42**

*Resolution of Crohn's disease. **(a, b)** $^{111}$In WBC scan of abdomen, original study. **(c, d)** Repeat study 2 months later.*

*On the original 2-hour study there is intense white cell localization in a large loop of bowel, extending across the midline to the left loin. There are much less marked areas of uptake in the right iliac fossa and in the pelvis. After 24 hours the uptake in the loop of bowel is much less marked, and the activity is in the pelvis. The scan findings are typical of active inflammatory bowel disease. The repeat study after 2 months of treatment shows only slightly increased tracer uptake in both the right and left pelvis, which is associated with bowel. The scan findings are in keeping with mild inflammatory bowel disease, and there has been a marked improvement since the previous study.*

*Differentiation between inflammatory bowel disease and abscess*

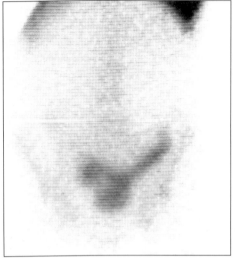
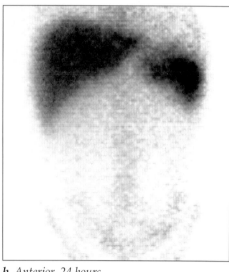

*a  Anterior, 2 hours*      *b  Anterior, 24 hours*

**Fig. 9.43**

*Inflammatory bowel disease. (a) $^{111}$In WBC scan of abdomen, showing tracer uptake in the pelvis. (b) Same view at 24 hours, showing considerable resolution.*

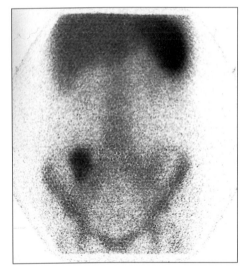
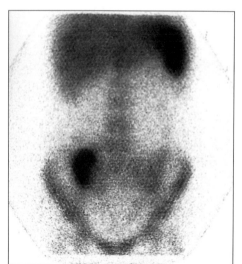

*a  Anterior, 3 hours*      *b  Anterior, 24 hours*

**Fig. 9.44**

*This patient with known Crohn's disease was admitted with right iliac fossa pain and swinging pyrexia. The $^{111}$In WBC scan at 3 hours (a) shows accumulation of WBC in the right iliac fossa. At 24 hours there has been further accumulation at this site (b), confirming Crohn's abscess.*

• On the $^{111}$In WBC scan inflammatory bowel disease shows early uptake of tracer, with subsequent dispersion because of migration of white cells, whereas an abscess will show progressively increased tracer uptake over 24 hours.
• Non-specific bowel activity at 24 hours with $^{99m}$Tc WBC scan may lead to problems of interpretation, and if an abscess is suspected, $^{111}$In WBC should be used.

# GASTROINTESTINAL TRACT STUDIES: CLINICAL APPLICATIONS

## *Abdominal infection*
### *Subphrenic abscess*

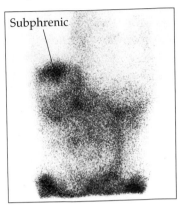

*a Anterior, ⁶⁷Ga*

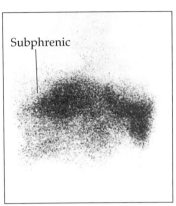

*b Anterior, ⁹⁹ᵐTc colloid*

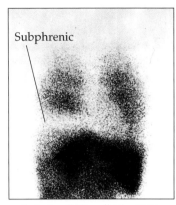

*c Anterior, ⁹⁹ᵐTc colloid + ⁹⁹ᵐTc MAA*

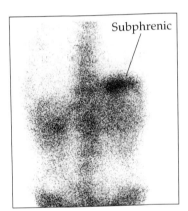

*d Posterior, ⁶⁷Ga*

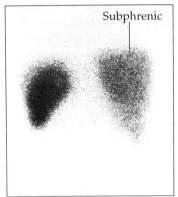

*e Posterior, ⁹⁹ᵐTc colloid*

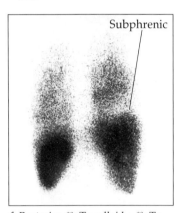

*f Posterior, ⁹⁹ᵐTc colloid + ⁹⁹ᵐTc MAA*

**Fig. 9.45**

*(a–f) Scan views of chest and abdomen.*

*This is an example of a subphrenic abscess in a patient following abdominal surgery for a perforated duodenal ulcer. There was postoperative fever, but no clear indication as to the site of origin of the presumed infection. Although labelled white cells would have been the radiopharmaceutical of choice, this scan could not be performed immediately, since ¹¹¹In was not available, so gallium-67 (⁶⁷Ga) was chosen as an alternative. Note how the use of ⁹⁹ᵐTc colloid and ⁹⁹ᵐTc macroaggregates of albumin (MAA) helps to outline the abscess.*

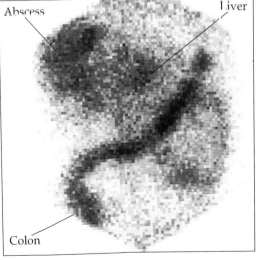

*a Anterior*

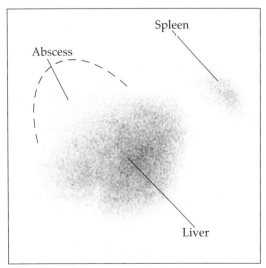

*b Anterior*

**Fig. 9.46**

*(a) 48-hour ⁶⁷Ga study of abdomen. (b) Liver scan.*

*This patient presented with a PUO, raised ESR and raised white cell count. The ⁶⁷Ga scan shows increased tracer uptake corresponding to the upper right lobe of the liver. A subphrenic abscess was subsequently confirmed by ultrasound and successfully drained. Note the activity in the transverse colon on the ⁶⁷Ga study (a) and the decreased tracer uptake in the right lobe at the site of the abscess in the liver scan (b).*

## Subhepatic abscess

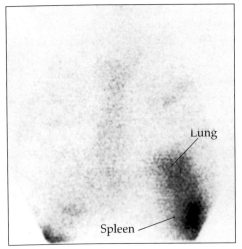

*a Anterior*

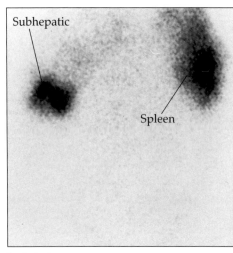

*b Anterior*

### Fig. 9.47

**(a)** [111]In WBC *24-hour view of the chest and abdomen.* **(b)** *View of abdomen.*

This patient developed a postoperative abdominal infection. There is abnormal white cell accumulation in the subhepatic area in the region of the gall bladder. In addition, there is some tracer uptake in the left lower chest. This patient had a confirmed abscess in the subhepatic region, and the lung uptake represented an associated chest infection.

## Abdominal abscesses

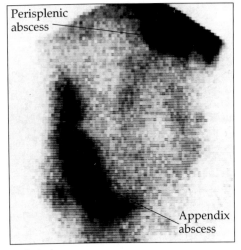

*a Anterior*

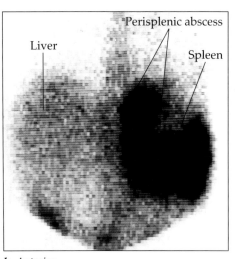

*b Anterior*

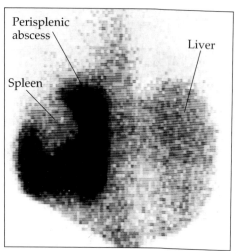

*c Posterior*

### Fig. 9.48

[67]Ga scan: **(a)** lower abdomen; **(b)** upper abdomen; **(c)** upper abdomen.

This patient was a 21-year-old woman who was admitted to hospital because of a history of pain in the left shoulder and left costal margin lasting several weeks. On admission she was found to have tenderness over the left costal margin, with slight swelling, and also swinging pyrexia associated with rigor. There was also a mass present in the right iliac fossa. The [67]Ga scan shows massive abnormal tracer accumulation in the left hypochondrium apparently surrounding the spleen. There is further abnormal uptake in the right iliac fossa. The liver/spleen scan was normal. This patient was found to have subphrenic and perisplenic abscesses in addition to an appendix abscess.

# GASTROINTESTINAL TRACT STUDIES: CLINICAL APPLICATIONS

## *Investigation of pyrexia of unknown origin (PUO)*

*Importance of delayed views with $^{111}$In WBC*

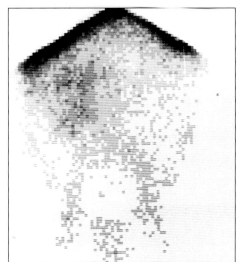 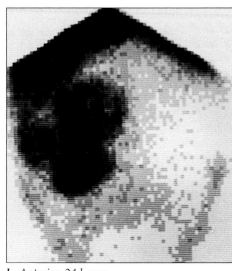

*a  Anterior, 2 hours*   *b  Anterior, 24 hours*

**Fig. 9.49**

*(a, b)* $^{111}$*In* WBC *scan of abdomen.*
On the early image there is some accumulation of tracer in the right side of the abdomen, but the 24-hour image shows clear-cut massive uptake. This elderly patient developed pyrexia following a right hemicolectomy, and the scan findings were due to a large abscess.

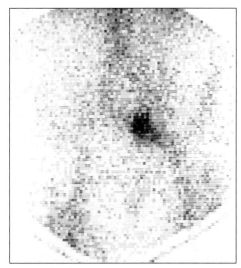 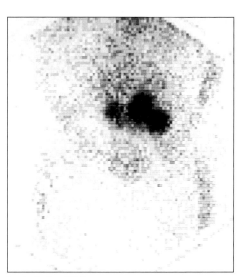

*a  Anterior, 2 hours*   *b  Anterior, 24 hours*

**Fig. 9.50**

*(a, b)* $^{111}$*In* WBC *scan of abdomen.*
The initial study shows focal tracer uptake to the left of the midline in the lower abdomen. However, the 24-hour image shows lobulated extensive uptake. This 60-year-old woman presented with PUO and raised white cell count. There were no clinical localizing features, but an abscess was suspected. The early study would have confirmed infection, but the full extent of the problem was not apparent until 24 hours.

**It is only rarely that an early $^{111}$In WBC study will be negative when the 24-hour study is positive, but the 24-hour scan is essential for full evaluation of a septic focus.**

## GASTROINTESTINAL TRACT STUDIES: CLINICAL APPLICATIONS

### Intrapelvic infection

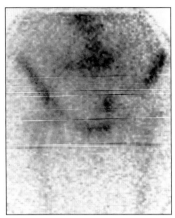 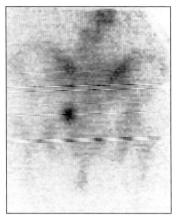

*a Anterior*　　　　*b Posterior*

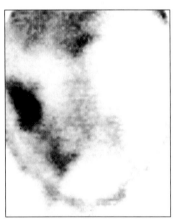 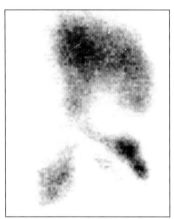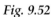

*a Anterior*　　　　*b Right lateral*

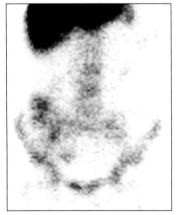 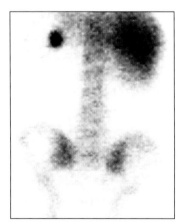

*a Anterior*　　　　*b Posterior*

**Fig. 9.51**

**(a, b)** $^{111}$In WBC 24-hour scan of pelvis.
　The patient was a 61-year-old woman who had two episodes of septicaemia. She was known to have both gall bladder and diverticular disease. The white cell scan shows a single focus of increased tracer uptake in the left pelvic area, lying posteriorly. This study identified an abscess in the left posterior lower pelvis.

**Fig. 9.52**

**(a, b)** $^{111}$In WBC 24-hour scan view of pelvis.
　This study identifies large focus of tracer uptake in the right iliac region, extending into the pelvis. This man had a pyrexia and abdominal tenderness following gastrectomy. The lateral view shows that the abscess is lying anteriorly, but with some posterior extension.

**Fig. 9.53**

**(a, b)** $^{111}$In WBC 24-hour scan of abdomen.
　This patient had previously received treatment for lymphoma, and subsequently developed fever and abdominal pain. The $^{111}$In study shows focal accumulation in the right iliac fossa at the site of an abscess. Note also the focus on the posterior view, left upper abdomen, which was due to a splenunculus which had grown after a previous staging splenectomy.

 **A false negative study for infection may occur when:**

- the patient is receiving steroids
- the patient is immunosuppressed by chemotherapy
- effective antibiotic therapy is being given.

## Infected abdominal viscera
### Infected pancreatic pseudocyst

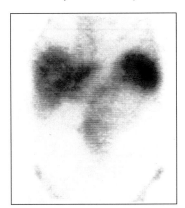

Anterior

**Fig. 9.54**

$^{111}In$ WBC 24-hour scan of abdomen.

There is tracer uptake seen centrally, extending into the left of the abdomen. The scan findings were due to an infected pancreatic pseudocyst.

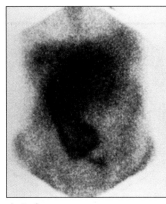

Anterior

**Fig. 9.55**

$^{67}Ga$ 48-hour scan of abdomen.

There is a very large area of abnormal $^{67}Ga$ accumulation in the abdomen to the right of the midline, extending up to the right hypochondrium. The centre of this area shows relatively less tracer accumulation than the periphery. This is a further example of an infected pancreatic pseudocyst.

### Infected kidney

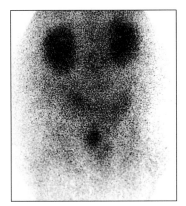

Posterior

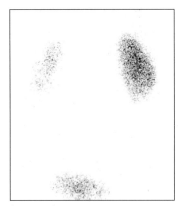

a  Posterior

b  Posterior

**Imaging with $^{67}Ga$ earlier than 48 hours** may show some renal uptake, and should not be reported as renal infection. However, renal uptake at 72 hours is always abnormal.

**Fig. 9.56**

$^{67}Ga$ 48-hour scan of abdomen and pelvis.

The patient was a 68-year-old woman who was being investigated for PUO. The $^{67}Ga$ study shows diffuse bilateral renal uptake. The scan findings were due to asymptomatic pyelonephritis.

**Fig. 9.57**

(a) $^{67}Ga$ 48-hour scan of abdomen. (b) DMSA scan of abdomen.

The $^{67}Ga$ study shows intense uptake of tracer in the left kidney and diffuse but less marked uptake in the right kidney. The DMSA study shows very poor uptake of tracer in the left kidney. The scan findings were due to right-sided pyelonephritis and a left-sided perinephric abscess.

# GASTROINTESTINAL TRACT STUDIES: CLINICAL APPLICATIONS

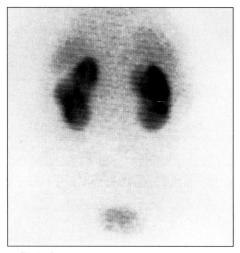

*a* Posterior

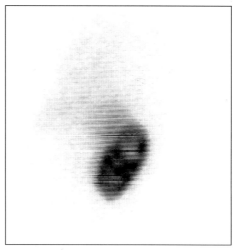

*b* Left lateral

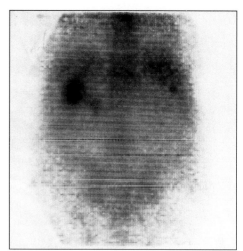

*c* Posterior

### Fig. 9.58

*(a, b)* DMSA *study. (c)* [67]*Ga 48-hour scan of abdomen.*

*This patient presenting with fever and left loin pain had an ultrasound examination which showed a mass in the left kidney of indeterminate pathology. The* DMSA *scan also demonstrates the space-occupying lesion. Note that this is best recognized on the left lateral view. The* [67]*Ga scan clearly shows focal uptake corresponding to this lesion, which, in the clinical context, made an intrarenal abscess the most likely diagnosis.*

### Fig. 9.59

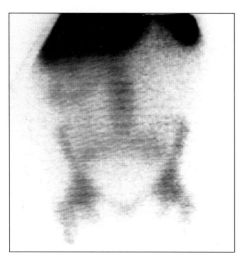

*a* Anterior

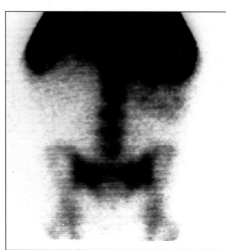

*b* Posterior

*(a, b)* [111]*In* WBC *24-hour scan of abdomen.*

*This patient had renal failure caused by polycystic kidneys. She was on the waiting list for a renal transplant and was being investigated for recurrent pyrexia. The white cell scan shows a large, diffuse area of increased tracer uptake in the right hypochondrium. This patient had an infected right polycystic kidney. She therefore underwent nephrectomy before renal transplantation.*

# 9.5.3   Gastrointestinal tract bleeding studies

With the use of modern endoscopy techniques, the localization of gastrointestinal bleeding usually presents little difficulty. Nevertheless, in problematic cases the use of $^{99m}$Tc-labelled red blood cells (RBC) may contribute significantly to the management of a patient who is actively bleeding. It is important that the usual investigation of upper and lower gastrointestinal endoscopy be performed prior to the red cell study.

A $^{99m}$Tc RBC bleeding study may be useful in two ways:

• To assist in the localization of the site of bleeding by the position of an accumulation of labelled red cells in the abdomen and by the general configuration of tracer in the gut lumen. This will also assist in the choice of mesenteric vessel to catheterize first if angiography is performed.

• The RBC bleeding study may be used to decide on the best time for angiography. The latter must be performed rapidly after the bleeding study becomes positive. Angiography, performed to localize a bleeding site, is only successful when bleeding is fast enough to visualize a 'spurt' of contrast (1–2 ml/minute). A RBC bleeding study will be positive at bleeding rates of 0.5 ml/min.

## *Normal gastrointestinal tract bleeding study*

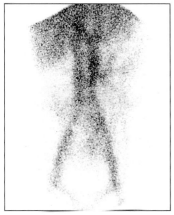

*a  2 minutes*

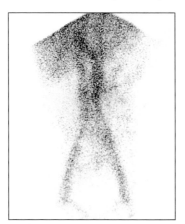

*b  10 minutes*

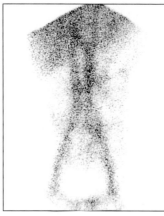

*c  20 minutes*

*Fig. 9.60*

*(a–f) $^{99m}$Tc RBC study.*
  *This is a normal study with no evidence of any active gastrointestinal bleeding. Although it is a good quality study, note that, with time, there is increasing tracer activity in the bladder caused by free pertechnetate.*

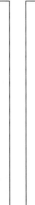
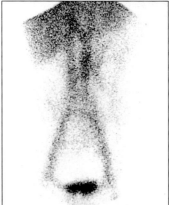

*d  35 minutes*

*e  45 minutes*

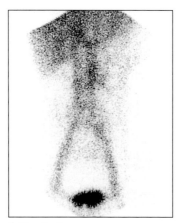

*f  50 minutes*

## *Acute gastrointestinal bleeding*
### *Small bowel*

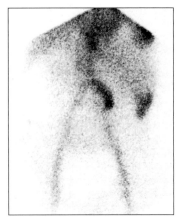

*a  Anterior, 5 minutes*

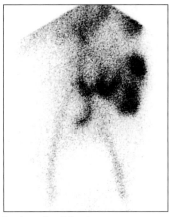

*b  Anterior, 25 minutes*

### Fig. 9.61

**(a, b)** ⁹⁹ᵐTc RBC study of the abdomen.

The patient was a 53-year-old woman with gastrointestinal bleeding. There is early accumulation of labelled red cells in the left flank which progresses rapidly over the 25 minutes of the study. This is a strongly positive study with high probability of acute localized bleeding, most likely in the small bowel.

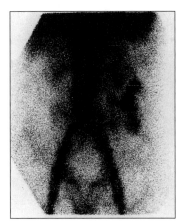

*a  3 minutes*

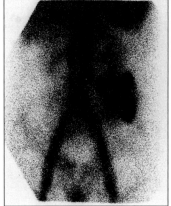

*b  10 minutes*

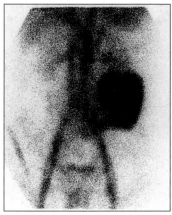

*c  35 minutes*

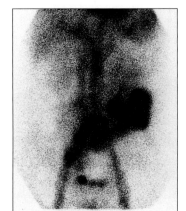

*d  40 minutes*

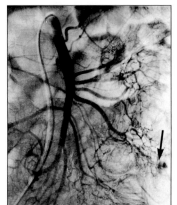

*e*

### Fig. 9.62

**(a–d)** ⁹⁹ᵐTc RBC study. **(e)** Arteriogram.

The patient was a 43-year-old man with gastrointestinal bleeding. The bleeding study shows evidence of accumulation of labelled red cells in the left side of the abdomen, probably originating in the jejunum and extending distally thereafter. The arteriogram shows injection into the superior mesenteric artery, and there is an area of angiodysplasia involving one of the jejunal branches (arrow).

## GASTROINTESTINAL TRACT STUDIES: CLINICAL APPLICATIONS

### Large bowel

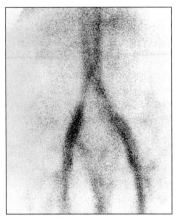 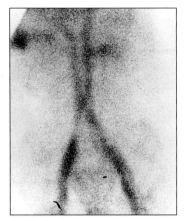 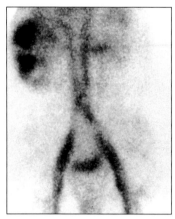 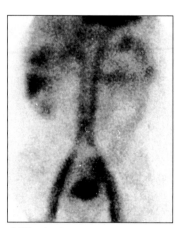

*a 2 minutes*   *b 15 minutes*   *c 25 minutes*   *d 35 minutes*

**Fig. 9.63**

*(a–d)* ⁹⁹ᵐTc RBC study.

The patient was a 64-year-old man with gastrointestinal bleeding. There is tracer accumulation visualized in the right upper quadrant of the abdomen. Activity is clearly visualized by 15 minutes, and there is subsequent accumulation and passage across the abdomen. This is a positive study which indicates active bleeding, the site of origin being most likely in the upper ascending colon.

### Sigmoid

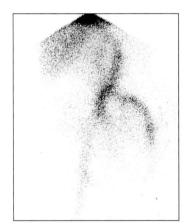
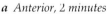
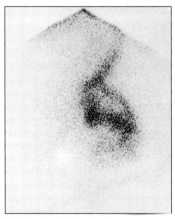

*a Anterior, 2 minutes*   *b Anterior, 35 minutes*

**Fig. 9.64**

*(a, b)* ⁹⁹ᵐTc RBC study.

The patient was a 81-year-old woman with gastrointestinal bleeding. On the 35-minute image there is clear-cut abnormal accumulation of red cells lying within the pelvis, most probably in the sigmoid colon. The site of bleeding is likely to be the descending colon. Note on the initial image that the aorta is somewhat tortuous, with marked tortuosity of the internal iliac vessels, and the suggestion of some change in diameter of the mid-portion of the right external iliac artery. These findings reflected arteriosclerotic vessels.

## *Timing of studies*

*First study*

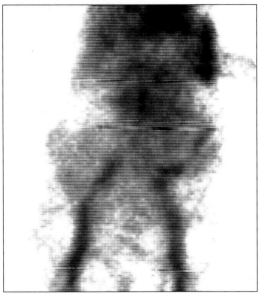

*a  2 minutes*

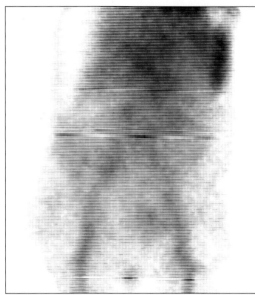

*b  30 minutes*

*Second study*

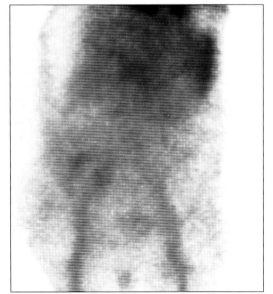

*c  5 minutes*

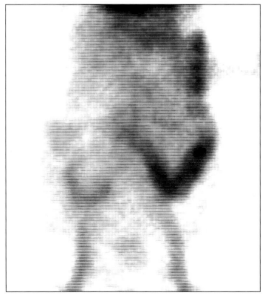

*d  60 minutes*

*Fig. 9.65*

*(a, b) First study equilibrium images. (c, d) Second study equilibrium images.*

*This patient with incidental splenomegaly was admitted following a gastrointestinal haemorrhage. The ⁹⁹ᵐTc RBC study was performed on the following day, at a time when the patient was no longer actively bleeding. This initial study was negative. Note the large splenic blood pool. However, the patient re-bled 3 days later, and the study at that time was strongly positive, showing accumulation of labelled red cells in the descending colon, both confirming the presence of active bleeding and localizing its probable site.*

- For a positive ⁹⁹ᵐTc RBC study, the patient must be actively bleeding.
- A positive study is likely to be obtained if bleeding is greater than 0.5 ml/minute. However, this will depend a great deal on the intestinal transit time, which will permit a smaller 'pool' of blood to be identified if it is slower.

## False localization of site of bleeding

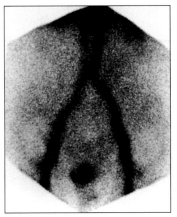
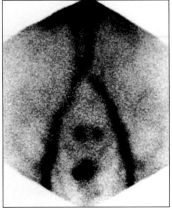
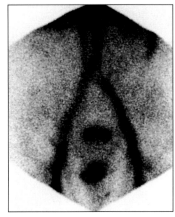
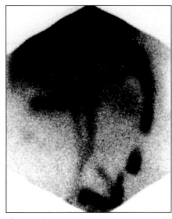

*a 2 minutes*    *b 10 minutes*    *c 20 minutes*    *d 30 minutes*

**Fig. 9.66**

*(a–d)* ⁹⁹ᵐTc RBC study.

   *On the 2-minute image there is a focus of tracer activity seen in the pelvis; this is too early to be in the bladder, and is most probably located in the rectum. On the 20-minute image tracer uptake is seen in the left hypochondrium at splenic flexure, and on the 30-minute image tracer is seen in the transverse colon. This elderly man was bleeding profusely from the ascending colon.*

**In the presence of profuse haemorrhage, gastrointestinal transit time may be very rapid. Therefore, unless imaging is continuous, labelled RBCs may be seen at a considerable distance distally from the true site of bleeding.**

## Incidental finding

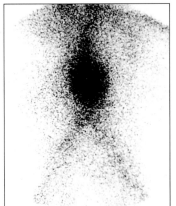
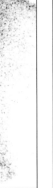
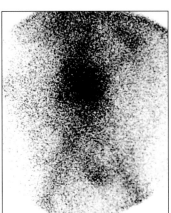
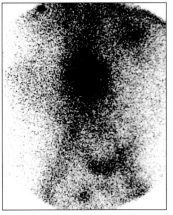
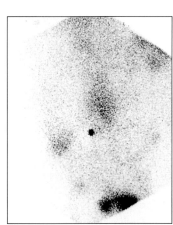

*a Anterior, 30 seconds*    *b Anterior, 2 minutes*    *c Anterior, 5 minutes*    *d Anterior, 70 minutes*

**Fig. 9.67**

*(a–d)* ⁹⁹ᵐTc RBC study of abdomen.

   *The patient was a 62-year-old man with alcoholic cirrhosis and gastrointestinal bleeding. During the first passage of activity through the abdomen, the upper aorta is dilated, with a large area of blood pool lying just above the aortic bifurcation. Between 2 and 5 minutes there is progressive accumulation of activity in the left side of the pelvis, approximately in the position of the sigmoid colon. However, on the 70-minute image there is an additional focal area of tracer in the right iliac fossa. The findings represent an aortic aneurysm and there is also bleeding, probably in the region of the rectosigmoid junction, with further intermittent bleeding in the right iliac fossa, possibly in the region of the caecum or lower ascending colon.*

## 9.5.4   Ectopic gastric mucosa studies

### Detection of ectopic gastric mucosa

$^{99m}$Tc pertechnetate ($^{99m}$TcO$_4$) is taken up by gastric mucosa, and forms the basis of the imaging study to detect sites of ectopic mucosa.

### Sites of gastric mucosa

*Normal*
- Stomach

*Ectopic*
- Meckel's diverticulum
- Lower oesophagus (Barrett's ulcer)
- Reduplication cyst

### Ectopic gastric mucosa: normal study

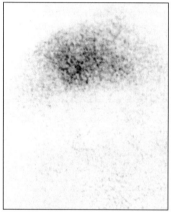

*a  0–30 seconds*

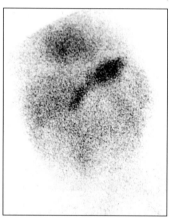

*b  2 minutes*

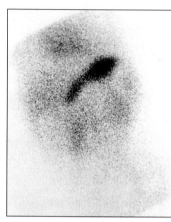

*c  5 minutes*

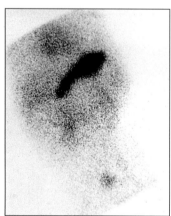

*d  10 minutes*

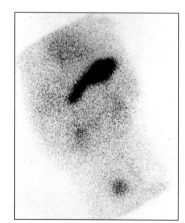

*e  15 minutes*

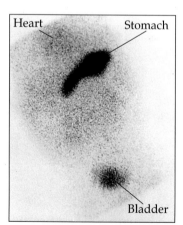

*f  25 minutes*

*Fig. 9.68*

*(a–f)* $^{99m}TcO_4$ *study.*
  *This is an ectopic gastric mucosa study in a 6-month-old child with recurrent bleeding. There is no ectopic site of pertechnetate accumulation, and the study is negative.*

*Ectopic gastric mucosa: abnormal study*

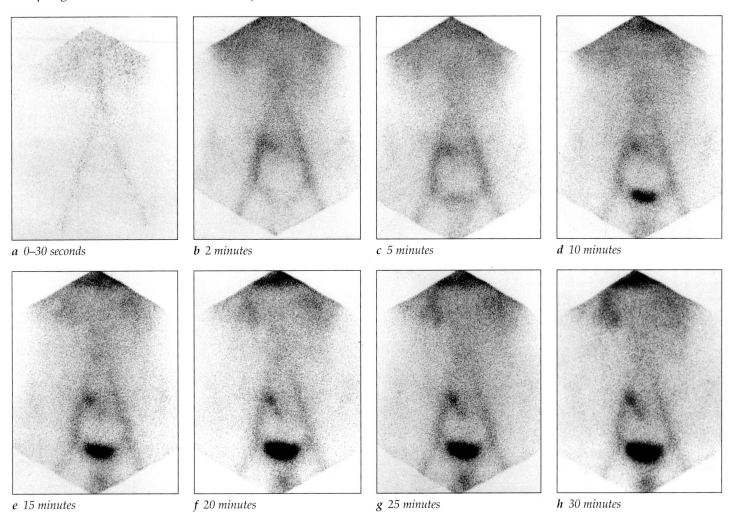

*a 0–30 seconds*  *b 2 minutes*  *c 5 minutes*  *d 10 minutes*

*e 15 minutes*  *f 20 minutes*  *g 25 minutes*  *h 30 minutes*

**Fig. 9.69**

**(a–h)** $^{99m}TcO_4$ study.

The patient was a 16-year-old girl with Meckel's diverticulum. There is a clear focus of increased tracer uptake seen to the right of the midline in the lower abdomen. This scan indicates Meckel's diverticulum, which was surgically proven.

## GASTROINTESTINAL TRACT STUDIES: CLINICAL APPLICATIONS

*False positive gastric mucosa study*

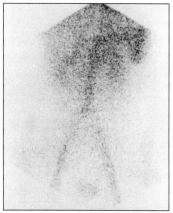

*a Anterior, 0–30 seconds*

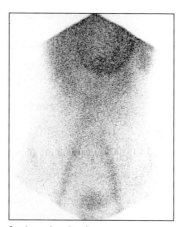

*b Anterior, 2 minutes*

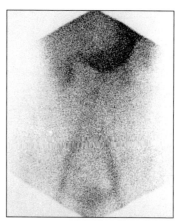

*c Anterior, 5 minutes*

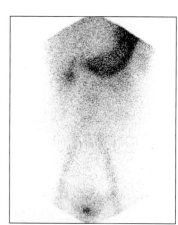

*d Anterior, 10 minutes*

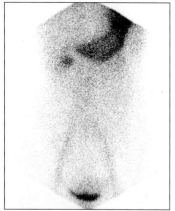

*e Anterior, 15 minutes*

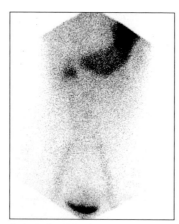

*f Anterior, 20 minutes*

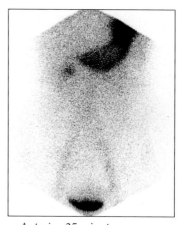

*g Anterior, 25 minutes*

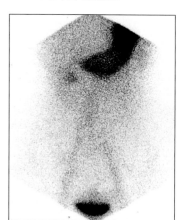

*h Anterior, 30 minutes*

**Fig. 9.70**

**(a–h)** $^{99m}TcO_4$ *study.*

The patient was a 16-year-old girl. As expected, the stomach is clearly visualized, but from the 5-minute view a focus of increased tracer uptake is seen in the upper right abdomen. This intensity increases to about 20 minutes and then starts to fade. This is a false positive scan result caused by tracer accumulation in the dilated right renal pelvis.

- Meckel's diverticulum is most common in children.
- Meckel's diverticulum without gastric mucosa rarely bleeds, and will not be detected using this method.
- Renal excretion of tracer is the commonest cause of a false positive scan result.

# CHAPTER 10

# MISCELLANEOUS STUDIES

## CHAPTER CONTENTS

# 10.1 LOCALIZATION OF INFECTION AND INFLAMMATION: RADIOPHARMACEUTICALS

Patients frequently present clinically with a problem of suspected infection and inflammation, but with no clearly defined site of origin. It is in precisely this situation that radionuclide studies are most useful. However, a further investigation (ultrasound, CT, etc) is usually necessary to confirm the presence of inflammation, increase specificity and improve anatomical localization.

Three radiopharmaceuticals are routinely available for such studies, and each has advantages and disadvantages:

- Gallium-67 ($^{67}$Ga) citrate
- Indium-111 ($^{111}$In) labelled leucocytes ($^{111}$In WBC)
- Technetium-99m ($^{99m}$Tc) labelled leucocytes ($^{99m}$Tc WBC).

*Table 10.1   Indications and choice of radiopharmaceutical*

| | |
|---|---|
| Pyrexia of unknown origin (PUO) | $^{67}$Ga is used, since it covers a wider spectrum of disease. If a pyogenic infection is clinically likely then $^{111}$In WBC should be used, especially if the white cell count is elevated |
| Postoperative infection and fever | $^{111}$In WBC is the first choice, especially if infection in the abdomen is suspected, since some confusion may arise from the normal bowel activity with $^{67}$Ga and $^{99m}$Tc WBC |
| Bone and orthopaedic prostheses infection | $^{67}$Ga is probably the first choice, unless an acute infection with elevated white cell count is present, when $^{111}$In WBC or $^{99m}$Tc WBC may be better |
| Sarcoidosis | $^{67}$Ga is used, since $^{111}$In WBC or $^{99m}$Tc WBC do not usually accumulate in this inflammatory condition |

*Table 10.2   Comparison of the radiopharmaceuticals $^{67}$Ga, $^{111}$In and $^{99m}$Tc WBC*

| | Advantages | Disadvantages |
|---|---|---|
| $^{67}$Ga | Non-specific—will detect both infection and inflammation | Usually takes 48 hours to make a diagnosis<br>Difficult in the abdomen because of normal bowel accumulation<br>Requires bowel preparation |
| $^{111}$In WBC | More specific for infection<br>Faster—may identify site of infection in 2–3 hours<br>Particularly low background activity in the abdomen | Expensive and difficult labelling technique<br>Difficult around the spleen because of high splenic accumulation<br>High splenic radiation dose |
| $^{99m}$Tc WBC | Excellent image quality<br>Lower splenic radiation dose than $^{111}$In | Expensive and difficult labelling technique<br>Difficult around spleen because of high splenic accumulation<br>Non-specific bowel activity after 3 hours. Lowers sensitivity for detection of intra-abdominal abscesses |

## 10.2 LOCALIZATION OF INFECTION AND INFLAMMATION: NORMAL SCANS AND VARIANTS

## 10.2.1 Normal ⁶⁷Ga study

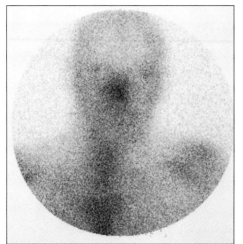

*a Anterior, 72 hours*

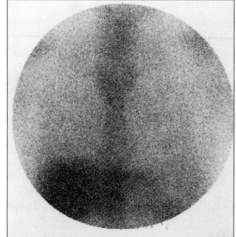

*b Anterior, 72 hours*

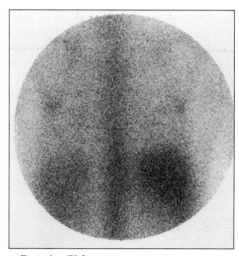

*c Posterior, 72 hours*

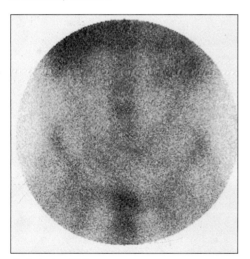

*d Anterior, 72 hours*

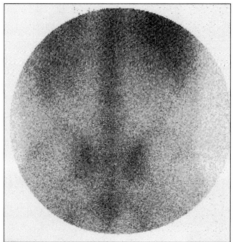

*e Posterior, 72 hours*

### Fig. 10.1

*Normal ⁶⁷Ga scan: (a) head; (b, c) chest; (d–g) abdomen.*

*The scan shows normal biodistribution in the bone, liver, spleen and bowel. Faint visualization of the lacrimal glands (a) may also be normal. Note the change in pattern of activity in the abdomen between 72 hours (d,e) and 96 hours (f,g), confirming that activity is located in the bowel.*

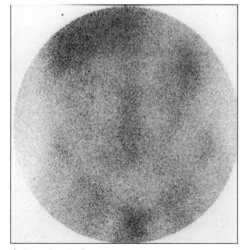

*f Anterior, 96 hours*

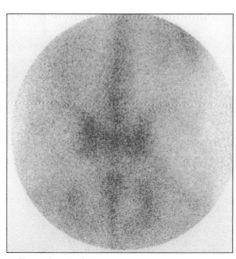

*g Posterior, 96 hours*

**Bowel preparation of the patient helps to reduce ⁶⁷Ga activity** within the bowel. A delayed abdominal view at 96 hours will aid in interpreting abdominal activity.

## 10.2.2 Normal ¹¹¹In WBC study

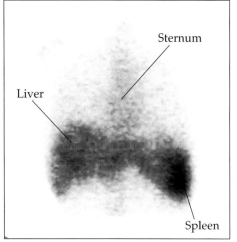

*a Anterior*

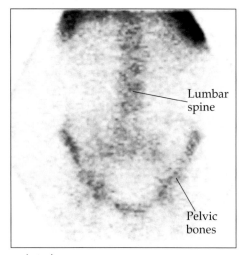

*c Anterior*

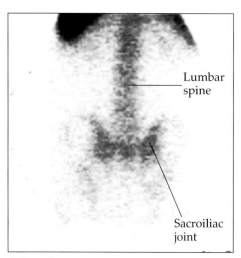

*b Posterior*

*d Posterior*

*Fig. 10.2*

*Normal ¹¹¹In WBC study: (a) anterior view of abdomen and chest; (b) posterior view of abdomen and chest; (c) anterior view of abdomen and pelvis; (d) posterior view of abdomen and pelvis.*

## 10.2.3 Normal ⁹⁹ᵐTc WBC study

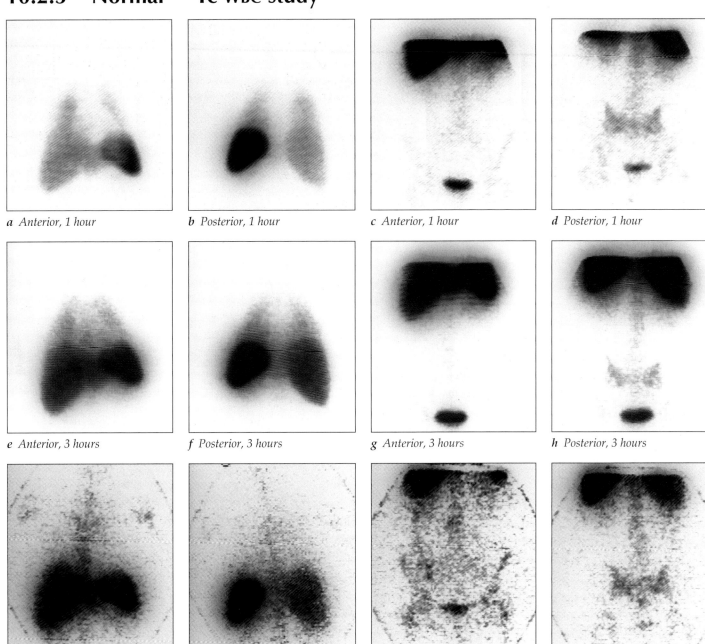

*a Anterior, 1 hour*   *b Posterior, 1 hour*   *c Anterior, 1 hour*   *d Posterior, 1 hour*

*e Anterior, 3 hours*   *f Posterior, 3 hours*   *g Anterior, 3 hours*   *h Posterior, 3 hours*

*i Anterior, 24 hours*   *j Posterior, 24 hours*   *k Anterior, 24 hours*   *l Posterior, 24 hours*

*Fig. 10.3*

*Normal ⁹⁹ᵐTc HMPAO WBC study. 1 hour images: (a, b) chest; (c, d) abdomen. 3 hour images: (e, f) chest; (g, h) abdomen. 24 hour images: (i, j) chest; (k, l) abdomen.*
 *Note the lung activity at 1 hour, which is clearing by 3 hours. No uptake is seen in the abdomen until 24 hours.*

**Lung activity should clear during the study. If it does not, the WBC may have been damaged (activated) during the labelling process.**

## 10.2.4    Artefacts and variants

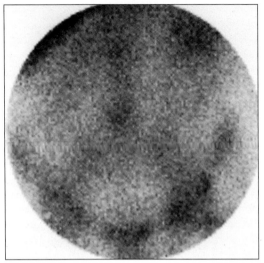

*a  Anterior, 72 hours*

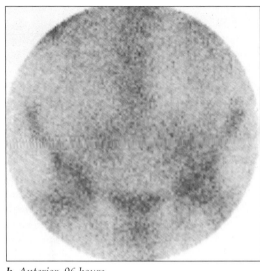

*b  Anterior, 96 hours*

*Fig. 10.4*

$^{67}$Ga *study.*

*The anterior abdominal view at 72 hours* (**a**) *demonstrates a mid-line focus of activity in the abdomen. At 96 hours* (**b**) *the focal abnormality is not seen, confirming that it was non-significant bowel activity.*

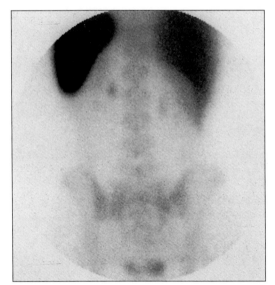

*a  Posterior, 1 hour*

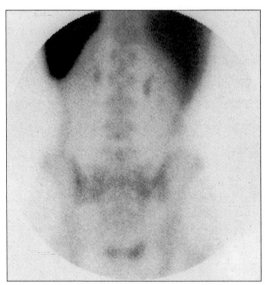

*b  Posterior, 3 hours*

*Fig. 10.5*

$^{99m}$Tc WBC *study.*

*At both 1 hour* (**a**) *and 3 hours* (**b**) *post-injection two foci of activity are seen on the posterior abdominal views corresponding to the renal pelves. These foci should not be mistaken for focal sepsis.*

# 10.3 LOCALIZATION OF INFECTION AND INFLAMMATION: CLINICAL APPLICATIONS

The clinical applications of imaging sites of infection and inflammation are listed below, and examples of the various clinical problems are given on subsequent pages.

**10.3.1 Infection**
Pneumonia
Tuberculosis
Lung abscess
Abdominal abscess
Infected renal cysts
Osteomyelitis
Infected wounds

**10.3.2 Sarcoidosis**
Clinical use of $^{67}$Ga scanning in sarcoidosis
Pulmonary sarcoidosis
Lacrimal and salivary glands
Systemic sarcoidosis
Meningeal sarcoidosis

# 10.3.1 Infection

## *Pneumonia*

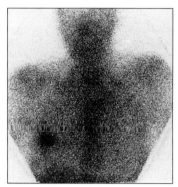

*a Anterior*

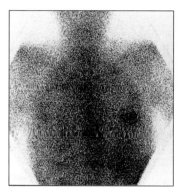

*b Posterior*

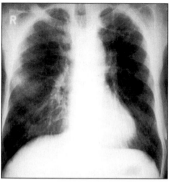

*c*

### Fig. 10.6

*(a, b)* $^{67}$Ga 24-hour scan of chest. *(c)* Chest x-ray.

The patient was a 77-year-old man with pneumonic illness. There is a focal area of increased $^{67}$Ga accumulation in the right side of the chest anteriorly. This corresponds to rather ill-defined peripheral shadowing in the right mid-zone in the chest x-ray. This patient was known to have Felty's syndrome with a previous splenectomy. He was found to have an infection with an uncommon Gram-positive aerobic organism (Nocardia asteroides).

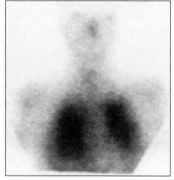

*a Anterior*

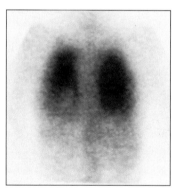

*b Posterior*

### Fig. 10.7

*(a, b)* $^{67}$Ga 48-hour scan of chest.

The patient was a 43-year-old man who was receiving chemotherapy for lymphoma. He developed a pyrexia, and the $^{67}$Ga study was performed to localize the site of infection. The study shows diffused lung uptake, and the findings were due to infection with pneumocystis. The chest x-ray was normal.

## *Tuberculosis*

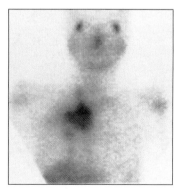

*Anterior*

### Fig. 10.8

$^{67}$Ga scan of chest.

In this case of pulmonary tuberculosis there is abnormal $^{67}$Ga uptake in the right side of the upper mediastinum and both lacrimal glands.

## Lung abscess

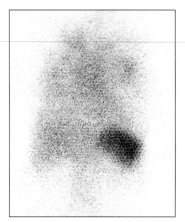

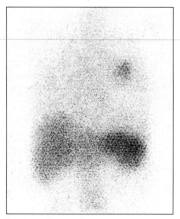

*a  Anterior, 4 hours*

*b  Anterior, 24 hours*

*Fig. 10.9*

$^{111}$In WBC *study: anterior views of the chest at* **(a)** *4 hours and* **(b)** *24 hours.*

*This patient was a 24-year-old female drug abuser admitted with a swinging pyrexia. The* $^{111}$In WBC *scan shows focal accumulation at 4 hours in the left upper chest, becoming more pronounced at 24 hours. A chest x-ray confirmed a lung abscess.*

**The diffuse lung activity at 4 hours in Fig. 10.9 is a common observation with WBC imaging and is caused by either damage to WBC during preparation or physiological margination in the lung vasculature.**

## Abdominal abscess

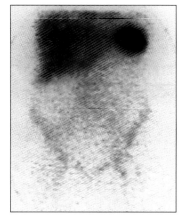

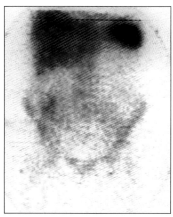

*a  Anterior, 3 hours*

*b  Anterior, 24 hours*

*Fig. 10.10*

$^{111}$In WBC *study: anterior views of the abdomen at* **(a)** *3 hours and* **(b)** *24 hours.*

*This patient was a 73-year-old woman admitted 3 weeks following abdominal surgery for carcinoma of the caecum with a swinging pyrexia, but no localizing features. The* $^{111}$In WBC *study at 3 hours appears normal, but at 24 hours a focal area of WBC accumulation is seen in the right iliac fossa. Ultrasound confirmed an abscess at this site.*

## Infected renal cysts

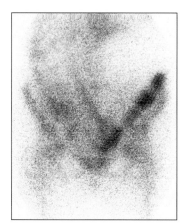

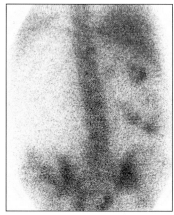

*a  Anterior*

*b  Posterior*

*Fig. 10.11*

**(a, b)** $^{67}$Ga *study.*

*This patient was a 50-year-old woman with known polycystic disease of the kidneys who presented with acute abdominal discomfort and pyrexia. The* $^{67}$Ga *study shows large photon-deficient areas in the abdomen corresponding to the renal cysts, with an area of* $^{67}$Ga *accumulation in the region of the right kidney seen on anterior and posterior views corresponding to infected cysts within one polycystic kidney.*

# Osteomyelitis

## Infected prosthesis

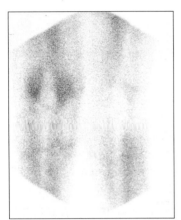

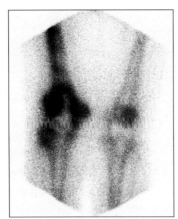

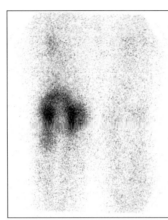

*a Equilibrium*

*b Delayed*

*c* $^{67}$Ga

### Fig. 10.12

*(a, b)* $^{99m}$Tc *bone scan of knees.*
*(c)* $^{67}$Ga *scan.*

The patient was a 72-year-old woman with bilateral knee replacement and increasing pain and swelling of the right knee. The $^{99m}$Tc bone scan study demonstrates increased blood pool and bone uptake surrounding the right knee prosthesis. $^{67}$Ga uptake confirms infection in the right prosthesis.

## Infected pin and plate

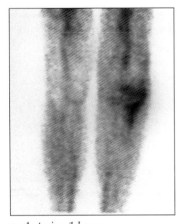

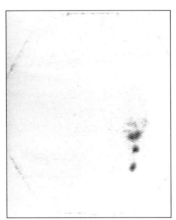

*a Anterior, 1 hour*

*b Anterior, 24 hours*

### Fig. 10.13

$^{99m}$Tc WBC *study of anterior legs at* *(a)* *1 hour and* *(b)* *24 hours.*

The patient was a 27-year-old man with a history of a recent road traffic accident and a fractured left tibia which had been pinned and plated. The pain had become progressively severe and a $^{99m}$Tc WBC study shows abnormal WBC accumulation, which at 24 hours is seen to correspond to the fixation screw sites, confirming infection.

# Infected wounds

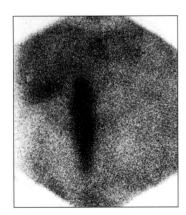

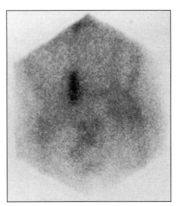

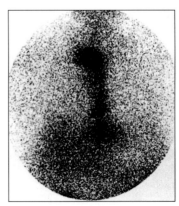

*a*

*b*

*c*

### Fig. 10.14

*(a) Upper right paramedian scar. (b) Lower right paramedian incision. (c) Infected sternal split following coronary artery bypass.*

# 10.3.2 Sarcoidosis

## Clinical use of $^{67}$Ga scanning in sarcoidosis

- Confirmation of the initial diagnosis
- Assessment of the extent of disease
- Identification of a suitable site for biopsy
- Follow-up to assess response to treatment
- Interpretation of x-ray
- Fibrosis versus active disease.

## Pulmonary sarcoidosis

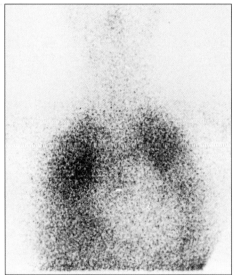

a Anterior

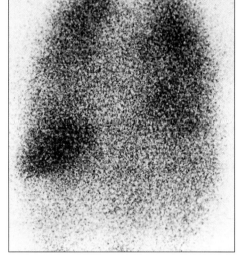

b Posterior

**Fig. 10.15**

*(a, b)* $^{67}$*Ga 48-hour scan of chest.*
  *Note the diffuse uptake of tracer over both lung fields in this case of sarcoidosis. Note also the abnormal uptake in the spleen.*

## Comparison of pulmonary sarcoidosis and tuberculosis

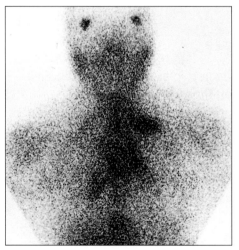

Anterior

**Fig. 10.16**

$^{67}$*Ga scan of chest.*
  *In this case of sarcoidosis there is abnormal tracer accumulation in both hilar areas, both lacrimal glands, the left supraclavicular fossa, and probably also the right supraclavicular fossa.*

## LOCALIZATION OF INFECTION AND INFLAMMATION: CLINICAL APPLICATIONS

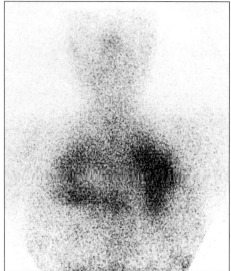

*a  Anterior*

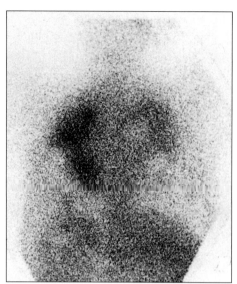

*b  Posterior*

### Fig. 10.17

*⁶⁷Ga 48-hour scan of chest.*
    *In this case of tuberculosis there is abnormal tracer accumulation in the thorax, but this is much more irregular when compared with the case illustrated in Fig. 10.15.*

 When considering the differential diagnosis between pulmonary sarcoidosis and tuberculosis, asymmetrical tracer uptake is an indication of tuberculosis. With sarcoidosis, hilar or diffuse lung involvement is most often seen, but these are only general guidelines.

## Lacrimal and salivary glands

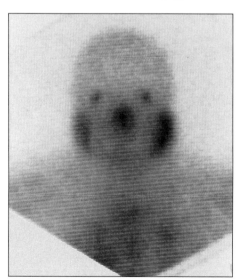

### Fig. 10.18

*⁶⁷Ga scan of head and neck.*
    *The patient was a 38-year-old woman with sarcoidosis. There is striking increased tracer uptake in the lacrimal and parotid glands.*

 The finding of increased uptake in lacrimal and parotid glands is strongly suggestive of sarcoidosis, although not diagnostic.

## *Systemic sarcoidosis*

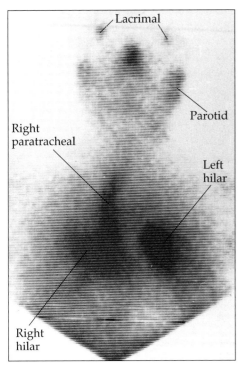

*a Anterior*

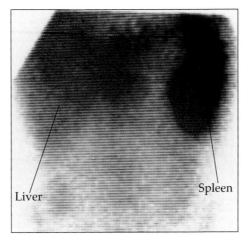

*b Anterior*

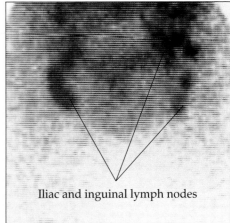

*c Anterior*

**Fig. 10.19**

⁶⁷Ga study: *(a)* head, neck and chest; *(b)* abdomen; *(c)* pelvis.
The patient was a 26-year-old man presenting with fever and weight loss, with marked hilar enlargement on a chest x-ray.

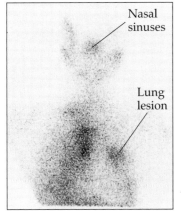

*a Anterior*

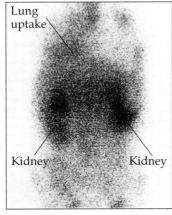

*b Anterior*

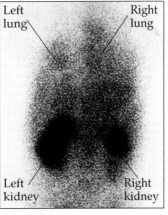

*c Posterior*

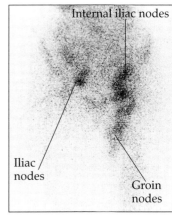

*d Anterior*

**Fig. 10.20**

⁶⁷Ga scan: *(a)* chest and head; *(b)* abdomen; *(c)* chest and abdomen; *(d)* pelvis.
A further case of systemic sarcoidosis. Although this 36-year-old woman had extensive disease with multiorgan involvement, she was relatively asymptomatic, and the physicians managing her case decided not to treat her with steroids. She presented 1 year later in renal failure and subsequently required haemodialysis.

# LOCALIZATION OF INFECTION AND INFLAMMATION: CLINICAL APPLICATIONS

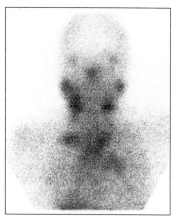 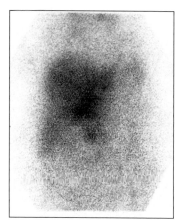

*a Anterior*    *b Anterior*

### Fig. 10.21

67Ga scan: *(a)* chest; *(b)* abdomen.

   This patient was a 60-year-old woman with known pulmonary sarcoid and lymphadenopathy. The ⁶⁷Ga study demonstrates intense uptake in the salivary glands, infraclavicular lymph nodes, left hilum and abdominal nodes.

## Meningeal sarcoidosis

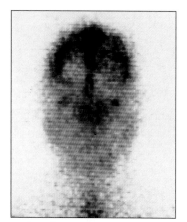 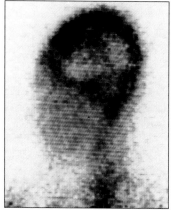

*a Anterior*    *b Lateral*

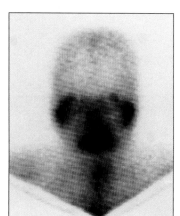 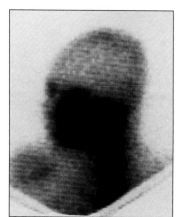

*c Anterior*    *d Lateral*

### Fig. 10.22

⁶⁷Ga scan of the face and skull: *(a)* lacrimal, parotid and meningeal uptake; *(b)* meningeal uptake; *(c, d)* same views after treatment, showing persistent activity in the lacrimal glands, but markedly decreased uptake in the meninges.

   This patient presented with recurrent headaches and a diagnosis of benign intracranial hypertension. A ⁶⁷Ga scan was performed for a PUO. The incidental finding showed uptake in the above sites, and a diagnosis of sarcoidosis was made. The CT scan was negative, but meningeal biopsy confirmed the diagnosis, and the patient responded to corticosteroid therapy.

## 10.4  LYMPHATIC AND LYMPH NODE IMAGING: NORMAL SCANS/RADIOPHARMACEUTICALS

The lymphatics and lymph nodes may be imaged by the subcutaneous injection of small colloid particles labelled with ⁹⁹ᵐTc in the tissues drained by the lymphatic system which is being investigated. The radiopharmaceuticals used are ⁹⁹ᵐTc human serum albumen microcolloid and ⁹⁹ᵐTc antimony sulphide microcolloid. Although such studies are capable of demonstrating the functionally active nodes, they have not found widespread application in most clinical situations.

### 10.4.1  Normal lymph node study

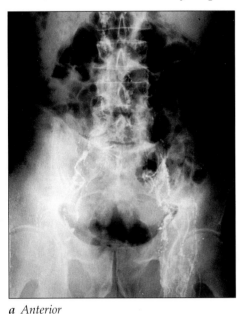

*a Anterior*

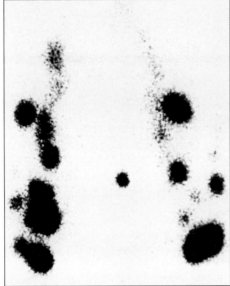

*b Anterior*

*Fig. 10.23*

*(a) Lipiodol lymphangiogram. (b) 2-hour lymph node study: anterior view of pelvis and femora, showing the inguinal and iliac lymph nodes.*

Note that the main disadvantage of radionuclide lymph node scanning is that it is usually not possible to say whether a lymph node is absent or replaced by tumour, because of anatomical variability.

### 10.4.2  Normal lymphoscintogram

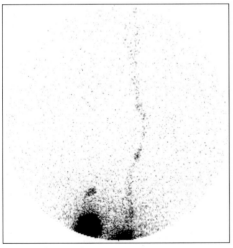

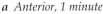

*a Anterior, 1 minute*

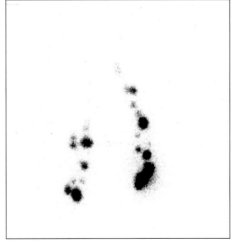

*b Anterior, 1 hour*

*c Anterior, 90 minutes*

*Fig. 10.24*

*(a) Activity is seen to be entering the lymphatics immediately after injection into the toe web space. (b) At 1 hour post-injection symmetrical activity is seen in the lymphatics of the thighs. (c) At 90 minutes post-injection activity is seen in the pelvic and abdominal nodes.*

# 10.5 LYMPHATIC AND LYMPH NODE IMAGING: CLINICAL APPLICATIONS

The clinical applications and the problems and advantages of lymph node scanning are listed below, and examples of the various clinical problems are given on subsequent pages.

10.5.1   Tumour infiltration of lymph nodes
10.5.2   Lymphoedema
         Unilateral lymphoedema
10.5.3   Traumatic injury

## Indications for lymphatic and lymph node imaging

- Investigation of suspected lymphoedema of the lower limbs
- As an alternative to a lymphangiogram in the investigation of lymph node disease, when a lymphangiogram is technically not possible
- Identification of the extent of lymph nodes, to assist in the planning of radiotherapy fields
- Investigation of lymph node replacement of the internal mammary chain in breast cancer.

*Table 10.3   Advantages and disadvantages of lymph node scanning*

| Advantages | Disadvantages |
|---|---|
| Non-invasive | Variation in normal anatomy makes interpretation of lymph node uptake difficult |
| Requires minimal co-operation | 30% of tests will be inconclusive |
| Physiological | |
| Applicable to lower limbs and thoracic chain | |
| Repeatable | |

## 10.5.1    Tumour infiltration of lymph nodes

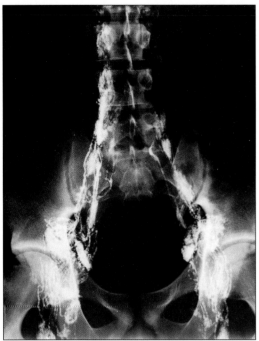

*a*

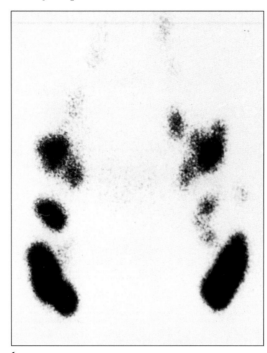

*b*

**Fig. 10.25**

*(a) Lymphangiogram, showing enlarged abnormal lymph nodes. (b) Lymph node scan, showing poor or absent uptake in some of the lymph nodes.*

*This case of prostatic carcinoma illustrates the difficulty of knowing whether poor or absent uptake is due to small or absent lymph nodes or tumour replacement.*

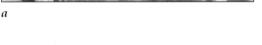

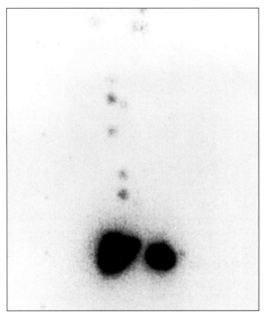

**Fig. 10.26**

*Anterior chest view following injection into both rectus sheaths.*

*Note the internal mammary nodes on the right but absent lymph node visualization on the left. This patient has left-sided breast tumour with internal mammary lymph node replacement.*

*Table 10.4    Criteria of abnormality*

Markedly asymmetrical tracer uptake

Presence of focal defects

Ballooning in size of lymph node groups

Mottled appearance of lymph nodes

## 10.5.2    Lymphoedema

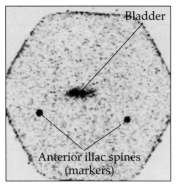

*a  Anterior*

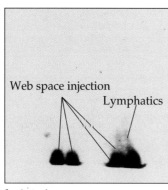

*b  Anterior*

### *Fig. 10.27*

*Anterior views: (a) pelvis; (b) legs.*

*In this case no progression of colloid is seen. The patient had bilateral lymphoedema caused by congenital absence of lymphatics (Milroy's disease).*

## *Unilateral lymphoedema*

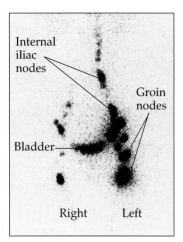

*a  Anterior*

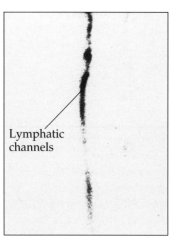

*b  Anterior*

### *Fig. 10.28*

*(a, b) Lymphatic and lymph node scans: (a) pelvis; (b) legs.*

*The scan shows a dilated lymphatic channel in the right leg (abnormal side) with poor visualization of the draining lymph nodes (a). Compare this with the normal left side where the nodes are shown clearly and there is clearance of tracer from the lower leg. This patient had a long history of swelling of the right leg, of unknown aetiology.*

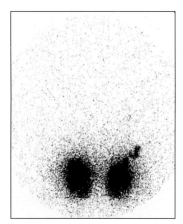

*a  Anterior, 2 minutes*

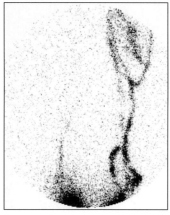

*b  Anterior, 30 minutes*

### *Fig. 10.29*

*Lymphoscintogram of the feet and calves: (a) 2 minutes post-injection; (b) 30 minutes post-injection.*

*This patient presented with a long history of swelling of the right calf. She had no history of trauma or deep vein thrombosis. The lymphoscintogram shows minimal activity in the lymphatics of the right calf. The lymphatic channels of the left calf are clearly seen at 30 minutes.*

## 10.5.3  Traumatic injury

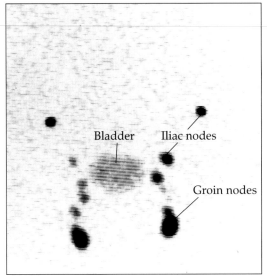

*a* Anterior

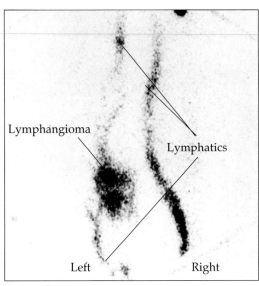

*b* Posterior

**Fig. 10.30**

*Lymphatic and lymph node scan: (**a**) pelvis; (**b**) calf. There is normal lymph node visualization, but on the left side there is a 'pool' of tracer.*

*This 28-year-old woman complained of left side ankle swelling. She had previously been injured at hockey and developed a traumatic lymphangioma in the left calf.*

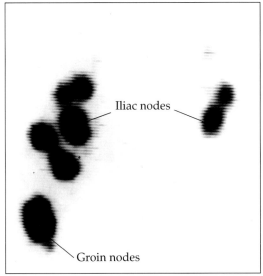

*a* Anterior

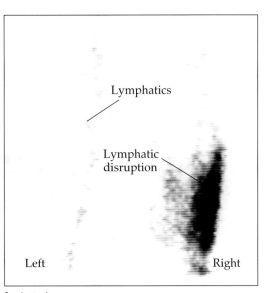

*b* Anterior

**Fig. 10.31**

*Lymphatic and lymph node scan: (**a**) pelvis; (**b**) legs. There is normal passage of tracer and lymph node visualization on the right. On the left there is delay, with 'pooling' in the calf.*

*This man received a traumatic injury to the calf followed by swelling of the ankle. The study shows leakage from the disrupted lymphatics.*

## 10.6 SCROTAL IMAGING: ANATOMY/RADIOPHARMACEUTICALS

Blood flow imaging of the scrotum employing a first pass and equilibrium imaging technique using $^{99m}$Tc pertechnetate ($^{99m}$TcO$_4$) is a simple, rapid method for assessing the scrotal and testicular blood supply. $^{99m}$TcO$_4$ is injected as a bolus after thyroid blockade with oral potassium perchlorate.

Torsion of the testis is due to rotation of the testis on the spermatic cord, causing the blood supply of the testes to be cut off. This leads to acute pain, and is a surgical emergency, since the chance of recovery of the testis after 4–6 hours of acute torsion is less than 20%, whereas surgical treatment in the early stages is usually successful. The main differential diagnosis is acute infective epididymo-orchitis, which is treated conservatively. The aim of diagnosis is to detect all cases of torsion, even if that means that a small number of cases of epididymitis will be operated on unnecessarily.

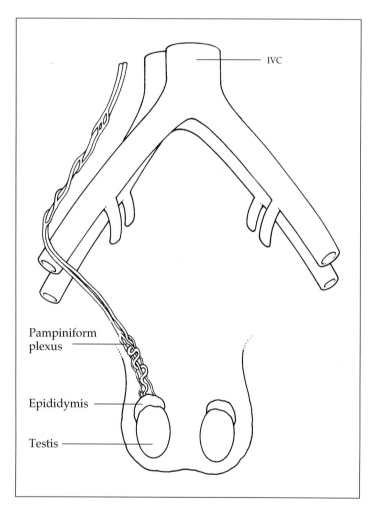

*Fig. 10.32*

*Anatomy of the testis and its blood supply.*

IVC

Pampiniform plexus

Epididymis

Testis

# 10.7 SCROTAL IMAGING: CLINICAL APPLICATIONS

The clinical applications of scrotal imaging are listed below, and examples of the various clinical problems are given on subsequent pages.

# 10.7.1 Torsion

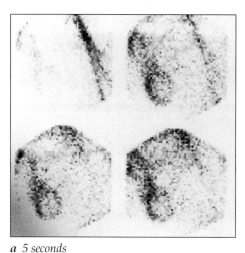 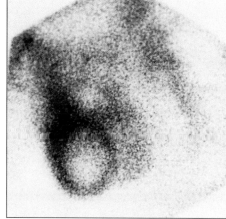

*a 5 seconds*  *b Equilibrium*

**Fig. 10.33**

***Case 1 (a)** 5-second images during the first pass study, showing increased blood flow around the testis. **(b)** Equilibrium phase image, showing increased blood pool around the right testis with a photon-deficient area within it.*

# 10.7.2 Epididymo-orchitis

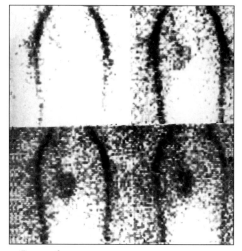 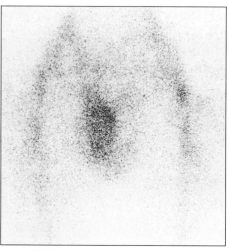

*c 5 seconds*  *d Equilibrium*

***Case 2 (c)** 5-second images during the first pass study, showing increased blood flow to the right side of the scrotum. **(d)** Equilibrium phase image, showing generalized increased blood pool on the right side.*

*In both cases the patients presented after 24 hours of testicular pain. Case 1 shows that delayed torsion may result in inflammatory changes in response to the avascular testis. This appearance may also be seen with epididymo-orchitis; however, bearing in mind the cost of errors, it is advisable to diagnose a torsion whenever there is a photon-deficient centre. Case 2 shows diffuse blood flow and blood pool with no photon-deficient centre.*

 **The increased flow patterns seen in torsion and inflammatory epididymitis are non-specific, and may be seen in other conditions such as tumours and trauma. This emphasizes that the report is much more clinically relevant when combined with clinical findings.**

## 10.7.3 Comparison of testicular torsion and epididymo-orchitis

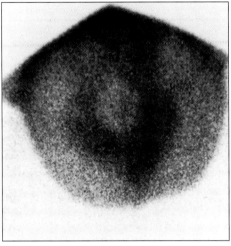 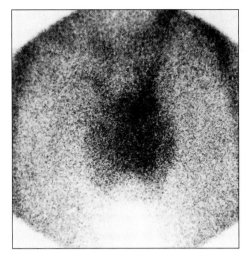

*a Testicular torsion*    *b Epididymo-orchitis*

**Fig. 10.34**

*(a) Testicular torsion: equilibrium phase image, showing a photon-deficient area centrally corresponding to the tender testis on the right side with some inflammatory reaction around it. (b) Epididymo-orchitis: equilibrium phase image, showing generalized increased blood supply to the left side of the scrotum caused by inflammation of both epididymis and testis.*

*In both cases the patients were boys who presented with acute pain in the scrotum of less than 4 hours' duration. The study enabled the testicular torsion to be relieved and avoided operating unnecessarily on the infected epididymis.*

*Table 10.5    Scan appearances of testicular torsion and epididymo-orchitis*

| Pathology | Scan appearance |
| --- | --- |
| Early torsion | Decreased blood flow with a central photon-deficient area |
| Late torsion | Increased blood flow with a central photon-deficient area |
| Epididymo-orchitis | Increased blood flow with no central photon-deficient area |

## 10.7.4   Traumatic injury

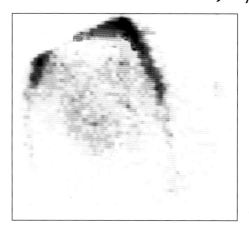

*a* 8 seconds

*b* 14 seconds

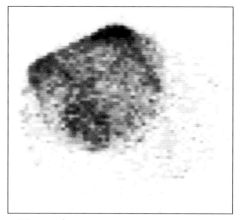

*c* 20 seconds

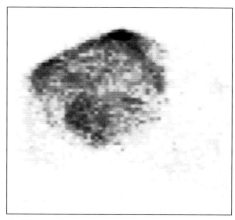

*d* 26 seconds

**Fig. 10.35**

*Dynamic testicular study: (a) 8 seconds;*
*(b) 14 seconds; (c) 20 seconds; (d) 26*
*seconds.*

  *This study shows increased blood flow to*
*the right of the scrotum. This patient had*
*sustained a traumatic injury to the*
*scrotum on a building site.*

# 10.8 LACRIMAL DRAINAGE STUDIES: ANATOMY/RADIOPHARMACEUTICALS

The functional integrity of the lacrimal drainage system can be assessed by visualizing the clearance of a small volume of radiopharmaceutical placed in the conjunctival sac into the lacrimal sac, duct and the nasal cavity.

Following the instillation of a drop of $^{99m}$Tc rhenium colloid onto the conjunctival sac, the material spreads over the globe of the eye by capillary action, thus labelling tears and outlining the drainage pathways. Sequential images are obtained, and normally drainage into the nose is seen within the first few minutes.

The standard imaging technique, namely an x-ray dacrocystogram (DCG), requires intubation of the canaliculi and manual injection of contrast to fill the tear duct. If gross distortion of the anatomy exists, or if infection is present, intubation may be difficult or, indeed, contraindicated. Further, an injection under pressure is not physiological, and may therefore not reflect the true functional state of the tear pump mechanism.

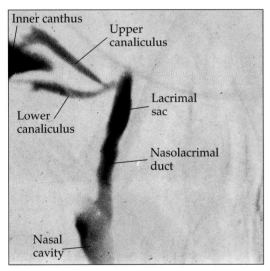

*a*

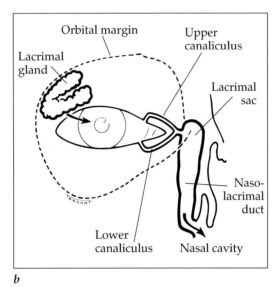

*b*

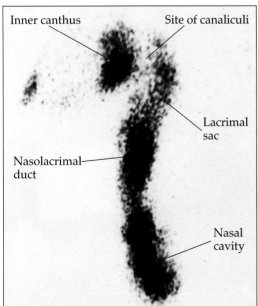

*c*

## Fig. 10.36

*(a) X-ray DCG. (b) Diagram of normal anatomy.*
*(c) Radionuclide lacrimal drainage scan 7*
*minutes after instillation of tracer into the eye.*

# 10.9 LACRIMAL DRAINAGE STUDIES: NORMAL SCANS

*Case 1*

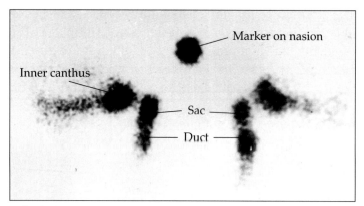
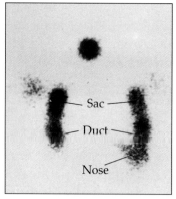
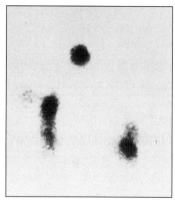

*a 1 minute*        *b 3 minutes*        *c 6 minutes*

*Case 2*

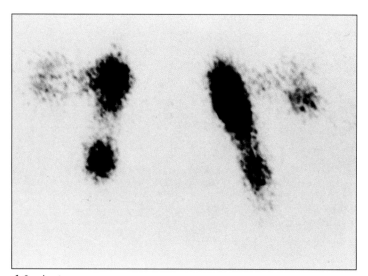

*d 2 minutes*        *e 6 minutes*

**Fig. 10.37**

*Normal lacrimal drainage scans.*
*   **Case 1 (a)** 1 minute after tracer instillation. This shows tracer already in both lacrimal sacs and early filling of the ducts.
*(b)* 3-minute image. Further filling of lacrimal sacs and ducts and nasal activity on the left. *(c)* 6-minute image. Further normal drainage.
*   **Case 2 (d)** 2-minute image. *(e)* 6-minute image.
*   Slight physiological differences may exist in normal subjects, as demonstrated in the above two cases.

# 10.10  LACRIMAL DRAINAGE STUDIES: CLINICAL APPLICATIONS

The clinical applications of lacrimal drainage studies
are listed below, and examples of the various clinical
problems are given on subsequent pages.

10.10.1  **Unilateral obstruction**
10.10.2  **Bilateral obstruction**
10.10.3  **Two potential pitfalls in interpretation**
         Tearing
         Lax lower eyelid

## 10.10.1  Unilateral obstruction

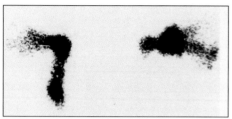

*a* 2 minutes

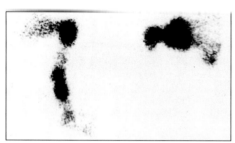

*b* 10 minutes

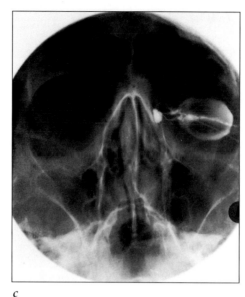

*c*

**Fig. 10.38**

*Lacrimal drainage study. (**a**) Normal drainage into the lacrimal sac and duct is seen on the right. There is tracer accumulation in the inner canthus on the left, with only a small amount of tracer present in the sac. (**b**) The right side drains well. The left side shows a little more tracer in the sac, but this is not reaching the duct (**c**) Left DCG, showing obstruction in the mid-portion of the lacrimal sac.*

*This man presented with left-sided epiphora with a lacrimal duct which was patent to syringing. The lacrimal drainage study confirms a functional obstruction. Because the drainage study was positive, a DCG was undertaken; this demonstrates the site of obstruction.*

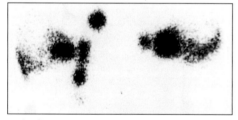

*a* 1 minute

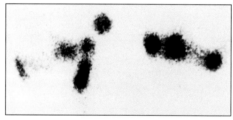

*b* 3 minutes

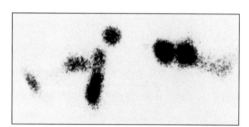

*c* 8 minutes

**Fig. 10.39**

*Lacrimal drainage study. (**a**) 1-minute image, showing rapid filling on the right system, but delayed filling on the left. (**b**) 3-minute image, showing further filling on the right, with only slow accumulation of tracer into the left sac. (**c**) 8-minute image, with no further drainage.*

*This patient had a left-sided obstruction causing epiphora. The right side is normal, and the apparent delay in the lower part of the sac, as demonstrated on the drainage scan, is a common variant which does not indicate obstruction. The key is the rate of entry into the sac and duct, which can be seen to be very rapid in the first image.*

# 10.10.2 Bilateral obstruction

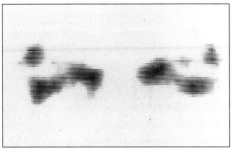 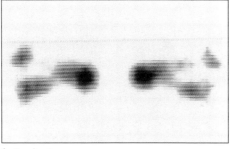 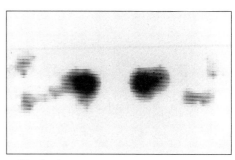

*a* 1 minute          *b* 3 minutes          *c* 12 minutes

***Fig. 10.40***

*Lacrimal drainage study. **(a)** 1-minute image, showing tracer entering the upper sac bilaterally. **(b)** 3-minute image, showing further filling of the upper sac. **(c)** 12-minute image, showing further filling, but with no drainage from the sac.*

*This patient presented with bilateral epiphora, and the study confirms bilateral obstruction of the drainage system.*

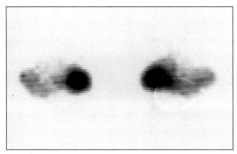 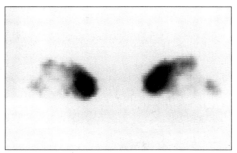

*a* 2 minutes          *b* 12 minutes

***Fig. 10.41***

*Lacrimal drainage study. **(a)** 2-minute image, showing tracer in the inner canthus bilaterally. **(b)** 12-minute image. Tracer remains in the inner canthus, with no passage into the sac.*

*A further case of bilateral epiphora, showing clear failure of the drainage system. However, since there is no passage at all of tracer into the sac, the problem may be proximal, eg common canaliculi or punctae.*

 **When obstruction is diagnosed, the tracer should be washed out physically to reduce the radiation dose to the eye. This is minimal for a normal system, but may be several hundred times higher in an obstructed system which is not irrigated.**

# 10.10.3 Two potential pitfalls in interpretation

## *Tearing*

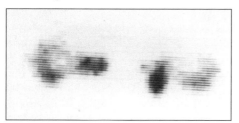

*a  1 minute*

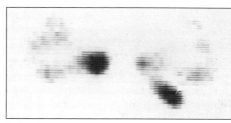

*b  3 minutes*

*Fig. 10.42*

*(a, b) Lacrimal drainage study.*
   *There is apparent filling of the lacrimal sac on the left in the first minute, with further drainage at 3 minutes. In fact, there is complete left-sided obstruction, and the 'drainage' is a tear from the inner canthus. Note the angle at which activity is seen, since this never occurs with a normal sac and duct.*

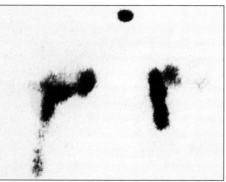

*a  1 minute*

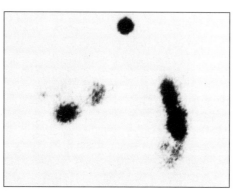

*b  3 minutes*

*Fig. 10.43*

*(a, b) Lacrimal drainage study.*
   *This is a case of right-sided obstruction. Once again, tearing from the pool of tracer is seen, on this occasion on the 1-minute image. The 3-minute image, however, shows apparent drainage from the conjunctival sac. If the image with the tear had been missed, it might have been concluded that there had been good drainage.*

 **It is important to image continuously and look for visualization of the sac as well as clearance of tracer from the eye.**

## *Lax lower eyelid*

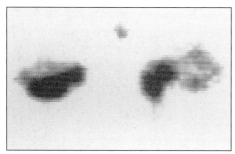

*a  1 minute*

*Fig. 10.44*

*(a, b) Lacrimal drainage study.*
   *In this case there is no lacrimal sac filling on the right side. However, the tracer is pooling in the lower conjunctival sac; in fact, the drainage system is normal, but there is failure of the tear pump mechanism because of a lax lower eyelid.*

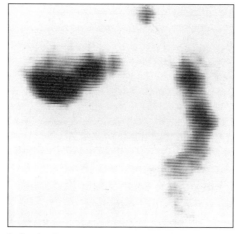

*b  3 minutes*

 **The lacrimal drainage scan provides more functional information than an x-ray DCG because:**
- **It tests the whole system—a DCG requires catheterization of the canaliculus for injection of dye**
- **Unlike the DCG, the tracer is not instilled under pressure.**

# 10.11  BONE MARROW IMAGING: ANATOMY/PHYSIOLOGY/RADIOPHARMACEUTICALS

Bone marrow has two main functions:

- The reticuloendothelial macrophage function
- The haemopoietic (red cell production) function.

Both of these functions may be imaged with radionuclides. The radiopharmaceuticals used for imaging are:

- Reticuloendothelial function—$^{99m}$Tc tin or antimony colloid, small particle albumin colloid or mini-microsphere
- Red cell function—$^{52}$Fe.

Iron $^{52}$Fe is a cyclotron-produced radioisotope and is limited for practical purposes to those centres possessing a positron gamma camera. It will therefore not be considered further here.

In a normal individual, and in most disease processes, the distribution of reticulo-endothelial and haemopoietic cells is identical. In performing imaging studies with $^{99m}$Tc colloid preparations, reticuloendothelial function is therefore presumed to match the red cell function. The use of colloid preparation has the additional advantage of allowing imaging of the liver and spleen to be performed at the same time, and this may often provide further useful information to the haematologist.

The patient must be imaged for a fixed time after a fixed dose of radiopharmaceutical per kilogram weight or surface area has been given, to permit semiquantitative assessment of images in serial studies, or comparisons between patients.

*Table 10.6   Distribution of active bone marrow*

| Adults | | Children |
|---|---|---|
| **Axial skeleton** | **Appendicular skeleton** | Extent depends on age. In the newborn active marrow extends along the full length of the limbs. In childhood marrow retracts until the adult pattern is reached by the age of 10. |
| Vertebral bodies | Proximal one-third of | |
| Pelvis | femora and humeri | |
| Sternum | | |
| Scapulae | | |
| Skull | | |

# 10.12   BONE MARROW IMAGING: NORMAL SCANS

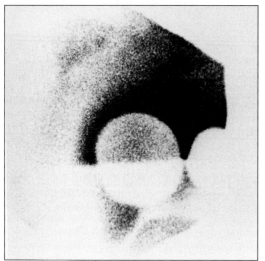

*a Anterior*

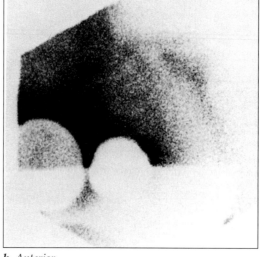

*b Anterior*

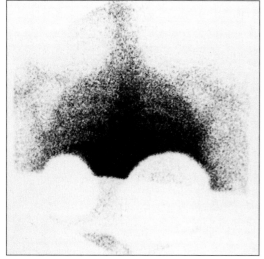

*c Posterior*

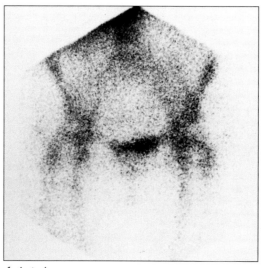

*d Anterior*

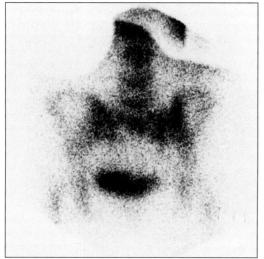

*e Anterior*

### Fig. 10.45

*Normal bone marrow scan: (a) right shoulder; (b) left shoulder; (c) thoracic spine; (d) pelvis; (e) pelvis.*

*Normal marrow is seen in the axial skeleton (spine and pelvis), skull and humeral heads, and reaches approximately to the upper third of the femoral shaft.*

# 10.13  BONE MARROW IMAGING: CLINICAL APPLICATIONS

The clinical applications of bone marrow imaging are listed below, and examples of the various clinical problems are given on subsequent pages.

(For the use of bone marrow imaging in the investigation of neoplastic disease see Chapter 4.)

**Assessment of marrow extension**
Polycythaemia rubra vera
Chronic haemolytic anaemia
Potential pitfalls
Myelofibrosis

# Assessment of marrow extension

## Polycythaemia rubra vera

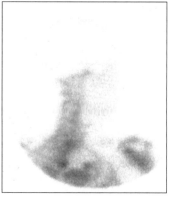

*a Anterior*

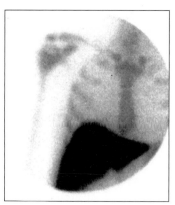

*b Anterior*

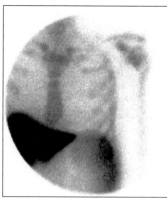

*c Posterior*

**Fig. 10.46**

$^{99m}Tc$ nanocolloid scan:
*(a)* anterior skull; *(b)* anterior thorax; *(c)* posterior thorax; *(d)* posterior chest; *(e)* posterior abdomen; *(f)* anterior pelvis; *(g)* posterior pelvis; *(h)* anterior thighs.

This patient was a 73-year-old man with known polycythaemia rubra vera. The study demonstrates active marrow in the axial skeleton extending down the humeri and femora. The spleen is somewhat enlarged.

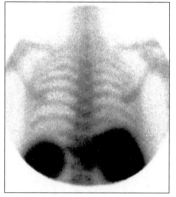

*d Posterior*

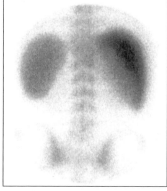
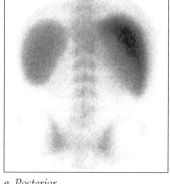

*e Posterior*

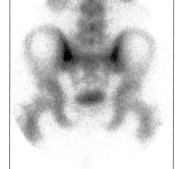

*f Anterior*

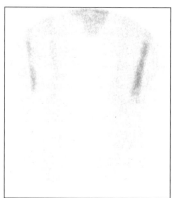

*g Posterior*

*h Anterior*

- **Bone marrow extension is very non-specific and may been seen in:** polycythaemia; haemolytic anaemia; chronic anaemia caused by blood loss; megaloblastic anaemia ($B_{12}$, folate); leukaemia, lymphoma and some cancers.
- **A marrow scan is rarely diagnostic alone. It must be interpreted in the light of known clinical and haematological findings.**

## *Chronic haemolytic anaemia*

*Marrow scan*

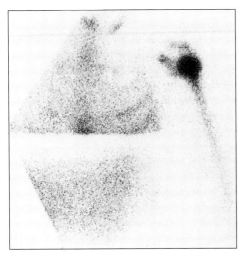

*a Anterior*

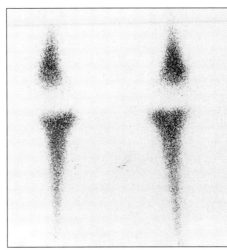

*b Anterior*

*c Anterior*

*Bone scan*

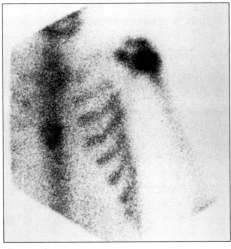

*d Anterior*

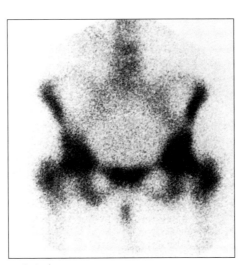

*e Anterior*

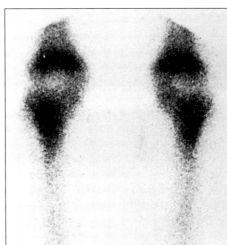

*f Anterior*

**Fig. 10.47**

*Bone marrow images: (a) left anterior chest; (b) anterior pelvis and femora; (c) tibiae; with corresponding bone scan views (d–f).*

*This patient had bone pain, and the bone scan was performed first. The bone scan and marrow appearances are due to chronic haemolytic anaemia. Note: (1) the extension of bone marrow down the humerus (a); (2) the very active 'globular' humeral head on the bone scan (d); (3) the extension of bone marrow down the femora (b); (4) the very active femoral head and trochanters (e); (5) the extension of marrow below the knees—there is none in the epiphyses or patella (c); (6) the identical pattern on the bone scan.*

## *Potential pitfalls*

### Aplastic anaemia

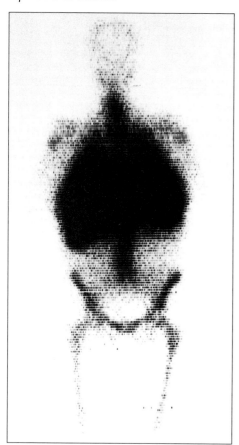

*a Anterior*

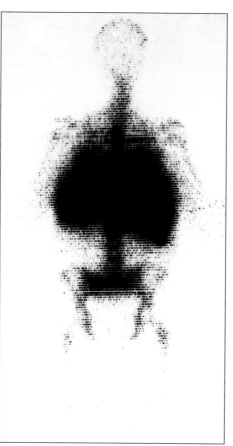

*b Posterior*

**Fig. 10.48**

*(a, b) Bone marrow scan. There is some evidence of peripheral extension of bone marrow.*

*The patient was a 54-year-old woman who presented with tiredness and dyspnoea of recent onset. She was found to be anaemic. The marrow scan suggests marrow hyperplasia, but the final diagnosis was aplastic anaemia.*

• The one important haematological disease which results in total mismatch between reticulo-endothelial function and red cell production is aplastic anaemia.

### Marrow hyperplasia

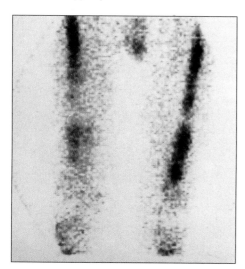

**Fig. 10.49**

*Peripheral extension caused by marrow hyperplasia may occasionally be very irregular, giving the appearance of focal replacement.*

# BONE MARROW IMAGING: CLINICAL APPLICATIONS

## *Myelofibrosis*

### *Myelofibrosis: early disease*

Myelofibrosis may be a long-term complication of polycythaemia rubra vera. It is important to detect the onset of this, especially if $^{32}$P or cytotoxic therapy is being considered.

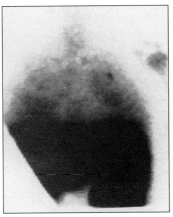

*a Anterior*

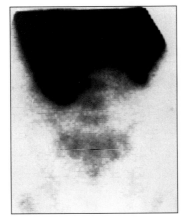

*b Posterior*

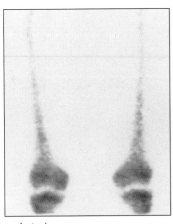

*c Anterior*

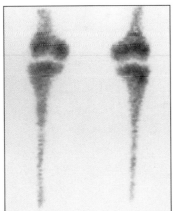

*d Posterior*

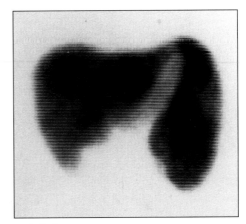

*e Anterior*

*f Anterior*

*g Anterior*

### Fig. 10.50

**(a)** *Anterior and* **(b)** *posterior views of chest, showing poor central marrow uptake. Note the massive spleen.* **(c)** *Anterior and* **(d)** *posterior views of pelvis. The marrow can be seen but the activity is low in proportion to the marrow extension.* **(e)** *Anterior view of femora and* **(f)** *anterior view of tibiae, showing massive extension of bone marrow.* **(g)** *Anterior liver/spleen view, showing the massively enlarged spleen.*

# BONE MARROW IMAGING: CLINICAL APPLICATIONS

## *Myelofibrosis: established disease*

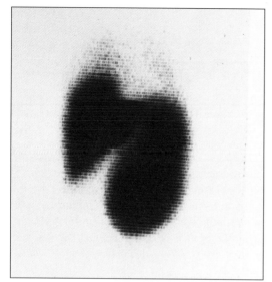

*a* Anterior

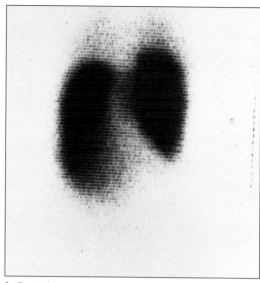

*b* Posterior

**Fig. 10.51**

*(a, b)* *Whole-body marrow scan, showing enormous splenomegaly but with virtual absence of bone marrow activity. This is the classical appearance of myelofibrosis, with almost complete replacement of marrow.*

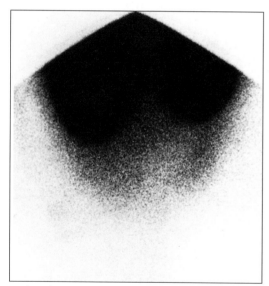

*a* Anterior

*b* Posterior

**Fig. 10.52**

*(a, b)* *Pelvic views of a bone marrow scan optimized in an attempt to show marrow uptake. Only a faint area of marrow uptake is seen.*

*This patient presented with anaemia and splenomegaly and was found to have myelofibrosis.*

# INDEX